RECENT ADVANCES IN PROSTATE CANCER AND BPH

RECENT ADVANCES IN PROSTATE CANCER AND BPH

The Proceedings of the IV Congress on Progress and Controversies in
Oncological Urology (PACIOU IV), held in Rotterdam, The Netherlands, April 1996

Edited by Fritz H. Schröder

*This publication is sponsored as an
educational service by Schering AG*

The Parthenon Publishing Group
International Publishers in Medicine, Science & Technology

NEW YORK   LONDON

Library of Congress Cataloging-in-Publication Data
Congress on Progress and Controversies on Oncological
Urology (4th : 1996 : Rotterdam. Netherlands)
    Recent advances in prostate cancer and BPH : the
proceedings of the IV Congress on Progress and
Controversies on Oncological Urology (PACIOU IV),
held in Rotterdam, The Netherlands, April 1996/
edited by F. H. Schröder.
        p.   cm.
    Includes bibliographical references and index.
    ISBN 1-85070-784-7
    1. Prostate—Cancer—Congresses.
    2. Prostate—Hypertrophy—Congresses.
I. Schröder, F. H. II. Title.
    [DNLM: 1. Prostatic Neoplasms—congresses.
2. Prostatic Hyperplasia—congresses. WJ 752 C749r
1997]
RC280.P7C64 1996
616.99′463—dc21
DNLM/DLC
for Library of Congress   96-44493
                                               CIP

British Library Cataloguing-in-Publication Data
Recent advances in prostate cancer and BPH
    1. Prostate—Cancer—Congresses.
    2. Prostate—Hypertrophy—Congresses.
    3. Prostate—Cancer—Treatment—Congresses.
    4. Prostate—Hypertrophy—Treatment—
    Congresses.
I. Schröder, F. H.
616.9′94′63
ISBN 1-85070-784-7

Published in North America by
The Parthenon Publishing Group Inc.
One Blue Hill Plaza
PO Box 1564, Pearl River
New York 10965, USA

Published in the UK and Europe by
The Parthenon Publishing Group Limited
Casterton Hall, Carnforth
Lancs. LA6 2LA, UK

Copyright © 1997 The Parthenon Publishing Group

First published 1997

Typeset by AMA Graphics Ltd., Preston, UK
Printed and bound in the UK by
The Bath Press, Bath

Contents

Section 6 PSA and the Early Detection of Prostate Cancer

Section 7 Management of Locally Confined Prostate Cancer

List of principal contributors

F. E. Alexander
Department of Public Health Sciences
Clinical Epidemiology
University of Edinburgh
Teviot Place
Edinburgh EH8 9AG
Scotland

C. H. Bangma
Department of Urology
Erasmus University & Academic Hospital
    Rotterdam
Dr. Molewaterplein 40
3015 GD Rotterdam
The Netherlands

J. L. H. R. Bosch
Department of Urology and Academic
    Hospital
Rotterdam-Dijkzigt
AZR-D, H1073
Dr. Molewaterplein 40
3015 GD Rotterdam
The Netherlands

M. K. Brawer
Department of Urology, RL-10
University of Washington
Seattle, WA 98108
USA

O. W. Brawley
Early Detection & Community Oncology
    Program
Division of Cancer Prevention & Control
National Cancer Institute
Bethesda, MD 20892
USA

H. B. Carter
Department of Urology
Marburg 403
Johns Hopkins Hospital
600N Wolfe Street
Baltimore, MD 21287
USA

G. W. Chodak
The Prostate & Urology Center
Weiss Memorial Hospital
4646 North Marine Drive
Chicago, IL 60614
USA

G. R. Dohle
Department of Urology
Erasmus University & Academic Hospital
    Rotterdam
Dr. Molewaterplein 40
3015 GD Rotterdam
The Netherlands

M. Gleave
D-9, 2733 Heather Street
Vancouver Hospital & Health Sciences Centre
Vancouver, B. C. V5Z 3J5
Canada

G. J. Gormley
Merck Research Laboratories
P.O. Box 2000
Rahway
New Jersey 07065
USA

J. Hugosson
Department of Urology
Östra University Hospital
S-41685 Göteborg
Sweden

P. Iversen
Department of Urology D 2112
Righospitalet
Blegdamsvej 9
DK-2100 Copenhagen O
University of Copenhagen
Denmark

R. A. Janknegt
Department of Urology
University Hospital Maastricht
P.. Box 5800
6202 AZ Maastricht
The Netherlands

K. H. Kurth
University of Amsterdam
Department of Urology
Meibergdreef 9
1105 AZ Amsterdam
The Netherlands

F. Labrie
Laboratory of Molecular Endocrinology
Prostate Cancer Research Unit
CHUL Research Unit
2705 Boul. Laurier, Québec
Canada G1V 4G4

H. Lilja
Department of Clinical Chemistry
Lund University
University Hospital, Malmö
S-205 02 Malmö
Sweden

G. J. Miller
Department of Urology
St. Radboud University Hospital
P.O. Box 9101
6500 HB Nijmegen
The Netherlands

M. S. Morton
Tenovus Cancer Research Centre
Tenovus Building
Heath Park
Cardiff CF4 4XX
Wales

J. L. Mostwin
Marburgh 401C
Johns Hopkins Hospital
Baltimore, MD 21287-2411
USA

R. P. Myers
Mayo Clinic
200 First Street, SW
Rochester, MN 55905
USA

J. C. Nickel
Department of Urology
Queen's University
Kingston General Hospital
Kingston
K7L 2V7
Canada

J. B. W. Rietbergen
Department of Urology
Erasmus University & Academic Hospital
    Rotterdam
P.O. Box 1738
3000 DR Rotterdam
The Netherlands

J. A. Schalken
Department of Urology
University Hospital Nijmegen
Geert Grooteplein 16
P.O. Box 9101
6500 HB Nijmegen
The Netherlands

F. Schreiter
Urological Department
General Hospital Hamburg-Harburg
Eissendorfer Pferdeweg 52
D-21075 Hamburg
Germany

F. H. Schröder
Department of Urology
Erasmus University & Academic Hospital
   Rotterdam
P.O. Box 1738
3000 DR Rotterdam
The Netherlands

P. H. Smith
Consultant in Urology
Department of Urology
St. James's University Hospital
Leeds LS9 7TF

U. W. Tunn
Urologische Klinik
Städtische Kliniken Offenbach
Starkenburgring 66
63069 Offenbach
Germany

P. J. Van Cangh
Department of Urology
University of Louvain Medical School
Saint Luc University Hospital
10 Avenue Hippocrate
1200 Brussels
Belgium

E. Varenhorst
Associate Professor
Department of Surgery/Urology
County Hospital
S-601 82 Norrköping
Sweden

A. L. Zietman
Genito-Urinary Oncology Unit
Department of Radiation Oncology
Massachusetts General Hospital
Harvard Medical School
Boston, MA 02114
USA

Foreword

F. H. Schröder

The present issue on 'Recent Advances in Prostate Cancer and BPH' represents the proceedings of the fourth Dutch congress on 'Progress and Controversies in Urological Oncology'. The volume, just as previous contributions, is meant to give an update of recent developments in the field of prostatic disease, mainly BPH and prostate cancer.

A major effort has been made to have this book appear very rapidly. As an editor I am very grateful to all those who have been involved in this successful endeavor. This excellent cooperation has allowed publication of this volume within only a few months. This guarantees that in a time of very fast developments in medical sciences the individual chapters can serve as an update and a reference for a number of years. This was exactly the purpose.

The subjects of this book do not represent another attempt to cover the main stream of clinical research in the field of BPH and prostate cancer. An attempt has been made, next to general reviews, to select items that are at the cutting edge of development or even at the stage of hypothesis building. Preventive strategies, in agreement with justified public demand, play a more and more important role in the field. Their design is difficult in a situation where epidemiological leads are not clear cut. Drugs such as 5α-reductase inhibitors, which may play a role in the prevention of prostatic disease in the future, remain of great interest.

The issue of early diagnosis and management of prostate cancer deserves and has received a central role in this issue. Nowhere are opinions as discrepant as in this field. While the preliminary results of the European Randomized Study of Screening for Prostate Cancer seem to document its feasibility, the ethical justification of screening for prostate cancer and even of a scientific study in this field remains a subject of intense discussion in the absence of clear data documenting the effectiveness and usefulness of early treatment.

It is disturbing to see that quality-of-life considerations only now become an important point of view in the management of prostatic disease, especially of early and metastatic prostate cancer. How do patients on average experience the natural course of the diseases under consideration? How does treatment impact on well-being and daily life? Is aggressive management always necessary? Can endocrine treatment be 'minimally invasive' and be upstaged following the course of the disease? Does every patient with advanced disease have to have the full effects of endocrine management? These questions and many others are dealt with in the present volume.

On behalf of the authors and the Scientific and Organizing Committee of 'Progess and Controversies in Oncological Urology IV' I wish you much pleasure in reading.

1

BPH – Definition and Management

Benign prostatic hyperplasia: characteristics of the disease observed in the general population

1

J. L. H. R. Bosch

Introduction

Although there is no conscencus on an exact case definition for benign prostatic hyperplasia (BPH), there is agreement that advancing age, symptoms of prostatism, prostate volume increase and bladder outflow obstruction constitute the most important characteristics of clinical BPH[1]. An increased prostate volume or benign prostatic enlargement may or may not be due to histological BPH, but in most cases it is. Bladder outflow obstruction may or may not be due to the benign prostatic enlargement. The collection of non-specific so-called 'symptoms of prostatism' which more recently are called 'lower urinary tract symptoms'[2] likewise may or may not be caused by BPH. Only a minority of the patients who are treated with a clinical diagnosis of BPH show all these characteristics. It is clear that different combinations of these characteristics can result in a wide spectrum of clinical pictures. It is not clear whether these should all be treated in the same manner. Most probably they should not.

The parameters most often used to assess these characteristics are the international prostate symptom score (IPSS)[3], prostate volume as measured by transrectal ultrasound, level of prostate specific antigen (PSA), urinary flow rate and post-void residual urine volume. A community-based population study conducted in men between 55 and 74 years of age in Rotterdam has revealed interesting data about the occurrence of the aforementioned characteristics of BPH in the general population.

Prostate volume

Cross-sectional data from this Rotterdam community-based study[4] have shown that 95% of men of 55–74 years have a prostate volume of more than 20 cm^3. The percentages of men with prostatic volumes above 30, 40 and 50 cm^3, respectively, increase with age. Slightly more than half of the male population have a volume of more than 30 cm^3, about a quarter have a volume of more than 40 cm^3 and a bit more than one-eighth have volumes of more than 50 cm^3 (Figure 1).

The frequency distributions of the total prostate volume and of the transition zone volume in these men are both skewed towards larger volumes. An approximately normal distribution is found when the logarithmic values for volume are considered. This indicates that prostate growth does not seem to be a linear process. The average growth of the total prostate volume in this cross-sectional study is 2% per year, resulting in an average doubling time of the total prostate volume of 35 years. The average growth of the transition zone volume in this cross-sectional study was 3.5% per year, resulting in an average doubling time of 20 years. There was only a minor increase of the peripheral zone volume with advancing age.

Prostate volumes measured by transrectal ultrasound in these men are larger than volumes measured at autopsy. The absolute difference increased from 7 cm^3 among men 55–59 years old to 12 cm^3 among those 70–74 years old, whereas the relative difference varied between 21 and 28% for the same age strata.

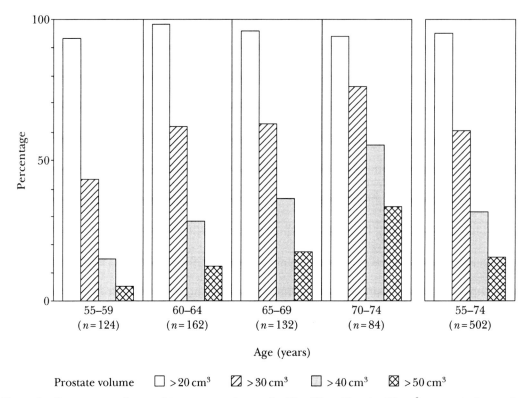

Figure 1 Percentages of men with prostate volume of > 20, > 30, > 40 and > 50 cm³, respectively, per 5-year stratum and for the entire population of men between 55 and 74 years

This disqualifies the long-used autopsy data as reference values for prostate volume or weight. These data are important for the definition of benign prostatic enlargement.

The shape of the prostatic area of greatest transverse diameter in the axial plane (increased roundness), which is expressed by the width-to-height ratio, correlates poorly with age. Body mass index is hardly associated with prostate size in a community-based population. A longitudinal study of prostate volume in a community-based sample of men is needed to determine the proportion of men who have a faster-than-average growth of the prostate.

Lower urinary tract symptoms

The IPSS is equivalent to the seven-item American Urological Association symptom score[5], which has been adopted by the World Health Organization after addition of one disease-specific quality of life question[3]; this question results in a separate quality of life score. This numerical symptom scoring system grades the presence of seven symptoms on a discrete scale of 0 (symptom never present) to 5 (symptom always present). The seven symptoms graded can be described as incomplete emptying, increased frequency, intermittency, urgency, weak stream, hesitancy and nocturia. The possible value range for this score is between 0 and 35 points. A subdivision of men into three symptom classes has been proposed[5], resulting in groups with minor (IPSS 0–7), moderate (IPSS 8–19) and severe (IPSS 20–35) symptoms.

The disease-specific quality of life question was phrased as follows: 'If you were to spend the rest of your life with your urinary condition just the way it is now, how would you feel about that?', and the answering scale ranged from 0 (delighted) to 6 (terrible).

Symptom frequency

A cumulative frequency plot of the international prostate symptom scores in this community-based population of men of 55–74 years[6] shows that 6% are severely symptomatic, as evidenced by a score of 20 or more points, and that 24% are moderately symptomatic, as evidenced by a score of between 8 and 19 points. The percentage of men who are severely symptomatic, that is those with an IPSS of 20 or more, remains surprisingly constant at about 6% in the 5-year strata between 55 and 74 years. The percentage of men with moderate complaints increases somewhat with age (Figure 2).

The relevance of the subdivision in mildly, moderately and severely symptomatic groups is confirmed by the relationship between the total IPSS subgroups and the results of the disease-specific quality of life question that is appended

to the IPSS. There was a good correlation between the total IPSS and the score of this single quality of life question ($r = 0.74$; $p = 0.001$). We also found that 31% of men were 'delighted', 24% were 'pleased', 29% were 'mostly satisfied' and 10% felt 'about equally satisfied and dissatisfied' about their urinary condition. Few men were 'mostly dissatisfied' (5%) or felt 'unhappy' (1%). No man scored 6, i.e. 'terrible'.

During an intake interview, answers to questions of a demographic nature and medical and surgical history were recorded. The median IPSS of the men who answered 'yes' or 'no' to the global intake question of whether they had any voiding complaints was 13.5 and 3.0, respectively ($p < 0.0001$). The quality of life score of the men who answered 'yes' or 'no' to the question of whether they had any voiding complaints was 3.0 and 1.0, respectively ($p < 0.0001$). Overall, 82% of the men gave a negative answer to the first part of this question. This contrasts with the results of the more detailed symptom questionnaire (IPSS). Only 12% of the men had a score of 0, i.e. they were asymptomatic. This indicates that men tolerate a certain level of symptom frequency without complaint.

Scores for individual symptoms

If the presence of a symptom is defined as having a score of 1 or more for that particular symptom, then the seven symptoms in the total group of men of 55–74 years were present in the following order of frequency[6]: nocturia, 75%; increased frequency, 60%; weak stream, 47%; urgency, 31%; incomplete emptying, 30%; intermittency, 28%; and hesitancy, 15%.

When results of the scores on the individual questions were subdivided into three classes of severity, i.e. slight, moderate and severe, on the basis of a score of 0–1, 2–3 and 4–5, respectively for that particular symptom, then the percentages of men respectively suffering moderately and severely from one particular symptom are

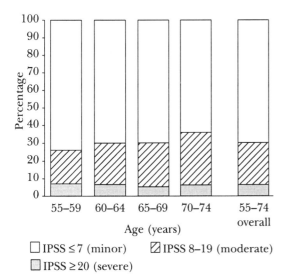

Figure 2 Frequency distribution of men with no or minor, moderate or severe symptoms for the four consecutive 5-year age strata and the entire population of men between 55 and 74 years

as follows: weak stream, 14% and 18%; increased frequency, 21% and 11%; nocturia, 25% and 4%; urgency, 11% and 8%; intermittency, 10% and 7%; incomplete emptying, 8% and 7%; and hesitancy, 5% and 4%. In general there are more men who complain moderately than men who complain severely of a particular symptom, except for the symptom 'weak stream'.

It is interesting to note that for all symptoms except urgency, the prevalence of men suffering severely from one particular symptom is higher in the age group of 55–59 years than in the group of 60–64 years. Nocturia is a very prevalent symptom: the percentage of men who wake up to void at least once every night rises from 63% between 55 and 59 years to 83% between 70 and 74 years of age (with an average of 75% between 55 and 74 years).

The individual questions of the IPSS were examined for the relationship to age. Although the prevalence of the symptoms nocturia, increased frequency, weak stream and incomplete emptying seems to increase somewhat with age, only the prevalence of nocturia increases significantly with age between 55 and 74 years ($p = 0.002$).

Scores on individual questions correlated with the physiological parameter for which it is assumed that it measures the same variable

The 'feeling of incomplete emptying' was poorly correlated[6] with residual urine volume ($r = 0.14$; $p = 0.01$). This question, however, may be difficult to interpret. An increased frequency may give the person the false impression that he has not emptied his bladder sufficiently, because he has to void again soon after the previous micturition. Five per cent (14/271) of the men without significant post-void residual urine volume (≤ 50 ml) claimed to have a feeling of incomplete emptying more than half of the time or almost always.

Intermittency was weakly correlated with total flow time divided by total voiding time ($r = -0.20$; $p < 0.001$).

The symptom weak stream was weakly correlated with the peak flow rate ($r = -0.19$; $p < 0.001$) and with the average flow rate ($r = -0.22$; $p < 0.001$). Nine per cent (9/105) of the men with a peak flow rate of ≥ 15 ml/s claimed to have a weak stream more than half of the time or almost always.

Hesitancy was poorly correlated with the time before flow actually commenced after the patient had been informed that the flow recorder was started ($r = 0.13$, $p = 0.0081$).

Prostate specific antigen

The 502 men without prostate cancer and PSA level of < 10 ng/ml were stratified by international prostate symptom score subgroups[7], as follows: those with no or minor symptoms (IPSS 0–7; $n = 318$), those with moderate symptoms (IPSS 8–19; $n = 120$) and those with severe symptoms (IPSS 20–35, $n = 30$). This stratification resulted in significant differences ($p = 0.002$) in median PSA values between IPSS strata. Further analysis showed that the median PSA value in the group with no or minor complaints (1.1 ng/ml) differed significantly ($p = 0.005$) from the median value in the group with moderate complaints (1.3 ng/ml), and also significantly ($p = 0.02$) from the median value in the group with severe complaints (1.8 ng/ml). These differences, although statistically significant, are not helpful clinically in the diagnostic work-up of patients with lower urinary tract symptoms.

Physiological parameters related to BPH

Peak flow rate

In a community-based sample of men studied in Olmsted County in Minnesota, USA, the peak flow rate decreased by about 2 ml/s per decade on average[8]. These data are cross-sectional, like the prostate size data, and do not represent changes over time in individual men. It is important to note that more than 50% of the men over 65 had peak flow rates below 15 ml/s. In the Scottish community study of Garraway and colleagues[9], the decrease per decade was between 0.3 and 1.7 ml/s. An interesting finding in the follow-up examination of the Scottish men was that 36% of the men who initially had a peak flow rate below 15 ml/s raised their peak flow rate above this cut-off point after 1 year of follow-up[10].

In the Rotterdam study, we found poor correlations between the age and physiological measurements such as flow rate (-0.08; p NS) and post-void residual urine volume (0.12; $p < 0.05$)[11].

Post-void residual urine volume

A post-void residual urine volume of more than 50 ml was found in 30% of all men aged between 70 and 74 years[12]. However, only 10% of these men had a post-void residual volume greater than 100 ml. Between 55 and 64 years of age, 12% of the men had post-void residual volume greater than 50 ml, and this was 18% between 65 and 69 years. Men with significant amounts of residual urine are therefore relatively uncommon in the community (Table 1).

Definition of clinical BPH

As a first step to generate a practical case definition of BPH[13], we could study the influence of the inclusion of different possible parameters that could be combined in a definition and of different cut-off values for these parameters. This was applied in this community-based population of men between 55 and 74 years. By making several combinations of the parameters prostate volume, symptom score, peak flow rate, post-void residual volume and the disease-specific quality of life score that is included in the IPSS and using various different cut-off values for these parameters, 28 possible definitions for clinical BPH were formulated. Only those eight case-definitions that resulted in a statistically significant increase of the prevalence of BPH with advancing age were

Table 1 Mean and median values and inter-quartile ranges obtained for post-void residual urine volume in four consecutive 5-year age strata in a community-based population of men without prostate cancer or a history of prostate operation

Age (years)	n	Post-void residual urine volume (ml)		
		Mean ± SE	Median	Inter-quartile range
55–59	76	22 ± 5	0	0–17
60–64	100	17 ± 5	0	0–0
65–69	90	25 ± 5	0	0–35
70–74	60	31 ± 7	0	0–53
Total	326	23 ± 3	0	0–21

Table 2 Percentage of men (mean and 95% confidence interval) in four consecutive 5-year age strata with clinical benign prostatic hyperplasia (BPH) according to the following case definition: clinical BPH is present if total prostate volume is > 30 cm^3 and IPSS is > 7

Age	n	Mean	95% CI
55–59	120	10	5–17
60–64	159	22	16–29
65–69	132	22	15–31
70–74	83	28	18–39
p-value			0.003

Table 3 Percentage of men (mean and 95% confidence interval) in four consecutive 5-year age strata with clinical benign prostatic hyperplasia (BPH) according to the following case definition: clinical BPH is present if total prostate volume is > 30 cm^3 and IPSS is > 7 and peak flow rate is < 10 ml/s and post-void residual volume is > 50 ml

Age	n	Mean	95% CI
55–59	76	1	0.03–7
60–64	100	2	0.2–7
65–69	90	3	1–9
70–74	60	8	3–18
p-value			0.03

accepted as valid definitions, since the most important determinant of BPH occurrence is age.

The highest age-specific prevalence rates were found by using a case-definition of prostate volume of > 30 cm^3 combined with an IPSS of > 7. The prevalence increased from 10% between 55 and 59 to 28% between 70 and 74 years (Table 2).

The lowest age-specific prevalence rates were found with a case-definition of prostate volume of > 30 cm^3 *and* an IPSS of > 7 *and* a peak flow rate of < 10 ml/s *and* a post-void residual volume of > 50 ml. The prevalence increased from 1% between 55 and 59 to 8% between 70 and 74 years (Table 3).

The prevalence rates became very low when the post-void residual volume was introduced as an additional parameter. The impact of the addition of flow rate as an additional parameter besides prostate volume and symptoms was very limited.

The most important conclusion should be that the true prevalence of benign prostatic hyperplasia in the community is unknown, but that the reported prevalence depends very much on the case-definition that is used. Before accepting a case-definition as the most appropriate definition, it is necessary to conduct a prospective study to determine the men who will eventually require treatment and to correlate this information with the different possible case-definitions.

References

1. Hald, T. (1989). Urodynamics in benign prostatic hyperplasia: a survey. *Prostate* (Suppl.), **2**, 69–77
2. Abrams, P. (1994). A critique of scoring systems. In Kurth, K. H. and Newling, D. W. W. (eds.) *Benign Prostatic Hyperplasia: Recent Progress in Clinical Research and Practice*, EORTC Genitourinary Group Monograph 12, pp. 109–23. (New York: Wiley-Liss)
3. Mebust, W., Roizo, R., Schröder, F. and Villers, A. (1992). Correlations between pathology, clinical symptoms and the course of the disease. In Cockett, A. T., Aso, Y., Chatelain. C., Denis, L., Griffiths, K., Khoury, S. and Murphy, G. (eds.) *Proceedings of the International Consultation on Benign Prostatic Hyperplasia*, pp. 53–62. (Channel Islands: SCI)
4. Bosch, J. L. H. R., Hop, W. C. J., Niemer, A. Q. H. L., Bangma, C. H., Kirkels, W. J. and Schröder, F. H. (1994). Parameters of prostate volume and shape in a community-based population of men 55 to 74 years old. *J. Urol.*, **152**, 1501–5
5. Barry, M. J., Fowler, F. J., O'Leary, M. P., Bruskewitz, R. C., Holtgrewe, H. L., Mebust, W. K., Cockett, A. T. K. and the measurement committee of the American Urological Association (1992). The American Urological Association symptom index for benign prostatic hyperplasia. *J. Urol.*, **148**, 1549–57
6. Bosch, J. L. H. R., Hop, W. C. J., Kirkels, W. J. and Schröder, F. H. (1995). The International Prostate Symptom Score in a community-based sample of men between fifty-five and seventy-four years of age. Prevalence and correlation of symptoms with age, prostate volume flow rate and residual urine volume. *Br. J. Urol.*, **75**, 622–30
7. Bosch, J. L. H. R., Hop, W. C. J., Kirkels, W. J. and Schröder, F. H. (1995). Prostate specific antigen in a community-based sample of men without prostate cancer: correlations with prostate volume, age, body mass index and symptoms of prostatism. *Prostate*, **27**, 241–9
8. Girman, C. J., Panser, L. A., Chute, C. G., Oesterling, J. E., Barret, D. M., Chem, C. C., Arrighi, H M., Guess, H. A. and Lieber, M. M. (1993). Natural history of prostatism: urinary flow rates in a community-based study. *J. Urol.*, **150**, 887–92
9. Garraway, W. M., Collins, G. N., and Lee, R. J. (1991). High prevalence of benign prostatic hyperplasia in the community. *Lancet*, **388**, 469–71
10. Garraway, W. M., Armstrong, C., Auld, S., King, D. and Simpson, R. J. (1993). Follow-up of a cohort of men with untreated benign prostatic hyperplasia. *Eur. Urol.*, **24**, 313–18

11. Bosch, J. L. H. R., Niemer, A. Q. H. L., Kirkels, W. J. and Schröder, F. H, (1994). Signs and symptoms of benign prostatic hyperplasia in men screened for prostatic carcinoma. In Kurth, K. H. and Newling, D. W. W. (eds.) *Benign Prostatic Hyperplasia: Recent Progress in Clinical Research and Practice*, EORTC genitourinary group monograph 12, pp. 97–107. (New York: Wiley-Liss)

12. Bosch, J. L. H. R. (1995). Postvoid residual urine in the evaluation of men with benign prostatic hyperplasia. *World J. Urol.*, **13**, 17–20

13. Bosch, J. L. H. R., Hop, W. C. J., Kirkels, W. J. and Schröder, F. H. (1995). Natural history of benign prostatic hyperplasia: appropriate case definition and estimation of its prevalence in the community. *Urology*, **46** (Suppl. 3A), 34–40

New and old interventions in benign prostatic hyperplasia: an update

2

P. H. Smith

Introduction

During this century prostatectomy has been transformed from a major open surgical intervention to a routine transurethral procedure suitable for all but the most seriously ill patients. The mortality rate has fallen to less than 1% and incontinence (which was not uncommon 30 years ago) is now rarely seen following the operation. Within the last 30 years the decreasing morbidity has resulted in the operation being offered to those whose symptoms are less severe and of shorter duration. In such patients the results have been not as satisfactory as in patients with severe obstruction or acute retention[1].

In the 1980s the medical profession became uncomfortably aware that middle-aged men in good general health with only moderate degrees of obstruction with some frequency by day or by night did not take kindly to a procedure that did not relieve them of all their symptoms and that included complications such as a recurrence rate of 2% per year, a 1% incidence of urethral stricture, a 5% chance of impotence and a 50% risk of retrograde ejaculation.

In 1989 Mebust and co-workers[2] reviewed 3885 patients following transurethral prostatectomy. Although the mortality rate was only 0.2%, the immediate postoperative morbidity was 18%, including failure to void, the need for blood transfusion, clot retention and genitourinary infection. In this series 93 patients (2.4%) were discharged from hospital with indwelling urethral catheters (usually associated with a hypotonic bladder).

In the same year Roos and colleagues[3] noted that the incidence of a second prostatectomy was between three and six times as common after transurethral than after open surgery. They also noted a relative risk of 1.45 of death from transurethral as compared with open prostatectomy.

In the UK Doll and associates[4] reported a much higher mortality rate (2.8%) than did Mebust and colleagues[2], but a similar rate of postoperative complications (17%). They also carried out a more prolonged follow-up, reporting that approximately one-quarter of the patients experienced persisting symptoms. They noted that obstructive symptoms were alleviated slightly more frequently than irritative symptoms and that, after 6–12 months, 12% of patients were troubled either by urinary tract infection or incontinence.

The recognition that prostatectomy did not cure all symptoms attributed to prostatic hypertrophy resulted in a re-assessment of the indications for the operation and a search for alternative means of treatment. The change was swift and reductions in the numbers of prostatectomies were already being recorded by Mebust and co-workers[2] and Holtgrewe and colleagues[5] at the end of the last decade.

The issues raised led to the formation of the International Prostate Health Council and to an intercontinental initiative by interested urologists in Europe, Japan and the United States of America under the patronage of the World Health Organization, known as the International Consultation on Benign Prostatic Hyperplasia (BPH). This group has now held three meetings, in 1991, 1993 and 1995, from which have emerged guidelines for symptom assessment, investigation and therapy including drug therapy and the alternative forms of treatment. The document *Recommendations of the International Concensus Committee* is now available in 12 languages.

Assessment of the patient

Symptom score

From an analysis of the different symptom scoring systems has emerged the International Prostate Scoring System (IPSS – Figure 1). This has now been validated and has been translated into many languages. The use of this single-page *pro forma* provides a simple means of assessing the severity of the patient's symptoms whilst the last question concerning his willingness or otherwise to accept his quality of life at the time of the assessment acts as a very good guide to our understanding of the patient's need for active intervention.

Patient : ______ DOB : ______ ID : ______ Date of assessment : ______

INTERNATIONAL PROSTATE SYMPTOM SCORE (IPSS)							
	Not at all	Less than 1 time in 5	Less than half the time	About half the time	More than half the time	Almost always	
1. Over the past month, how often have you had a sensation of not emptying your bladder completely after you finished urinating?	0	1	2	3	4	5	
2. Over the past month, how often have you had to urinate again less than two hours after you finished urinating?	0	1	2	3	4	5	
3. Over the past month, how often have you found you stopped and started again several times when you urinated?	0	1	2	3	4	5	
4. Over the past month, how often have you found it difficult to postpone urination?	0	1	2	3	4	5	
5. Over the past month, how often have you had a weak urinary stream?	0	1	2	3	4	5	
6. Over the past month, how often have you had to push or strain to begin urination?	0	1	2	3	4	5	
	None	1 time	2 times	3 times	4 times	5 or more times	
7. Over the past month, how many times did you most typically get up to urinate from the time you went to bed at night until the time you got up in the morning?	0	1	2	3	4	5	
Total IPPS Score S =							

QUALITY OF LIFE DUE TO URINARY SYMPTOMS							
7. If you were to spend the rest of your life with your urinary condition just the way it is now, how would you feel about that?	Delighted	Pleased	Mostly satisfied	Mixed about equally satisfied and dissatisfied	Mostly Dissatisfied	Unhappy	Terrible
	0	1	2	3	4	5	6
Quality of Life assessment index QOL =							

Figure 1 International Prostate Scoring System

Investigation

Apart from a careful history and physical examination, including assessment of the prostate by digital rectal examination, urologists are advised to test the urine by dipstick, to exclude the presence of urinary infection, to determine the renal function by serum creatinine measurement and to check the residual urine. This is most simply done by transabdominal ultrasound where this is available. Ultrasound examination of the upper tract and cystoscopy are not advised as routine investigations. It is also important to check the maximum urinary flow rate (Q_{max}, in ml/s) on two occasions with a voided volume greater than 150 ml. A test for prostate specific antigen (PSA) is also indicated in patients with a life expectancy of 10 years or more in whom a diagnosis of prostate cancer would change the treatment plan.

Significance of symptoms

The increasing interest in BPH has prompted surveys of urological symptoms in local communities. Ball and co-workers[6] showed that urological symptoms potentially attributable to prostatic enlargement resolved spontaneously in 25% of patients. Garraway and associates[7] surveyed 1627 men aged 40–79 years in Scotland and defined prostatic hyperplasia as a prostate gland more than 20 g in weight in the presence of symptoms of urinary dysfunction and/or a peak flow rate of < 15 ml/s without evidence of malignancy. Of 410 men who satisfied the criteria for BPH, 51% reported that their symptoms interfered with at least one of a number of selected activities of daily living as compared with 28% of men who did not have the condition. They concluded that there was considerable unmet need and that a substantial number of middle-aged and elderly men living in the UK might benefit from assessment and treatment for this condition.

These two approaches were quite different and the authors have drawn differing conclusions. Some think that the search for the male with symptoms is an appropriate public health measure that should be encouraged, since the symptoms may well be relieved by drug therapy. Others believe that such a proposal is premature, since such patients are not seriously ill and do not have a life-threatening condition.

In the UK, hospital doctors have been encouraged to set up shared care initiatives in which patients in the community can easily be assessed by standard forms and investigations in a nurse-led clinic. The general practitioners are not uniformly enthusiastic about this approach, since their workload is already demanding and the cost implications of prolonged drug treatment are considerable. The matter is not yet resolved.

Choosing a treatment

In a patient whose symptoms are believed to arise from the prostate gland, urologists are increasingly cautious about suggesting transurethral resection as the first approach. The fact that symptoms improve spontaneously in 25% of patients is one factor. Another is related to the urodynamic findings which show that a further 25% have bladder failure as their primary problem, whilst almost 50% have detrusor instability responsible for frequency and urgency. This subject is well reviewed by Abrams and colleagues[8]. Increasingly, it seems appropriate to investigate carefully before choosing surgery as the form of therapy.

Abrams and associates[8] believe that the term 'prostatism' should be replaced by 'lower urinary tract symptoms', since this description implies the need for continuing assessment and investigation leading to a definitive diagnosis. In such circumstances urodynamic evaluation is obviously appropriate for anyone whose symptoms are not clearly obstructive. The development of a more precise diagnosis allows therapy to be targeted more specifically.

Economic issues are also of importance and have been well reviewed by Holtgrewe and co-workers[9]. They costed watchful waiting, finasteride, α-blocker therapy, transurethral and open prostatectomy. The costs in the USA for the initial treatment and 1 year of follow-up

Table 1 Average costs of treatment for benign prostatic hyperplasia. United States 1985–89[9]

Therapy	Cost of treatment and 1-year follow-up ($)	Cost of second year ($)
Watchful waiting	1162	640
Finasteride	1326	788
Alpha-blocker	1395	845
Transurethral prostatectomy	8606	360
Open prostatectomy	12 788	69

(including expected complications) together with the cost of continuing this treatment are listed in Table 1. From this table it can be seen that watchful waiting or drug therapy – even allowing for the failure rate – is cost-effective over a period of 10–15 years. If the cost of surgery is less, as in the UK, the balance is different. Some relevant points in relation to the different options are considered below.

Non-surgical options

Watchful waiting Once the patient has been assessed and found to have symptoms that are not particularly troublesome – normal renal function, no significant residual urine and a normal PSA – it is possible to consider reassurance rather than active intervention. If this approach is acceptable to the patient, re-evaluation will be required every 6–12 months. If this is carried out, 25% of patients improve spontaneously, 50% have symptoms that are reasonably static and 25% experience deterioration of symptoms, demanding some form of active treatment.

Drug therapy Alpha-blockers and inhibitors of 5α-reductase are increasingly used for patients with moderate symptoms, for which relief is required. The cost of the different drugs is reflected in the pricings shown in Table 1. The use of the two differing types of drugs has increased dramatically, there being a three-fold increase in prescriptions of α-blockers from 1992 to 1994 and a six-fold increase in prescriptions for finasteride during the same period.

Although both groups of drugs produce a 30–40% reduction in symptom score and an increase in flow rates of 30–40%, the changes in detrusor pressure are relatively small. In randomized placebo-controlled trials, both types of drug have demonstrated the benefit of the active agent over placebo. In general the benefit is modest, although it appears to be maintained over periods of 3–4 years at least.

In addition to the α-blockers and inhibitors of 5α-reductase, several other agents are freely available within Europe, including pollen extract (Cernilton®), *Seronoa repens*, *Pygeum africanum* and mepartricin[10]. In view of the known placebo effect of drug therapy in BPH it is evident that these agents must be evaluated in placebo-controlled randomized double-blind clinical trials before they can be recommended. Some trials are now under way.

Non-medical therapies

Balloon dilatation is no longer recommended, and hyperthermia is also thought to be ineffective[11]. All forms of treatment which are effective and durable depend upon stenting or heat in one of its forms. The information on these forms of treatment comes largely from the *Third International Consultation on BPH*[12].

Urethral stents

Temporary stents have been available for some years and are designed to be inserted in such a way that the bladder neck is maintained in the open position whilst the external sphincter remains intact. Some of the stents available are listed in Table 2. They are relatively easy to insert and can be most effective in restoring

Table 2 Characteristics of intraurethral stents[12]

Stent	Expansion	Caliber	Length (mm)	Composition	Indwelling time
Temporary					
Urospiral	fixed caliber	21F	40–80	stainless steel	up to 12 months
Prostakath	fixed caliber	21F	35–95	gold-plated stainless steel	up to 12 months
Intraurethral catheter	fixed caliber	16F	40–60	polyurethane	up to 6 months
Memokath	heat expandable	22F	35–95	nickel–titanium	up to 36 months
Prostacoil	self expanding	24/30F	40–80	nickel–titanium	up to 36 months
Biofix	fixed caliber	24F	45–75	polylactic polymer	up to 6 months
Permanent					
Urolume/Wallstent	self expanding	42F	20–40	superalloy	permanent
Memotherm	heat expandable	42F	15–80	nickel–titanium	permanent
Ultraflex	self expandable	42F	20–60	elastalloy (nickel–titanium)	permanent

Table 3 Voiding symptoms following use of Prostakath in 318 patients (J. Nordling, personal communication)

Symptom	None	Moderate	Severe
Stress incontinence	244	20	17
Urge	155	79	46 (incontinent)
Frequency	162	63	45
Nocturia	205 (0–1)	62 (2–3)	12 (> 3)
Emptying problems	259	15	8
Urethral bleeding	271	9	2
Local discomfort	262	13	7

micturition to a patient who is unfit for operation or who for some reason refuses surgical intervention. Complications include migration, local irritation and persisting frequency and urgency. The complications in 318 patients treated with the Prostakath are shown in Table 3 (J. Nordling, personal communication). Similar complications are seen with other stents.

Biodegradable stents

Within the last 2 years biodegradable stents have become available. These are made of polyglycolide or polylactide polymers and last for a period of 1–6 months, depending upon the type of stent selected. They are likely to find a use in the prevention of urinary retention after laser prostatectomy, thermoablation and high-intensity focused ultrasound use. As the stents degrade, they are passed in the urine.

Permanent stents

These are designed to remain permanently *in situ* and to be incorporated within the urethral lining. If any part of the stent projects into the bladder, it cannot be incorporated and subsequent calcification is likely to form upon it. If the stent is inserted below the bladder neck, it will become incorporated but will not be effective. An additional problem is that the stent is effectively cylindrical, but the prostatic urethra is not. Even the bladder neck is not totally regular in outline, and the prostatic urethra is angulated and has varying dimensions. It is therefore very difficult to guarantee that the whole of a stent, however carefully positioned, will be incorporated. The permanent stents available are shown in Table 2. As yet there is little clinical experience with the Ultraflex® stent and most with the Urolume®, made of a superalloy. The Memotherm® stent is made of a woven nickel titanium alloy and is heat expandable. This makes it simple both to insert and to remove, since the alloy expands when heated and contracts when cooled.

In a European randomized trial in which 60 patients with urodynamic evidence of bladder outflow obstruction were randomized to treatment with the Urolume (34 patients) or TUR (26 patients), the stent has so far proved as effective as prostatectomy in reducing symptoms and increasing the flow rate[13]. Similar changes in symptom score and flow rate were found at a 3-year follow-up of 49 patients in a North American study group. Those with prostatism had a more acceptable flow rate (approximately 15 ml/s) than did those treated because of retention of urine (approximately 11 ml/s)[14].

Thermotherapy

With this form of treatment the aim is to destroy prostatic tissue, without damaging the surrounding structure. The temperature must be raised to 44°C or more to allow coagulation necrosis to occur.

Most information has come from the Prosatron® (Technomed Medical Systems). Other devices include the ECP®, Prostalund® (Dantec), T3® (Urologix), Thermex® (Direx Medical Systems) and Urowave® (Dornier Medical Systems). Whilst it is possible to monitor the intra-prostatic temperature directly by means of interstitial thermometry, it is more usual to monitor the urethral and rectal temperatures to ensure that neither exceeds 44.5°C. The position of the treatment device must be monitored regularly during therapy to be certain that it is not displaced.

In conventional thermotherapy the temperature within the prostate lies between 45 and 55°C. Clinical studies have shown that thermotherapy of this type produces a significant reduction in symptom score (by 50–75% with reductions in both irritative and obstructive symptoms) and an increase in flow rate of between 50 and 60%. The effect is significantly superior to sham therapy[15].

In a randomized study the reduction in symptom score and residual volume were similar, whether the patient was treated by prostatectomy or thermotherapy. The increase in flow rate was, however, much greater in the patients treated by prostatectomy (approximately 125 vs. 50%)[16].

In another study in which thermotherapy was compared to sham treatment it was notable that the symptom score fell by almost 30% whilst the peak flow rate increased by more than 25% in those receiving sham treatment[17]. This placebo effect must be taken into account whenever drug therapy or newer forms of treatment are being evaluated.

Using the newer high-temperature thermotherapy (Thermex, T3, Prostatron 2.5) the temperature in the prostate is likely to be between 60 and 70°C. Such patients need to be catheterized in the post-treatment period – often for several days – and they have some discomfort. As a consequence of the greater destruction, however, the increase in peak flow is likely to be between 50 and 70% compared with 20–30% for the low-temperature therapy.

Low-temperature thermotherapy produces symptomatic improvement in the majority of patients, with a modest improvement in flow rate. The higher-energy thermotherapy produces a much greater increase in the flow rate at the price of post-treatment discomfort and the need for catheterization or the use of a temporary stent. This form of treatment is *not* likely to be suitable for the patient with significant enlargement of his middle lobe.

Transurethral needle ablation

In this technique adjustable needles are passed into the prostatic substance under direct vision. Adjustable shields on the needles minimize the chance of damage to the urethral mucosa. Once the device is in position, low-level radiofrequency (RF energy power) from a special stimulator generates temperatures in excess of 80°C within the substance of the prostate. Power of 4–15 W is applied for 5 min, the temperature in the prostate being recorded by thermosensors on the end of the shields and the tip of the catheter. The prostate is treated on each side, starting 1 cm distal to the bladder neck and at 1-cm intervals between there and the veru montanum. It is common to leave a urethral catheter *in situ* for 1–2 days and for the patient to be given antibiotics and anti-inflammatory agents for approximately 5 days. Hematuria and mild dysuria are to be expected, together with retention of urine in approximately 30% of patients. From five separate clinical studies it appears that there is a 60–70% reduction in symptom score, a 50–70% increase in peak flow and a 30–40% reduction in detrusor pressure at peak flow within 6 months of the procedure[18]. Transurethral needle ablation has recently been shown to be effective in relieving acute retention of urine in 30 of 38 treated patients[19].

The advantage of this technique is that it is relatively minor, can be provided on an outpatient basis and uses a relatively cheap and portable generator. It is accepted that longer-term follow-up and further randomized studies will be required before its true place can be evaluated.

High-intensity focused ultrasound

In this technique a beam of ultrasound is focused at a selected depth within the body, resulting in a high temperature with immediate death of the cellular elements within the focus of the beam. The prostate is treated transrectally with one transducer used for imaging and another for therapy in one system, or a single transducer in the other, in which the transducer can adopt an imaging or therapeutic mode[20]. The patient requires general or spinal anesthesia, a suprapubic catheter and a urethral catheter, to allow the exact identification of the urethra, bladder neck and veru montanum during imaging.

Once the optimal position is obtained the transducer is immobilized with a locking arm device and treatment is given, to destroy the tissue adjacent to the prostatic urethra. Treatment with 1000–3000 W/cm^2 over an ellipsoidal length of 10–30 mm is used. Necrosis without cavitation is produced at temperatures of 80–200°C.

Following treatment the symptom score decreases by 50% or more, whilst the peak flow rate improves by up to 50%. In 25% of patients cystic cavities are seen within the prostate. This technique is not yet fully developed and its final role in the management of BPH remains to be decided.

Laser prostatectomy

The use of laser energy to coagulate or vaporize prostatic tissue has attracted increasing interest this decade. With the initial device know as transurethral ultrasound-guided laser-induced prostatectomy (TULIP) the energy was delivered to the prostate through a balloon, which distended the urethra and compressed the prostatic lobes. The mechanism of delivery was controlled by transrectal ultrasound. Following initial encouraging results, the technique has been changed, to allow the delivery of laser energy through conventional endoscopes. A contact technique is used, in which the fiber is applied to the surface of the prostate; a non-contact technique may be used, in which the energy is delivered without touching the surface of the gland; and an interstitial technique is used, in which the fiber is passed into the prostate prior to delivery of the energy.

The contact technique requires high energy delivered for a short time, e.g. 100 W for 1 s, and produces tissue vaporization without charring if contact is not prolonged.

With the non-contact technique the energy is absorbed into the tissue, producing coagulation necrosis. With this technique one might use 25 W for 4 s or for a period of time that will induce a visible grayish-white change in the tissue.

With interstitial therapy there is coagulation necrosis, with very low wattage used in as many sites as are needed. Constant laser power of 5–7 W for approximately 10 min produces the maximal coagulation volume[21].

The attraction of laser prostatectomy is the concept that one can destroy prostatic tissue with minimal blood loss over a short period of time, using a technique that is suitable for outpatient therapy or overnight stay.

In practice, as with the other forms of therapy, it is possible to reduce the symptom score

by 50–70% and to increase the mean peak flow rates by 50–60%. These results, which are durable for at lest a year, have been obtained in an American study that used 40 W for 40 s at the 3 and 9 o'clock positions and 40 W for 30 s at the 6 and 12 o'clock positions[22]. In a study in the UK, 60 W for 60 s was used at 2, 5, 7 and 10 o'clock positions[23]. In each study treatment was repeated closer to the bladder neck in patients with the larger prostates, and in the UK study treatment was given for 30–60 s at the 6 o'clock position if a middle lobe was prominent[23,24].

Despite the great clinical and commercial interest, this form of treatment has not yet displaced prostatectomy, perhaps in part because the vaporization technique is time-consuming, whilst the non-contact technique, which produced coagulation necrosis, is associated with the need for catheterization and significant postoperative pain and discomfort lasting often in excess of 4 weeks.

Although the true role for laser prostatectomy has not yet been found, it is clearly advantageous for those in poor general health and in those with coagulation disorders. Its future role is likely to be determined in part by the degree of postoperative discomfort and in part by the cost of the procedure, since the majority of lasers are more expensive than a traditional resectoscope and the majority of laser fibers, unlike resectoscope loops, are for single use only. In two recent papers Keoghane and colleagues[25,26] have commented, from 148 patients treated by transurethral resection ($n = 72$) or contact laser ($n = 76$) that the results were similar but that the laser treatment was more expensive, because of the theater consumables.

Transurethral electrovaporization of the prostate

This technique is a modified form of cystodiathermy in which a conventional rollerball electrode or specially designed electrode is used to coagulate and vaporize the prostate. A very high energy of up to 250 W is used with a cutting current, and 60 W for coagulation. If the electrode is moved slowly over the prostatic tissue it causes vaporization with hemostasis and allows gradual destruction with repeated passes of the ball or other device[27].

Patients are catheterized for up to 24 h and appear to have a much more trouble-free postoperative course than after laser prostatectomy that uses coagulation necrosis (the non-contact technique).

This approach in which the surgeon uses a technique with which he is familiar, is naturally appealing, as is the fact that the cost of the equipment is much less than that involved in laser prostatectomy. As yet the limitations, if any, of this technique and the long-term durability are unknown.

Transurethral prostatectomy

Though unchallenged for 40–50 years, the place of prostatectomy has been questioned carefully within the last decade. The debate has been in part about the suitability of the patient for the operation and in part about the suitability of the operation for the patient. Most patients are fit for prostatectomy, but not all need it. Once they are aware that the problem is not due to cancer, many patients are happy to live with their symptoms, at least for the time being. Others are willing to consider drug therapy and some express preferences for the newer forms of treatment, particularly laser therapy – usually without fully understanding the state of development of laser surgery or that of the other alternatives.

Transurethral prostatectomy or transurethral incision of the bladder neck and prostate is more appropriate for those with obstructive rather than irritative symptoms. Recognizing that approximately a quarter of the patients presenting are not obstructed, Cetinel and colleagues[28] have recommended that pressure flow studies be performed in all patients in whom the irritative symptoms are dominant, in the hope of minimizing surgical intervention. Clearly it is important to select only those patients who can benefit from surgery, since careful selection is likely to reduce the numbers of patients whose symptoms are not completely relieved. At the present time it seems that pros-

tatectomy completely relieves symptoms in only 75% of patients[29,30].

Unless operation is vital because of severe symptoms or retention of urine, the temptation is to suggest no active treatment. Wasson and co-workers[31] have compared transurethral surgery with watchful waiting for patients with moderate symptoms of benign hyperplasia. Of 556 men studied (280 undergoing surgery and 276 in the watchful waiting group) it was clear that surgery was more effective than watchful waiting (no therapy) in improving symptoms and in minimizing the need for subsequent treatment. In the surgery group there was an 8% failure rate, including a 1% incidence of a residual urine volume greater than 350 ml, a 1% incidence of doubling of the serum creatinine level and of urinary incontinence. Although 'treatment failure' was approximately twice as high in the group undergoing watchful waiting (20% of cases), the problems could be relieved in the majority of patients in this group by transurethral prostatectomy. This seems to show that the approach of watchful waiting is likely to be satisfactory (though without complete relief of symptoms) in approximately 80% of patients for a period of 3 years at least.

Those favoring transurethral prostatectomy draw attention to the fact that none of the alternatives offer such a great improvement in symptom scores, flow rate, reduction in bladder pressure and residual urine as does the operation. The more conservative emphasize the relative safety of watchful waiting and the possibility of symptom relief from drug therapy.

It is nearly always possible to improve upon a procedure which had for many years been regarded as effective and Klimberg and associates[32] have now reported the results of outpatient transurethral resection of the prostate at a urological ambulatory surgery center in 125 selected patients. Only five were subsequently transferred to hospital (because of hematuria in three, fever in one and cardiac dysrhythmia in one). No patient required hospitalization after being discharged from the ambulatory surgery center. This approach offers the advantages of prostatectomy with minimal inpatient stay and, if it proves to be applicable for the majority of patients and in the majority of centers, it is likely that prostatectomy will retain its pre-eminence.

Discussion

The last 10 years have seen a growing curiosity and caution amongst urologists managing patients with BPH. It is now recognized that a structured history, examination and routine investigation to exclude urinary infection, uremia and residual urine, and to determine the flow rate, are helpful in selecting the most appropriate initial treatment. Patients with symptoms that are primarily irritative should almost certainly be investigated by urodynamics before prostatectomy is considered. Those in whom surgery is an option, despite a peak flow of > 10 ml/s, should also be investigated urodynamically to identify that 25% whose problem is primarily that of bladder failure rather than of obstruction.

Once the diagnosis has been made and cancer has been excluded, the patient with minor symptoms and a peak flow rate of 15 ml/s or more does not necessarily need active treatment. For the patient with moderate symptoms and a peak flow rate of 10–15 ml/s it is likely that drug therapy will prove adequate in many cases. For those with more severe symptoms of an obstructive nature and a peak flow rate of < 10 ml/s, surgical intervention is still likely to be required and also to be appropriate[33].

Increasing use is being made of the α-blockers and the inhibitors of 5α-reductase in relieving symptoms and improving flow rates in those whose problems are not severe. If the drug therapy is satisfactory for the patient it may be wise to discontinue it at intervals, to reveal the 25% of patients whose symptoms improve spontaneously and to restrict continuous drug therapy to those for whom it is mandatory.

The development of stents, thermotherapy, thermoablation, transurethral needle ablation, high-intensity focused ultrasound, laser therapy and electrovaporization has been far more rapid than many urologists would have expected 10 years ago. So far none of the newer devices has been subject to the regulatory controls demanded of pharmaceutical companies wishing to introduce new products and none has yet established a place as a natural successor to transurethral prostatectomy. The increasing sophistication of the alternative forms of treatment offers a number of opportunities. These are, however, counterbalanced by the changes in the urologists' attitude towards surgical intervention and by their attempts further to improve the technique of transurethral resection itself.

Most urologists believe that further development of the other alternative techniques is required before they can be recommended for general use. These improvements must come as a consequence of technical development and from the results of prospective randomized clinical trials.

The recommendations of the International Concensus Committee of the *3rd International Consultation on BPH* refer to the evaluation of new treatment modalities. Their suggestions are printed below.

Technological treatment modalities

(1) Studies should meet the clinical research criteria proposed by the WHO-sponsored *International Consultation on BPH*.

(2) Outcome measurements should employ the response criteria proposed by the *International Consultation on BPH*.

(3) All studies must be randomized and controlled and include at least 1 year of follow-up. Whenever appropriate, results should be stratified with regard to predictors of treatment outcome (age, surgical risk factors, baseline symptom score, maximum flow rate and other measures of obstruction and prostate size (if relevant).

(4) The new treatment technologies must be tested against appropriate controls:
  (a) Technologies aiming to imitate the tissue-ablative effect of transurethral prostatectomy should be compared with transurethral prostatectomy.

(b) Technologies not claiming such tissue-ablative effect should be tested against a sham (placebo treatment arm). An additional transurethral prostatectomy arm as a treatment standard is to be encouraged.

(5) Studies should include analysis of the morbidity of the various treatment options studied.

(6) Pilot studies should allow a tentative cost analysis. If results prove the treatment efficacious, then a cost-effectiveness study should be undertaken.

Pharmacological management of BPH

(1) Studies should meet the clinical research criteria proposed by the WHO-sponsored *International Consultation on BPH.*

(2) Outcome measurements should employ response criteria proposed by the *International Consultation on BPH.*

(3) All phase II and III studies must be randomized, controlled and include a follow-up of at least 1 year following the expected time of onset of response. Studies should be conducted under double-blind conditions. Whenever appropriate, results should be stratified with regard to predictors of treatment outcome (age, surgical risk factors, baseline symptom score, maximum flow rate and other measures of obstruction and prostate size (if relevant)).

(4) Pharmacological treatments for BPH must be compared with an appropriate control. The most appropriate control is a placebo-treated group. Comparison of results of the study with published results of other treatment modalities is encouraged.

(5) Studies should include an analysis of the morbidity of the pharmacological management. The morbidity of pharmacological management should be compared to placebo and to established surgical therapies.

(6) Pilot studies should allow a tentative cost analysis. If results prove the treatment efficacious, then a cost-effectiveness study should be undertaken.

For all existing or emerging treatment modalities

For all existing or emerging treatment modalities, long-term studies should be conducted to demonstrate:

(1) Continued effectiveness and safety.

(2) Continued effectiveness relative to available treatment options.

(3) Cost-effectiveness related to available treatment options.

If these recommendations are implemented in full, the profession and the patients will be much better informed in 10 years' time than they are now, and thus in a much better position to discuss and agree upon the most appropriate treatment for the individual patient. Whether such a discussion will conclude that transurethral prostatectomy continues to be the best way of relieving prostatic obstruction remains to be seen.

Acknowledgement

I should like to thank Mrs S. Cordingley for her help in the preparation of this paper.

References

1. Neal, D. E. (1990). Prostatectomy – an open or closed case. *Br. J. Urol.*, **66**, 449–54

2. Mebust, W. K., Holtgrewe, H. L., Cockett, A. T. K., Peters, P. C. and the Writing Com-

mittee (1989). Transurethral prostatectomy: immediate and postoperative complications. A cooperative study of 13 participating institutions evaluating 3,885 patients. *J. Urol.*, **141**, 243–7

3. Roos, N. P., Wennberg, J. E., Malenka, D. J., Fisher, E. S., McPherson, K., Andersen, T. F., Cohen, M. M. and Ramsey, E. (1989). Mortality and reoperation after open and transurethral resection of the prostate for benign prostatic hyperplasia. *N. Engl. J. Med.*, **320**, 1120–4

4. Doll, H. A., Black, K., McPherson, K., Flod, A. B., Williams, G. B. and Smith, J. C. (1992). Mortality, morbidity and complications following transurethral resection of the prostate for benign prostatic hypertrophy. *J. Urol.*, **147**, 1566–73

5. Holtgrewe, H. L., Mebust, W. K., Dowd, J. B., Cockett, A. T. K., Peters, P. C. and Proctor, C. (1989). Transurethral prostatectomy: practice aspects of the dominant operation in American urology. *J. Urol.*, **141**, 248–53

6. Ball, A. J., Feneley, R. C. C. and Abrams, P. H. (1981). The natural history of untreated 'prostatism'. *Br. J. Urol*, **49**, 683–8

7. Garraway, W. M., Russell, E. B. A. W., Lee, R. J., Collins, G. N., McKelvie, G. B., Hehir, M., Rogers, A. C. N. and Simpson, R. J. (1993). Impact of previously unrecognized benign prostatic hyperplasia on the daily activities of middle-aged and elderly men. *Br. J. Gen. Prac.*, **43**, 318–21

8. Abrams, P., Bruskewitz, R., de la Rosette, J., Griffiths, D., Koyanagi, T., Nordling, J., Park Y.-C., Schäfer, W. and Zimmern, P. (1996). The diagnosis of bladder outlet obstruction: urodynamics. In Cockett, A. T. K., Khoury, S., Aso, Y., Chatelain, C., Denis, L., Griffiths, K. and Murphy, G. (eds.) *The Third International Consultation on Benign Prostatic Hyperplasia (BPH)*, pp. 297–368. (Paris: SCI)

9. Holtgrewe, H. L., Ackerman, R., Bay-Neilson, H., Boyce, P., Carlsson, P., Coast, J., Frohneberg, D. H., Mazeman, E., Standaert, B., Tajima, A., Thibault, P. and Viens-Bitker, C. (1996). Economics of BPH. In Cockett, A. T. K., Khoury, S., Aso, Y., Chatelain, C., Denis, L., Griffiths, K. and Murphy, G. (eds.) *The Third International Consultation on Benign Prostatic Hyperplasia (BPH)*, pp. 51–70. (Paris: SCI)

10. Fitzpatrick, J. M., Braeckman, J., Denis, L., Dreikorn, K., Khoury, S., Levin, R. and Perrin, P. (1996). The medical management of BPH with agents other than hormones or alpha-blockers. In Cockett, A. T. K., Khoury, S., Aso, Y., Chatelain, C., Denis, L., Griffiths, K. and Murphy, G. (eds.) *The Third International Consultation on Benign Prostatic Hyperplasia (BPH)*, pp. 489–95. (Paris: SCI)

11. Abbou, C. C., Payan, C., Viens-Bitker, C., Richard, F., Boccon-Gibod, L., Jardin, A., Beurton, D., Le Duc, A., Fermanian, J., Thibault, P. and the French BPH Hyperthemia Group (1995). Transrectal and transurethral hyperthemia versus sham treatment in benign prostatic hyperplasia: a double blind randomized multicentre trial. *Br. J. Urol.*, **76**, 619–24

12. Smith, P. H., Conort, P., de la Rosette, J., Devonec, M., Fitzpatrick, J., Jonas, V., Leduc, A., Marberger, M., McLeod, D., Milroy, E., Nordling, J., Schulman, C. C., Tazaki, H., Williams, G. and Yachia, D. (1996). Other non-medical therapies. In Cockett, A. T. K., Khoury, S., Aso, Y., Chatelain, C., Denis, L., Griffiths, K. and Murphy, G. (eds.) *The Third International Consultation on Benign Prostatic Hyperplasia (BPH)*, pp. 575–603. (Paris: SCI)

13. Chapple, C. R., Rosario, D. J., Wasserfallen, M. and Woo, H. H. (1995). A randomised study of the Urolume stent vs prostate surgery. *J. Urol.*, **153**, 436A

14. Defalco, A., Oesterling, J. E., Epstein, H. and the North American Urolume Study Group (1995). The North American experience with the Urolume endourethral prosthesis as a treatment for BPH: three year results. *J. Urol.*, **153**, 436A

15. De Wildt, M. J. A. M., Hubregtse, M., Ogden, C., Carter, S. St. C., Debruyne, F. M. J. and de la Rosette, J. J. M. C. H. (1996). A 12-month study of the placebo effect in transurethral microwave thermotherapy. *Br. J. Urol.*, **77**, 221–7

16. Dahlstrand, C., Walden, M., Geirsson, G. and Pettersson, S. (1995). Transurethral microwave therapy versus transurethral resection for benign prostatic hyperplasia; a prospective randomised study with a three year follow up. *Br. J. Urol.*, **76**, 614–18

17. Blute, M. L., Patterson, D. E., Segura, J. W., Hellerstein, D. K. and Tomera, K. M. (1994). Transurethral microwave thermotherapy versus sham; a prospective double blind randomised study. *J. Urol.*, **151**, 415A

18. Schulman, C. C. and Zlotta, A. R. (1995). Transurethral needle ablation of the prostate for treatment of BPH: early clinical experience. *Urology*, **45–1**, 28–33

19. Zlotta, A. R., Peny, M.-O., Matos, C. and Schulman, C. C. (1996). Transurethral needle ablation of the prostate: clinical experience in patients in urinary retention. *Br. J. Urol.*, **77**, 391–7

20. Madersbacher, S. and Marberger, M. (1995). Therapeutic application of ultrasound in urology. In Marberger, M. (ed.) *Application of Newer Forms of Therapeutic Energy in Urology*, pp. 115–36. (Oxford: ISIS Medical Media)

21. McCullough, D. L. (1966). Laser prostatectomy: free beam and contact techniques. *Curr. Opin. Urol.*, **6**, 10–13
22. Muschter, R. (1996). Interstitial laser therapy. *Curr. Opin. Urol.*, **6**, 34–8
23. Cowles, R., Kabalin, J. and Childs, S. (1996). A prospective randomised comparison of transurethral resection to visual laser ablation of the prostate for the treatment of benign prostatic hyperplasia. *Urology*, in press
24. Anson, K., Nawrocki, J. and Buckley, J. (1996). A multicentre randomised prospective study of endoscopic laser ablation versus transurethral resection of the prostate. *Urology*, in press
25. Keoghane, S. R., Cranston, D. W., Lawrence, K. C., Doll, H. A., Fellows, G. J. and Smith, J. C. (1996). The Oxford Laser Prostate Trial: a double blind randomised controlled trial of contact vaporisation of the prostate against transurethral resection: preliminary results. *Br. J. Urol.*, **77**, 382–5
26. Keoghane, S. R., Lawrence, K. C., Gray, A. M. and Chappell, D. B. (1996). The Oxford Laser Prostate Trial: economic issues surrounding contact laser prostatectomy. *Br. J. Urol.*, **77**, 386–90
27. Te, A. E. and Kaplan, S. A. (1996). Electrovaporisation of the prostate. *Curr. Opin. Urol.*, **6**, 2–9
28. Cetinel, B., Turan, T., Talat, Z., Yalcin, V., Alici, B. and Solok, V. (1994). Update evaluation of benign prostatic hyperplasia: when should we offer prostatectomy? *Br. J. Urol.*, **74**, 566–71
29. Doll, H. A., Black, N. A., Flood, A. B. and McPherson, K. (1993). Patient-perceived health status before and up to 12 months after transurethral resection of the prostate for benign prostatic hypertrophy. *Br. J. Urol.*, **71**, 297–305
30. Emberton, M., Neal, D. E., Black, N., Fordham, M., Harrison, M., McBrien, M. P., Williams, R. E., McPherson, K. and Devlin, H. B. (1996). The effect of prostatectomy on symptom severity and quality of life. *Br. J. Urol.*, **77**, 233–47
31. Wasson, J. H., Reda, D. J., Bruskewitz, R. C., Elinson, J., Keller, A. M. and Henderson, W. G. (1995). A comparison of transurethral surgery with watchful waiting for moderate symptoms of benign prostatic hyperplasia. *N. Engl. J. Med.*, **332**, 75–9
32. Klimberg, I. W., Locke, D. R., Leonard, E., Madore, R. and Klimberg, S. R. (1994). Outpatient transurethral resection of the prostate at a urological ambulatory surgical center. *J. Urol.*, **151**, 1547–9
33. Jensen, K. M.-E. and Andersen, J. T. (1990). Urodynamic implications of benign prostatic hyperplasia. *Urologe A.*, **29**, 1–4

Interactive Voting System

1 If you are 60 years of age, have some difficulty in micturition, a sterile urine, normal creatinine level, a peak flow of 12 ml per second and a residual urine volume of 30 ml, would you prefer to be treated with:

Response	Option
68%	Watchful waiting.
28%	Drugs.
2%	Stents.
0%	Thermotherapy.
2%	Thermoablation/TUNA/HIFU/Laser.

Number of votes: 123

2 If you have marked difficulty in micturition, a sterile urine, normal creatinine level, peak flow of 9 ml per second and a residual urine volume of 75 ml, would you prefer to be treated by:

38%	Drugs.
2%	Stents.
52%	TUR.
6%	Laser/Vapotrode.
2%	Thermoablation.

Number of votes: 121

Update on the use of finasteride in benign prostatic hyperplasia: long-term results

3

J. C. Nickel for the PROSPECT study group* and J. T. Andersen for the SCARP study group*

Introduction

The symptoms of benign prostatic hyperplasia (BPH) appear to result, in part, as a consequence of the progressive enlargement of the prostate gland that occurs in men as they age[1]. Although surgical resection of the prostate gland has always been the traditional therapy for BPH, effective medical therapy has now become an important therapeutic option[2].

Growth and regulation of prostate size is dependent on androgens, primarily dihydrotestosterone[3]. Finasteride, a synthetic azasteroid, is a potent and specific inhibitor of 5α-reductase, an intracellular enzyme that converts testosterone to dihydrotestosterone[4]. A 12-month, double blind, placebo-controlled study[5] evaluated the safety and efficacy of finasteride for the treatment of BPH. After 12 months of therapy, the prostate volume was reduced, the urinary flow rate increased and symptoms improved in a significant number of patients, with a very low incidence of side effects. Since medical therapy for this chronic and progressive disease is potentially for life, long-term efficacy and safety data are required. Some data are available for patients from this large controlled 12-month trial who were followed in an open extension study and continued to receive finasteride, regardless of their original study therapy[6]. In this subset of patients the therapeutic benefit of finasteride after year 1 was maintained and disease progression appeared to have been halted. This extension study also demonstrated that finasteride was well tolerated and that there was no evidence of tachyphylaxis of effect. Such an analysis of efficacy has been criticized, because the study cohort was probably made up predominantly of responders[7]. The absence of a placebo group beyond 12 months did not allow a direct comparison between finasteride treatment and placebo. The results of two new studies[8,9], evaluating the long-term safety and efficacy of finasteride compared to placebo in the treatment of patients with moderate symptoms of BPH over a 2-year period, are now available.

Two-year randomized placebo-controlled studies

The SCARP and PROSPECT studies were large multi-center, double-blind, placebo-controlled trials, comparing finasteride treatment to placebo treatment in patients with moderate symptoms of BPH. In the SCARP study, patients were enrolled at 59 centers in five Scandinavian countries, and in the PROSPECT study, patients were enrolled at 28 centers across Canada (Table 1).

---

*See appendix for list of members

Inclusion criteria were similar in both studies (Table 2). Eligible patients entered a 1-month single-blind placebo run-in period following which the patients were randomized to receive finasteride 5 mg once daily or placebo, for 24 months.

Study endpoints for both trials were: (1) changes in symptoms attributable to BPH; (2) changes in urine flow rates; and (3) changes in prostate volume. The evaluation procedures for both SCARP and PROSPECT were similar and are listed in Table 3. In both studies the analysis was based on the all-patients-treated approach. Patients who withdrew were included by the last observation on treatment used for all time points subsequent to withdrawal. Analysis of variance models were used to compare treatment groups for symptom scores, urinary flow rates, prostate volumes and safety parameters.

Results

The baseline values for age, symptom score, maximum uroflow and prostate volumes were not statistically significantly different between placebo and finasteride groups. The baseline characteristics were similar in both the SCARP and PROSPECT studies and were compatible with moderate BPH. The results from the SCARP study have been recently published[8] and can be presented in this review. The PROSPECT study is currently under revision for publication and the results cannot be presented in a review format until the entire study has been published in the primary medical journal (personal communication with journal editors).

The mean prostate volume in the control group increased progressively over the two year study period in SCARP (+11.5%) and a similar increase was noted in PROSPECT. The finasteride group, on the other hand, experienced a progressive decrease in mean prostate volume (−19.2% in SCARP; confirmed in PROSPECT). The difference between groups in both studies was statistically significant ($p < 0.01$).

The changes in maximum urinary flow rate from baseline at 2 years for the placebo and finasteride treated groups respectively was

Table 1 The SCARP and PROSPECT studies

	Location	Centers	Patients		
			Total	Placebo	Finasteride
SCARP	Scandinavia	59	707	354	353
PROSPECT	Canada	28	613	303	310

Table 2 The inclusion criteria for the SCARP and PROSPECT studies

(1)	At least two symptoms scored in the moderate range, but not more than two symptoms scored at the severe end of the scale, on a symptom questionnaire (modified Boyarsky questionnaire)
(2)	An enlarged prostate by digital rectal examination
(3)	A peak urinary flow rate of 5–15 ml/s on two separate occasions obtained on a voided volume of
(4)	> 150 ml
(5)	Prostate specific antigen level of < 10 ng/ml
	Post-void residual volume of < 150 ml

Table 3 Evaluation procedures for the SCARP and PROSPECT studies

(1)	*Symptoms:* modified Boyarsky symptom questionnaire
(2)	*Urinary flow rate:* urinary flow rate meter (Urodyn 1000™, Dantec, Copenhagen, Denmark and Mahwah, NJ)
(3)	*Residual volume:* portable ultrasonic scanner (Bladderscan BVI™, Diagnostic Ultrasound Corporation, Kirkland, Washington)
(4)	*Prostate volume:* transrectal ultrasound examination (SCARP: 416/707; PROSPECT: 562/613)

−0.3 ml/s and +1.5 ml/s for the SCARP study. An identical trend was demonstrated for the PROSPECT study. The difference between the two groups at the termination of the study was statistically significant ($p < 0.01$) in both studies.

In both the SCARP and PROSPECT studies, a small improvement in total symptom score was observed in the placebo group during the first year, however over the second year of the study the symptoms worsened in this group and returned to baseline values. The finasteride group in both studies continued to show improvement over the two year study resulting in a change in total symptom score of −2.0 in the SCARP study (similar degree of improvement confirmed in the PROSPECT study). The difference between the two groups in both studies was statistically significant ($p < 0.05$) at 12 months and even more so by 24 months ($p < 0.01$).

The overall drop out rate over the 24 months was 18.4% for the SCARP study (slightly higher for the PROSPECT study). The proportions of patients who discontinued for various reasons during the trial were similar in both placebo and finasteride groups in both studies, although more patients dropped out of the placebo group because of adverse events and/or insufficient response compared to the finasteride group. The incidence of serious and non-serious adverse events were similar in both groups. Although there was no difference in the frequency of urogenital adverse events, when adverse events related to sexual function were analyzed separately, there were more men with ejaculatory disorders and impotence in the finasteride treated group in both studies. A *post-hoc* analysis found that more patients in the placebo groups developed urinary retention (SCARP and PROSPECT) and required prostate surgery (PROSPECT) than that reported in the finasteride groups.

Comment

Prostatic enlargement is one definite component of symptomatic BPH[10]. The condition is a chronic disease and usually progresses over time[11]. Finasteride, a drug that is intended to reverse the progression of BPH, theoretically needs to be prescribed for life. These studies were undertaken to evaluate the safety and efficacy of finasteride compared to placebo over 2 years. This type of long-term study is necessary for any medication that is recommended for potential lifetime treatment of symptomatic BPH.

These two 24-month, double-blind, placebo-controlled, randomized studies of the safety and efficacy of finasteride in patients with moderate symptoms of BPH, although similar, were independent and carried out by investigators in different corners of the world. Yet they both demonstrate the persistence of the therapeutic effect of 5α-reductase inhibition over a 2-year term, as viewed from the triple perspective of prostate size, uroflow measurements and patient symptoms. It also confirms that a significant placebo effect on BPH symptoms, which was observed in earlier studies, may persist for at least a year. The data demonstrate that the natural history of untreated BPH is a gradual trend towards an increase in prostate size, whereas placebo treatment results in an initially improved uroflow and improvement of symptoms which gradually returns to near baseline values over 2 years. This placebo group would, of course, not accurately represent the natural history of BPH in men who are not treated or who are on watchful waiting, since the placebo groups in these trials are being actively treated with some expectation of improvement.

The long-term results confirm and extend observations from previous 6- and 12-month double-blind studies of finasteride and BPH[5,12]. The earlier studies showed significant improvements in symptom score, maximum urinary flow rate and prostate volume in finasteride-treated groups compared with placebo. These longer studies showed that finasteride treatment results in ongoing improvement in these parameters over 24 months. The prolonged placebo effect that was documented in these studies emphasizes the need for long-term, double-blind, placebo-controlled trials if any medical therapy for BPH is to be reliably assessed.

The patients in the two long-term studies presented here had moderate symptoms of BPH and a uroflow consistent with presumably mild or moderate bladder outlet obstruction. In usual clinical practice, such patients are observed (watchful waiting), treated pharmacologically or offered prostate surgery. Since the baseline symptoms in this population are in the mild-to-moderate range, modest improvement can be clinically appreciated by the patients as a successful therapeutic outcome. The treatment objective for this type of patient should aim to minimize risk while relieving and possibly preventing as many symptoms or complications as possible. Finasteride specifically and mechanistically reduced the volume of the prostate and improved most patients' symptoms and urinary flow rates. It was generally well tolerated and associated with good compliance and a low incidence of side effects (slightly higher incidence of reversible sexual dysfunction compared to placebo).

Finasteride has now been evaluated in two double-blind placebo-controlled trials over a 2-year period. On the basis of the results from these large, independent long-term studies, we conclude that finasteride is an effective long-term alternative to watchful waiting and offers an effective medical therapeutic option.

References

1. Guess, H. A. (1992). Benign prostatic hyperplasia: antecedents and natural history. *Epidemiol. Rev.*, **14**, 131–53
2. Osterling, J. E. (1995). Benign prostatic hyperplasia: medical and minimally invasive treatment options. *N. Engl. J. Med.*, **332**, 99–109
3. Walsh, P., Madden, J., Harrod, M. *et al.* (1974). Familial incomplete male pseudohermaphroditism type 2: decreased dihydrotestosterone formation in pseudovaginal perineoscrotal hypospadias. *N. Engl. J. Med.*, **291**, 944–9
4. Bruchovsky, N. and Wilson, J. (1968). The conversion of testosterone to 5-alpha-androstane-17-beta-ol-3-one by rat prostate *in vivo* and *in vitro*. *J. Biol. Chem.*, **243**, 2012–21
5. Gormley, G. J, Stoner, E., Bruskewik, R. C. *et al.* (1992). The effect of finasteride in men with benign prostatic hyperplasia. *N. Engl. J. Med.*, **327**, 1185–91
6. Stoner, E. (1994). Three-year safety and efficacy data on the use of finasteride in the treatment of benign prostatic hyperplasia. *Urology.*, **43**, 284–94
7. Lepor, H. (1994). Editorial comment. *Urology*, **43**, 292–3
8. Anderson, J., Ekman, P., Wolf, H. *et al.* (1995). Can finasteride reverse the progress of benign prostatic hyperplasia? A two year placebo-controlled study. *Urology*, **46**, 631–7
9. Nickel, J. C., Fradet, Y., Boake, R. *et al.* (1995). Longterm effects of finasteride vs. placebo in the treatment of patients with moderate symptoms of benign prostatic hyperplasia (BPH). *Can. J. Urol.*, **2**, A50
10. McNeal, J. E. (1984). Morphology and biology of benign prostatic hyperplasia. In Bruckovsky, N., Chapdelaine, A. and Neumann, F. (eds.) *Regulation of Androgen Action. Proceedings of an International Symposium*, pp. 23–30. (Montreal, Berlin: R. Bruckner)
11. Jacobsen, S. J., Girman, C. J, Guess, H. A. *et al.* (1996). Natural history of prostatism: longitudinal changes in voiding symptoms in community-dwelling men. *J. Urol.*, **155**, 595–600

Appendix

Members of the PROSPECT study group are:

J. C. Nickel, Y. Fradet, R. Boake, P. Pommerville, J. P. Perreault, S. Afridi, M. Elhilali, J. Simard, L. Goldenberg, W. Orovan, L. Sullivan, R. Norman, I. Reid, S. Herschorn, J. Trachtenberg, J. Collins, G.Beland, P. Bertrand, E. Ramsey, D. Pharand, A. Vallieres, J. Williams, H. Fenster, P. Feero, R. Barr, N. Struthers, J. Pike

Members of the SCARP study group are:

Denmark – J. T. Andersen, A. Bodker, O. Vedel, J. Nordling, A. L. Poulsen, J. Schou, V. Hvidt, J. B. Hansen, H. H. Meyhoff, J. Eldrup, D. Hartwell, H. Colstrup, P. Lyngdorf, A. Holm Nielsen, E. Larsen, H. Wolf, S. Walter, E. H. Larsen, E. Thybo, S. Mommsen, K. E. Brok, L. Palm, H. Genster, M. Andersen

Finland – P. Kauppinen, M. Rauvala, M. Kontturi, J. Hakkinen, T. Tammela, H. Tainio, O. Hynninen, J. Tiitinen, K. Lehtoranta, M. Ala-Opas, T. Lehtonen, I. Perttila, A. Petas, E. Rintala, R. Salminen, H. Juusela, E. Hansson, R. von Wendt, K. Tuhkanen, M. Talja, M. Nurmi, P. Puntala, J. Permi, V. M. Puolakka, J. Viitanen

Iceland – T. Gislason, G. V. Einarsson

Norway – L. M. Eri, S. Karlsen, P. Holme, S. M. Sivertsen, E. Steinsvik, E. Servoll, T. Urnes, P. A. Malme, T. E. Johansen, H. Omland, J. Nagelhus, S. E. Kloster, O. Skjeggestad, K. Vada, R. Mortensen.

Sweden – G. Nyberg, G. Pettersson, L. Wedman, S. Bratnel, P. Folmerz, B. Zackrisson, K. Dahlgren, A. Tillegard, G. Aus, S. Bergdahl, J. Hugosson, B. Holmquist, A. Ek, C. Rademark, P. Kristiansen, C. G. Hermansson, K. Pedersen, C. Oscarsson, B. Kihl, J. O. Olsson, L. Nelvin, K. H. Leissner, S. Lundstam, H. Hjertberg, E. Varenhorst, S. O. Andersson, J. E. Johansson, T. Windahl, R. Swartz, B. Ahlberg, S. Gedda, C. Anderstrom, A. Eddeland, R. Hansson, P. Stroberg, J. Adolfsson, P. Ekman, P. Bauer, H. Kleist, B. Storm, T. Ranch, H. Stravsnes, E. Brekkan, T. Eklund, L. Karlberg

Interactive Voting System

1 A 65-year-old male with stable angina and a past history of a stroke (now recovered) has progressive symptoms of prostatism: I-PSS 16; quality of life 5; serum creatinine 97; urine analysis negative; residual urine 60 ml; CMG-stable bladder; Q_{max} 10 ml/s; voiding pressure 75 mm H_2O at maximum flow; digital rectal examination > 50 g. What is your therapy of choice for this patient?

Response	Option
27%	Transurethral resection of the prostate.
6%	Open prostatectomy.
41%	Finasteride.
18%	Alpha-blocker.
8%	Watchful waiting.

Number of votes: 103

2 He was treated with finasteride 5 mg po qhs. Three months later he stated that he had a modest but noticeable improvement in his symptoms (I-PSS = 14). He reports no adverse effects. At this time, would you suggest?

83%	Continue finasteride.
4%	Stop finasteride and start an alpha-blocker.
13%	Talk patient into surgery.

Number of votes: 134

3 At 6 months the patient perceived a significant decrease in symptoms (I-PSS = 11) and his uroflow had increased to 13 ml/s. He was content with his mild-to-moderate symptoms (quality of life score, 2).
At this time, would you suggest?

75%	Continue finasteride indefinitely.
20%	Stop finasteride and reassess in 6 months.
2%	Stop finasteride and start an alpha-blocker.
3%	Talk patient into surgery.

Number of votes: 122

2

BPH and Prostate Cancer – Prevention

Combination therapy in localized prostate cancer

4

F. Labrie, L. Cusan, J.-L. Gomez, P. Diamond, A. Bélanger and B. Candas

As it is the second most frequent cause of cancer death in men in the Western world, prostate cancer has become a major health and social problem comparable to breast cancer. In the United States alone, 40 400 men are expected to die from prostate cancer in 1996[1], whereas the annual health care costs, mostly related to treatment of advanced and terminal disease, are estimated at $4.5 billion[2]. Since it is well recognized that the only opportunity for a significant reduction in prostate cancer deaths is treatment of localized disease before the appearance of metastases, it is surprising that screening and early treatment remain controversial, despite the convincing evidence accumulated during recent years, clearly supporting early diagnosis and treatment. Much progress has in fact been made by several groups on the rational use of prostate specific antigen (PSA) and transrectal ultrasonography of the prostate for earlier diagnosis of prostate cancer, and more efficient and well-tolerated curative therapies have been developed[3–15]. A highly efficient, easily applied and low-cost strategy for the detection of localized prostate cancer is now available[11].

Although limited information is available on the best choice of therapy for early-stage prostate cancer[16], it is well recognized that the only opportunity for a cure of prostate cancer is at an early stage, when the cancer is still localized to the prostate[9,16,17]. The main objective in the prostate cancer field should therefore be early diagnosis and treatment of organ-confined disease, since it is known that such patients treated by radical prostatectomy have a life expectancy comparable to that of men having no prostate cancer[17,18].

The most serious limitation to the curative approaches of prostate cancer presumed to be localized at diagnosis is that, in approximately 50% of cases, the cancer is found to have migrated outside the prostate at histopathological examination of the surgical specimen, thus making the surgery performed of questionable usefulness[19–25]. As an example, only 51% of 157 stage T_{1c} (non-palpable prostate cancers diagnosed by needle biopsy) were organ-confined (no capsular penetration), with 17% having positive margins[26]. Moreover, of 439 stage T_2 (palpable) cancers, organ-confined disease was limited to 34% of cases, and surgical margins were positive in 43% of cases. In another study[27], 70% of 60 stage T_{1c} cancers were organ-confined but 23% had positive margins. Such data indicate that a large proportion of stage T_{1c} tumors become incurable before they are diagnosed. If one could rely with confidence upon an accurate staging or grade of the tumor at diagnosis, the choice of treatment would be greatly facilitated. Unfortunately, although screening can at least double the proportion of organ-confined cancers, the high proportion of non-organ-confined cancers remains[12].

A possible means of improving the proportion of patients with organ-confined disease and cancer-negative margins at surgery was clearly suggested by the observation that patients treated by combination therapy with the use of a pure antiandrogen associated with medical or surgical castration for metastatic disease showed a much more rapid and marked regression of their cancer in the prostatic area compared with distant metastatic disease[28–30]. Moreover, it is well recognized that when recurrence of the disease occurs, progression of the cancer at the level of the prostate is a rare event; the bones are the usual site of progression. Since prostate cancer localized into the prostatic area is so highly sensitive to androgen deprivation, it is logical to use combination therapy to downstage prostate cancer in men diagnosed as having localized prostate cancer before performing radical surgical prostatectomy or radiotherapy.

Following an encouraging preliminary study[3], we have conducted a prospective and randomized clinical trial in order precisely to assess the potential advantages of neoadjuvant combination therapy with the pure antiandrogen flutamide and a luteinizing hormone releasing hormone (LHRH) agonist administered for 3 months before radical prostatectomy compared with surgery alone[12]. This report is an update of this first randomized trial which analyses the data on organ-confined disease and specimen-confined disease, and compares the final stage at histopathological examination of the surgical specimen with the clinical stage at diagnosis.

Methods

Patients

A total of 161 men aged between 46 and 72 years (Table 1) with histopathology-proven adenocarcinoma of the prostate took part in the study. All gave written informed consent, had a life expectancy of more than 10 years, and were diagnosed as having localized prostate cancer in the first prospective study of screening for prostate cancer performed in a randomly selected

Table 1 Effect of 3-month neoadjuvant combination therapy with the antiandrogen flutamide and an LHRH agonist on positive margins at radical prostatectomy in stages B and C prostate cancer

Group	Negative margins	Positive margins	Total
Control	47 (66.2%)	24 (33.8%)	71
Combination therapy	83 (92.2%)	7 (7.8%)	90
Total			161

χ^2 test: $p < 0.001$

population of men. This study was started in November 1988 in the Québec City area by the Laval University Prostate Cancer Detection Program (LUPCDP)[9].

Other information about staging, eligibility, randomization, radical prostatectomy, histology, follow-up and statistical analysis are as described[31,32].

Results

As shown in Table 1, the incidence of cancer-positive surgical margins was reduced highly significantly to only 7.8% (7/90) in the group of patients who received an LHRH superagonist and flutamide for 3 months before radical prostatectomy, compared with 33.8% (24/71) in the group of men who had no endocrine therapy before radical prostatectomy (χ^2 test, $p < 0.001$). Figure 1 shows that the decrease in cancer-positive surgical margins is of major amplitude at all stages of the disease except at stage B_0 and C_1. In fact, although cancer-positive margins were found in the surgical specimen in 25.5% of stage B_1, 58.8% of stage B_2 and 80% of stage C_2 control patients, the incidence of positive margins decreased to 2.3% in stage B_1, 10.8% in stage B_2 and 14.3% in stage C_2 patients who received combination therapy for 3 months before surgery.

It is then of particular interest to assess the final staging at histopathological examination of the specimen obtained at surgery compared with clinical staging at diagnosis and to determine the effect of combination therapy at each stage of the disease. Upstaging is particularly striking at stages B_1 and B_2 in the control (untreated) group. In fact, of 39 cancers originally classified as B_1, 21 showed a more advanced stage at surgery, including five with C_1 and ten with C_2 disease (Table 2). Similarly, of 17 cancers originally classified as B_2 disease in the control group, three became C_1, eight became C_2 and two became D_1 disease. On the other hand, it can also be seen in Table 2 that downstaging following neoadjuvant combination therapy was frequent at all stages of the disease: in fact, in the patients originally

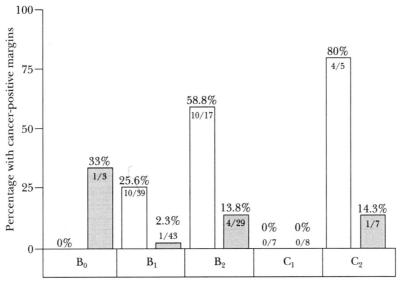

Figure 1 Effect of 3-month neoadjuvant combination therapy with flutamide and an LHRH agonist (shaded bars) on cancer-positive surgical margins at radical prostatectomy, compared with controls (open bars), according to the clinical stage at diagnosis. Data are expressed as percentage of patients in each group. The number within the bars indicates the number of patients having cancer-positive margins in each group[31]

Table 2 Effect of 3-month neoadjuvant combination therapy with flutamide and leuprolide acetate on the final histopathological stage at surgery, compared with the initial clinical stage at diagnosis. NC, no cancer[31]

| Original stage | n | Final histopathological stage at surgery | | | | | | |
		NC	B_0	B_1	B_2	C_1	C_2	D_1
Controls – untreated								
B_0	3	0	1	0	1	1	0	0
B_1	39	0	7	11	6	5	10	0
B_2	17	0	0	3	1	3	8	2
C_1	7	0	1	1	2	3	0	0
C_2	5	0	0	0	1	0	1	3
Three-month neoadjuvant combination therapy								
B_0	3	0	1	0	0	1	1	0
B_1	43	6	14	11	7	3	2	0
B_2	29	0	2	11	6	5	3	2
C_1	8	0	2	1	3	1	1	0
C_2	7	0	1	2	2	1	0	1

classified as having B_1 disease, 14 of 43 (32.5%) tumors originally classified as having a mean diameter of 1.0–1.5 cm decreased to < 1.0 cm, and no cancer was found in six patients after thorough examination of additional histological sections. Downstaging was seen in 13 of 29 (44.8%) of patients originally classified as having stage B_2 disease. Although the number of patients was small, the downstaging effect was particularly important in patients originally classified as having C_1 disease at diagnosis, with six of eight (75%) having downstaging, and in patients originally classified at diagnosis as stage C_2, with six of seven cancers (85.7%) being downstaged following neoadjuvant combination therapy.

Comparison of the initial clinical stage at diagnosis with the final stage at histopathological examination of the surgical specimen following radical prostatectomy can be seen in Figure 2. The downstaging effect of combination therapy is thus clearly seen at all stages of the disease,

except at stage B_0. The net advantages of combination therapy are illustrated in Figure 3; the final stage at surgery had, on average, worsened by 35.9% (14/39) in stage B_1 disease, 58.8% (10 of 17) in stage B_2 disease and 40% in stage C_2 disease in patients who had radical prostatectomy alone. The final stage of the disease, conversely, improved following combination therapy by 18.5% (8/43) in stage B_1 disease, 10.3% (3/29) in stage B_2 disease, 62.5% (5/8)

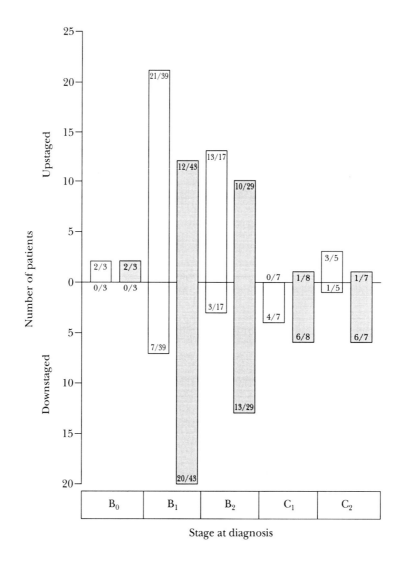

Figure 2 Effect of 3-month combination therapy with flutamide and an LHRH agonist (shaded bars) compared with controls (open bars) on the final histopathological stage at surgery vs. the clinical staging at diagnosis. Data are expressed as number of patients showing upstaging or downstaging in each group

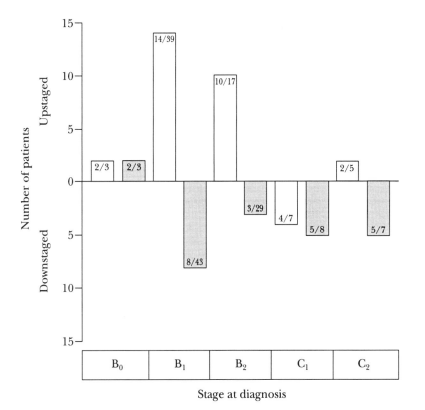

Figure 3   Net changes of stage between clinical staging at diagnosis and final staging of the histopathological examination of the specimen obtained at radical prostatectomy. The data presented are the difference between the number of patients who had upstaging and those in whom the disease was downstaged for each treatment group, according to the stage at diagnosis. Black bars, combination therapy with flutamide and an LHRH agonist; white bars, controls

in stage C_1 disease and 71.4% (5/7) in stage C_2 disease.

After 3 months of combination therapy, average upstaging decreased to 28.9% (26 of 90) in patients who received neoadjuvant combination therapy compared to 54.9% (39 of 71) in the control group. Thus, net upstaging (the difference between the number of patients who had upstaging and the number of those who had downstaging) occurred, on average, in 33.8% of control patients, whereas, in contrast, 21.1% of patients were downstaged at analysis of the surgical specimen in the group of patients who had combination therapy before surgery, for a net difference of 54.9% in favor of neoadjuvant combination therapy (Figure 4).

The net effect of neoadjuvant therapy on specimen-confined margins and organ-con-fined disease can be clearly seen in Figure 5 and Table 3. Since organ-confined disease has such an important prognostic value, it is of major interest to see in Figure 5a that organ-confined disease increased from 49.3% (35/71) in the control group to 77.8% (70/90) for a 57.8% improvement in the group of men who received neoadjuvant combination therapy. In fact, organ-confined disease increased from 61.5% (24/39) to 88.4% (38/43) in stage B_1 disease, from 23.5% (4/17) to 65.5% (19/29) in stage B_2 disease, from 57.1% (4/7) to 87.5% (7/8) in stage C_1 disease and from 20% (1/5) to 71.4% (5/7) in stage C_2 disease. On the other hand, specimen-confined disease or cancer-negative margins increased from 66.2% (47/71) in men who had radical prostatectomy alone to 92.2% (83/90) ($p < 0.001$) in those who received neoadjuvant combination therapy before radical prostatectomy (Figure 5b). There is thus a 57.8% increase in the incidence of organ-

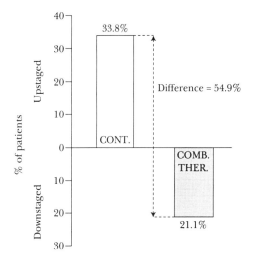

Figure 4 Net change of stage between initial staging at diagnosis and final staging at radical prostatectomy in control (CONT.) patients who had radical prostatectomy alone and those who received combination therapy (COMB. THER.) for 3 months before radical prostatectomy. Controls: 39/71 (54.9%) upstaged, 15/71 (21.1%) downstaged; combination therapy: 26/90 (28.9%) upstaged, 45/90 (50%) downstaged

confined disease following 3 months of neoadjuvant combination endocrine therapy compared to untreated men (Figure 5a) while the incidence of cancer-positive margins is 4.3-fold higher in the control group of untreated men (33.8% vs. 7.8%) (Figure 5b).

As shown in Table 4, serum PSA level measured at diagnosis in patients who did not receive combination therapy prior to surgery showed a correlation with the final stage determined by histopathological examination of the surgical specimen. Cancer was confined to the prostate in 58.5% of those who had a PSA level at diagnosis below or equal to 10 ng/ml, and this ratio dropped to 22.2% when PSA level was higher than 10 ng/ml at diagnosis (significant difference, $p < 0.02$). Although not statistically significant, a similar trend toward non-confined disease at higher serum PSA level was observed in patients who received the combination

Table 3 Effect of 3-month neoadjuvant combination therapy with flutamide and an LHRH agonist on organ-confined disease at radical prostatectomy in stages B and C prostate cancer

Group	Organ-confined	Not organ-confined	Total
Control	35 (49.3%)	36 (50.7%)	71
Combination therapy	70 (77.8%)	20 (22.2%)	90

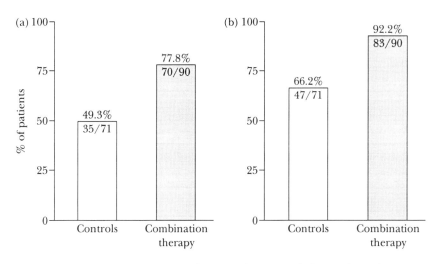

Figure 5 Effect of 3-month neoadjuvant combination therapy with flutamide and an LHRH agonist[31] on organ-confined disease (a) and specimen-confined disease (b) in stages B and C prostate cancer

therapy for 3 months (Table 5). Figure 6 clearly illustrates the fact that the risk of upstaging was related to the PSA level at diagnosis if no combination therapy was provided to the patients. The ratio of upstaged disease continuously rose from 30% to 33, 64, 70 and 100% in patients having a serum PSA level at diagnosis of 0–3, 3–5, 5–10, 10–15 and > 15 ng/ml, respectively. The rate of upstaging was higher than average (54.9%) for all those who had a PSA level above 5 ng/ml. Moreover, all of those patients who had a PSA level of > 15 ng/ml were upstaged from 62.5% organ-confined to 100% stage C or D disease. Eighty per cent of those upstaged to D_1 disease were above that threshold of 15 ng/ml.

Since serum PSA level has become such an important marker of prostate cancer growth, it is of interest to see in Figure 7 the changes in serum PSA level that occurred during the 3-month period of combination therapy before radical prostatectomy. Serum PSA level above the limit of detection was measured in only a few

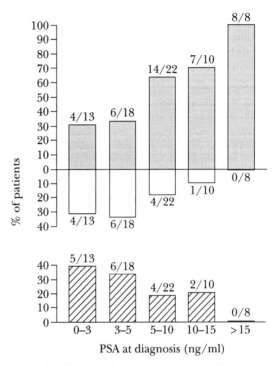

Figure 6   Change of stages versus serum PSA level at diagnosis. Percentages are relative to the total number of patients within the same PSA range. Black bars, upstaging; white bars, downstaging; hatched bars, no change

Table 4   Relationship between serum PSA concentration at diagnosis and frequency distribution of organ-confined disease in patients who did not receive combination therapy prior to the surgery

Serum PSA level at diagnosis	Organ-confined	Not organ-confined	Total
≤ 10 ng/ml	31 (58.5%)	22 (41.5%)	53
> 10 ng/ml	4 (22.2%)	14 (77.8%)	18
Total	35	36	71

Continuity-adjusted χ^2: $p < 0.02$

Table 5   Relationship between serum PSA concentration at diagnosis and frequency distribution of organ-confined disease in patients who received combination therapy for 3 months prior to the surgery

Serum PSA level at diagnosis	Organ-confined	Not organ-confined	Total
≤ 10 ng/ml	54 (80.6%)	13 (19.4%)	67
> 10 ng/ml	15 (65.2%)	8 (34.8%)	23
Total	69	21	90

Continuity-adjusted χ^2 not significant

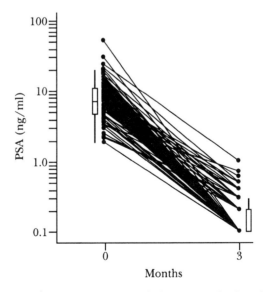

Figure 7   Serum PSA levels before and after 3 months of combination therapy

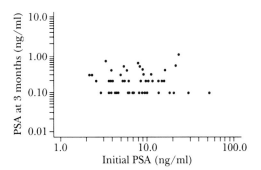

Figure 8 Serum PSA levels after 3 months of combination therapy vs. levels at diagnosis

patients, and no relationship with the PSA level at diagnosis could be identified (Figure 8). The mean serum PSA level at diagnosis of those with a level below and those with a level above 0.3 ng/ml after the 3 months of combination therapy were very similar to one another, being 9.4 ± 1.1 ng/ml and 10.8 ± 2.4 ng/ml (± SEM), respectively.

Comments

A possible means of improving the proportion of patients with organ-confined disease and cancer-negative margins at surgery was clearly suggested by the observation that patients with metastatic disease who were treated by combination therapy using a pure antiandrogen associated with medical or surgical castration showed a much more rapid and marked regression of their cancer in the prostatic area than with distant metastatic disease[29]. Moreover, it is well recognized that when recurrence of the disease occurs, progression of the cancer at the level of the prostate is a rare event; the bones are the usual site of progression. Since prostate cancer localized into the prostatic area is so highly sensitive to androgen deprivation, it appeared logical to use combination therapy to downstage prostate cancer in men diagnosed as having localized disease before performing radical prostatectomy or radiotherapy the first.

Following an encouraging preliminary study[3], we have conducted a prospective and randomized clinical trial in order to assess the potential advantages of neoadjuvant combination therapy with the pure antiandrogen flutamide and an LHRH agonist administered for 3 months before radical prostatectomy, compared with surgery alone[12].

Although the long-term effects of androgen deprivation achieved by neoadjuvant combination therapy on survival remain to be assessed by long-term follow-up of the patients, the present data show that prostate cancer cell death or apoptosis occurs at a relatively high rate in the prostatic area, under the influence of combination therapy: such cancer cell death leads to a relatively rapid downstaging of the disease.

The success of the present approach relies, to a large extent, on the availability of an efficient, low-cost and widely acceptable strategy to detect early-stage prostate cancer in the general population[9]. It is reasonable to expect that patients with localized disease at final histopathological staging following radical prostatectomy should have a life expectancy not unlike that of men of similar age with no prostate cancer.

The rationale for combination therapy before radiotherapy is to reduce the number of stem cells to be inactivated by radiation therapy. In the RTOG 8610 trial, in which combination therapy with flutamide and Zoladex® was given for 2 months before and 2 months during radiotherapy vs. radiotherapy alone, the clear advantages of combination therapy, with 3 years of follow-up, are indicated by disease-free survivals of 46% vs. 26%, respectively ($p = 0.0001$). In fact, in the RTOG 8610 trial, the combined therapy of flutamide + goserelin is to become the standard arm against which other modalities will be compared[33].

With no assumption other than surgical excision of organ-confined disease being equivalent to cure of the disease, screening is clearly a major factor able to decrease mortality due to prostate cancer. The simple use of screening could increase the number of patients potentially curable by about 125% compared to no screening, or from 20 to 45% of patients[11,12]. Neoadjuvant or preoperative combination endocrine therapy could potentially further increase the rate of curable disease up to 60–80%. The positive economic impact of such an approach on health care costs has been previously discussed[11,12]. The calculations performed leave little doubt that this strategy, based upon efficient screening and preoperative endocrine combination therapy, could play a key role in a successful fight against prostate cancer[34]. In fact, the progress at hand could have a major impact if performed by specialized facilities.

It must be remembered that a male has a 9–11% risk of developing clinically significant prostate cancer during his lifetime, and a 2.6–4.3% risk of dying from prostate[35]. Even patients with stage A₁ disease have a 10% chance of dying from prostate cancer if left untreated for 10 years[36]. The only possibility for a significant decrease of the death rate due to prostate cancer is early diagnosis and treatment. We should not further delay the use of the available screening and therapeutic technology while concentrating our research efforts on the development of more sensitive and reliable diagnostic procedures, more reliable and specific prognostic factors as well as improved therapy for this deadly disease. We are pursuing the first prospective randomized trial on prostate cancer screening, started in 1988, but the evidence gained during the last 5 years and summarized above clearly supports the benefits of early diagnosis and treatment. The Québec[9,11], European[37] and United States National Cancer Institute randomized screening studies should, if the problem of contamination of the control arm by spontaneous screening does not become too high, provide an important assessment of the impact of screening on morbidity and mortality. The convincing demonstration that excision of organ-confined prostate cancer by radical prostatectomy cures the disease and the clear evidence showing that screening can at least double the proportion of curable prostate cancers are extremely important findings that should already be used to the benefit of the patients. Neoadjuvant combination therapy for downstaging of cancer could well add significantly to screening, and the two approaches in combination could well offer a unique opportunity for highly significant progress.

As shown in the present study, downstaging of prostate cancer with 3-month combination therapy dramatically improves the results of radical prostatectomy, thus permitting 90% of patients found to have prostate cancer at first visit to become candidates for radical prostatectomy and nearly 100% of men at follow-up visits to have access to the same potentially curative treatment. However, to achieve such results, the detection strategy mentioned above must be followed[9]. Serum PSA level must be used as a pre-screening technique with the addition of digital rectal examination (DRE) when possible at the first visit; transrectal ultra sonography (TRUS) should be restricted to patients with serum PSA level above 3.0 µg/l and/or positive DRE[9,38]. We have in fact found that 88% of cancers could be detected by serum PSA level alone at first visit, and 97% of cancers could be detected by serum PSA level at follow-up visits. If annual or biennial serum PSA measurements are performed, it is expected that more than 90% of the cancers detected will be candidates for radical prostatectomy, thus making it possible, as demonstrated in the present study, to obtain cancer-negative surgical margins in 92% of cases or in more than 80% of the total population of men who develop prostate cancer detectable by serum PSA level and/or DRE. This is a complete reversal of the present situation without screening, in which 75% of the prostate cancers are not confined to the prostate at diagnosis, and only prolongation of life can be offered to the patients.

Although the effects of the present approach on survival remain to be determined by long-term follow-up, it is reasonable to expect that patients with localized disease at final histopathological staging following radical prostatectomy should have a life expectancy not unlike that of men of similar age with no prostate cancer[17,39]. It remains to be seen, however, whether cancer cell death or apoptosis induced by combination therapy in the prostatic area, as clearly demonstrated in the present study, occurs to the same extent at distant micrometastatic sites. The answer to this important question will also be provided by long-term follow-up of these patients.

Previous studies have shown that combination endocrine therapy decreases the total volume of the prostate and of the cancer[3,13,40–45]. The present data show, in the first randomized study, that neoadjuvant combination therapy leads not only to downsizing of the prostate and tumor but also to a true downstaging of prostate cancer. Lee and colleagues[13] have also clearly demonstrated that prostate cancer cell death is induced by combination therapy in the prostatic area.

The present data show that neoadjuvant combination therapy removes the previous serious limitation that 50% of men had a disease more advanced than expected at diagnosis when the final and true staging was obtained by histopathological examination of the surgical specimen. Following only 3 months of combination endocrine therapy, the stage of the disease was, on average, decreased by 23% compared to the initial staging at diagnosis. Such histopathological findings, which remain to be supported by long-term follow-up of the patients, offer the hope of a major improvement in the morbidity and mortality from prostate cancer.

As much as there is no doubt that androgen deprivation causes apoptosis or cell death of prostate cancer cells[46], it has also become clear that 3 months of neoadjuvant combination therapy is too short to cause optimal cell death. In fact, after 3 months of combination therapy, 22% of cancers remain not organ-confined (Figure 5a), thus leaving at least 22% of patients with no cure following radical prostatectomy. Moreover, one should take into account that 15% of organ-confined disease at surgery will ultimately show recurrence of the cancer as indicated by an elevation of serum PSA within 10 years[47]. Since there is a 15% risk of an increase in serum PSA within 10 years after radical prostatectomy in patients with organ-confined disease at surgery, it thus seems appropriate to reduce by 15% the probability of cure in patients who receive radical prostatectomy alone (50–

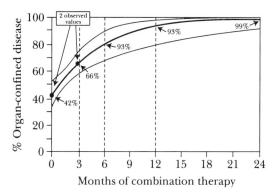

Figure 9 Estimate of optimal duration of combination therapy in localized prostate cancer

8 = 42%) as well as following 3 months of combination therapy (78–12 = 66%). Following 3 months of combination therapy, one can thus estimate that only 66% of patients should be cured while 44% can expect recurrence of the disease within 10 years.

Using these numbers, we have estimated the duration of combination therapy required to cause an optimal or near-100% rate of organ-confined disease. The calculations illustrated in Figure 9 are thus based upon the data obtained on organ-confined disease with and without 3 months of neoadjuvant combination therapy (Figure 5A). These calculations indicate the probability of organ-confined disease during the first 2 years + 95% confidence interval. For the reasons mentioned above, we have assumed that 15% of organ-confined disease at surgery will ultimately lead to recurrence of the disease as indicated by an elevation of PSA within 10 years[47].

With no neoadjuvant combination therapy, the predicted cure rate is estimated at 42% while it increases to 66% and 79% following 3 and 6 months of combination therapy. The estimated cure rate increases to 93% (79–98%) and 99% (91–99.9%) at 12 and 24 months, respectively, of combination therapy.

The previous choice of 3 months of neoadjuvant therapy[3] was motivated by the possibility of growth of prostate cancer under neoadjuvant combination therapy before proceeding to the removal of the prostate by radical prostatectomy. However, the data that have now accumulated convincingly show that localized prostate cancer does not progress for many years under combination therapy alone (Labrie *et al.*, unpublished data). A duration of combination therapy up to 2 years is also supported by the data obtained in an analogous cancer, namely breast cancer, where a 20% increase in survival at 5 years was measured in women who received Tamoxifen for 2 years or more[48]. A duration of treatment much longer than 3 months is also supported by our data obtained on serum PSA and positive biopsies performed 12 and 24 months following radiation therapy associated with neoadjuvant and adjuvant combination therapy administered for a total of 3 or 10.5 months. Much better results, although not yet reaching 100%, were obtained with 10.5 months compared to 3 months of combination therapy[49].

Although the choice of 3 months of neoadjuvant combination therapy has permitted to prove the marked induction of apoptosis and downstaging of localized prostate cancer[3,12,31,40–45], it is also clear from the observations and calculations mentioned above that combination therapy should be given for up to 2 years for optimal chances of success. This estimate is based upon the best scientific evidence gained from both prostate and breast cancer responses to androgen and estrogen deprivation, respectively[31,48,49]. It is equally clear

that the best results are obtained with maximal androgen blockade with a pure antiandrogen: monotherapy or a lower degree of androgen blockade cannot achieve the similar level of apoptosis with the added risk of development of androgen-insensitive clones. It is in fact well known that suboptimal androgen blockade causes the development of tumors which have become irresponsive to combination therapy applied later at time of progression.

The expected rate of organ-confined disease has been calculated assuming that the benefit of the combination treatment would asymptotically reach 100% according to a mono-exponential improvement with a non-zero initial value. The equation therefore reads: % organ-confined = 1 -A* exp(-Alpha*Duration) where A is fixed by the initial value which is given by the % organ-confined disease with no treatment (1-A = 49.3% ± 5.9). The time constant is derived from the rate of organ-confined disease at 3 months (77.8% ± 4.4). These data are available from a previous clinical trial (31)[1] and standard deviations are calculated using the normal distribution approximation for rates. Confidence intervals of the model predictions were further obtained by Monte-Carlo simulation.

---

[1]The data obtained at time of surgery in Labrie *et al.*[31] have been reduced by 15% to take into account the 15% of PSA failure following 10 years for organ-confined disease[47]

References

1. Parker, S. L., Tong, T., Bolden, S. and Wingo, P. A. (1996). Cancer statistics 1996. *CA Cancer J. Clin.*, **65**, 5–27
2. Brown, M. L., Fintor, L. and Newman-Horm, P. A. (1993). The economic burden of cancer. *J. Natl. Cancer Inst.*, **85**, 351
3. Monfette, G., Dupont, A. and Labrie, F. (1989). Temporary combination therapy with flutamide and Tryptex as adjuvant to radical prostatectomy for the treatment of early stage prostate cancer. In Labrie, F., Lee, F. and Dupont, A. (eds.) *Early Stage Prostate Cancer: Diagnosis and Choice of Therapy*, pp. 41–51. (New York: Excerpta Medica)
4. Lee, F., Torp-Pedersen, S. T., Siders, D., Littrup, P. J. and McLeary, R. D. (1989). Transrectal ultrasound in the diagnosis and staging of prostatic carcinoma. *Radiology*, **170**, 609–15
5. Cooner, W. H., Mosley, B. R. Jr, Rutherford, C. L. R., Beard, J. H., Pond, H. S., Terry, W. J.,

Igel, T. C. and Kidd, D. D. (1990). Prostate cancer detection in a clinical urological practice by ultrasonography, digital rectal examination and prostate-specific antigen. *Urology*, **143**, 1146–54

6. Whitmore, W. (1990). Natural history of low-stage prostatic cancer and the impact of early detection. *Urol. Clin. North Am.*, **17**, 689–97
7. Oesterling, J. E. (1991). Prostate specific antigen: a critical assessment of the most useful tumor marker for adenocarcinoma of the prostate. *J. Urol.*, **145**, 907–23
8. Catalona, W. J., Smith, D. S., Ratliff, T. L., Dodds, K. M., Coplen, D. E., Yuan, J. J., Petros, J. A. and Andriole, G. L. (1991). Measurement of prostate-specific antigen in serum as a screening test for prostate cancer. *N. Engl. J. Med.*, **324**, 1156–61
9. Labrie, F., Dupont, A., Suburu, R., Cusan, L., Tremblay, M., Gomez, J. L. and Emond, J. (1992). Serum prostatic specific antigen (PSA) as prescreening test for prostate cancer. *J. Urol.*, **147**, 846–52
10. Lee, F., Littrup, P. J., Loft-Christensen, L. Jr, Kelly, B. S., McHugh, T. A., Siders, D. B., Mitchell, A. E. and Newby, J. E. (1992). Predicted prostate specific antigen results using transrectal ultrasound gland volume. *Cancer*, **70** (Suppl.), 211–20
11. Labrie, F., Dupont, A., Suburu, R., Cusan, L., Gomez, J. L., Koutsilieris, M., Diamond, P., Emond, J., Lemay, M. and Têtu, B. (1993). Optimized strategy for detection of early stage, curable prostate cancer: role of prescreening with prostatic-specific antigen. *Clin. Invest. Med.*, **16**, 426–41
12. Labrie, F., Dupont, A., Cusan, L., Gomez, J. L., Diamond, P., Koutsilieris, M., Suburu, R., Fradet, Y., Lemay, M., Têtu, B., Emond, J. and Candas, B. (1993). Downstaging of localized prostate cancer by neoadjuvant therapy with flutamide and lupron: the first controlled and randomized trial. *Clin. Invest. Med.*, **16**, 511–21
13. Lee, F., Siders, D. B., Newby, J. E., McHugh, T. A. and Solomon, M. H. (1993). The role of transrectal ultrasound-guided staging biopsy and androgen ablation therapy prior to radical prostatectomy. *Clin. Invest. Med.*, **16**, 458–70
14. Littrup, P. J., Goodman, A. C. and Mettlin, C. J. (1993). The benefit and cost of prostate cancer early detection. The Investigators of the American Cancer Society–National Prostate Cancer Project. *CA Cancer J. Clin.*, **43**, 143–9
15. Mettlin, C. (1993). Early detection of prostate cancer following repeated examinations by multiple modalities: results of the American Cancer

Society National Prostate Cancer Detection Project. *Clin. Invest. Med.*, **16**, 440–7
16. Kolata, G. (1987). Prostate cancer consensus hampered by lack of data. *Science*, **236**, 1626–7
17. Walsh, P. C. and Jewett, H. J. (1980). Radical surgery for prostatic cancer. *Cancer*, **45**, 1906–11
18. Jewett, H. J., Bridge, R. W., Gray, G. F. Jr and Shelley, W. M. (1968). The palpable nodule of prostatic cancer. Results 15 years after radical excision. *J. Am. Med. Assoc.*, **203**, 403–6
19. Brawer, M. K. and Lange, P. H. (1990). Adjuvant therapy after radical prostatectomy. *Probl. Urol.*, **4**, 461–72
20. Gibbons, R. P., Correa, R. J. Jr, Brannen, G. E. and Weissman, R. M. (1989). Total prostatectomy for clinically localized prostate cancer: long-term results. *J. Urol.*, **141**, 564–6
21. Lange, P. H. and Narayan, P. (1983). Understaging and undergrading of prostate cancer. Argument for postoperative radiation as adjuvant therapy. *Urology*, **21**, 113–18
22. Catalona, W. J. and Stein, A. J. (1982). Staging errors in clinically localized prostatic cancer. *J. Urol.*, **127**, 452–6
23. Veenema, R. J., Gursel, E. O. and Lattimer, J. K. (1977). Radical retropubic prostatectomy for cancer: a 20-year experience. *J. Urol.*, **117**, 330–1
24. Elder, J. S., Jewett, H. J. and Walsh, P. C. (1982). Radical perineal prostatectomy for clinical stage B2 carcinoma of the prostate. *J. Urol.*, **127**, 704–6
25. Boxer, R. J., Kaufman, J. J. and Goodwin, W. E. (1977). Radical prostatectomy for carcinoma of the prostate: 1951–1976. A review of 329 patients. *J. Urol.*, **117**, 208–13
26. Epstein, J. I., Walsh, P. C., Carmichael, M. and Brendler, C. B. (1994). Pathologic and clinical findings to predict tumor extent of nonpalpable (stage T1c) prostate cancer. *J. Am. Med. Assoc.*, **271**, 368–74
27. Stormont, T. J., Farrow, G. M., Myers, R. P., Blute, M. L., Zincke, H., Wilson, T. M. and Oesterling, J. E. (1993). Clinical stage B0 or T1c prostate cancer: nonpalpable disease identified by elevated serum prostate-specific antigen concentration. *Urology*, **41**, 3–8
28. Labrie, F., Dupont, A., Bélanger, A., Cusan, L., Lacourcière, Y., Monfette, G., Laberge, J. G., Emond, J., Fazekas, A. T. A., Raynaud, J. P. and Husson, J. M. (1982). New hormonal therapy in prostatic carcinoma: combined treatment with an LHRH agonist and an antiandrogen. *J. Clin. Invest. Med.*, **5**, 267–75
29. Labrie, F., Dupont, A. and Bélanger, A. (1985). Complete androgen blockade for the treatment of prostate cancer. In de Vita, V. T., Hellman, S. and Rosenberg, S. A. (eds.) *Important Advances*

in Oncology, pp. 193–217. (Philadelphia: J. B. Lippincott)

30. Labrie, F., Bélanger, A., Dupont, A., Luu-The, V., Simard, J. and Labrie, C. (1993). Science behind total androgen blockade: from gene to combination therapy. *Clin. Invest. Med.*, **16**, 475–92

31. Labrie, F., Cusan, L., Gomez, J. L., Diamond, P., Suburu, R., Lemay, M., Tetu, B., Fradet, Y. and Candas, B. (1994). Down-staging of early stage prostate cancer before radical prostatectomy: the first randomized trial of neoadjuvant combination therapy with Flutamide and a luteinizing hormone-releasing hormone agonist. *Urology*, **44**, 29–37

32. Vaillancourt, L., Têtu, B., Fradet, Y., Dupont, A., Gomez, J., Cusan, L., Suburu, E. R., Diamond, P., Candas, B. and Labrie, F. (1996). Effect of neoadjuvant endocrine therapy (combined androgen blockade) on normal prostate and prostatic carcinoma. *Am. J. Surg. Pathol.*, **20**, 86–93

33. Radiation Therapy Oncology Group (1994). Phase III trial of androgen suppression before and during radiation therapy for locally advanced prostatic cancer: abstract report of RTOG 8610. *Prostate*, **5**, 2–3

34. Labrie, F. (1994). Intracrinology and cancer therapy. *Science Watch*, **5**, 3–8

35. Boring, C. C., Squires, T. S., Tong, T. and Montgomery, S. (1994). Cancer statistics 1994. *CA Cancer J. Clin.*, **44**, 7–26

36. Epstein, J. I., Paull, G., Eggleston, J. C. and Walsh, P. C. (1986). Prognosis of untreated stage A1 prostatic carcinoma: a study of 94 cases with extended followup. *J. Urol.*, **136**, 837–9

37. Schröder, F. H., Denis, L., Kirkels, W. J., Koning, H. J. and de Standaert, B. (1994). European randomized study of screening for prostate cancer. *Cancer*, in press

38. Labrie, F., Dupont, A., Simard, J., Luu-The, V. and Bélanger, A. (1993). Intracrinology: the basis for the rational design of endocrine therapy at all stages of prostate cancer. *Eur. Urol.*, **24** (Suppl. 2), 94–105

39. Brendler, C. B. and Walsh, P. C. (1992). The role of radical prostatectomy in the treatment of prostate cancer. *CA Cancer J. Clin.*, **42**, 212–22

40. Solomon, M. H. (1990). Radical prostatectomy following androgen blockade. In Lee, F. and McLeary, R. L. (eds.) Proceedings of the *5th International Symposium on Transrectal Ultrasound in the Diagnosis and Management of Prostate Cancer*, p. 100. (Chicago: University Press)

41. Schulman, C. C. and Sassine, A. N. (1993). Neoadjuvant hormonal deprivation before radical prostatectomy. *Clin. Invest. Med.*, **16**, 523–31

42. Fair, W. F., Aprikian, A. G., Cohen, D., Sogani, P. and Reuter, V. (1993). Use of neoadjuvant androgen deprivation therapy in clinical localized prostate cancer. *Clin. Invest. Med.*, **16**, 516–22

43. Labrie, F. (1991). Endocrine therapy for prostate cancer. *Endocrinol. Metab. Clin. North Am.*, **20**, 845–72

44. Solomon, M. H., McHugh, T. A., Dorr, R. P., Lee, F. and Siders, D. B. (1993). Hormone ablation therapy as neoadjuvant treatment to radical prostatectomy. *Clin. Invest. Med.*, **16**, 532–8

45. Andros, E. A., Danesghari, F. and Crawford, E. D. (1993). Neoadjuvant hormonal therapy in stage C carcinoma of the prostate. *Clin. Invest. Med.*, **16**, 510–15

46. Kerr, J. F., Wyllie, A. H. and Currie, A. R. (1972). Apoptosis: a basic biological phenomenon with wide-ranging implications in tissue kinetics. *Br. J. Cancer*, **26**, 239–57

47. Partin, A. W., Pound, C. R., Clemens, J. Q., Epstein, J. I. and Walsh, P. C. (1993). The John Hopkins Experience after 10 Years. *Urol. Clin. North Amer.*, **20**, 713–25

48. The Scottish Trial. (1987). *Lancet*, **ii:** 171–5

49. Labrie, F., Gomez, J. L., Laverdiere, J., Cusan, L., Diamond, P., Suburu, E. R., Lemay, M. and Candas, B. (1996). Benefits of neoadjuvant and adjuvant complete antiandrogen therapy associated with curative radiation therapy in early stages prostate cancer: preliminary report of prospective and randomized study. *Proc. Endocrin Society Meeting*, San Francisco, No. OR57–6, p. 732

Interactive Voting System

1 Prostate cancer cell death is better achieved with longer treatment and more efficient androgen blockade.

Response	*Option*
76%	Yes.
24%	No.

Number of votes: 99

5α-Reductase inhibition in the treatment of prostate cancer

5

G. J. Gormley

Is there a role for the use of 5α-reductase inhibitors in the treatment of prostate cancer? This question is frequently raised when consideration is given to evolving strategies for treatment of this disease. To date, information is not available to answer this question completely, but there are data to support further efforts to define an appropriate role. The rationale for considering a 5α-reductase inhibitor is summarized in Table 1. Prostate cancer is derived from an endocrine-sensitive organ and is itself hormonally dependent. In 1941, Huggins and Hodges elegantly established the importance of circulating androgens on the growth and spread of prostate cancer[1]. This fundamental discovery, for which they were awarded the Nobel prize in medicine, led to the understanding that depriving prostate cancer cells of androgens could alter the clinical course of the disease and in some cases result in cure. For many years after the work of Huggins and Hodges, it was believed that testosterone, secreted from both the testis and the adrenal gland, was responsible for maintenance of the prostate gland and was a promoter of carcinogenesis. Almost a decade ago, Pollard and colleagues established that the incidence of lobund Wistar rats developing prostate cancer was influenced by exposure to the car-

cinogen methyl-nitroso urea and testosterone in a dose-dependent manner[2].

The importance of testosterone as a direct promoter of prostate cancer has been greatly influenced by the work of two independent laboratories who described the genetic syndrome of 5α-reductase deficiency[3,4]. Affected individuals with this disorder are unable to convert testosterone into the 5α-reduced metabolite dihydrotestosterone (DHT). Male offspring are born with ambiguous genitalia, a microphallus, hypospadias and an underdeveloped prostate gland. With the increased testosterone secretion at puberty, masculinization of the external genitalia occurs, but the prostate gland remains underdeveloped. These observations established DHT as the active androgen modulating prostate growth and physiology.

Since the discovery of the 5α-reductase deficiency, much has been learned about this enzyme system. The 5α-reductase enzyme is a membrane-bound NADPH-dependent protein that metabolizes testosterone to DHT within androgen-dependent target cells (Figure 1). When testosterone from testicular or adrenal sources arrives at an androgen-dependent target cell (such as the prostate), it can bind directly to the androgen receptor or be converted to DHT. DHT can then bind to the same androgen receptor, but with greater affinity compared to testosterone. This metabolic step results in an amplification of androgen action, leading to increased activation of androgen response elements within the genome of androgen-dependent cells. In the rat, 5α-reductase appears to be controlled by a feed-forward mechanism mediated by DHT levels which

Table 1 5α-Reductase inhibitors in prostate cancer

Growth of the prostate is androgen-dependent
Androgens are promoters of prostate cancer
5α-Reductase inhibition leads to:
   regression of the hyperplastic prostate
   suppression of androgen-dependent tumor
     growth
   suppression of serum PSA levels in men with
     prostate cancer
5α-Reductase activity is decreased in Japanese men

induces 5α-reductase enzyme activity and mRNA expression[5]. Recently, two isoenzymes of 5αR-reductase have been characterized, cloned and localized in human tissues[6–8] (Figure 2). The gene for the type 1 isozyme (5αR-1) has been localized to the short arm of chromosome 5 and is found in highest concentrations in skin and liver[9]. The gene for the type 2 isozyme (5αR-2) has been localized to the short arm of chromosome 2 and is found in highest concen-

trations in liver and genital tissue, including the prostate[10,11].

Recent epidemiological data support the role of 5α-reductase activity in the development of prostate cancer. The human SRD5A2 gene encodes the type 2 5α-reductase enzyme. African–American men appear to have a unique family of 121–131 bp alleles not found in men with lower lifetime risk of prostate cancer such as Asian–Americans and non-Hispanic whites[12]. In another report, 5α-reductase activity in Japanese men was found to be lower than in white or African–American men[13]. Therefore, expression of the gene or activity of the 5α-reductase enzyme may contribute to differences in lifetime risk for prostate cancer.

Recognizing the importance of the 5α-reductase enzyme system to prostate physiology, several groups made intensive efforts, leading to the development of specific 5α-reductase inhibitors aimed at the treatment of both benign and malignant disease of the prostate. The first inhibitor to be developed was finasteride, a structural analog of testosterone which selectively

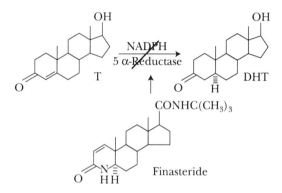

Figure 1 Conversion of testosterone to dihydrotestosterone (DHT) inhibited by finasteride

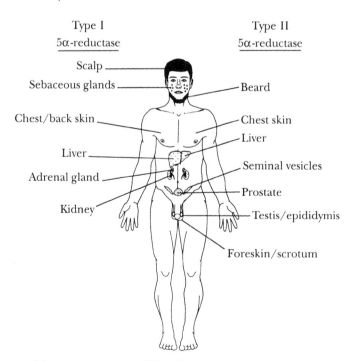

Figure 2 Localization of the two isoenzymes of 5α-reductase

inhibits the 5αR-2 isoenzyme without inhibiting the 5αR-1 enzyme system or interfering with androgen receptor binding. DHT appears to be essential for prostatic growth, since men with 5α-reductase deficiency have atrophic prostate glands throughout their lives, despite normal or elevated levels of testosterone in adulthood. These findings suggest that specific inhibitors of type 2 5α-reductase could be used to decrease DHT formation within the prostate and cause involution of the hyperplastic tissue. This hypothesis has been proven to be correct. The effect of finasteride on intraprostatic androgen concentrations has been described[14] and is summarized in Figure 3.

In studies of men with enlarged prostates from benign prostatic hyperplasia (BPH), treatment with finasteride has led to 20% reductions in total volume within 1 year[15] and 27% reductions within 3 years[16]. These data confirm the importance of DHT in hyperplastic growth of the benign prostate gland and establish reversibility of this process when DHT is removed. Recently several human prostate cancer cell lines including PC3[17], DU145[17], PCEW[18] and LnCap[19] have demonstrated a dose-dependent inhibition of cell growth by finasteride. The data on finasteride's effect on LnCap cells is summarized in Figure 4. In contrast, one study was unable to demonstrate an effect of finasteride on the dunning tumor in nude mice[20].

The first clinical study reported with a 5α-reductase inhibitor in the treatment of prostate cancer involved 28 men with untreated stage D disease[21]. Treatment with 10 mg of finasteride or placebo per day for six weeks resulted in a 15% reduction in serum levels of prostate specific antigen (PSA). Those patients who remained on therapy for 3 months had a 20% reduction with no serious adverse experiences. This study established the fact that the metabolic effects of finasteride in men with prostate cancer were similar to those seen in men with BPH[22, 23] and that reductions in DHT were not compensated for by increases in serum testosterone levels. However, the modest reduction in PSA suggested limited efficacy in advanced disease, so this trial was not continued.

Because advanced disease was recognized as relatively insensitive to 5α-reductase inhibition, the concept of combining an antiandrogen with finasteride evolved. The rationale for this combination is shown in Figure 5. By blocking the production of DHT with finasteride, an antiandrogen may be more effective since testosterone is the weaker androgen. In a small uncontrolled study, ten men with intact sexual function and stage C or D prostate cancer were treated with the combination of finasteride and

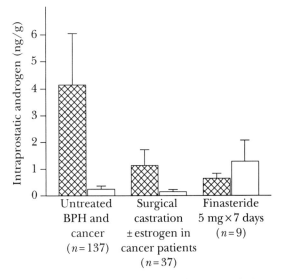

Figure 3 Effect of finasteride in three populations of patients on intraprostatic androgen concentration. Hatched bars, dihydrotestosterone; white bars, testosterone. Whiskers indicate standard deviation. From reference 14

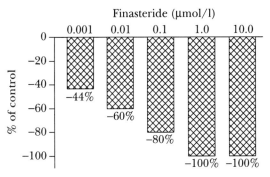

Figure 4 Effect of finasteride on the growth rate of LnCap cells. From reference 19

flutamide. Serum PSA levels fell from a baseline mean of 34.3 ng/ml to 3.8 ng/ml in 3 months (89% decrease from baseline) with eight of the ten men remaining sexually potent[24]. This work was later extended to 39 patients with similar results[25].

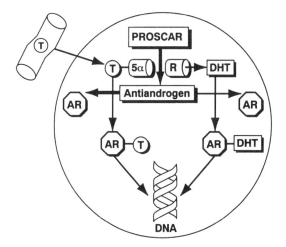

Figure 5 Mechanism of action of PROSCAR (finasteride) vs. antiandrogens. T, testosterone; 5αR, 5α-reductase; DHT, dihydrotestosterone; AR, androgen receptor

In the most comprehensive study published to date, 120 men with detectable PSA levels following radical prostatectomy who were previously untreated with any hormonal therapy were treated with 10 mg finasteride or placebo for 1 year[26]. The rationale for this study was based on the observation that a rising PSA level is usually the first sign of relapse following prostatectomy. The goal was to slow the rate of rise in PSA in the hopes of delaying recurrence. In this study, a significant delay in PSA rise was seen in 1 year compared to placebo (Figure 6), with continued suppression detectable up to 3 years in the open label extension study (Figure 7). There were numerically fewer recurrences in the finasteride group, but these differences from placebo were not statistically significant.

In summary, the 5α-reductase enzyme plays a very specific but critical role in prostate physiology. This specificity provides an opportunity to utilize inhibitors to interfere with pathological processes such as benign prostatic hyperplasia and prostate cancer. In the case of benign prostatic hyperplasia the utility has been widely established, but in prostate cancer much work remains to be done.

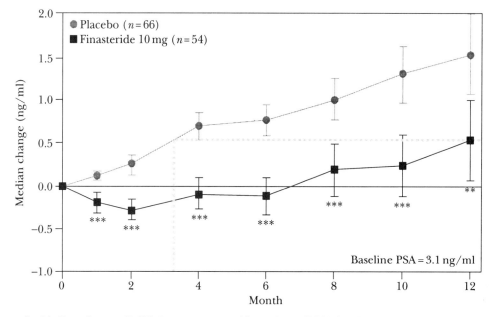

Figure 6 Median change ($\pm$ SE) in prostate specific antigen (PSA) level for all patients in the first year. ***$p \leq 0.001$; **$p \leq 0.01$, placebo vs. finasteride

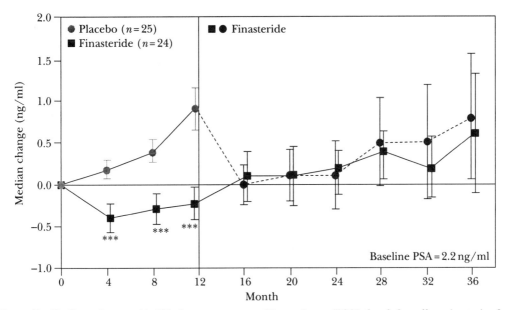

Figure 7 Median change (± SE) in prostate specific antigen (PSA) level for all patients in 3 years. ***$p < 0.001$, placebo vs. finasteride

References

1. Huggins, C. and Hodges, C. V. (1941). Studies on prostatic cancer; effect of castration, of estrogen and of androgen injection on serum phosphatases in metastatic carcinoma of prostate. *Cancer Res.*, **1**, 293–7

2. Pollard, M., Luckert, P. H. and Snyder, D. L. (1989). The promotional effect of testosterone on induction of prostate cancer in MNU-sensitized L-W rats. *Cancer Lett.*, **45**, 209–12

3. Imperato-McGinley, J., Guerrero, L., Gautier, T., and Peterson, R. E. (1974). Steroid 5α-reductase deficiency in man: an inherited form of male pseudohermaphroditism. *Science*, **186**, 1213–15

4. Walsh, P. C., Madden, J. D., Harrod, M. J., Goldstein, J. L., MacDonald, P. C. and Wilson, J. D. (1974). Familial incomplete male pseudohermaphroditism, type 2. Decreased dihydrotestosterone formation in pseudovaginal perineoscrotal hypospadias. *N. Engl. J. Med.*, **291**, 944–9

5. George, F. W., Russell, D. W. and Wilson, J. D. (1991). Feed forward control of prostate growth: dihydrotestosterone induces expression of its own biosynthetic enzyme steroid 5α-reductase. *Proc. Natl. Acad. Sci. USA*, **88**, 8044–7

6. Andersson, S., Bishop, R. W. and Russell, D. W. (1989). Expression cloning and regulation of steriod 5α-reductase, an enzyme essential for male sexual differentiation. *J. Biol. Chem.*, **264**, 16249–55

7. Andersson, S. and Russel, D. W. (1990). Structural and biochemical properties of cloned and expressed human and rat steroid 5α-reductase. *Proc. Natl. Acad. Sci. USA*, **87**, 3640–4

8. Moore, R. J. and Wilson, J. D. (1976). Steroid 5α-reductase in cultured human fibroblasts: biochemical and genetic evidence for two distinct enzyme activities. *J. Biol. Chem.*, **251**, 5895–900

9. Jenkins, E. P., Hsieh, C.-L., Milatovich, A. *et al.* (1991). Characterization and chromosomal mapping of a human steroid 5α-reductase gene and pseudogene and mapping of the mouse homologue. *Genomics*, **11**, 1102–12

10. Thigpen, A. E., Davis, D. L., Milatovich, A. *et al.* (1992). Molecular genetics of steroid 5α-reductase 2 deficiency. *J. Clin. Invest.*, **90**, 799–809

11. Thigpen, A. E., Davis, D. L., Gautier, T., Imperato-McGinley, J. and Russell, D. W. (1992). The molecular basis of steroid 5α-reductase deficiency in a large Dominican kindred. *N. Engl. J. Med.*, **327**, 1216–19

12. Reichardt, J. K. V., Makridakis, N., Henderson, B. E., Yu, M. C., Pike, M. C. and Ross, R. K. (1995). Genetic variability of the human

SRD5A2 gene: implications for prostate cancer risk. *Cancer Res.*, **55**, 3973–5

13. Ross, R. K., Shimizu, H., Bernstein, L., Stanczyk, F. Z., Henderson, B. E., Lobo, R. A. and Pike, M. C. (1992). 5α-Reductase activity and risk of prostate cancer among Japanese and US white and black males. *Lancet*, **339**, 887–9

14. Geller, J. and Sionit, L. (1992). Castration-like effects on the human prostate of a 5α-reductase inhibitor, finasteride. *J. Cell Biochem.*, **16H**, 109–12

15. Gormley, G. J., Stoner, E., Bruskewitz, R. C. *et al.* (1992). The effect of finasteride in men with benign prostatic hyperplasia. *N. Engl. J. Med.*, **327**, 1185–91

16. Stoner, E. and Members of the Finasteride Study Group (1994). Three year safety and efficacy data on the use of finasteride in the treatment of benign prostatic hyperplasia. *Urology*, **43**, 284–94

17. Bologna, M., Muzi, P., Biordi, L., Festuccia, C. and Vicentini, C. (1992). Antiandrogens and 5α-reductase inhibition of the proliferation rate in PC3 and DU145 human prostatic cancer cell lines. *Curr. Ther. Res.*, **51**, 799–813

18. Henschel, T., Kuhn, R., Schafhauser, W. and Schrott, K. M. (1994). *XLVI Kongreß der Deutschen Gesellschaft für Urologie*, E.V. Abstr. S34, August. (Germany: Springer-Verlag)

19. Bologna, M., Muzi, P., Biordi, L., Festuccia, C. and Vicentini, C. (1995). Finasteride dose-dependently reduces the proliferation of the LnCap human prostatic cancer cell line *in vitro*. *Urology*, **45**, 282–90

20. Brooks, J. R., Berman, C., Hguyen, H., Prahalada, S., Primka, R. L., Rasmusson, G. H. and Slater, E. E. (1991). Effect of castration, DES, flutamide, and the 5α-reductase inhibitor, MK-906, on the growth of the Dunning rat prostatic carcinoma, R-3327. *Prostate*, **18**, 215–27

21. Presti, J. C., Fair, W. R., Andriole, G., Sogani, P. *et al.* (1992). Multicenter, randomized, double-blind, placebo controlled study to investigate the effect of finasteride (MK-906) on stage D prostate cancer. *J. Urol.*, **148**, 1201–4

22. Gormley, G. J., Stoner, E., Rittmaster, R. *et al.* (1990). Effects of finasteride (MK-906), a 5α-reductase inhibitor, on circulating androgens in male volunteers. *J. Clin. Endocrinol. Metab.*, **70**, 1136–41

23. Finasteride Study Group (1993). Finasteride (MK-906) in the treatment of benign prostatic hyperplasia. *Prostate*, **22**, 291–9

24. Fleshner, N. E. and Trachtenberg, J. (1993). Treatment of advanced prostate cancer with the combination of finasteride plus flutamide: early results. *Eur. Urol.*, **24** (Suppl. 2), 106–12

25. Fleshner, N. E., Fair, W. R. and Trachtenberg, J. (1995). Further experience with sequential androgen blockade. *J. Urol.*, **153**, Abstr. 882, p. 449A

26. Andriole, G., Lieber, M., Smith, J., Soloway, M. *et al.* (1995). Treatment with finasteride following radical prostatectomy for prostate cancer. *Urology*, **45**, 491–7

Interactive Voting System

---

1   Which of the following is not true?

Response   *Option*
29%   Finasteride inhibits the growth of a hormone-insensitive cell line.
10%   African–American men appear to have a unique SRD5A2 allele for type II 5α-reductase.
48%   Castration lowers intra-prostatic DHT more than finasteride.
13%   Combining an anti-androgen with a 5α-reductase inhibitor is likely to interfere with the effect of antiandrogen

Number of votes: 89

2   What tissue does not contain 5α-reductase type II?

29%   Liver.
30%   Scalp skin.
3%   Testis.
4%   Prostate.
34%   Andrenal gland.

Number of votes: 109

Chemoprevention of prostate cancer and the Prostate Cancer Prevention Trial*

6

O. W. Brawley and I. M. Thompson

The impact of prostate cancer is substantial. This has led to aggressive screening for and aggressive treatment of prostate cancer. There is, of course, significant controversy regarding the utility of both prostate cancer screening and prostate cancer treatment[1]. Both are active areas of investigation and the goal of reducing prostate cancer morbidity and mortality continues to elude modern medicine. An approach deserving consideration is the chemoprevention of prostate cancer.

Sporn and colleagues originally used the term 'chemoprevention' in 1976[2]. Chemoprevention is defined as the use of natural or synthetic chemical agents to reverse, suppress, or prevent carcinogenic progression to invasive cancer[3]. Although the chemoprevention of cancer may be a relatively new concept, the concept of using a drug to prevent a chronic disease is not new. Drugs are used to treat hypertension chemoprevent cardiovascular and renal disease. In a similar manner the medical treatment of hypercholesterolemia is chemoprevention of cardiovascular disease, and many postmenopausal women take estrogens to chemoprevent osteoporosis.

Cancer chemoprevention has attracted great interest. If it is to be developed most economically, the strategies tested should target the most common cancers and those individuals at high risk for these cancers. Chemoprevention of several cancers is now a real possibility, and chemoprevention of prostate cancer may be possible[3].

This paper describes leads in prostate cancer chemoprevention and the Prostate Cancer Prevention Trial[4-6]. This Prostate Cancer Prevention Trial is sponsored by the United States National Cancer Institute. It began accruing subjects in the fall of 1993 and will continue till 2006. Its primary purpose is to determine whether prolonged treatment with a 5α-reductase inhibitor will decrease an individual's risk for development of prostate cancer or the progression of small indolent cancers to larger potentially aggressive ones.

Biologic basis of cancer chemoprevention

The strategy of chemoprevention is strongly linked to the concept that carcinogenesis is a process[3,7]. The process begins with a genetic alteration called initiation. Promotion is the part of the process leading to phenotypical change of cells and ultimately to loss of replication, control, metastasis and invasiveness. Progression is the portion of the process in which cancerous cells form malignant tumor with increased morphologic change. Initiation can occur due to a hereditary

---

*Opinions expressed are those of the authors and do not necessarily reflect the views of the United States Army nor the U. S. Department of Health and Human Service

51

genetic alteration or acquired genetic damage due to the action of physical, viral or chemical carcinogens. Promotor influences are usually a physical or chemical force. Some influences can act as initiator and promoter. Other forces encourage progression of promoted cells.

Effective cancer chemoprevention agents interfere with the factors causing cancer initiation, promotion, or progression[7]. Prostate cancer is ideal for chemoprevention because it is a disease with a high histologic prevalence, a low rate of clinical progression, and it occurs in older men when competing causes of mortality are high. Indeed one does not have to prevent cancer from developing to have significant impact, one must only delay progression of a prostatic tumor for just a few years to have significant positive impact.

Potential chemopreventive agents generally have antimutagenic, antioxidant or antiproliferative activity. Agents being investigated include initiation inhibitors that induce enzymes that detoxify carcinogens (flavonoids and isothiocyanates); antioxidants that scavenge reactive oxygen species (*N*-acetylcysteine); and inhibitors of enzymes that activate carcinogens (butylated hydroxyanisole). Agents that inhibit promotional influences include inhibitors of DNA synthesis and cellular proliferation such as the non-steroidal anti-inflammatory agents calcium and selenium. Angiogenesis inhibitors such as thalidomide may also be effective.

Cancer chemoprevention is still largely theoretical and is not yet established in clinical practice. Well designed clinical trials will have to be completed to demonstrate efficacy. Chemoprevention trials are usually large, long-term, randomized, placebo-controlled and double-bind. The size and design of chemoprevention trials usually allows for study of multiple end-points. A number of chemoprevention trials have been completed in the fields of the upper aerodigestive tract, colon, skin, bladder, breast and cervical cancers, with surprising and valuable results[3,7].

Is prostate cancer a preventable disease?

The prostate cancer mortality rate varies markedly among populations and cultures around the world[8]. It has been noted that Japanese and Chinese men who migrate from Asia to the United States and adopt American habits have higher prostate cancer mortality rates and risks of prostate cancer death than men in their native country[9–12]. Descendants of these Asian men have mortality rates equivalent to those of white Americans. These studies suggest that an environmental influence acquired when adopting American habits or lost when giving up Japanese habits are causal co-factors or promoters of clinically significant (lethal) prostate cancer. The removal of the acquired promoter influence or the adoption of the anti-promoter influence may prevent prostate cancer.

The promotional influences on prostate cancer probably act over a period of years. Autopsy studies of men dying of trauma and heart disease find that multiple small microscopic foci of prostate cancer are common in early to mid-adulthood[13]. This suggests that the window of opportunity for inhibiting prostate cancer promotion is decades long.

One of the most obvious differences among cultures is diet, and the relationship between diet and prostate cancer has been of great interest[8,14–18]. The dietary factor most widely studied is fat intake. Populations with diets high in fat have higher relative risks for prostate cancer mortality[19–26]. Studies have also shown that populations with diets high in fibre and presumably lower in fat have lower incidences of prostate cancer[27–35]. The protective effect of a low-fat diet may lie in its alteration of circulating androgen levels. Reduction of dietary fat intake leads to reduction in urinary and serum androgens.

A trial to determine whether a low-fat diet would decrease the prostate cancer risk would take decades to carry out and involve thousands of men. A low-fat diet can, of course, be advocated without definitive proof of prostate cancer prevention, because of its known collateral health benefits.

Hormonal therapy

Androgenic stimulation is vital to prostate biology. Castration of males in childhood and early adulthood prevents benign prostatic hyperplasia and prostate cancer[36,37]. Removal of androgenic stimulation leads to a decrease in prostate weight. Castration has been utilized in treatment of severe prostatism for nearly a century[38] and the hormonal sensitivity of prostate cancer has been exploited in treatment for more than 50 years[38].

It has been suggested that populations with greater androgenic stimulation of the prostate may be more prone to develop clinically significant prostate cancer[39,40]. Studies testing this hypothesis vary widely in their results, because this is a difficult matter to study[39]. Androgens other than testosterone may be responsible for androgenic stimulation of the prostate, and serum androgen levels may not correlate with intraprostatic androgen activity. Several studies have found no difference in baseline circulating testosterone levels in prostate cancer patients when compared to controls, and other studies have found a positive correlation between androgen levels and prostate cancer risk[41–44]. Barrett-Connor and colleagues studied 1008 men for 14 years and found a positive dose–response correlation for plasma androstenedione level and the development of prostate cancer[45]. Meikle and colleagues observed a higher sex hormone binding globulin level in men with prostate cancer when compared to controls and found that prostate cancer patients had a higher testosterone conversion rate than did non-cancer patients[46].

Differences in mean androgenic activity amongst populations may explain varying risks of prostate cancer mortality. Ross and co-workers observed a higher circulating testosterone concentration in African-American men when compared to white American men[47]. African-American men have a two-fold increased prostate cancer mortality rate than

white Americans. Ross and colleagues have also found higher levels of 3α, 17β-androstenediol glucuronide and androsterone glucuronide in black and white American men when compared to Japanese men[48]. It is believed that 3α, 17β-androstenediol glucuronide and androsterone glucuronide are markers of 5α-reductase activity.

The role of dietary fat in the etiology of human prostate cancer can be linked to the concept that androgenic stimulation causes prostate cancer. Populations with higher androgen levels tend to have higher average amounts of fat in their diet[18]. Higher levels of dietary fat cause higher bioavailability and production of sexual hormones[49–51]. The precise mechanisms are not well defined, but it is known that plasma concentrations of fatty acids are responsive to dietary fat, and these levels, in turn, correlate with concentrations of bioavailable sex steroids[52]. Fatty acids inhibit binding of gonadal steroids to serum sex hormone binding globulin, causing greater bioavailability of gonadal hormones[53]. In addition, a low-fat, high-fiber diet decreases the enterohepatic circulation of gonadal hormones, resulting in increased fecal excretion of gonadal hormones and the lowering of serum levels of gonadal hormones[54].

In animal models, androgens promote cell proliferation and inhibit prostate cell death[55]. Importantly, almost all animal models of prostate carcinogenesis require exogenous androgen administration to induce prostate cancer[56,57]. Although the precise role of androgens in the etiology of human prostate cancer is unclear, the above facts taken as a whole suggest that prostate cancer requires androgenic stimulation and that it can be prevented if androgenic reduction, inhibition or blockade can be applied.

The common hormonal treatments that remove androgens or block their cellular effects have side effects that significantly limit their usefulness as chemopreventives. A key point in prostate cancer biology makes a tolerable reduction possible in androgenic stimulation of the prostate. The more potent and major androgen in the normal prostate is dihydrotestosterone and not testosterone[58,59]. The enzyme 5α-reductase is a nuclear-membrane-bound NADPH-dependent Δ3-ketosteroid 5α-oxidoreductase. Its primary function is to convert testosterone to the more potent dihydrotestosterone[59,60] (Figure 1). Dihydrotestosterone is 8–10 times more potent an androgen than testosterone[58,59]. In essence the function of 5α-reduction is to amplify the androgenic effect of testosterone. 5α-Reductase can now be blocked with minimal toxicity.

In humans, dihydrotestosterone promotes development of prostate cells and benign prostatic hyperplasia (BPH), and possibly serves as a promoter for prostate cancer. An observation of nature documents the key role that 5α-reductase and dihydrotestosterone play in prostate development and prostate cancer[61,62]. Males with inherited homozygous 5α-reductase deficiency are pseudohermaphrodites with female or ambiguous external genitalia until puberty. The normal increase in testosterone production at puberty induces development of a small phallus and virilization. After puberty, individuals with the enzyme deficiency usually become morphologically and functionally normal males, although they never develop acne or male-pattern baldness. Men deficient in 5α-reductase have underdeveloped prostates and do not develop

prostate cancer, even though they maintain normal serum testosterone levels after puberty. No other illnesses are associated with 5α-reductase deficiency, and females with the inherited enzyme deficiency have no known medical sequelae[61,63].

There are two 5α-reductase isoenzymes. 5α-Reductase-1 is present at very low levels in a number of tissues and 5α-reductase-2 is found in high amounts in androgen-sensitive cells of the skin, liver and prostate[63]. The testes and adrenal glands secrete testosterone into the bloodstream. In the normal prostate, a substantial portion of testosterone diffusing into 5α-reductase-containing cells is irreversibly converted to dihydrotestosterone.

Finasteride (Proscar®) was approved by the United States Food and Drug Administration in 1992 for the treatment of benign prostatic hyperplasia[64]. Preclinical and clinical studies have demonstrated that 7 days of finasteride 5 mg daily causes a 70% decrease in serum levels of dihydrotestosterone, with an 8–10% increase in serum testosterone. This dosing causes intraprostatic dihydrotestosterone levels to decrease by more than 90%. Intraprostatic testosterone levels do increase by a small factor. Finasteride therapy causes an estimated overall decrease in androgenic stimulation of the prostate of more than 75%[59,60].

5α-Reductase inhibition and prostate cancer

A cancer preventive manipulation need not have antitumor activity in order to be effective. Several studies using prostate tumor in tissue culture or rodent implant models have shown that 5α-reductase inhibition inhibits and prevents the progression of some prostate cancers[65–67]. PC-82 is a moderately differentiated human prostatic adenocarcinoma cell line. Its growth in mice is inhibited when 5α-reductase inhibitors are administered. Enzyme inhibitors also suppress growth of implanted hormone-sensitive Dunning R-3327G rat prostate tumor[68–70].

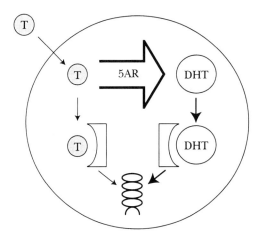

Figure 1 5α-Reductase (5AR) in the prostate cell. T, testosterone; DHT, dihydrotestosterone

Most available rodent carcinogenesis models are not ideally suited for testing the 5α–reductase cancer prevention hypothesis. These models involve pulse doses of a chemical carcinogen followed by chronic administration of androgens[51,57]. The exogenous androgen can override the effect of finasteride. Indeed, the fact that androgen administration is necessary to promote prostate cancer development in laboratory animals is in itself supportive of the theory that decreasing androgenic stimulation can lower prostate cancer risk. Recently Tsukamoto and colleagues demonstrated that finasteride therapy can decrease prostate cancer prevalence in an F344 rat model[71]. In this study rats were administered an initiator and chronic low-dose testosterone propionate. Rats administered finasteride or the androgen receptor blocker Casodex® had a lower prevalence of prostate cancer development when compared to controls[71].

In human trials, finasteride induces a small decline in prostate specific antigen (PSA) in men with widely metastatic disease. The clinical significance of this decline is probably minimal, but it does indicate some anticancer activity[72]. Andriole and colleagues[73] evaluated the long-term effect of finasteride vs. placebo on serum PSA levels of men with measurable serum PSA after prostatectomy. Over a period of 1 year, those men treated with finasteride experienced a delayed increase in PSA when compared to those given a placebo. Importantly, among those with recurrence, there was no affect on initial response to subsequent hormonal therapies[73].

An effective cancer chemopreventive agent must be administered in a tolerable fashion with minimal if any side effects. Benefits beyond cancer prevention are desirable in any chemoprevention effort. Finasteride has few side effects[64,74,75]. It is widely used throughout the world; indeed nearly a million men in the age group at risk from prostate cancer take the drug daily to treat benign prostatic hyperplasia. It is conceivable that it might be more effective in the prevention of BPH.

The Prostate Cancer Prevention Trial

In 1991 the Division of Cancer Prevention and Control of the National Cancer Institute convened a multidisciplinary group of scientists to assess the possibility of a prostate cancer prevention study. The trial was developed over the next 2 years and began accruing subjects in the autumn of 1993. The hypothesis of the trial is that a prolonged finasteride-induced decrease in androgenic stimulation of the prostate will inhibit or retard the progression of prostate cells through the carcinogenic process, resulting in a decreased period prevalence of diagnosed prostate cancer.

This is a randomized placebo-controlled trial involving 18 000 men, aged 55 or above, and in good health[5,6] (Figure 2). Each subject will be treated for 7 years. The actual trial will span approximately 10 years, with all participants followed for life. Prostatic digital rectal examination must not be suggestive of malignancy. Subjects can have an enlarged prostate, but should not have symptoms of prostatism so

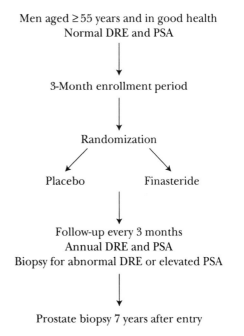

Men aged ≥ 55 years and in good health
Normal DRE and PSA

3-Month enrollment period

Randomization

Placebo   Finasteride

Follow-up every 3 months
Annual DRE and PSA
Biopsy for abnormal DRE or elevated PSA

Prostate biopsy 7 years after entry

Figure 2 Protocol for the Prostate Cancer Prevention Trial. DRE, digital rectal examination of the prostate; PSA, prostate specific antigen

severe that a transurethral resection of the prostate (TURP) is thought to be necessary in the near future. The PSA level must be < 3.0 ng/ml (by Hybritech, normal is usually considered to be < 4.0 ng/ml). This is an attempt to be as sure as possible that men entering the trial do not have prostate cancer.

Subjects undergo digital rectal examination and serum PSA measurement on an annual basis. Because finasteride decreases serum PSA level and there are concerns about inter-assay PSA variability, all PSA values are analyzed at a central laboratory and corrected numerical values are reported to the patients and physicians. An algorithm has been worked out to minimize the risk of a detection bias (to assure that both arms of the study have an equal number of blind sextant prostatic biopsies to evaluate malignancy due to PSA abnormality)[76]. Further to assure as little bias as possible, all subjects are asked to undergo transrectal ultrasound examination and prostate biopsy after 7 years on the study. The trial design has a 90% power to detect a 25% reduction in prostate cancer period prevalence.

This trial allows for more than just assessment of finasteride in the prevention of cancer. It allows for the prevention of BPH and prevention of the need for TURP. This study will yield information on prostate cancer screening, particularly the use of the measurement of changing PSA level over time in men in the finasteride and the placebo groups. There is some evidence that 5α-reductase inhibition may increase the specificity of PSA screening for prostate cancer[77,78]. Annual serum samples are being preserved, so that promising future tests may be evaluated. The trial is also an opportunity to obtain tissue and history, enhancing the opportunity to understand benign and malignant prostate pathologies.

References

1. Woolf, S. H. (1995). Screening for prostate cancer with prostate-specific antigen. *N. Engl. J. Med.*, **333**, 1401–5
2. Sporn, M. B., Dunlop, N. M. and Newton, D. L. (1976). Prevention of chemical carcinogenesis by vitamin A and its synthetic analogs (retinoids). *Fed. Proc.*, **35**, 1332–8
3. Lippman, S. M., Benner, S. E. and Ki Hong, W. (1994). Cancer chemoprevention. *J. Clin. Oncol.*, **12**, 851–73
4. Feigl, P., Blumenstein, B., Thompson, I. M., Crowley, J., Wolf, M., Kramer, B S. *et al.* (1995). Design of the Prostate Cancer Prevention Trial (PCPT). *Controlled Clin. Trials*, **16**, 150–63
5. Brawley, O. W., Ford, L. G., Thompson, I. M., Perlman, J. A. and Kramer, B. S. (1994). 5-Alpha-reductase inhibition and prostate cancer prevention. *Cancer Epidemiol. Biomarkers Prev.*, **3**, 177–82
6. Thompson, I. M., Feigl, P. and Coltman, C. (1995). Chemoprevention of prostate cancer with finasteride. In DeVita, V., Hellman, S. and Rosenberg, S. (eds.) *Important Advances in Oncology*, pp. 57–76. (Philadelphia: J. B. Lippincott)
7. Sporn, M. B. (1991). Carcinogenesis and cancer: different perspectives on the same disease. *Cancer Res.*, **51**, 6215–18
8. Pienta, K. J. and Esper, P. S. (1993). Current concepts regarding the epidemiology of prostate cancer. *Ann. Int. Med.*, **118**, 793–803
9. Meikle, A. W. and Smith, J. A. (1996). Epidemiology of prostate cancer. *Urol. Clin. North Am.*, **17**, 709–18
10. Shimizu, H., Ross, R. K., Bernstein, L., Yatani, R., Henderson, B. E. and Mack, T. M. (1991). Cancers of the prostate and breast among Japanese and white immigrants in Los Angeles County. *Br. J. Cancer*, **63**, 963–6
11. Muir, C. S., Nectoux, J. and Staszewski, J. (1991). The epidemiology of prostate cancer. Geographical distribution and time-trends. *Acta Oncol.*, **30**, 133–40
12. Flanders, W. D. (1984). Review: prostate cancer epidemiology. *Prostate*, **5**, 621–9
13. Sakr, W. A., Hass, G. P., Cassin, B. F., Pontes, J. E. and Crissman, J. D. (1993). The frequency of carcinoma and intraepithelial neoplasia of the prostate in young male patients. *J. Urol.*, **150**, 379–85

14. Dunn, J. E. (1975). Cancer epidemiology in populations of the United States. *Cancer Res.*, **35**, 3240–5

15. Haenszel, W. and Kurihoro, M. (1969). Studies of Japanese migrants. *J. Natl. Cancer Inst.*, **40**, 43–68

16. Yu, H., Harris, R. E., Gao, R. and Wynder, E. L. (1991). Comparative epidemiology of cancers of the colon, rectum, prostate and breast in Shanghai, China versus the United States. *Int. J. Epidemiol.*, **20**, 76–81

17. Muir, C. S., Nectoux, J. and Staszewski, J. (1991). The epidemiology of prostate cancer. Geographical distribution and timetrends. *Acta Oncol.*, **30**, 133–40

18. Pienta, K. J. and Esper, P. S. (1993). Is dietary fat a risk factor for prostate cancer? *J. Natl. Cancer Inst.*, **85**, 1538–41

19. Kolonel, L. N., Nomura, A. M. Y., Hinds, M. W., Hirohata, T., Hankin, J. H. and Lee, J. (1983). Role of diet in cancer incidence in Hawaii. *Cancer Res.* (Suppl.), **43**, 2397–402

20. Lew, E. A. and Garfinkel, L. (1979). Variations in mortality by weight among 750,000 men and women. *J. Chronic Dis.*, **32**, 563–76

21. Severson, R. K., Grove, J. S., Nomura, A. M. and Stemmerman, G. N. (1988). Body mass and prostatic cancer: a prospective study. *Br. Med. J.*, **297**, 713–15

22. Kaul, L., Heshmat, M. Y., Kovi, J., Jackson, M. A., Jackson, A. G. and Jones, G. W. (1987). The role of diet in prostate cancer. *Nutr. Cancer*, **9**, 123–8

23. Severson, R. K., Nomura, A. M. Y., Grove, J. S. and Stemmerman, G. N. (1989). A prospective study of demographics, diet, and prostate cancer among men of Japanese ancestry in Hawaii. *Cancer Res.*, **49**, 1857–60

24. Berg, J. W. (1975). Can nutrition explain the pattern of international epidemiology of hormone-dependent cancers? *Cancer Res.*, **35**, 3345–50

25. Armstrong, B. and Doll, R. (1975). Environmental factors and cancer incidence and mortality in different countries with special reference to dietary practices. *Int. J. Cancer*, **15**, 617–31

26. Rose, D. P. Boyar, A. P. and Wynder, E. L. (1986). International comparisons of mortality rates for cancer of the breast, ovary, prostate, and colon, and per capita food consumption. *Cancer*, **58**, 2363–71

27. Rotkin, I. D. (1977). Studies in the epidemiology of prostatic cancer: expanded sampling. *Cancer Treat. Rep.*, **61**, 173–80

28. Hutchinson, G. B. (1976). Epidemiology of prostatic cancer. *Semin. Oncol.*, **3**, 151–9

29. Slattery, M. L., Schumacher, M. C., West, D. W., Robinson, L. M., French, T. K. (1990). Food consumption trends between adolescent and adult years and subsequent risk of prostate cancer. *Am. J. Clin. Nutr.*, **52**, 752–7

30. Snowdon, D. A., Phillips, R. L and Choi, W. (1984). Diet, obesity, and risk of fatal prostate cancer. *Am. J. Epidemiol.*, **120**, 244–50

31. Mettlin, C., Selenskas, S., Natarajan, N. and Huben, R. (1989). Beta-carotene and animal fats and their relationship to prostate cancer risk. A case control study. *Cancer*, **64**, 605–12

32. Mills, P. K., Beeson, W. L., Phillips, R. L. and Fraser, G. E. (1989). Cohort study of diet, life-style, and prostate cancer in Adventist men. *Cancer*, **64**, 598–604

33. Hirayama, T. (1979). Epidemiology of prostate cancer with special reference to the role of diet. *Natl. Cancer Inst. Monogr.*, **53**, 149–155

34. Heshma, M. Y., Kaul, L., Kovi, J., Jackson, M. A., Jackson, A. G. and Jones, G. W. (1985). Nutrition and prostate cancer: a case–control study. *Prostate*, **6**, 7–17

35. Ohno, Y., Yoshida, O., Oishi, K., Yamabe, H. and Schröeder, F. (1988). Dietary beta-carotene and cancer of the prostate: a case–control study in Kyoto, Japan. *Cancer Res.*, **48**, 1331–6

36. Wynder, E. R., Mabuchi, K. and Whitmore, W. (1971). Epidemiology of cancer of the prostate. *Cancer*, **28**, 344–68

37. Hovenian, M. S. and Deming, C. L. (1948). The heterologous growth of cancer of the human prostate. *Surg. Gynecol. Obset.*, **86**, 29–35

38. Huggins, C. and Hodges, C. V. (1941). Studies on prostate cancer I: The effect of castration of estrogen and of androgen injection on serum phosphatases in metastatic carinoma of the prostate. *Cancer Res.*, **1**, 293–7

39. Ross, R. K. (1990). The hormonal basis of prostate cancer. *Proc. Annu. Meet. Am. Assoc. Cancer Res.*, **31**, 457–8

40. Montie, J. E. and Pienta, K. J. (1994). Review of the role of androgenic hormones in the epidemiology of benign prostatic hyperplasia and prostate cancer. *Urology*, **43**, 892–9

41. Meikle, W. and Stanish, W. M. (1982). Familial prostatic cancer risk and low testosterone. *J. Clin. Endocrinol. Metab.*, **54**, 1104–8

42. Ghanadian, R., Puah, K. M. and O'Donohue, E. P. M. (1979). Serum testosterone and dihydrotestosterone and dihydrotestosterone in carcinoma of the prostate. *Br. J. Cancer*, **39**, 696–9

43. Hammond, G. L., Kontturi, M. and Vihko, R. (1978). Serum steroids in normal males and patients with prostatic diseases. *Clin. Endocr.*, **9**, 113–21

44. Comstock, G. W., Gordon, G. B. and Hsing, A. W. (1993). The relationship of serum dehy-

droepiandrosterone and its sulfate to subsequent cancer of the prostate. *Cancer Epidemiol. Biomarkers Prev.*, **2**, 219–21

45. Barrett-Connor, E., Garland, C., McPhillips, J. B., Khaw, K. T. and Wingard, D. L. (1990). A prospective, population-based study of androstenedione, estrogens, and prostatic cancer. *Cancer Res.*, **50**, 169–73

46. Meikle, A. W., Smith, J. A. and Stringham, J. D. (1987). Production, clearance, and metabolism of testosterone in men with prostatic cancer. *Prostate*, **10**, 25–31

47. Ross, R. K., Berstein, L., Judd, H., Hanisch, R., Pike, M. and Henderson, B. (1986). Serum testosterone levels in healthy young black and white men. *J. Natl. Cancer Inst.*, **76**, 45–8

48. Ross, R. K., Berstein, L., Lobo, R. A., Shimizu, H., Stanczyk, F. Z. and Pike, M. (1992). 5-alpha-reductase activity and risk of prostate cancer among Japanese and US white and black males. *Lancet*, **339**, 887–9

49. Hamalainen, E., Adlercreutz, H. and Puska, P. (1984). Diet and serum hormones in healthy men. *J. Steroid Biochem.*, **20**, 459–64

50. Coffey, D. S. (1979). Physiological control of prostatic growth. In *Prostate Cancer, an Overview*, UICC workshop on prostatic cancer, 1978, vol. 48, pp. 4–23. (Geneva: International Union Against Cancer)

51. Noble, R. L. (1959). The development of prostatic adenocarcinoma in Nb rats following prolonged sex hormone administration. *Cancer Res.*, **19**, 1125–39

52. Bruning, P. F. and Bonfrer, J. M. G. (1989). Free fatty acid concentrations correlated with the available fraction of estradiol in human plasma. *Cancer Res.*, **46**, 2606–9

53. Street, C., Howell, R. J. S. and Perry, L. (1989). Inhibition of binding of gonadal steriods to serum binding proteins by non-esterified fatty acids: the influence of chain length and degree of unsaturation. *Acta Endocrinol.*, **120**, 175–9

54. Pusater, D. J., Roth, W. T., Ross, J. K. and Shultz, T. D. (1990). Dietary and hormonal evaluation of men at different risks for prostate cancer: plasma and fecal hormone–nutrient interrelationships. *Am. J. Clin. Nutr.*, **51**, 371–7

55. Kyprianou, N. and Isaacs, J. T. (1988). Activation of programmed cell death in the rat ventral prostate after castration. *Endocrinology*, **122**, 552–62

56. Nobel, R. L. (1977). The development of prostatic adenocarcinoma in NB rats following prolonged sex hormone adminsistration. *Cancer Res.*, **37**, 1929

57. Shirai, T., Tamano, S., Kato, T., Iwasaki, S., Takahashi, S. and Ito, N. (1991). Induction of invasive carcinomas in the accessory sex organs other than the ventral prostate of rats given 3,2′-dimethyl-4-aminobiphenyl and testosterone propionate. *Cancer Res.*, **51**, 1264–9

58. Grino, P., Griffin, J. and Wilson, J. (1990). Testosterone at high concentrations interacts with the human adrogen receptor similarly to dihydrotestosterone. *Endocrinology*, **126**, 1165–72

59. Geller, J. (1990). Effect of finasteride, a 5 alpha-reductase inhibitor on prostate tissue androgens, and prostate specific antigen. *J. Clin. Endocrinol, Metab.*, **71**, 1552–5

60. McConnell, J. D., Wilson, J., George, F. W., Geller, J., Pappas, F. and Stoner, E. (1992). Finasteride, an inhibitor of 5 alpha-reductase suppresses prostatic dihydrotestosterone in men with benign prostatic hyperplasia. *J. Clin. Endrocrinol. Metab.*, **74**, 505–8

61. Petersen, R. E., Imperato-McGinley, J., Gautier, T. and Sturla, E. (1977). Male pseudohermaphroditism due to steriod 5 alpha reductase deficiency. *Am. J. Med.*, **62**, 170–91

62. Imperato-McGinley, J., Guerrero, L., Gautier, T. and Petersen, R. E. (1974). Steriod 5 alpha-reductase deficiency in man: an inherited form of male pseudohermaphroditism. *Science*, **186**, 1213–15

63. Anderson, S., Berman, D. M., Jenkins, E. P. and Russell, D. W. (1991). Deletion of steriod 5 alpha-reductase-2 gene in male pseudohermaproditism. *Nature (London)*, **354**, 159

64. Gormley, G., Stoner, E., Bruskewitz, R., Imperato-McGinley, J., Walsh, P. C., McConnell, J. D. *et al.* (1992). The effect of finasteride in men with benign prostatic hyperplasia. *N. Engl. J. Med.*, **327**, 1185–91

65. Kadoham, N., Karr, J. P., Murphy, G. P. and Sandberg, A. A. (1984). Selective inhibition of prostatic tumor 5 alpha-reductase by a 4-methyl-4-aza steriod. *Cancer Res.*, **44**, 4947–54

66. Petrow, V., Padilla, G. M., Mukherji, S. and Marts, S. A. (1984). Endocrine dependence of prostatic cancer upon dihydrotestosterone and not upon testosterone. *J. Pharm. Pharmacol.*, **36**, 352–3

67. Bologna, M., Muzi, P., Biordi, L. and Pestuccia, C. V. (1992). Antiandrogens and 5 alpha-reductase inhibition of the proliferation rate in PC3 and DU145 human prostatic cancer cell lines. *Curr. Ther. Res.*, **5**, 799–813

68. Damber, J. E., Bergh, A., Daehlin, L., Petrov, V. and Landstrom, M. (1992). Effect of 6-methylene progesterone on growth, morphology, and blood flow of the Dunning R3327 prostatic adenocarcinoma. *Prostate*, **20**, 187–90

69. Lamb, J. C., English, H., Levandoski, P. L., Rhodes, G. R., Johnson, R. K. and Isaccs, J. R. (1992). Prostatic involution in rats induced by novel 5 alpha-reductase inhibitor, SK and F 105657: role for testosterone in the androgenic response. *Endocrinology*, **130**, 685–94

70. Brooks, J. R., Berman, C. and Nguyen, H. (1991). Effect of castration, DES, flutamide, and the 5-alpha-reductase inhibitor, MK-906, on the growth of the Dunning rat prostatic carcinoma, R3327. *Prostate*, **18**, 215–27

71. Tsukamoto, S., Adaza, H., Imada, S., Koiso, K., Tomoyuki, S., Ideyama, Y. *et al.* (1995). Chemoprevention of rat prostate carcinogenesis by use of finasteride or casodex. *J. Natl. Cancer Inst.*, **87**, 842–3

72. Presti, J. C., Fair, W. R., Andriole, G., Sogani, P. C., Seidman, F. D., Ng, J. *et al.* (1992). Multicenter, randomized, double-blind, placebo controlled study to investigate the effect of finasteride (MK-906) on stage D prostate cancer. *J. Urol.*, **148**, 1201–4

73. Andriole, G., Lieber, M. D., Smith, J. A., Soloway, M., Schroeder, F., Kadmon, D. *et al.* (1995). Treatment with finasteride following radical prostatectomy for prostate cancer. *Urology*, **45**, 491–7

74. Stoner, E. and The Finasteride Study Group (1994). Three year safety and efficacy data on the use of finasteride in the treatment of benign prostatic hyperplasia. *Urology*, **43**, 284–94

75. Rittmaster, R. (1994). Finasteride. *N. Engl. J. Med.*, **330**, 120–5

76. Thompson, I. M., Coltman, C., Brawley, O. W. and Ryan, A. (1995). Chemoprevention of prostate cancer. *Semin. Urol.*, **13**, 122–9

77. Guess, H. A.. Heyse, J. F. and Gormley, G. (1993). The effect of finasteride on prostate-specific antigen in men with benign prostatic hyperplasia. *Prostate*, **22**, 31–7

78. Stoner, E., Round, E., Ferguson, D., Gormley, G. and The Finasteride Study Group (1994). Clinical experience of the detection of prostate cancer in patients with BPH treated with finasteride. *J. Urol.*, **151**, 1296–300

Interactive Voting System

1 Do you believe androgenic stimulation is important to prostate carcinogenesis?

Response	Option
87%	Yes.
13%	No.

Number of votes: 54

2 If a drug reduces prostate cancer and the need for transurethral resection of the prostate by 20%, would you use it?

63%	Yes.
37%	No.

Number of votes: 87

Western diet and prostate cancer: does the available evidence justify dietary advice?

M. S. Morton, N. Blacklock, L. Denis and K. Griffiths

7

Introduction

The large differences in the incidence of certain types of cancer between different populations direct attention to the possible influence of dietary factors on the biological processes concerned with carcinogenesis. Estimates of the number of cancers attributable to dietary habit have varied in studies[1,2], but tend to be around 30–35%, although the evidence is not precise, and Doll and Peto[3] suggest a range of 10–70%. In a recent comprehensive review of diet in relation to cancer etiology, Miller and colleagues[4] considered that appropriate dietary changes could decrease the incidence of certain cancers by up to 68%. They suggested that such decreases were largely attainable by reducing fat intake and increasing fruit and vegetable consumption. Such a concept is controversial[5,6], with much of the controversy bearing on the relationship between dietary fat intake and cancer risk[5,7].

Cancer of the prostate belongs to a group of diseases that are referred to as 'Western diseases', which would also include breast and colorectal cancer, cardiovascular disease and osteoporosis – so-called because of their prevalence in affluent Western countries and regions of Europe and North America, compared with Asian countries. 'Western diseases' have previously been associated with dietary fat as a causative factor, and only recently has it been recognized that there may be constituents of the more-vegetarian Asian diet that protect against the development of these diseases, and it is a lack of such constituents in the Western diet, rather than the high fat content, which may be the important factor.

The concept is therefore that certain components in the Asian diet, and possibly also in that of the Mediterranean area, are protective against the development of those diseases that are so prevalent in the more affluent Western countries. This chapter explores the relationship between diet and cancer of the prostate and cites specific components of Asian and vegetarian diets that appear to have a restraining influence on cancer development.

Geographical differences in prostate cancer incidence

Prostate cancer is now one of the most commonly diagnosed cancers in the West[8–10]. World-wide, the incidence is rising annually by approximately 2–3%[11,12]. In North American men prostate cancer is now the second most commonly diagnosed cancer after skin cancer, and the second most common cause of death from cancer after that of the lung. An estimated 200 000 new cases were diagnosed in the United States in 1995, and 40 000 died from the disease that year[13].

Epidemiological studies have demonstrated considerable geographical variation in the age-adjusted incidence of cancer of the prostate[14,15]. However, autopsy studies reveal that the incidence of latent carcinoma of the prostate, microscopic foci of cancer cells, is the same in men of all races, from both East and West[16]. The incidence of the clinically malignant disease is highest in the black North American male[11,17], some 30-fold greater than in Japanese men[11], and 120 times greater than seen in

Chinese men in Shanghai[9,18-20]. The incidence rate for cancer of the prostate in Japan is now rising[9,21], and for Japanese migrants to North America the mortality rate increases to half that of the indigenous population within one or two generations[22,23]. The epidemiological phenomena observed in migrating populations appear sufficiently quickly to suggest that dietary and environmental factors, rather than genetic factors, are responsible.

Benign prostatic hyperplasia (BPH) is also reported to be more common in elderly men from Western countries than in their counterparts from the East[24]. The prevalence of microscopic BPH, an early clinical event in the development of the disease, is, however, the same in men of all races[25].

Prostate cancer and BPH are clinically manifest in men over the age of 50. With the prevalence of both diseases later in life, the increasing life-expectancy, world-wide, suggests that BPH and cancer of the prostate will become serious health-care problems. This further highlights the importance of current research into disease prevention.

Diet and cancer

General considerations

The Western diet is high in animal fat and protein and refined carbohydrate and low in fiber-rich foodstuffs. In contrast, the low-fat diet of the less developed Asian communities is rich in starches, legumes, fruit and vegetables – many of which have a high fiber content[15,26,27].

In general the Western diet is deficient in fiber, which is considered to be protective against colorectal cancer. Burkitt[28,29] noted a low incidence of colorectal cancer in East Africa, where a high fiber diet is consumed. Animal and experimental studies support the concept that high dietary fiber protects, not only against colorectal cancer[30], but also against other cancers such as mammary cancer[31].

Vegetables are a source of fiber, but their protective role[32,33] may also be attributable to other constituents. Evidence[34,35] suggests that certain non-nutrient components of plant products, vegetables and fruits play a preventive role in various carcinogenic processes particularly relating to endocrine cancers such as of the breast and prostate, and also colorectal cancer[32,33,36].

Dietary fat and prostate cancer

Several studies have established a positive correlation between prostatic cancer occurrence and mortality and *per capita* fat consumption[37]. In addition, strong correlations are reported between prostate cancer mortality rates and those of other cancers, such as those of the breast and ovary, suspected of being associated with fat intake[38].

In The United States Health Professionals Follow-up Study, total fat consumption was directly, though not significantly, related to the risk of advanced prostatic cancer. The association was mainly related to animal fat and was not found with vegetable fat. Red meat consumption had the strongest association with prostate cancer risk[39]. Positive correlations have been reported for animal fat in other studies[40,41]. However, other investigations in Hawaii failed to find this relationship[42-44], and dietary fat had no influence on the incidence of prostate cancer in animal model systems[45,46].

Most epidemiological studies do, however, support the hypothesis that prostate cancer risk is increased by high levels of dietary fat[38], and of 13 case-controlled studies, ten have shown positive evidence. Overall, there is evidence that the risk of prostate cancer is increased by a diet high in calories, animal fat and meat. Unfortunately, a few of these studies failed to adjust for total caloric intake and also made little or no reference to fruits, vegetables and cereals, rich sources of both dietary fiber and other non-nutrient components that are present in the typical Asian diet[26].

Vitamins and prostate cancer

A recent study suggests that the risk of prostate cancer is increased by vitamin A[38]. Among

23 000 Finnish smokers entered into a randomized study comparing intake of β-carotene vs. placebo, a higher rate of prostate cancer was observed in the β-carotene group (16.3 per 10 000) compared to the placebo group (13.2 per 10 000). A similar positive association was demonstrated only in men aged 70 years or more[47], and others report that vitamin A intake, as retinol or β-carotene, is either unrelated to prostate cancer risk[48–50] or protective[51].

A protective effect for vitamin D has recently been reported following the measurement of 1,25-dihydroxyvitamin D_3 in the serum of men in California[52]. In this case-controlled study, the mean serum levels of this vitamin were 1.81 pg/ml lower in cases than in controls. Although this was statistically significant, the long-term storage of the samples must cast some doubt on the overall significance of this finding. Studies *in vitro* have shown antiproliferative effects of 1,25-dihydroxyvitamin D_3 on primary cultures of human prostatic cells[53].

A marked negative association between risk of prostate cancer and intake of vitamin E has also been demonstrated. Among men randomized to α-tocopherol (50 mg daily) there were 99 cases of prostate cancer (11.7 per 10 000) compared to 151 (17.8 per 10 000) cases in men receiving the placebo[54].

Vegetables, fruit and cereals and prostate cancer

The long-term studies of 265 118 adults by Hirayama in Japan[55–57] demonstrated that daily consumption of green–yellow vegetables was an important protective factor against cancers of the stomach and prostate, as well as other 'Western diseases'. Green–yellow vegetables were defined as containing more than 600 μg of carotene/100 g, and included pumpkin, carrots, spinach, green lettuce and green asparagus. The standardized mortality rate for cancer of the breast was also reported to be lower when there was an increase in the consumption of soya bean paste soup and soya milk. Hirayama[55] speculated that β-carotene and possibly other components of soya beans and vegetables were implicated in the reduction of mortality.

A case–control study on the effects of diet on breast cancer risk in Singapore[58] indicated that red meat intake was a predisposing factor. However, soya protein, β-carotene and polyunsaturated fatty acids were reported to be protective components of the diet.

Both the investigations in Japan[55] and Singapore[58] suggested a protective influence of soya bean products as well as β-carotene on breast cancer risk and drew attention to components of certain vegetables, present in the traditional Asian diet, that may also influence carcinogenesis. A study of Japanese men in Hawaii reported that increased consumption of both rice and tofu were associated with a decreased risk of prostate cancer[42]. Tofu and other soya-based foods are rich sources of isoflavonoid phytoestrogens[59]. Several investigators have also demonstrated significant, strong negative correlations between mortality from prostate cancer and dietary intake of cereals[60,61]. Cereals contain precursors of the mammalian lignans, another group of dietary phytoestrogens[59]. Furthermore, a cohort study of diet, life-style and prostate cancer in Seventh-Day Adventist men revealed that increasing consumption of beans, lentils, peas, tomatoes, raisins, dates and other dried foods were all associated with significantly decreased prostate cancer risk[40]. The Mediterranean-style diet is considered to be protective against the endocrine cancers[62,63] and features a low animal fat and meat content, with a high intake of fresh fruit, vegetables and pasta. Fresh fruit, citrus fruits and raw vegetables were found to be protective against many cancers, including that of the prostate, in several Italian studies[64–66]. Many fresh fruits and vegetables also contain high concentrations of flavonoids, some of which also have estrogenic properties[67].

Estrogenic substances in plants

The presence in plants of non-steroidal substances with estrogenic activity has been recognized for some time. Many hundreds of plants manifest some degree of estrogenic activity[68,69].

Soya bean and red clover are members of the Leguminosae family and are a major source of isoflavonoids[69–71]. Soya is consumed daily in large amounts in a number of forms in China and Japan and in Asia generally. Many foods of plant origin contain varying amounts of isoflavonoids, flavonoids and lignans. Some of these polyphenolic phytoestrogens possess weak estrogenic activity and therefore the potential for exerting an influence on hormone-dependent cancers such as those of the breast and prostate[59].

Soya beans contain the glycoside conjugates of the isoflavonoids genistein and daidzein, which can be metabolized by gut bacteria to the aglycones, genistein and daidzein (Figure 1). Genistein can be further metabolized to the non-estrogenic *p*-ethylphenol and daidzein is converted to the estrogenic isoflavan, equol (Figure 1). The aglycones and their metabolites are then absorbed and appear in blood and urine, primarily as glucuronide conjugates, and also sulfates[59]. Daidzein and genistein were isolated from soya beans more than 60 years ago[72]; 100 g fat-free soya beans may yield up to 300 mg genistein[73]. Generally the presence of isoflavonoids in plants is limited to legumes, although they have recently been identified in beer and bourbon[74,75] and may be more widely distributed than was previously thought.

Lignans are another group of polyphenolic plant compounds[69,76]. The plant precursors, matairesinol and secoisolariciresinol, are metabolized after ingestion by intestinal microflora to give rise to the weakly estrogenic enterolactone and enterodiol (Figure 2), respectively. The lignans are absorbed from the gut to appear in blood and other body fluids[59]. The lignans are widely distributed in nature and precursors are found in many cereals, grains, fruits and vegetables, but the richest source is linseed (flaxseed) and other oilseeds such as sesame[77].

The flavonoids are closely related in structure to the isoflavonoids, the former having a 2-phenylchroman nucleus and the latter a 3-phenylchroman nucleus[67]. Recently several commonly occurring plant flavonoids have been shown to possess weak estrogenic activity[67].

Unlike isoflavonoids, the flavonoids are ubiquitous in nature, and are found in high concentration in many fruits, vegetables and crop species. In particular, apigenin and kaempferol (Figure 3), both of which are estrogenic, are regarded as two of the major flavonoids, because of their common occurrence among plants, and their significant concentrations when they are present. Apigenin, for example, is found in the leaves, seeds and fruits of flowering plants, with up to 7% of dry weight in leafy vegetables. Tea-leaves are an excellent source of apigenin[67].

Isoflavonoids and lignans are normal constituents of body fluids and have been identified in most animal[59] and human body fluids by gas chromatography–mass spectrometry. They are present in urine[78,79], plasma[80], saliva[81] and semen[82]. Analysis of expressed prostatic fluid found that enterolactone and equol were

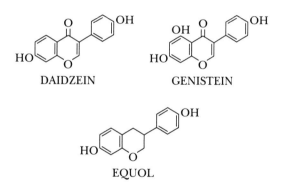

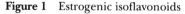

Figure 1 Estrogenic isoflavonoids

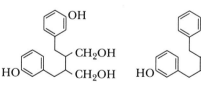

Figure 2 Estrogenic lignans

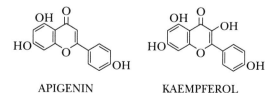

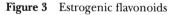

Figure 3 Estrogenic flavonoids

64

constituents[81], suggesting that dietary estrogens can accumulate in the prostate.

The levels of isoflavonoids are high in the urine and plasma of the Japanese and Chinese[83,84], whose traditional foodstuffs contain large amounts of soya in the form of bean curd (tofu), soya bean milk, miso and tempeh. The concentration of lignans is high in the urine of vegetarians[79], whose diet contains whole-grain cereals, vegetables and fruits. In Western subjects fed 40 g soya daily, the urinary excretion of equol was found to increase 1000-fold above control levels[71,85]. The concentrations of flavonoids in plasma and urine of different populations have yet to be determined and is an obvious program for future research. However, as tea, fruit and vegetables are the principal sources of flavonoids, it is probable that Asians, with their high consumption of tea, and vegetarians have significant circulating levels of these compounds.

The data relating to the incidence of prostate cancer, already quoted, show that considerable protection is afforded to Japanese and Chinese men and also to vegetarians who have a lower incidence of prostate cancer than the general population in the West. This may be attributable to their intake of phytoestrogens.

Biological properties of isoflavonoids, flavonoids and lignans and their relevance to the prevention of prostate cancer

Estrogenic activity

The mammalian lignans enterolactone and enterodiol, the isoflavonoids daidzein, genistein, coumestrol and equol and the flavonoids apigenin, kaempferol and phloretin all possess weak estrogenic activity[67,86,87]. Some antiestrogenic properties have also been described[88]. As weak estrogens, they compete with estradiol for binding to the nuclear estrogen receptor[89] and also stimulate the synthesis of sex hormone binding globulin (SHBG) in the liver[90].

The growth, development and function of the prostate is dependent on the concentration of testosterone in plasma. Although testosterone is the most important plasma androgen, it is the concentration of the free, non-protein-bound form that is the biologically available moiety[91–94]. For the young adult male, approximately 98% of plasma testosterone is bound to SHBG and other transport proteins[95–97], 2% is free, and it is this biologically available fraction that passively diffuses into the prostate target cells. An increase in the concentration of SHBG, following ingestion of phytoestrogens, for example, reduces the free fraction of testosterone.

Vegetarian[98] and Japanese and Chinese[99] men have higher plasma levels of SHBG and lower concentrations of free testosterone[98] than Western omnivores.

Inhibition of 5α-reductase

Within the prostate, testosterone is metabolized to 5α-dihydrotestosterone (DHT) by the 5α-reductase enzyme[100] primarily located on the nuclear membrane. DHT has an approximately five-fold greater affinity than testosterone for the intracellular androgen receptor protein and is the active intracellular androgen in prostate cells[101–103].

Isoflavonoids and lignans[104] inhibit 5α-reductase and also 17β-hydroxysteroid dehydrogenase. This latter enzyme system catalyzes the reversible interconversion of 17β-hydroxy and 17-oxo steroids and may have a significant influence on the metabolism of both androgens and estrogens.

The activity of 5α-reductase was assessed in cultured genital skin fibroblast monolayers. At a concentration of 100 μmol/l, the lignan enterolactone, and the isoflavonoids equol, genistein, biochanin A and daidzein were all inhibitors of 5α-reductase. A 'cocktail' of eight compounds, 10 μmol/l each, also inhibited the 5α-reductase activity by more than 70%. In this whole-cell assay, the dietary compounds, like finasteride, are more efficient inhibitors of the 5α-reductase 2 isozyme.

Lower levels of 5α-reductase activity have been observed in young Japanese men in comparison to their Western counterparts[105]. It is likely that daily consumption of phytoestrogens results in a small but significant effect on the biological availability and metabolism of androgens such as testosterone and DHT, which may relate to the lower incidence of prostate cancer in Asians. It is also of interest that synthetic 5α-reductase inhibitors, such as finasteride, are currently employed in the treatment of BPH and are being assessed as chemopreventive agents in early prostate cancer[106].

Inhibition of the aromatase enzyme

Approximately one-third of the plasma estrogens in the human male is synthesized and secreted by the testes. The remainder is derived from the peripheral conversion of the adrenal C19-steroids, dehydroepiandrosterone (DHA) and androstenedione, by the aromatase enzyme system in adipose and muscle tissue. In a similar manner to plasma testosterone, it is the free non-protein-bound estradiol fraction that diffuses into the prostate cells.

As a man ages, declining testicular activity and increasing aromatization sustain the level of the plasma free estradiol-17β concentration relative to the falling level of free testosterone[97,107,108]. This enhanced mid-life 'estrogenic stimulus' has been considered to be responsible for the increased level of plasma SHBG at this time. This change in the estrogen/androgen balance may well be a predominant factor in the induction of stromal hyperplasia of the prostate, mediated through a synergistic action between estradiol-17β and DHT.

Adlercreutz and colleagues[109] have recently shown that enterolactone is an inhibitor of the aromatase enzyme, with an IC_{50} of 14 μmol/l. The lignan enterolactone was found to bind to, or near to, the active site of the aromatase, thereby competing with the androgen substrate of the enzyme.

In studies at the Tenovus Cancer Research Centre, inhibition of the aromatase enzyme was assessed with the use of cultured genital skin fibroblast monolayers as a model system[110]. The release of ^3H_2O following the conversion of [^3H]1β-androstenedione to estrone was monitored. At a concentration of 100 μmol/l, the lignans enterolactone and enterodiol, and the isoflavonoids biochanin A, genistein and equol, were all moderate inhibitors of aromatase. Interestingly, a 'cocktail' containing all of the eight compounds investigated, at a concentration of 10 μmol/l each, inhibited the aromatase activity in this system by 35%.

A concept might be that naturally ubiquitous weak dietary estrogens, in the Asian and Mediterranean male, influence the pathogenesis of clinical BPH by directly inhibiting the growth-promoting effect of DHT and estradiol-17β on the stromal tissue of their 'aging' prostate glands.

Inhibition of tyrosine-specific protein kinases

Tyrosine kinases are necessary for the function of several growth factor receptors, including those for epidermal growth factor, platelet-derived growth factor, insulin and insulin-like growth factors[111]. In addition, several retroviral oncogenes such as *src, abl, fps, yes, fes* and *ros,* code for tyrosine-specific protein-kinases[112]. Tyrosine phosphorylation plays an important role in cell proliferation and cell transformation and tyrosine kinase-specific inhibitors may well be used an anticancer agents[113,114]. The isoflavonoid genistein has been shown to be a specific inhibitor of tyrosine kinase activity[115]. In addition, the flavonoids apigenin and kaempferol reverse the transformed phenotypes of v-H-*ras* NIH3T3 cells, an effect mediated via inhibition of tyrosine kinase[116].

Furthermore, genistein induces apoptosis in human breast tumor cells[117], inhibits invasion of murine mammary carcinoma cells[118] and enhances adhesion of endothelial cells[119].

Inhibition of DNA topoisomerases

DNA topoisomerases are enzymes that alter the conformation of DNA and are crucial to cell division[120]. By a process involving strand cleavage, strand passage and religation, these enzymes are able to untangle supercoiled DNA.

Genistein is a potent inhibitor of these enzymes and is considered to act by stabilization of a putative 'cleavable complex' between DNA and the topoisomerase enzyme[121]. The flavonoids quercetin, fisetin and morin also inhibit DNA topoisomerases I and II, while kaempferol inhibits only DNA topoisomerase II[122]. Inhibition of the topoisomerases is now the target for the design of new anticancer drugs. In addition, genistein is cytostatic, arresting cell cycle progression in G2-M[123,124], and induces apoptosis in immature human thymocytes by inhibiting DNA topoisomerase II[121]. The flavonoid apigenin induces morphological differentiation and G2-M arrest in rat neuronal cells[125].

Inhibition of angiogenesis

Angiogenesis, or neovascularization, involves the generation of new capillaries, a process invoking the proliferation and migration of endothelial cells. Normally the process is restricted to wound healing, but it is also enhanced in association with cancer growth. Folkman and co-workers[126–128] report that new capillary blood vessels are necessary for a cancer to expand beyond 2 mm in size. Angiogenesis therefore exercises an important role in cancer progression and is essentially seen as the growth towards a focus of cancer, of capillary sprouts and columns of endothelial cells from pre-existing capillaries. The process is probably promoted by the production of growth factors by the cancer cells; fibroblast growth factor (FGF), or members of the FGF family, are recognized as potent angiogenic agents. Genistein inhibits angiogenesis and endothelial cell proliferation[129]. In wound healing, the process is regulated by a balance between angiogenic factors and restraining factors such as transforming growth factor-β (TGF-β). Restraining the process of angiogenesis could inhibit cancer progression; cortisone and heparin treatment has been reported to suppress the metastatic capacity of experimental tumors by this means[127]. Significantly, genistein may have a similar influence. These effects may relate to the inhibition of the tyrosine kinase-associated FGF receptor[115].

Antioxidant activity

Flavonoids, isoflavonoids and lignans are all polyphenolic compounds and can function as effective antioxidants and radical scavengers. Compounds such as quercetin and cyanidin have antioxidant potentials four times that of Trolox™, the vitamin E analog. Removing the *ortho*-dihydroxy substitution, as in kaempferol, for example, or reducing the 2,3 double bond in the C-ring, as in catechin or epicatechin, decreases the antioxidant activity by more than 50%, although these structures are still more effective than α-tocopherol or ascorbate[130]. In addition, flavonoids such as catechin inhibit the oxidation of low-density lipoprotein, an effect consistent with the ability of some flavonoids of similar structure to inhibit lipoxygenases[131].

Inhibition of tumorigenesis

Soya-bean isoflavones and lignans inhibit experimental carcinogenesis in a wide variety of systems. Of 26 animal studies in which diets containing soya or soya bean isoflavones were employed, 17 (65%) reported protective effects[132]. No studies reported that soya intake increased tumor development. Most of the studies reporting no inhibition of tumorigenesis employed soya protein isolate (SPI), the preparation of which includes treatment with strong alkali and is responsible for a 4–6-fold reduction in isoflavone concentration[73].

Many *in vitro* tumor model systems are also growth-inhibited by isoflavonoids and lignans, including those for both breast and prostate cancers[133,134]. Genistein and biochanin A, the precursor of genistein, inhibit, in culture, the growth of androgen-dependent and androgen-independent prostatic cancer cells[134].

In addition, isoflavonoids and flavonoids inhibit the bioactivation of potent chemical carcinogens. Biochanin A inhibits the metabolic activation of benzo[a]pyrene[135] and the flavonoid catechins from green and black tea inhibit the activation of the potent tobacco carcinogen 4-(methylnitrosoamino)-1-(3-pyridyl)-

1-butanone (NNK) and subsequent lung tumorigenesis in A/J mice[136].

Phytoestrogens and chemoprevention

This presentation advances the concept that certain dietary factors are responsible for the differences in prostatic cancer incidence and mortality between East and West. The large amounts of isoflavonoids, flavonoids and lignans in the Asian diet and their specific properties may restrain the processes of carcinogenesis and suppress the development of cancer of the prostate.

The first strategy of prevention would be health education, specifically directed to the occurrence, morbidity and mortality associated with prostatic cancer and the vulnerability of Western people consuming a Western diet. Dietary advice on the lines of lesser dependence on animal protein and fat and a greater consumption of vegetables, especially legumes, fruit and cereals, would follow. More specifically, soya should be introduced into the diet. With the reluctance of individuals to change as fundamental a habit as diet, dietary supplementation with isoflavonoids and lignans, to be taken along with the customary foods, may be beneficial. There have already been successful trials of a prototype supplement at the Tenovus Cancer Research Centre.

The objectives of dietary change with isoflavonoid/lignan supplementation in the Western environment will be to achieve plasma and urine levels of these compounds equivalent to those observed in Asian men and women who consume traditional foods. Initial monitoring of the effectiveness of this intervention, with the use of plasma and urine samples, may well be necessary.

A strategy of health education is equally necessary in Asian countries to ensure the knowledge of the existing health benefits of their traditional soya-based diet. This is particularly necessary when population groups in Asia acquire any degree of affluence, since this is readily detected by the fast-food industries, always eager to expand into new areas. As a result, Asians are persuaded away from their traditional foods.

It remains to be determined whether these isoflavonoids, flavonoids and lignans exercise their biological effect as antioxidants, antiestrogens or, indeed, as weak estrogens. Tamoxifen, as a weak estrogen, can effectively suppress early breast cancer lesions; concomitantly, as an estrogen, it can provide a beneficial influence with regard to cardiovascular disease and osteoporosis in women. Hormone replacement therapy, which is essentially low-dose estrogen therapy, controls menopausal problems, such as hot flushes, and provides longer-term benefits in restraining cardiovascular disease and osteoporosis. It is noteworthy that menopausal Japanese women have a lower frequency of hot flushes than their Western counterparts[137] which presumably could be attributable to their soya-based diet and its weak estrogen content.

Whilst there are these benefits, and others, for the menopausal and postmenopausal women from such dietary intervention, there might be concern amongst men for possible occurrence of undesirable side effects, such as feminization phenomena from these weak estrogenic influences. Such fears are natural, but reassuringly answerable by the absence of such phenomena in the vast male population of Asia, consuming, life long, a traditional soya diet. All of the evidence suggests that the Asian male eating traditional food lives all aspects of a healthy male life and is abundantly fertile, whilst at the same time enjoying a significantly reduced risk of prostatic malignancy as well as other benefits, already observed, which may well be linked with his dietary style.

Chemopreventive trials that use various dietary constituents may be difficult and expensive to establish. Some adverse side effects may emerge from current lack of knowledge or understanding of biological processes, but if the aim of such studies is to evaluate the influence of enhancing the concentrations of particular isoflavonoids or lignans in the study groups merely to the predetermined levels of the Asian people, then it would be hoped that any side effects would be minimal.

Acknowledgements

The authors are grateful for the generous financial support of South Glamorgan Area Health Authority and Tenovus Cancer Research Organisation. We are also indebted to Mrs Pat Davies for the expert typing of this manuscript.

References

1. Wynder, E. and Gori, G. (1977). Contribution of the environment to cancer incidence: an epidemiological study. *J. Natl. Cancer Inst.*, **58**, 825–32
2. Higginson, J. and Muir, C. (1979). Environmental carcinogenesis: misconceptions and limitations to cancer control. *J. Natl. Cancer Inst.*, **63**, 1291–8
3. Doll, R. and Peto, R. (1981). The causes of cancer: quantitative estimates of avoidable risks of cancer in the United States today. *J. Natl. Cancer Inst.*, **66**, 1191–308
4. Miller, A. B., Berrino, F., Hill, M., Pietinen, P., Riboli, E. and Wahrendorf, J. (1994). Diet in the aetiology of cancer: a review. *Eur. J. Cancer*, **30A**, 207–20
5. Skrabanek, P. (1994). Invited viewpoints. *Eur. J. Cancer*, **30A**, 220–1
6. McMichael, A. J. (1994). Invited viewpoints. *Eur. J. Cancer*, **30A**, 221–3
7. Anon. (1992). Diet and breast cancer. *Nature (London)*, **359**, 76
8. Silverberg, E., Boring, C. C. and Squires, T. S. (1990). *Cancer statistics. A Cancer Journal for Clinicians*, **40**, 9–26
9. Zaridze, D. G., Boyle, P. and Smans, M. (1984). International trends in prostatic cancer. *Int. J. Cancer*, **33**, 223–30
10. Sondik, E. (1988). Incidence, survival and mortality trends in prostate cancer in the United States. In Coffey, D. S., Resnick, M. I., Dorr, F. A. and Karr, J. P. (eds.) *A Multidisciplinary Analysis of Controversies in the Management of Prostate Cancer*, pp. 9–16. (New York: Plenum Press)
11. Dhom, G. (1991). Epidemiology of hormone-dependent tumors. In Voigt, K. D. and Knabbe, C. (eds.) *Endocrine Dependent Tumors*, pp. 1–42. (New York: Raven Press)
12. Boyle, P. (1994). Evolution of an epidemic of unknown origin. In Denis, L. (ed.) *European School of Oncology Monograph Prostate Cancer 2000*, pp. 5–11. (Heidelberg: Springer-Verlag)
13. Boring, C. C., Squires, T. S. and Tong, T. (1994). *Cancer Statistics. A Cancer Journal for Clinicians*, **44**, 7–26
14. Muir, C. S., Waterhouse, J. A. H., Mack, T., Powell, J. and Whelan, S. (eds.) (1987). *Cancer Incidence in Five Continents*, vol. V, IARC Scientific Publications, No. 88. (Lyon: IARC)
15. Armstrong, B. E. and Doll, R. (1975). Environmental factors and cancer incidence and mortality in different countries with special reference to dietary practices. *Int. J. Cancer*, **15**, 617–31
16. Breslow, N., Chan, C. E., Dhom, G., Drury, R. A. B., Franks, L. M., Gellei, B., Lee, Y. S., Lundberg, S., Sparke, B., Sternby, N. H. and Tulinius, H. (1977). Latent carcinoma of the prostate at autopsy in seven areas. *Int. J. Cancer*, **20**, 680–8
17. Zaridze, D. G. and Boyle, P. (1987). Cancer of the prostate: epidemiology and aetiology. *Br. J. Urol.*, **59**, 493–503
18. Skeet, R. G. (1976). Epidemiology of urological tumours. In Williams, D. I. and Chisholm, G. D. (eds.) *Scientific Foundations of Urology*, vol. II, pp. 199–211. (London: William Heineman Medical Books)
19. Miller, G. J. (1988). Diagnosis of stage A prostatic cancer in the People's Republic of China. In Coffey, D. S., Resnick, M. I., Dorr, F. A. and Karr, J. P. (eds.) *A Multidisciplinary Analysis of Controversies in the Management of Prostate Cancer*, pp. 17–24. (New York: Plenum Press)
20. Parkin, D. M., Muir, C. S., Whelan, S., Gao, Y. T., Ferlay, J. and Powell, J. (eds.) (1992). *Cancer Incidence in Five Continents*, vol. VI, IARC Scientific Publication No. 120. (Lyon: IARC)
21. Boyle, P., Levi, F., Lucchini, F. and La Vecchia C. (1993). Trends in diet-related cancers in Japan: a conundrum. *Lancet*, **324**, 752
22. Haenzel, W. and Kurihara, M. (1968). Studies of Japanese migrants. I. Mortality from cancer and other diseases among Japanese in the United States. *J. Natl. Cancer Inst.*, **40**, 43–68
23. Shimizu, H., Ropp, R. K., Bernstein, L., Yatani, R., Henderson, B. E. and Mack, T. H. (1991). Cancers of the breast and prostate among Japanese and white immigrants in Los Angeles County. *Br. J. Cancer*, **63**, 963–6
24. Ekman, P. (1989). BPH epidemiology and risk factors. *Prostate*, Suppl. **2**, 23–33

25. Isaacs, J. T. and Coffey, D. (1989). Etiology and disease process of benign prostatic hyperplasia. *Prostate*, Suppl. **2**, 33–50

26. Adlercreutz, H. (1990). Western diet and Western diseases: some hormonal and biochemical mechanisms and associations. *Scand. J. Clin. Lab. Invest.*, **50** (Suppl. 201), 3–23

27. Slavin, J. L. (1994). Epidemiological evidence for the impact of whole grains on health. *Crit. Rev. Food Sci. Nutr.*, **34**, 427–34

28. Burkitt, D. P. (1971). Epidemiology of cancer of the colon and rectum. *Cancer*, **28**, 3–13

29. Trowell, H. C. and Burkitt, D. P. (1983). In *Western Diseases: their Emergence and Prevention*. (London: Edward Arnold)

30. Reddy, B. S. and Cohen, L. A. (eds.) (1986). *Diet, Nutrition and Cancer: a Critical Evaluation.* (Boca Raton, FL: CRC Press)

31. Rose, D. P. (1990). Dietary fibre, phytoestrogens, and breast cancer. *Nutrition*, **8**, 47–51

32. Trock, B., Lanza, E. and Greenwald, P. (1990). Dietary fibre, vegetables, and colon cancer: critical review and meta-analysis of the epidemiological evidence. *J. Natl. Cancer Inst.*, **82**, 650–61

33. Macquart-Moulin, G., Riboli, E., Cornee, J., Charnay, B., Berthezene, P. and Day, N. (1986). Case–control study on colorectal cancer and diet in Marseilles. *Int. J. Cancer*, **38**, 183–91

34. Steinmetz, K. and Potter, J. (1991). Vegetables, fruit and cancer. I. Epidemiology. *Cancer Causes Control*, **2**, 325–57

35. Steinmetz, K. and Potter, J. (1991). Vegetables, fruit and cancer. II. Mechanisms. *Cancer Causes Control*, **2**, 427–42

36. Ingram, D. M., Nottage, E. and Roberts, T. (1991). The role of diet in the development of breast cancer: a case–control study of patients with breast cancer, benign epithelial hyperplasia and fibrocystic disease of the breast. *Br. J. Cancer*, **64**, 187–91

37. Wynder, E. L., Mabuchi, K. and Whitmore, W. F. (1971). Epidemiology of cancer of the prostate. *Cancer*, **28**, 344–60

38. Boyle, P. and Zaridze, D. G. (1993). Risk factors for prostate and testicular cancer. *Eur. J. Cancer*, **29A**, 1048–55

39. Giovannuucci, E., Rimm, E. B., Colditz, G. A., Stampfer, M. J., Ascherio, A., Chute, C. C. and Willett, W. C. (1993). A prospective study of dietary fat and risk of prostate cancer. *J. Natl. Cancer Inst.*, **85**, 1571–9

40. Mills, P. K., Beeson, W. L., Phillips, R. L. and Frazer, G. E. (1989). Cohort study of diet, lifestyle and prostate cancer in Adventist men. *Cancer*, **64**, 598–604

41. Le Marchand, L., Kolonel, L., Wilkens, L. R., Myers, B. C. and Hirohata, T. (1994). Animal fat consumption and prostate cancer: a prospective study in Hawaii. *Epidemiology*, **5**, 276–82

42. Severson, R. K., Nomura, A. M., Grove, A. S. and Stemmerman, G. N. (1989). A prospective study of demographics, diet and prostate cancer among men of Japanese ancestry in Hawaii. *Cancer Res.*, **49**, 1857–60

43. Stemmerman, G. N., Nomura, A. M. and Heilbrun, L. K. (1985). Cancer risk in relation to fat and energy intake among Hawaii Japanese: a prospective study. *Int. Symp. Princess Takamatsu Cancer Res. Fund*, **16**, 265–74

44. Kolonel, L. N., Hankin, J. H., Nomura, A. M. and Chu, S. Y. (1981). Dietary fat intake and cancer incidence among five ethnic groups in Hawaii. *Cancer Res.*, **41**, 3727–8

45. Kroes, R., Beems, R. B., Bosland, M. C., Bunnick, G. S. and Sinkeldam, E. J. (1986). Nutritional factors in lung, colon and prostate cancer in animal models. *Fed. Proc.*, **45**, 136–41

46. Simopoulos, A. P. (1987). Nutritional cancer risks derived from energy and fat. *Med. Oncol. Tumor Pharm.*, **4**, 227–39

47. Kolonel, L. N., Hankin, J. H. and Yoshizawa, C. N. (1987). Vitamin A and prostate cancer in elderly men: enhancement of risk. *Cancer Res.*, **47**, 2982–5

48. Paganini-Hill, A., Chao, A., Ross, R. and Henderson, B. E. (1987). Vitamin A, betacarotene and risk of prostate cancer: a prospective study. *J. Natl. Cancer Inst.*, **79**, 443–8

49. Hsing, A. W., McLauhglin, J. K., Schuman, L. M., Bjelke, E., Gridley, G., Wascholder, S., Chien, T. and Blot, W. J. (1990). Diet, tobacco use and fatal prostate cancer: results from the Lutheran Brotherhood Study. *Cancer Res.*, **50**, 6836–40

50. Ross, R. K., Shimuzu, H., Paganini-Hill, A., Honda, G. and Henderson, B. E. (1987). Case-controlled studies of prostate cancer in blacks and whites in Southern California. *J. Natl. Cancer Inst.*, **78**, 869–74

51. Ohno, Y., Yoshida, O., Oishi, K., Yamabe, H. and Schroeder, F. H. (1988). Dietary beta-carotene and cancer of the prostate: a case-controlled study in Kyoto, Japan. *Cancer Res.*, **48**, 1331–6

52. Corder, E. H., Guess, H. A., Hulka, B. S., Friedman, G. D., Sadler, M., Vollmer, R. T., Lobaugh, B., Drezner, M. K., Vogelman, J. H. and Orentreich, N. (1993). Vitamin D and prostate cancer: a prediagnostic study with stored sera. *Cancer Epidemiol. Biomarkers Prev.*, **2**, 467–72

53. Peehl, D. M., Skowronski, R. J., Leung, G. K., Wong, S. T., Stamey, T. A. and Feldman, D. (1994). Anti-proliferative effects of 1,25-dihy-

droxyvitamin D$_3$ on primary cultures of human prostatic cells. *Cancer Res.*, **54**, 805–10

54. Anon. (1995). The effect of vitamin E and beta-carotene on the incidence of lung cancer and other cancers in smokers. The Alpha-Tocopherol, Beta-Carotene Cancer Prevention Study Group. *N. Engl. J. Med.*, **330**, 1029–35

55. Hirayama, T. (1986). A large scale cohort study on cancer risks by diet – with special reference to the risk reducing effects of green–yellow vegetable consumption. In Hayashi, Y. *et al.* (eds.) *Diet, Nutrition and Cancer*, pp. 41–53. (Utrecht: Japan Science Society Press, Tokyo/VNU Science Press)

56. Hirayama, T. (1979). Epidemiology of prostate cancer with special reference to the role of diet. *Monographs Natl. Cancer Inst.*, **53**, 149–55

57. Hirayama, T. (1992). Life-style and cancer: from epidemiological evidence to public behavior change to mortality reduction of target cancers. *Monographs Natl. Cancer Inst.*, **12**, 65–74

58. Lee, H. P., Gourley, L., Duffy, S. W., Esteve, J., Lee, J. and Day, N. E. (1991). Dietary effects on breast cancer risk in Singapore. *Lancet*, **337**, 1197–200

59. Setchell, K. D. R. and Adlercreutz, H. (1988). Mammalian lignans and phytooestrogens. Recent studies on their formation, metabolism and biological role in health and disease. In Rowland, I. R. (ed.) *Role of Gut Flora in Toxicity and Cancer*, pp. 315–45. (London: Academic Press)

60. Kodama, M. and Kodama, T. (1990). Interrelation between Western type cancers and non-Western type cancers as regards their risk variations in time and space. II. Nutrition and cancer risk. *Anticancer Res.*, **10**, 1043–9

61. Rose, D. P., Boyar, A. P. and Wynder, E. L. (1986). International comparisons of mortality rates for cancer of the breast, ovary, prostate and colon and *per capita* food consumption. *Cancer*, **58**, 2363–71

62. Block, G., Patterson, B. and Subar, A. (1992). Fruit, vegetables and cancer prevention: a review of the epidemiological evidence. *Nutr. Cancer*, **18**, 1–29

63. Negri, E., La Vecchia, C., Franceschi, S., D'Avanzo, B. and Parazzini, F. (1994). The role of vegetables and fruit in cancer risk. In Hill, M. J., Giacosa, A. and Caygill, C. P. J. (eds.) *Epidemiology of Diet and Cancer*, pp. 327–34. (Chichester: Ellis Horwood)

64. Buiatti, E., Palli, D., Dc Carli, A., Amodori, D., Avellini, C., Bianchi, S., Biserni, R., Cipriani, F., Collo, P., Giacosa, A., Marubini, E., Puntoni, R., Vindigni, C., Fraumeni, J. F. and Blot, W. J. (1989). A case–control study of gastric cancer and diet in Italy. *Int. J. Cancer*, **44**, 611–16

65. Buatti, E., Palli, D., De Carli, A., Amadori, D., Avellini, C., Bianchi, S., Bonaguri, C., Cipriani, F., Collo, P., Giacosa, A., Marubini, E., Minacci, C., Puntoni, R., Russo, A., Vindigni, C., Fraumeni, J. F. and Blot, W. J. (1990). A case–control study of gastric cancer and diet in Italy. II. Association with nutrients. *Int. J. Cancer*, **45**, 896–901

66. La Vecchia, C., De Carli, A., Negri, E. and Parazzini, F. (1988). Epidemiological aspects of diet and cancer: a summary review of case–control studies from Northern Italy. *Oncology*, **45**, 364–70

67. Miksicek, R. J. (1993). Commonly occurring plant flavonoids have estrogenic activity. *Molec. Pharmacol.*, **44**, 37–43

68. Bradbury, R. B. and White, D. C. (1954). Oestrogens and related substances in plants. *Vitam. Horm.*, **12**, 207–33

69. Price, K. R. and Fenwick, G. R. (1985). Naturally occurring oestrogens in food – a review. *Food Add. Contam.*, **2**, 73–106

70. Verdeal, K., Brown, R. R., Richardson, T. and Ryan, D. S. (1980). Affinity of phytoestrogens for estradiol-binding proteins and effect of coumestrol on growth of 7,12-dimethylbenz(a) anthracene-induced rat mammary tumors. *J. Natl. Cancer Inst.*, **64**, 285–90

71. Axelson, M., Sjovall, J., Gustafsson, B. E. and Setchell, K. D. R. (1984). A dietary source of the non-steroidal oestrogen equol in man and animals. *J. Endocrinol.*, **102**, 49–56

72. Walz, E. (1931). Isoflavon-und Sapogenin-Glucoside in Sojahispida. *Justus Liebigs Annal. Chem.*, **489**, 118–55

73. Coward, L., Barnes, N. C., Setchell, K. D. R. and Barnes, S. (1993). Genistein, daidzein, and their β-glycoside conjugates: antitumor isoflavones in soybean foods from American and Asian diets. *J. Agric. Food Chem.*, **41**, 1961–7

74. Rosenblum, E. R., Campbell, I. M., van Thiel, D. H. and Gavaler, J. S. (1992). Isolation and identification of phytoestrogens from beer. *Alcoholism, Clin. Exp. Res.*, **16**, 843–5

75. Van Thiel, D. H., Galvao-Teles, A., Monteiro, E., Rosenblum, E. and Gavaler, J. S. (1991). The phytoestrogens present in de-ethanolised bourbon are biologically active: a preliminary study in postmenopausal women. *Alcoholism, Clin. Exp. Res.*, **15**, 822–3

76. Rao, C. B. S. (ed.) (1978). *The Chemistry of Lignans*, pp. 1–377. (Waltair, India: Andra University Press and Publications)

77. Thompson, L. U., Robb, P., Serraino, M. and Cheung, F. (1991). Mammalian lignan

production from various foods. *Nutr. Cancer*, **16**, 43–52

78. Kelly, G. E., Nelson, C., Waring, M. A., Joannou, G. E. and Reeder, A. Y. (1993). Metabolites of dietary (soya) isoflavones in human urine. *Clin. Chim. Acta*, **223**, 9–22

79. Adlercreutz, H., Fotsis, T., Bannwart, C., Wahala, K., Makela, T., Brunow, G. and Hase, T. (1986). Determination of urinary lignans and phytoestrogen metabolites, potential antiestrogens and anticarcinogens, in urine of women on various habitual diets. *J. Steroid Biochem.*, **25**, 791–7

80. Morton, M. S., Wilcox, G., Wahlquvist, M. L. and Griffiths, K. (1994). Determination of lignans and isoflavonoids in human female plasma following dietary supplementation. *J. Endocrinol.*, **142**, 251–9

81. Finlay, E. M. H., Wilson, D. W., Adlercreutz, H. and Griffiths, K. (1991). The identification and measurement of 'phyto-oestrogens' in human saliva, plasma, breast aspirate or cyst fluid, and prostatic fluid using gas chromatography–mass spectrometry. *J. Endocrinol.*, **129** (Suppl.), 49

82. Dehennin, L., Reiffsteck, A., Joudet, M. and Thibier, M. (1982). Identification and quantitative estimation of a lignan in human and bovine semen. *J. Reprod. Fert.*, **66**, 305–9

83. Adlercreutz, H., Honjo, H., Higashi, A., Fotsis, T., Hamalainen, E., Hasegawa, T. and Okada, H. (1991). Urinary excretion of lignans and isoflavonoid phytoestrogens in Japanese men and women consuming traditional Japanese diet. *Am. J. Clin. Nutr.*, **54**, 1093–100

84. Adlercreutz, H., Markkanen, H. and Watanabe, S. (1993). Plasma concentrations of phyto-oestrogens in Japanese men. *Lancet*, **342**, 1209–10

85. Setchell, K. D. R., Borriello, S. P., Hulme, P., Kirk, D. N. and Axelson, M. (1984). Non-steroidal oestrogens of dietary origin: possible roles in hormone-dependent disease. *Am. J. Clin. Nutr.*, **40**, 569–78

86. Pope, G. S. and Wright, H. G. (1954). Oestrogenic isoflavones in red clover and subterranean clover. *Chem. Ind.*, 1019–20

87. Bickoff, E. M. (1961). Estrogen-like substances in plants. In Hissaw, F. L. (ed.) *Physiology of Reproduction*, pp. 93–118. Proceedings of the 22nd Animal Biology Colloquium. (Corvallis: Oregon State University Press)

88. Waters, A. P. and Knowler, J. T. (1982). Effect of a lignan (HPMF) on RNA synthesis in the rat uterus. *J. Reprod. Fert.*, **66**, 379–81

89. Martin, P. M., Horwitz, K. B., Ryan, D. S. and McGuire, W. L. (1978). Phytoestrogen interaction with estrogen receptors in human breast cancer cells. *Endocrinology*, **103**, 1860–7

90. Adlercreutz, H., Hockerstedt, K., Bannwart, C., Bloigu, S., Hamalainen, E., Fotsis, T. and Ollus, A. (1987). Effect of dietary components, including lignans and phytoestrogens on enterohepatic circulation and liver metabolism of estrogens and on sex hormone binding globulin (SHBG). *J. Steroid Biochem.*, **27**, 1135–44

91. Cunha, G. R., Chung, L. W. K., Shannon, J. M., Taguchi, O. and Fujii, H. (1983). Hormone-induced morphogenesis and growth: role of mesenchymal–epithelial interaction. *Recent Prog. Horm. Res.*, **39**, 559–95

92. Griffiths, K., Davies, P., Eaton, C. L., Harper, M. E., Turkes, A. and Peeling, W. B. (1991). Endocrine factors in the initiation, diagnosis and treatment of prostatic cancer. In Voigt, K.-D. and Knabbe, C. (eds.) *Endocrine Dependent Tumors*, pp. 83–130. (New York: Raven Press)

93. Coffey, D. S. (1990). In Khoury, S., Chatelain, C., Murphy, G. and Denis, L. (eds.) *The Structure and Function of the Prostate Gland and Sex Accessory Tissues in Prostate Cancer*, pp. 70–103. (Paris: FISS Publications)

94. Griffiths, K., Davies, P., Eaton, C. L., Harper, M. E., Peeling, W. B., Turkes, A. O., Turkes, A., Wilson, D. W. and Pierrepoint, C. G. (1987). Cancer of the prostate: endocrine factors. In Clark, J. R. (ed.) *Oxford Reviews of Reproductive Biology*, vol. 9, pp. 192–259. (Oxford: Clarendon Press)

95. Vermeulen, A., Rubens, R. and Verdonck, L. (1972). Testosterone secretion and metabolism in male senescence. *J. Clin. Endocrinol. Metab.*, **34**, 730–5

96. Rubens, R., Dhont, M. and Vermeulen, A. (1974). Further studies on Leydig cell function in old age. *J. Clin. Endocrinol. Metab.*, **39**, 40–5

97. Vermeulen, A., van Camp, A., Mattelaer, J. and De Sy, W. (1979) Hormonal factors related to abnormal growth of the prostate. In Coffey, D. S. and Isaacs, J. T. (eds.) *Prostate Cancer*, Technical Workshop Series, vol. 48, pp. 81–92. (Geneva: UICC)

98. Belanger, A., Locong, A., Noel, C., Cusan, L., Dupont, A., Prevost, J., Caron, S. and Sevigny, J. (1989). Influence of diet on plasma steroids and sex hormone-binding globulin levels in adult men. *J. Steroid Biochem.*, **32**, 829–33

99. Vermeulen, A. (1993). Metabolic effects of obesity in men. *Verhandelingen-Koninklijke Academie Voor Geneeskunde Van Belgie*, **55**, 393–7

100. Griffiths, K., Akaza, H., Eaton, C L., El Etreby, M., Habib, F., Lee, C., Partin, A. W., Coffey, D. S., Sciarra, F., Steiner, G. and Tenniswood, M. P. (1993). Regulation of prostatic growth. In

Cockett, A. T. K., Khoury, S., Aso, Y., Chatelain, C., Denis, L., Griffiths, K. and Murphy, G. (eds.) *The 2nd International Consultation on Benign Prostatic Hyperplasia (BPH)*, pp. 49–75. (Paris: S.C.I.)

101. Bruchovsky, N. and Wilson, J. D. (1968). The conversion of testosterone to 5-alpha-androstan-17-beta-ol-3-one by rat prostate *in vivo* and *in vitro*. *J. Biol. Chem.*, **243**, 2012–21

102. Bruchovsky, N. and Wilson, J. D. (1968). The intranuclear binding of testosterone and 5-alpha-androstan-17-beta-ol-3-one by rat prostate. *J. Biol. Chem.*, **243**, 5953–60

103. Anderson, K. H. and Liao, S. (1968). Selective retention of dihydrotestosterone by prostatic nuclei. *Nature (London)*, **219**, 277–9

104. Evans, B. A. J., Griffiths, K. and Morton, M. (1995). Inhibition of 5α-reductase and 17β-hydroxysteroid dehydrogenase in genital skin fibroblasts by dietary lignans and isoflavonoids. *J. Endocrinol.*, **147**, 295–302

105. Ross, R. K., Bernstein, L., Lobo, R. A., Shimuzu, H., Stanczyk, F. Z., Pike, M. C. and Henderson, B. E. (1992). 5-alpha-reductase activity and risk of prostate cancer among Japanese and US white and black males. *Lancet*, **339**, 887–9

106. Rittmaster, R. S. (1994). Finasteride. *N. Engl. J. Med.*, **330**, 120–5

107. Vermeulen, A. (1976). Testicular hormone secretion and aging in males. In Grayshack, J. T., Wilson, J. D. and Saherbenske, M. J. (eds.) *Benign Prostatic Hyperplasia*, DHEW publication No. (Washington: National Institute of Health) 76-1113, pp. 117–82.

108. Vermeulen, A., Deslypere, J. P. and Meirleir, K. (1989). A new look to the andropause: altered function of the gonadotrophs. *J. Steroid. Biochem.*, **32**, 163–5

109. Adlercreutz, H., Bannwart, C., Wahala, K., Makela, T., Brunow, G., Hase, T., Arosemena, P. J., Kellis, J. T. and Vickery, L. E. (1993). Inhibition of human aromatase by mammalian lignans and isoflavonoid phytoestrogens. *J. Steroid Biochem. Molec. Biol.*, **44**. 147–53

110. Evans, B. A. J., Griffiths, K. and Morton, M. (1995). Inhibition of aromatase in human genital skin fibroblasts by dietary isoflavonoids and lignans. Personal communication

111. Hunter, T. and Cooper, J. A. (1985). Protein tyrosine kinases. *Annu. Rev. Biochem.*, **54**, 897–930

112. Bishop, J. M. (1985). Cellular oncogenes and retroviruses. *Annu. Rev. Biochem.*, **52**, 301–54

113. Schlessinger, J., Schreiber, A. B., Levi, A., Lax, J., Liberman, T. and Yarder, Y. (1983). Regula- tion of cell proliferation by epidermal growth factor. *Crit. Rev. Biochem.*, **14**, 93–111

114. Kenyon, G. L. and Garcia, G. A. (1987). Design of kinase inhibitors. *Med. Res. Rev.*, **7**, 389–416

115. Akiyama, T., Ishida, J., Nakagawa, S., Ogawara, H., Watanaba, S.-I., Itoh, N., Shibuya, M. and Fukami, Y. (1987). Genistein, a specific inhibi- tor of tyrosine-specific protein kinases. *J. Biol. Chem.*, **262**. 552–5

116. Kuo, M. L., Lin, J. K., Huang, T. S. and Yang, N. C. (1994). Reversion of the transformed phenotypes of v-H-ras NIH3T3 cells by flavonoids through attenuating the content of phosphotyrosine. *Cancer Lett.*, **87**, 91–7

117. Kiguchi, K., Glesne, D., Chubb, C. H., Fujiki, H. and Huberman, E. (1994). Differential induc- tion of apoptosis in human breast cells by okadaic acid and related inhibitors of protein phosphatases 1 and 2A. *Cell Growth Differ.*, **5**, 995–1004

118. Scholar, E. M. and Toews, M. L. (1994). Inhibi- tion of invasion of murine mammary carcinoma cells by the tyrosine kinase inhibitor genistein. *Cancer Lett.*, **87**, 159–62

119. Tiisala, S., Majuri, M. L., Carpen, O. and Ren- konen, R. (1994). Genistein enhances the ICAM-mediated adhesion by inducing the ex- pression of ICAM-1 and its counter receptors. *Biochem. Biophys. Res. Comm.*, **203**, 443–9

120. Cummings, J. and Smyth, J. F. (1993). DNA topoisomerase I and II as targets for rational design of new anticancer drugs. *Ann. Oncol.*, **4**, 533–43

121. McCabe, M. J. Jr and Orrenius, S. (1993). Genistein induces apoptosis in immature human thymocytes by inhibiting topoisom- erase-II. *Biochem. Biophys. Res. Comm.*, **194**, 944–50

122. Constantinou, A., Mehta, R., Runyan, C., Rao, K., Vaughan, A. and Moon, R. (1995). Flavonoids as DNA topoisomerase antagonists and poisons: structure–activity relationships. *J. Nat. Prod.*, **58**, 217–25

123. Spinozzi, F., Pagliacci, M. C., Migliorati, G., Moraca, R., Grignani, F., Riccardi, C. and Ni- coletti, I. (1994). The natural tyrosine kinase inhibitor genistein produces cell cycle arrest and apoptosis in Jurkat T-leukemia cells. *Leuk. Res.*, **18**, 431–9

124. Matsukawa, Y., Marui, N., Sakai, T., Satomi, Y., Yoshida, M., Matsumoto, K., Nishino, H. and Aoike, A. (1993). Genistein arrests cell cycle progression at G2-M. *Cancer Res.*, **53**, 1328–31

125. Sato, F., Matsukawa, Y., Matsumoto, K., Nishino, H. and Sakai, T. (1994). Apigenin induces mor- phological differentiation and G-2M arrest in

rat neuronal cells. *Biochem. Biophys. Res. Comm.,* **204**, 578–84

126. Folkman, J., Watson, K., Ingber, D. and Hanahan, D. (1989). Induction of angiogenesis during the transition from hyperplasia to neoplasia. *Nature (London),* **339**, 58–61

127. Folkman, J. (1985). Toward an understanding of angiogenesis: search and discovery. *Perspect. Biol. Med.,* **29**, 10–36

128. Weidner, M., Semple, J. P., Welch, W. R. and Folkman, J. (1991). Tumour angiogenesis and metaplasia-correlation in invasive breast cancer. *N. Engl. J. Med.,* **324**, 1–8

129. Fotsis, T., Pepper, M., Adlercreutz, H., Fleischmann, G., Hase, T., Montesano, R. and Schweigerer, L. (1993). Genistein, a dietary-derived inhibitor of *in vitro* angiogenesis. *Proc. Natl. Acad. Sci. USA,* **90**, 2690–4

130. Rice-Evans, C. A., Miller, N. J., Bolwell, P. G., Bramley, P. M. and Pridham, J. B. (1995). The relative antioxidant activities of plant-derived polyphenolic flavonoids. *Free Radical Res.,* **22**, 375–83

131. Mangiapane, H., Thomson, J., Salter, A., Brown, S., Bell, G. D. and White, D. A. (1992). The inhibition of the oxidation of low density lipoprotein by (+)-catechin, a naturally occurring flavonoid. *Biochem. Pharmacol.,* **43**, 445–50

132. Messina, M. J., Persky, V., Setchell, K. D. R. and Barnes, S. (1994). Soy intake and cancer risk: a review of the *in vitro* and *in vivo* data. *Nutr. Cancer,* **21**, 113–30

133. Peterson, G. and Barnes, S. (1991). Genistein inhibition of the growth of human breast cancer cells: independence from estrogen receptors and the multi-drug resistant gene. *Biochem. Biophys. Res. Comm.,* **179**, 661–7

134. Peterson, G. and Barnes, S.(1993). Genistein and biochanin A inhibit the growth of human prostate cancer cells but not epidermal growth factor receptor tyrosine autophosphorylation. *Prostate,* **22**, 335–45

135. Chae, Y. H., Ho, D. K., Cassady, J. M., Cook, V. M., Marcus, C. B. and Baird, W. M. (1992). Effects of synthetic and naturally occurring flavonoids on metabolic activation of benzo[a]pyrene in hamster cell cultures. *Chem. Biol. Inter.,* **82**, 181–93

136. Shi, S. T., Wang, Z. Y., Smith, T. J., Hong, J. Y., Chen, W. F., Ho, C. T. and Yang, C. S. (1994). Effects of green tea and black tea on 4-(methylnitrosoamino)-1-(3-pyridyl)-1-butanone bioactivation, DNA methylation and lung tumorigenesis in A/J mice. *Cancer Res.,* **54**, 4641–7

137. Adlercreutz, H., Hamalainen, E., Gorbach, S. and Goldin, B. (1992). Dietary phyto-oestrogens and the menopause in Japan. *Lancet,* **339**, 1233

Interactive Voting System

1 Has the time come for dietary advice to prevent prostate cancer?

Response	*Option*
52%	Yes.
31%	No.
17%	No opinion.

Number of votes: 108

2 Which dietary advice would you consider, if at all?

6%	A low animal-fat diet.
12%	High fiber and plant estrogens.
7%	A dietary supplement.
63%	A combination of 1 and 2.
12%	None of the above.

Number of votes: 115

3 Can early minimal endocrine treatment prevent prostate cancer?

27%	Yes.
33%	No.
40%	No opinion.

Number of votes: 109

3

Post-radical Prostatectomy Incontinence and Impotence: Etiology, Evaluation, Trends and Treatment

Sexual function before and after radical prostatectomy: prevalence, etiology, diagnosis and management

G. R. Dohle

8

Introduction

Radical prostatectomy has been associated with a loss of sexual potency in the majority of cases, due to injury to the autonomic cavernous nerves. Since the introduction of the anatomical approach of the neurovascular bundles by Walsh and Donker[1], the nerve-sparing radical prostatectomy has become the operation of first choice in potent and sexually active men with an organ-confined prostatic carcinoma. Numerous series on the recovery of sexual potency after a nerve-sparing radical prostatectomy have been published since, showing a high rate of potency after the operation in a selected group of patients[2-7]. Most of these studies, however, involve sexually active young patients with an early-stage cancer and low cancer volume. Recently a Medicare-based report showed a much lower rate of potency after radical prostatectomy[8], questioning the feasibility of the nerve-sparing procedure in a general urological population.

We have reviewed the literature on sexual potency after radical prostatectomy. We also discuss the etiology, prognostic factors, diagnosis and current management of impotence after radical prostatectomy.

Materials and methods

A literature search of Medline 1980–96 was performed with the use of the following key words: sexual function, potency, impotence, erectile dysfunction, prostatic carcinoma, adenocarcinoma of the prostate and (nerve sparing) radical prostatectomy. Articles were reviewed containing the following information: age, sexual activity and potency before the operation, nerve-sparing radical prostatectomy (bilateral and unilateral), clinical stage, pathological stage (positive surgical margins), follow-up of at least 1 year, incontinence and strictures. Potency was defined as the ability to achieve unassisted intercourse with vaginal penetration. Of the 51 articles selected by Medline, only 21 articles met these criteria.

We also reviewed all articles on the etiology of erectile dysfunction; there were five of these articles. Neurogenic factors and vascular factors are discussed in detail.

The diagnosis of erectile dysfunction is discussed and the value of different diagnostic techniques are presented. Finally, the current management of erectile failure following radical prostatectomy with respect to sexual counselling, vacuum devices, intracavernosal injection therapy, vascular surgery and penile prosthesis is discussed.

Results

In a general urological practice the mean age of patients undergoing a radical prostatectomy is 60–70 years. Before the operation, potency is reported in 67–84% of cases. Selection criteria for performing a nerve-sparing radical prostatectomy were: normal erection before the operation and clinical diagnosis of stage A or B prostate cancer.

We have reviewed 21 articles on nerve-sparing radical prostatectomy. In most series a selection of patients are presented; usually only men who were potent before the operation and who had a nerve-sparing radical prostatectomy were evaluated. From most studies it is impossible to determine the results of the total group of patients who underwent operation. Fowler and colleagues[8] reported on a sample of Medicare patients who underwent radical prostatectomy in different institutions in the United States: from their survey it was concluded that in only 11% of patients erections were sufficient for intercourse. It is unknown how many of these 855 patients had a nerve-sparing radical prostatectomy.

From two large series[3,4], the number could be estimated of the total group of patients who underwent operation who were potent after the operation: Geary and co-workers[4] evaluated 459 men who were operated on between 1983 and 1991 and found potency in 51 cases (11%). Catalona and Basler[3] reported on 784 patients operated on between 1983 and 1992 and found potency in 173 cases (22%) of the total group.

In most series a correlation was found between the number of spared neurovascular bundles and the recovery of potency. In cases of bilateral nerve-sparing radical prostatectomy, potency was found in 31–76%. In cases of unilateral nerve-sparing radical prostatectomy, recovery of erection occurred in 13–56%. Table 1 summarizes the prevalence of potency after nerve-sparing radical prostatectomy.

More favorable results were usually achieved in younger patients with organ-confined disease[2,3]. Also, the data on sexual activity before

the operation showed good prognostic value[4]. In most series the number of spared neurovascular bundles was the single most important prognostic factor. Other related factors were: age, tumor stage, cancer volume, incontinence and strictures. In 12% of cases recovery of erections appeared after a follow-up of 1 year. In non-nerve-sparing radical prostatectomy, potency returned in 0–17%[2,5]. Orgasm was present in 80% of cases[4].

We have reviewed articles on the etiology of impotence after radical prostatectomy: neurogenic factors appeared to be the most common explanation for this feature. Arguments in favor of a neurogenic cause were: clear relation to the number of spared neurovascular bundles, absence of a history of vascular disease in most cases and a good response to low doses of intracavernosal treatment.

A vascular component was suggested in studies on duplex scanning before and after nerve-sparing radical prostatectomy: a decrease in peak systolic flow velocity and diameter of the cavernosal arteries was determined in 8/20 cases by Abosief and associates[9]. An explanation for this decrease was found in the cadaveric dissections of Breza and colleagues[10], who found accessory pudendal arteries in 7/10 cases originating from the obturator artery, the inferior vesical artery or the superior vesical artery. These accessory pudendal arteries were found to be anterolateral to the prostatic surface; they are usually injured during dissection. They supply additional blood to the cavernous bodies: in two cases the accessory pudendal artery was the main supply to the penis. Kim and co-workers[11] also found decreased penile blood

Table 1 Potency after radical prostatectomy. Results are separated into bilateral/unilateral/non-nerve-sparing

Reference	Patients (n)	Age (years)	Radical prostatectomy	Potency (%)
Quinlan et al. (1991)[2]	600	59	291/96/97	76/56/0
Catalona and Basler (1993)[3]	784	64	236/59/489	63/41/—
Geary et al. (1995)[4]	481	64	69/203/187	31/13/1
Leandri et al. (1992)[6]	620	68	106/—/514	71/—/—
Fowler et al. (1993)[8]	855	> 65	unknown	11/—/—
Drago et al. (1992)[7]	528	64	151/377/—	66/—/—
Davidson et al. (1996)[5]	188	63	42/17/24	43/24/17

flow on color Doppler ultrasound examination after radical prostatectomy, especially on the side where the nerve bundle had been sacrificed. These differences, however, were not statistically significant. No evidence for veno-occlusive dysfunction was found after radical prostatectomy in the ten studied cases. Polascik and Walsh[12] reported on the presence of accessory pudendal arteries in a series of 835 radical prostatectomies and found the accessory artery present in only 4% of cases. Preservation of the accessory pudendal artery did not significantly increase potency rates.

An evaluation of different diagnostic techniques has recently been published by Zimmern and colleagues[13]. In a group of 45 potent men, candidates for radical prostatectomy, biothesiometry, nocturnal penile tumescence registration (Rigiscan analysis) and color Doppler ultrasound were studied before the operation. Only color Doppler showed normal results in most patients (93%); both Rigiscan analysis and biothesiometry correlated poorly with the potency status of the investigated subjects.

Management of erectile failure after radical prostatectomy focuses primarily on intracavernosal injection therapy. Both papaverine/phentolamine mixtures and prostaglandin E_1 were effective treatments in 60–85% of cases[12,14]. Vacuum devices have also been applied successfully after radical prostatectomy. The combination of these therapies with sexual counselling increases acceptance by patient and partner and provides better long-term results. In cases of therapy failure, penile prosthesis can be offered.

Discussion

With the introduction of anatomical radical retropubic prostatectomy, Walsh[15] modified the operation to preserve erections by avoiding injury to the neurovascular bundles. Increasing numbers of nerve-sparing radical prostatectomies have been performed since. In numerous large retrospective series, the effectiveness of preserving sexual activity after this procedure has been shown. Recovery of sexual potency has become a realistic option for relatively young patients suffering from an organ-confined prostatic carcinoma[3,4]. The outcome of potency after the operation is mainly determined by age and the number of neurovascular bundles saved during surgery[2]. Since advanced tumor stage usually coincides with wide excision of one or both neurovascular bundles, potency rates in these cases are limited. In practice in many patients, a nerve-sparing procedure is not achieved and potency is usually lost.

Some concern was raised over the incidence of positive surgical margins with respect to nerve-sparing procedures. The number of positive surgical margins due to a nerve-sparing radical prostatectomy has been estimated as 2–3%[2,4]. Furthermore, the incidence of positive surgical margins in patients undergoing a radical retropubic prostatectomy was found to be not significantly different from that of patients undergoing standard radical prostatectomy. Positive surgical margins are probably determined by tumor extent rather than by the operative technique[2].

Etiology of impotence after radical prostatectomy is multifactorial. A strong correlation between the number of preserved neurovascular bundles and the recovery of potency is usually found. Younger patients in general need fewer preserved bundles to recover potency than older patients[2,3]. With increasing age, the nerve regeneration capacity decreases.

Vascular factors may also play a substantial role in aging men, since the operation potentially compromises the penile blood flow. More prospective studies on vascular involvement are required for full understanding of its role in post-radical prostatectomy impotence.

Diagnostic investigations in erectile failure are limited by the available treatment options. In practice a goal-directed approach, as proposed by Lue[16], is effective in most cases. Invasive diagnostic procedures should only be performed if they influence therapy choice. Since intracavernosal injections are effective in the majority of cases, diagnosis should be focused on this therapy initially. Color Doppler ultrasound studies in combination with administration of papaverine or prostaglandin

E_1 has shown to be a reliable test for vascular factors[13].

Conclusions

Nerve-sparing radical prostatectomy preserves potency in 31–76% of cases of sexually active men with organ-confined disease. However, in most cases of radical prostatectomy, a nerve-sparing procedure is not achieved and potency is usually lost. Prognostic factors for recovery of sexual potency are: number of spared neurovascular bundles, age, sexual activity before the operation, tumor stage, incontinence and strictures.

The etiology of impotence following radical prostatectomy is multifactorial, but neurogenic factors play a major role. Vascular factors may play a substantial role in selective cases, in which accessory internal pudendal arteries are the major supply for the cavernous bodies.

Color Doppler ultrasound appears to be the most reliable diagnostic test for impotence after radical prostatectomy. Most patients respond well to intracavernosal injections, indicating a neurogenic cause of the erectile dysfunction. A prospective study on the different factors involved in sexual potency after radical prostatectomy is mandatory.

References

1. Walsh, P. C. and Donker, P. J. (1982). Impotence following radical prostatectomy: insight into etiology and prevention. *J. Urol.*, **128**, 492–7

2. Quinlan, D. M., Epstein, J. I., Carter, B. S. and Walsh, P. C. (1991). Sexual function following radical prostatectomy: influence of preservation of neurovascular bundles. *J. Urol.*, **145**, 998–1002

3. Catalona, W. J. and Basler, J. W. (1993). Return of erections and urinary continence following nerve sparing radical retropubic prostatectomy. *J. Urol.*, **150**, 905–7

4. Geary, E. S., Dendinger, T. E., Freiha, F. S. and Stamey, T. A. (1995). Nerve sparing radical prostatectomy: a different view. *J. Urol.*, **154**, 145–9

5. Davidson, P. J. T., Van Den Ouden, D. and Schroeder, F. H. (1996). Radical prostatectomy: prospective assessment of mortality and morbidity. *Eur. Urol.*, **29**, 168–73

6. Leandri, P., Rossignol, G., Gautier, J. R. and Ramon, J. (1992). Radical retropubic prostatectomy: morbidity and quality of life. Experience with 620 consecutive cases. *J. Urol.*, **147**, 883–7

7. Drago, J. R., Badalament, R. A., York, J. P., Simon, J., Riemenschneider, H., Nesbitt, J. A. and Perez, J. (1992). Radical prostatectomy: OSU and affiliated hospitals' experience 1985–1989. *Urology*, **39**, 44–7

8. Fowler, F. J., Barry, M. J., Lu-Yao, G., Roman, A., Wasson, J. and Wennberg, J. E. (1993). Patient-reported complications and follow-up treatment after radical prostatectomy. *Urology*, **42**, 622–9

9. Abosief, S. R., Shinohara, K., Breza, J. and Narayan, P. (1994). Role of penile vascular injury in erectile dysfunction after radical prostatectomy. *Br. J. Urol.*, **73**, 75–82

10. Breza, J., Abosief, S. R., Orvis, B. R., Lue, T. F. and Tanago, E. A. (1989). Detailed anatomy of penile neurovascular structures surgical significance. *J. Urol.*, **141**, 437–43

11. Kim, E. D., Blackburn, D. and McVary, K. T. (1994). Post-radical prostatectomy penile blood flow: assessment with color doppler ultrasound. *J. Urol.*, **152**, 2276–9

12. Polascik, T. J. and Walsh, P. C. (1995). Radical retropubic prostatectomy: the influence of accessory pudendal arteries on the recovery of sexual function. *J. Urol.*, **153**, 150–2

13. Zimmern, P. E., Kaswick, J. and Leach, G. E. (1995). How potent is potent before nerve sparing radical retropubic prostatectomy? *J. Urol.*, **154**, 1100–1

14. Dennis, R. L. and McDougal, W. J. (1987). Pharmacological treatment of erectile dysfunction after radical prostatectomy. *J. Urol.*, **139**, 775–6

15. Walsh, P. C. (1986). Radical retropubic prostatectomy. In Walsh, P. C., Gittes, R. F., Perlmutter, A. D. and Stamey, T. A. (eds.) *Campbell's Urology*, pp. 2754–75. (Philadelphia: W.B. Saunders)

16. Lue, T. F. (1990). Impotence: a patient's goal-directed approach to treatment. *World J. Urol.*, **8**, 67–74

Anatomy and physiology of the external urethral sphincter: implications for preservation of continence after radical prostatectomy

9

R. P. Myers

The best result for complete urinary control after radical prostatectomy was reported at 99.5% for radical perineal prostatectomy (RPP)[1] and the worst result stands at only 13% continent after radical retropubic prostatectomy (RRP)[2]. Advances in the knowledge of pelvic floor and perineal anatomy are such that a very low rate of incontinence should be achievable with careful technique, and total incontinence should be a thing of the past. Despite advances, urinary incontinence is still a troubling complication for many surgeons[3]. The aim herein is to review the salient features of the anatomy and physiology as they relate to radical prostatectomy and the preservation of urinary control.

Unless the patient has a normal bladder and infravesical anatomy, no surgeon can expect a good result. Trabeculation from obstructive uropathy, e.g. benign prostatic hyperplasia (BPH) or stricture disease, may presage postoperative detrusor instability and wetting from continual urgency and urge incontinence. Similarly, prior definitive radiotherapy to the prostate for 'cure' can so change the bladder and continence zone that, despite meticulous technique, urinary control is forever elusive and pad dependence a matter of course for substantial numbers of patients[4].

The term 'intramural distal sphincter mechanism' was coined by Turner-Warwick[5] to connote the continence zone below the seminal colliculus (verumontanum = veru). Like Gil Vernet[6], he stressed the continuity of tissues associated with continence, not from apex of prostate to penile bulb (corpus spongiosum), but from veru to penile bulb. Tissue components of the sphincteric complex include the outer striated urethral sphincter (rhabdosphincter), which is the extrinsic mechanism. The urethral wall smooth muscle with elastic tissue and the urethral mucosa constitutes the intrinsic mechanism[7]. In the adult male, the striated sphincter surrounds the membranous urethra except for a tiny posterior fibrous tissue raphe that is in continuity with the perineal body. Thus, the striated muscle forms a continuous series of different horseshoe configurations about the membranous urethra[8]. The striated urethral sphincter is functional only from the apex of the prostate to the bulb and may exhibit increasing girth as one proceeds distally (Figure 1a), making the most distal sphincter in general functionally more significant.

In contrast to the rhabdosphincter, which stops at the prostate apex, the urethral wall smooth muscle and elastic tissue components extend the entire distance from veru to bulb (Figure 1b). It is this component that can be damaged by transurethral resection distal to the veru, and physiologically this is the important component with respect to urinary control: the striated urethral sphincter is not necessary. It is widely recognized that experimental paralysis of the striated sphincter induced by pudendal nerve block does not result in urinary incontinence[9], but damage to the urethral wall smooth

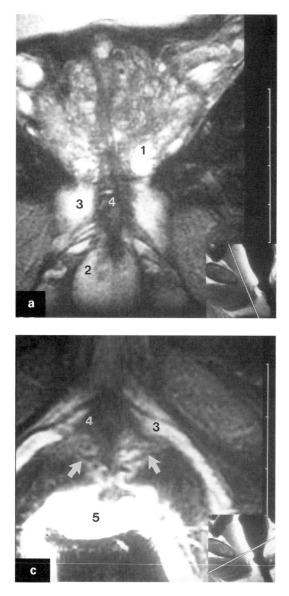

Figure 1 Endorectal coil magnetic resonance images of the prostate, membranous urethra and striated urethral sphincter. (a) Coronal cut through mid-striated urethral sphincter with sagittal inset for localization of coronal cut. Distance from apex of prostate to bulb approximately 2 cm. (b) Coronal cut, posterior to (a), to show urethral wall extending up into prostate apex to level of seminal colliculus (arrow). (c) Axial cut through membranous urethra at base of striated sphincter. Note stranding posterior to urethra, which probably represents deep transverse perineus (arrows). Sagittal inset shows angle of axial cut. 1, prostate; 2, bulb; 3, anterior recess of ischioanal fossa; 4, striated urethral sphincter; 5, endorectal coil

muscle and elastic tissue segment almost invariably does. The use of large resectoscope sheaths or sounds may cause, from overstretching, irreversible damage to the smooth muscle/elastic tissue architecture of this important urethral segment.

The mucosa does not possess any substantial sphincteric quality, but with its folds and the urethra in the collapsed state it provides, together with intact outer elements, a measure of flow resistance. An intact, healthy mucosa may be responsible for the success of submucosal collagen injection for the treatment of post-prostatectomy incontinence.

The goal in radical prostatectomy is to preserve all tissues responsible for continence. In addition to the above primary tissue, fascial support and the neurovascular structures serving the continence mechanism should be preserved whenever possible.

If an RPP is performed correctly, it is potentially superior to an RRP with respect to achieving urinary control. The reason for this lies in the fact that there is far less disturbance of the above-named tissues. There is no disturbance of the dorsal vein complex and anterior nerves[10], anterior arteries, prostatic venous plexus, or striated urethral sphincter. During the course of uneventful RPP, none of these structures are ever really seen or appreciated. The proper line of urethral transection is proximal to the most posterior midline prostate, which is retracted slightly to allow an approximately 0.5 cm cuff of urethral wall to remain intact with the urethral stump[11]. The only threat to continence, other than improper perineal entry and exposure, lies in malplacement of sutures during anastomosis,

gobbling up and destroying precious sphincter and urethra distal to the point of transection.

It is said that the anastomosis of the bladder to urethra in RPP is easy because the urethral stump is obvious, quite visible and a simple matter to expose for the placement of suture material; but this is not always the case. One straightforward anastomosis under the circumstances is a modified Vest anastomosis, bringing bladder neck sutures onto the perineum and tying them over a roll of soft sponge material (Figure 2). This maneuver places no sutures in a position to reduce functional residual urethral length by ensnaring striated urethral sphincter. The exposed posterior half of the urethra can be approximated with simple sutures to the bladder to close any posterior gap left by the

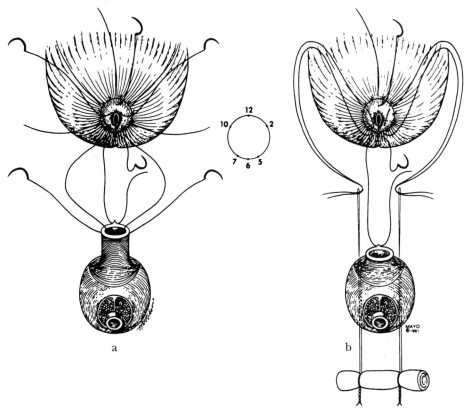

Figure 2 (a) Simple sutures at 2, 5, 6, 7, 10 and 12 o'clock of 00 chromic catgut after vesical neck plication and urinary bladder mucosal eversion in case of long membranous urethra. (b) Modified Vest technique: 00 chromic catgut simple sutures at 12 and 6 o'clock with lateral full bladder wall thickness sutures of monofilament, absorbable 0 polydioxanone brought out through perineum along side of short membranous urethra and tied over soft sponge material as traction

laterally placed Vest sutures after they have been tied over the sponge roll.

There would appear to be a minimum length of residual urethra for the establishment of continence at approximately 1 cm. At least 1.5 cm is optimal and residual length less than 1.5 cm seems to be associated with increasing degrees of stress incontinence. If there is any damage to the urethral wall (intrinsic mechanism) in addition to reduced length, the likelihood of total incontinence increases dramatically.

Magnetic resonance imaging (MRI) demonstrates that the membranous urethra with its coat of striated muscle sits within and is flanked by levator muscle of the pelvic diaphragm. The membranous urethra extends both above and below the pelvic diaphragm. Below the pelvic diaphragm on the way to the bulb, the membranous urethra is flanked by the anterior recess of each ischioanal fossa with its fibrofatty content including neurovascular tissue.

In RRP, the levator muscle is pushed laterally away from the prostatourethral junction after the endopelvic (supradiaphragmatic) fascia has been opened just lateral to the tendinous fascial arch of the pelvis. Once this is accomplished and urethral transection performed properly, the residual urethra will appear to extend superiorly above the pelvic diaphragm, and suture placement for anastomosis is facilitated and often aided by externally applied perineal pressure. The goal in the anterior dissection of RRP is to come down properly at the prostatourethral junction a few millimeters distal to the apex of the prostate, to expose the urethra. At the same time, the apical prostate must not be incised thereby jeopardizing a negative margin of resection by leaving residual cancer. Like RPP, the prostate in RRP can be retracted gently prior to urethral transection so that a 0.5-cm cuff of urethral wall is left with the visible striated urethral sphincter.

What confounds the anterior dissection of RRP, but not RPP, is variation in prostate shape at the apex[7,12,13]. In RPP, one has only to follow the obvious apical prostate boundary forward around the urethra, so that it makes no difference what contour is encountered. However, in RRP the presence of the anterolateral dorsal vein complex obfuscates the approach to the prostatomembranous urethral junction. Asymmetry and the presence of an anterior or posterior apical notch cannot be readily appreciated until the dorsal vein complex has been ligated and divided. If the dissection comes down too far distally, apical shape variations can be missed entirely. Furthermore, BPH and overlap of the membranous urethra by the prostate interfere with urethral exposure and tend to put the operator too far distally. This then may result in an inadvertently short urethral stump after urethral transection, with resultant urinary incontinence.

Retrograde urethrography is an inexpensive way to look at the anatomy associated with the distal continence zone. Such study provides quick assessment of the distance from veru to bulb, which is variable from about 1.2 cm to 3 cm (R. P. Myers, unpublished data). Placement of the veru within the prostatic urethra is variable with respect to the most distal posterior aspect of the prostate. At times, the distal border of the veru lies flush with the most distal prostate, in which case there is no urethral crest distal to the veru. Usually associated with the absence of BPH, this configuration is associated with very short membranous urethras and dissection at surgery must proceed with great caution. In order to leave sufficient length in the urethral stump, transection of the urethra has to be absolutely flush with the most posterior prostate. There is no way short of preoperative retrograde urethrography to know about this configuration. The endoscopic identification of this type of prostate is possible, but in general urethroscopy is not performed routinely prior to radical prostatectomy. It is clear that this type of prostate could be responsible for the fact that some patients are reported to be totally incontinent after surgery. The way to be wary is to perform retrograde urethrography on all patients prior to RRP. This should not be an issue for the patient undergoing RPP.

In a previously reported series[14], 172 consecutive patients underwent RRP for localized prostate cancer. Each patient underwent preoperative retrograde urethrography. Any patient with a veru-to-bulb length greater than 1.5 cm underwent a simple sutured mucosa-to-mucosa anastomosis, and any patient with a veru-to-bulb length of 1.5 cm or less, or who had a visibly short urethra at the time of surgery, underwent a modified Vest anastomosis (Figure 2). All patients were followed prospectively and each was asked to report the date when they stopped using a protective pad for postoperative wetting. This allowed the use of the Kaplan–Meier estimator to construct time in days from catheter removal to pad-free urinary continence (Figure 3a and b). A smooth asymptotic curve was achieved for the 170 evaluable patients showing 10% immediately dry on catheter removal, 35% at 2 weeks, 47% at 1 month, 81% at 4 months, 87% at 6 months and 94% at 1 year. By September 1991, there were only eight patients who required pads: six using one pad/day for minimal stress incontinence and two using two pads/day for mild stress incontinence. In follow-up, these patients tended not to improve after September 1991. Therefore, 5% of the 170 remained minimally pad-dependent. No patient experienced serious incontinence according to the above strategy for type of anastomosis based on estimating membranous urethral length either by preoperative retrograde urethrography or by intraoperative judgment as to available urethral stump length.

There were two additional findings: (1) time to pad-free continence was the same for the direct, sutured anastomosis ($n = 88$) as it was for the Vest anastomosis ($n = 82$); and (2) there was no influence in time to pad-free continence whether or not neurovascular preservation, either bilateral or unilateral, took place as compared to deliberate sacrifice of the neurovascular tissue left with the specimen as a result of wide resection (Figure 3c).

This study sought to establish the best possible continence rate by paying particular attention to the length of the membranous urethra. It was considered that patients with short membranous urethras might sustain less reduction of residual functional urethral length from damage due to suture material if they were

subjected to a Vest anastomosis than if they had undergone direct sutured anastomosis. The incidence of vesical neck contracture was higher at 10% with the Vest anastomosis than the direct anastomosis at 2%, presumably a function of

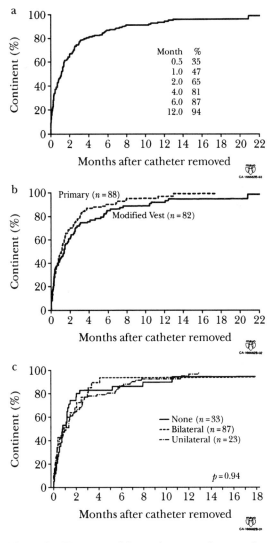

Figure 3 Time to pad-free urinary continence after radical retropubic prostatectomy: (a) all patients ($n = 170$); (b) primary suture anastomosis ($n = 88$) compared to modified Vest technique ($n = 82$); (c) comparison of bilateral, unilateral and no neurovascular preservation with respect to time to pad-free continence. Total does not account for 27 patients, because precise information about neurovascular preservation was not stated in surgical dictation

better mucosa-to-mucosa approximation in the direct anastomosis.

The tubular nature of the membranous urethra within its supporting fascia has been addressed and is a very important concept with respect to radical prostatectomy. MRI makes it patently clear that the concept of a 'urogenital diaphragm' or muscle sandwich[15] does not apply in the proper conduct of RRP. The classic description of a 'urogenital diaphragm' erroneously puts the entire striated urethral sphincter between two fascial plates – superior and inferior – the latter plate the perineal membrane. Illustrations of a urogenital diaphragm[16] are in gross error and bear no relationship to proper, artifact-free gross dissection and MRI in living subjects. Anastomotic techniques should not be guided by the concept of a urogenital diaphragm.

In summary, the obvious, simple key to a patient's achieving urinary control after either RRP or RPP is the least disturbance of the tissues related to urinary continence by the surgeon during surgery.

References

1. Hodges, C. V. (1977). Vesicourethral anastomosis after radical prostatectomy: experience with the Jewett modifications. *J. Urol.*, **118**, 209–10
2. Rudy, D. C., Woodside, J. R. and Crawford, E. D. (1984). Urodynamic evaluation of incontinence in patients undergoing modified Campbell radical retropubic prostatectomy: a prospective study. *J. Urol.*, **132**, 708–12
3. Fowler, F. J., Barry, M. J., Lu-Yao, G., Roman, A., Wasson, J. and Wennberg, J. E. (1993). Patient-reported complications and follow-up treatment after radical prostatectomy. *Urology*, **42**, 622–9
4. Lerner, S. E., Blute, M. L. and Zincke, H. (1995). Critical evaluation of salvage surgery for radio-recurrent/resistant prostate cancer. *J. Urol.*, **154**, 1103–9
5. Turner-Warwick, R. (1983). The sphincter mechanisms: their relation to prostatic enlargement and its treatment. In Hinman, F. Jr (ed.) *Benign Prostatic Hypertrophy*, pp. 809–28. (New York: Springer-Verlag)
6. Gil Vernet, S. (1968). *Morphology and Function of Vesico-prostato-urethral Musculature.* (Treviso: Canova)
7. Myers, R. P. (1994). Radical prostatectomy: pertinent surgical anatomy. *Atlas of Urol. Clin. North Am.*, **22**, 1–18
8. Myers, R. P. (1991). Male urethral sphincteric anatomy and radical prostatectomy. *Urol. Clin. North Am.*, **18**, 211–27
9. Krahn, H. P. and Morales, P. A. (1965). The effect of pudendal nerve anaesthesia on urinary continence after prostatectomy. *J. Urol.*, **94**, 282–5
10. Narayan, P., Konety, B., Aslam, K., Aboseif, S. Blumenfeld, W. and Tanagho, E. (1995). Neuroanatomy of external urethral sphincter: implications for urinary continence preservation during radical prostate surgery. *J. Urol.*, **153**, 337–41
11. Hudson, P. D. (1970). Perineal prostatectomy. In Campbell, M. F. and Harrison, J. H. (eds.) *Campbell's Urology*, pp. 2419–78. (Philadelphia: Saunders)
12. Myers, R. P., Goellner, J. R. and Cahill, D. R. (1987). Prostate shape, external striated urethral sphincter and radical prostatectomy: the apical dissection. *J. Urol.*, **138**, 543–50
13. Myers, R. P. (1994). Practical pelvic anatomy pertinent to radical retropubic prostatectomy. *AUA Update Series*, **13** (4), 26–32
14. Myers, R. P. (1995). Radical retropubic prostatectomy: balance between preserving urinary continence and achievement of negative margins. *Eur. Urol.*, **27** (Suppl. 2), 32–3
15. Colapinto, V. (1984). The anatomy of the distal urethral sphincters and the myth of the urogenital sandwich: Part 2. *J. Urol.*, **131**, 164A
16. Netter, F. H. (1989). *Atlas of Human Anatomy. Pelvis and Perineum*, plate 361. (New Jersey: Summit)

Incontinence after radical prostatectomy: a review of the urodynamic perspective

10

J. L. Mostwin

Introduction

Prior to the recent increase in surgical treatment of prostate cancer, post-prostatectomy incontinence was limited to men undergoing surgery for benign disease. Leakage was assumed to be due to sphincteric injury, and the appearance of an effective artificial urinary sphincter prosthesis all but eliminated research into basic mechanisms of post-prostatectomy incontinence. The rise of urodynamic specialization within urology permitted attention to be directed to the study of these patients. Many were found to have bladder dysfunction manifested by instability, poor compliance or reduced contractility. As urodynamic understanding of the pathophysiology of bladder outlet obstruction grew, it was felt that, in most cases, postoperative incontinence was due less to sphincteric damage than to bladder dysfunction, which was unmasked rather than caused by simple prostatectomy. More recent studies of incontinence after simple prostatectomy continue to support this widely held impression[1].

The availability of serum prostate specific antigen testing, transrectal guided sonographic needle biopsy and improved anatomic techniques in radical retropubic prostatectomy have led to a surge in radical prostatectomy with growing public awareness of the problem and demand for high-quality treatment preserving quality of life. Indeed, the raging battle over outcomes and quality of life determination in evaluation of treatments for what is widely held to be a slow-growing tumor of moderate life-threatening potential has sharpened the focus of concern on the two major postoperative complications of radical prostatectomy: impotence and incontinence.

Estimates of post-prostatectomy incontinence

In 1993, The American College of Surgeons (ACS) Commission on Cancer reviewed the reported results of 2122 patients treated by radical prostatectomy performed at 484 institutions in 1990 to obtain an overall impression of the success of surgical treatment for the disease[2]. These results were obtained from the treating physicians, not from patients themselves. The reported outcomes with respect to urinary continence are shown in Table 1.

In 1992, Fowler and colleagues[3] published the results of an outcomes study with considerably different results. In this series of Medicare patients (aged > 65) surveyed by mail, telephone and personal interview, over 30% reported currently wearing pads or clamps to

Table 1 Results of 2122 patients treated by radical prostatectomy at 484 institutions in 1990. Reports reviewed by American College of Surgeons Commission on Cancer[2]

Continence status	Patients	
	n	%
Complete control	1042	58.0
Occasional, no pads	415	23.1
Daily, two pads	201	11.2
Daily, more than two pads	73	4.1
Total incontinence	65	3.6

deal with wetness; over 40% said that they dripped urine when they coughed or when their bladders were full; 23% reported daily wetting of more than a few drops. Six per cent had surgery after the radical prostatectomy, to treat incontinence.

In an editorial reviewing both reports, Walsh[4] questioned the Medicare interview studies and considered the ACS results to show 81.1% complete continence. He noted that 40% of the men in the ACS series had stage C or D disease, which might reduce the opportunity for better postoperative continence. In reviewing several reports from centers with broad experience, he noted that the possibility of significant urinary incontinence was low (2–5%) and the need for artificial sphincter was rare (0–0.5%)[4]. In a further report of 593 consecutive patients treated at Johns Hopkins Hospital, complete urinary control was achieved in 92% and stress incontinence was present in 8%. There were 6% who wore one or fewer pads per day and stress incontinence was severe enough to require placement of an artificial sphincter in two men (0.3%). Of patients older than 70 years, 86% were completely dry[5]. In the most recent patients reported ($n = 700$), in 1993, no one required an artificial sphincter. Eight men with the most severe incontinence wore more than one pad per day[6].

Talcot and co-workers[7] reported that of 196 patients treated at Harvard University (75% of treated patients who returned a completed questionnaire), 39 (20%) felt that their postoperative urinary continence was excellent, the same as before surgery; 80 (41%) considered control good (no pads); 61 (31%) were fair (wore pads or some type of external appliances, but were not limited in social activities); and 16 (8%) reported poor control with continuous leaking and limitation of social activities.

Geary and associates[8] reported a higher general rate of incontinence at Stanford, determined by asking patients how many pads they wore. Of 458 patients with adequate follow-up to determine recovery of continence, 80.1% required no pads, 8.1% required one to two pads a day, 6.6% required three to five pads a day,

and 5.2% were totally incontinent 1 year or more after surgery. Incontinence was closely associated with postoperative urinary urgency.

A telephone interview was conducted with 247 men who had undergone radical retropubic prostatectomy from January 1990 to June 1993 at the University of Southern California in Los Angeles[9]. A total of 55% stated that they leaked some urine at least once a week; 9.9% felt that the leakage caused moderate to severe interference with daily activities; and 29.9% said that it was at least somewhat upsetting. Most patients wore none (59.9%) or one (14.5%) pad per day. A total of 73.7% of patients reported good to excellent quality of life; 79.1% said that they would recommend surgical treatment of prostate cancer.

There may be significant discrepancy between self-reported and objectively evaluated estimates of incontinence. Morten and associates[10] reported on the results of a 24-h pad test at various intervals after prostatectomy: incontinence was found in 8% of the patients prior to surgery, 79% 1 month after surgery, 64% 3 months after surgery and 43% 6 months after surgery. The proportions of patients reporting problems with continence were 25% prior to surgery, 92% 1 month after, 81% 3 months after and 50% 6 months after surgery. When directly questioned, 50% reported leaking only a few drops, a significant discrepancy between subjective perception and pad weights.

Prompted by the discrepancies between the Medicare report[11] and the reports from centers of excellence, Litweiler and colleagues[12] reviewed continence results from 467 radical prostatectomies performed by 22 different private attending urologists in a community hospital in Texas. Of those questioned by telephone survey by an independent interviewer, 23% had been continent since surgery, 18.2% achieved delayed continence and 58.5% were still incontinent at the time of interview. The majority of incontinent patients had stress incontinence (77.5%) while 59.8% had urge incontinence and 27.7% leaked only drops, and less than once a day. The authors concluded that these outcomes, better than the Fowler estimates, but not as good as the reports of centers of excellence, were more representative of what private practitioners in America could expect with their patients.

Estimates of post-prostatectomy continence may therefore vary widely, depending on how soon after surgery the results are reported, the experience of the operating surgeons and center reporting the results, the definitions of continence, the method of interview and record retrieval, and the consideration of subjective vs. objective results. Recalling these differences helps when urodynamic reports are reviewed.

Anatomical considerations and potential sources of injury

The sphincter of the male, its exact location and innervation, and the best ways to preserve its function remain an intense source of discussion and speculation.

It is generally agreed that the striated sphincter of the male consists of slow-twitch type I fibers, which are adapted for tonic closure and passive continence[13]. Levator ani muscles, which insert on the prostate and proximal urethra as these structures pass through the levator hiatus, consist of fast-twitch phasic type II muscles. These provide temporary elevation and interruption of the urinary stream. It is well known that this levator and contraction activity can reciprocally inhibit unstable bladder contractions, and the technique is widely taught to women with stress incontinence and bladder instability. It is also generally appreciated that many men with post-prostatectomy incontinence can interrupt their stream during voiding but have impaired passive continence, suggesting type I muscle injury.

Anatomical studies[14,15] have emphasized that the urethral sphincter is tubular and invests the urethra circumferentially from the pubis to the bladder neck, and that the frequently described planar diaphragm on which the prostate sits like a spinning toy top is imaginary. Recognizing the importance of these findings, Myers and co-workers[16] have drawn attention to the variability of prostatic apical anatomy and the possible

consequences of excessive sphincter ablation when dividing the prostate with a poorly developed anterior commissure evenly with the posterior margin of the gland. Myers has also suggested that some men may have congenitally short urethral sphincters, which may function well enough while supplemented by additional functional length of the prostatic urethra but, when shortened after prostatectomy, these urethrae may fall below a critical level of functional length[17]. Concern about apical surgical margins prevents widespread application of these insights at this time.

The innervation of the periurethral striated sphincters is by the pudendal nerve travelling beneath the levator ani to branch within the pelvis[18] and beneath the pubis[19]. The subpubic branches separate from the subpubic portion of the dorsal nerve of the penis after its separation from the pudendal nerve. The branches migrate in a retrograde manner toward the sphincteric urethra. Whether these fibers are motor or sensory has not been determined and their role in post-prostatectomy incontinence remains to be clarified. These fibers could easily be injured during excessive traction on the subpubic urethra at the time of apical dissection or during excessive cautery or suture placement when an attempt is being made to control bleeding from the dorsal vein complex.

Urodynamic studies: bladder or urethral dysfunction?

The primary role of urodynamic studies has been to determine whether bladder or sphincter dysfunction is responsible for post-prostatectomy incontinence. In reviewing published studies, it is essential to clarify whether patients who underwent radical prostatectomy for cancer were considered separately from those who underwent treatment for benign prostatic hyperplasia: the latter group is well known to suffer from more bladder dysfunction.

Walsh and co-workers[6] reviewed continence in a series of 700 consecutive radical prostatectomies. No-one was sufficiently incontinent to require an artificial sphincter. Eight men with the most severe incontinence requiring more than one pad per day were evaluated. The average bladder capacity was 450 ml. None had uninhibited bladder contractions. There was no correlation between potency and continence and no correlation between continence and preservation or removal of one or both neurovascular bundles. The authors concluded that anatomic factors rather than preservation of autonomic innervation were responsible for post-prostatectomy incontinence.

Chao and Mayo[20] reviewed the video-urodynamic records of 74 men referred for incontinence after radical prostatectomy. Of these, 57% had sphincter weakness alone; 39% had combined sphincter weakness and evidence of detrusor instability and/or decreased compliance. Only 4% had detrusor instability alone. Of the patients, 42% voided by abdominal straining without evidence of intrinsic bladder contraction. The authors concluded that detrusor abnormalities are rarely the sole cause of incontinence, with sphincter weakness being present in 96%.

In an electromyographic study of motor units of the periurethral striated sphincter in ten men after radical prostatectomy, seven of whom were continent, all showed evidence of loss of motor units and diminished electromyographic activity[21].

Hammerer and co-workers[22] performed thorough urodynamic evaluation in 53 of 88 men who underwent radical prostatectomy. The results are shown in Table 2. Although there were slight changes in bladder capacity and threshold for voiding, there was no statistically significant change in compliance. The dramatic findings concerned the changes in maximum urethral closure pressure and maximum voluntary urethral closure pressure. The authors noted additionally that incontinent men showed a significantly smaller functional profile length (21.5 vs. 29.9 mm) and a lower maximal urethral closure pressure (51.3 vs. 67.7 cmH_2O) than did continent men.

In contrast to the studies reviewed so far which provide urodynamic evidence that sphincteric incompetence is the most likely cause of incontinence after radical prostatectomy, several other studies have suggested that bladder dysfunction may be a significant factor.

Goluboff and associates[23] evaluated 56 men with post-prostatectomy incontinence, 31 after transurethral and 25 after radical prostatectomy. Detrusor instability alone was present in 34 patients (61%), including 24 (77%) after transurethral resection of the prostate and ten (40%) after radical retropubic prostatectomy. Stress incontinence alone was present in only three patients (5%), including one (3%) after transurethral resection of the prostate and two (8%) after radical retropubic prostatectomy. Detrusor instability with stress incontinence was present in 19 patients (34%), including six (19%) after transurethral resection of the prostate and 13 (52%) after radical retropubic prostatectomy. Of these 19 patients, four (21%)

Table 2 Urodynamic evaluation of 53 men who had undergone radical prostatectomy. From reference 22

Parameter	Preoperatively	6–8 weeks postoperatively	p-Value
Bladder volume (ml) at initial contraction	281 ± 97.7	225 ± 75.7	< 0.01
Maximum bladder volume (ml)	394.2 ± 116.9	306 ± 100	< 0.001
Compliance (ml/cmH$_2$O)	133.5 ± 104	73.2 ± 86.1	NS
Functional profile length (mm)	62 ± 11.3	26.2 ± 8.5	< 0.001
Maximum urethral closure (cmH$_2$O)	89.5 ± 26.5	64.9 ± 16.9	< 0.001
Maximum urethral closure (cmH$_2$O) during voluntary contraction	124.1 ± 42.2	103 ± 43.4	< 0.02
Residual urine volume (ml)	43.3 ± 56.6	6.1 ± 19.2	NS
Maximum flow rate (ml/s)	14.6 ± 7.3	21.5 ± 11.6	< 0.001

NS, non significant

had poorly compliant bladders. These authors concluded that detrusor instability was much more likely to be the cause of incontinence than was sphincteric weakness.

In an editorial comment regarding this report, Leach drew attention to the high prevalence of bladder instability and decreased compliance he had found in post-prostatectomy patients, many of whom had undergone radical prostatectomy[24,25]. Referring to a more recent prospective study of 26 men before and 3, 6 and 12 months after radical prostatectomy, he noted a high incidence of *de novo* bladder instability in the incontinent patients[26]. This would be in contrast to the findings in patients studied an average of 3.8 years after surgery in whom a much lower incidence of bladder dysfunction was found[20].

Could preoperative urodynamic testing improve surgical results by identifying patients at risk of developing postoperative bladder dysfunction? Aboseif and colleagues[27] examined 92 men preoperatively and followed them for a year after surgery. Two main groups of patients were found: group 1 ($n = 64$) patients with normal urodynamic findings, and group 2 ($n = 28$) patients with abnormal urodynamic findings. The latter group was further subdivided according to the abnormality: detrusor instability ($n = 12$), weak sphincter mechanism ($n = 9$) and detrusor and sphincter instability ($n = 7$). There was a substantial difference in the incidence of urinary incontinence between the two main groups, with only two patients with incontinence in group 1 (3%) vs. 11 patients in group 2 (39%). In addition, the incidence of incontinence in group 2 differed depending on the type of abnormality: the lower incidence occurred in patients with detrusor instability (17%) and the higher incidence in patients with both detrusor and sphincter instability (71%). Identification of sphincteric and bladder dysfunction preoperatively may indicate a high risk of urinary incontinence after radical prostatectomy; but should such patients be excluded from potentially curative treatment on the basis of preoperative urodynamic testing?

Experience with the artificial sphincter

Experience with the artificial sphincter for the treatment of post-prostatectomy incontinence would support the view that treatment of sphincteric incompetence alone can produce satisfactory results in the majority of patients. The experience suggests that the bladder function that may co-exist has been under-reported, or has not significantly affected the outcome with artificial sphincters.

In 75 unselected patients with post-prostatectomy incontinence, a follow-up of different patients with adverse features for implantation of an artificial sphincter, including 44 with bladder hyperactivity and 11 with previous radiation therapy, found that there was no significant difference between the patients with and those without adverse features with respect to satisfaction with urinary control[28].

Fishman and co-workers[29] reported on 112 men as part of a larger series, reporting 90% overall socially acceptable continence rates. Patients with post-prostatectomy incontinence were among those with the best success rates.

Malloy and colleagues[30] reported on 42 incontinent men treated with the AMS 800 sphincter, with a mean follow-up of 26.2 months. Thirty-two (76%) were completely continent. Four (9%) had minimal to moderate stress incontinence. Two (5%) were unable to manipulate the device secondary to physical and/or mental incapacity. Four (9%) required removal and two received successful replacements. There were no reports of bladder dysfunction.

Seventeen patients who were continent after AMS insertion were investigated by profilometry[31]. No bladder dysfunction was reported.

The model AMS 800 artificial urinary sphincter was implanted in 117 patients referred to the Mayo Clinic for urinary incontinence resulting from radical prostatectomy[32]. The indication for implantation was total incontinence in 107 patients and stress incontinence in ten. A follow-up questionnaire indicated a 90% significantly improved continence rate and a 90% satisfaction rate among patients. Sixty-four surgical revisions were required in 37 patients for mechanical malfunction. There were no reports of bladder dysfunction.

In 1985, Furlow and Barrett reported on late complications after implantation of an artificial sphincter[33]. Detrusor hyperreflexia was mentioned as a confounding factor, but no case reports were presented. Earlier they had reported their experience with the AS791 prosthetic sphincter in 66 patients with post-radical prostatectomy[34]. When the 22 patients who had previous pelvic radiation therapy were excluded, 41 (93%) were continent. Webster and Sihelnik[35] also reviewed the experience with a malfunctioning artificial sphincter. Detrusor hyperreflexia was mentioned in the differential diagnosis of complications causing post-implantation malfunction, but all the cases reviewed were of mechanical malfunction and there were no cases of bladder dysfunction described.

In 1984 Diokno and associates[36] reviewed the experience in 30 patients implanted before 1982, for a minimum follow-up of 1 year and an average follow-up of 3.7 years. Twenty-one (70%) had a functioning sphincter: 17 were continent and four required one pad per day. Erosion and infection were causes of malfunction. Bladder dysfunction was mentioned as a possible cause, but like the three previous studies, patients with severe bladder dysfunction might have been excluded from initial implantation. However, if one were to assume that unexpected bladder dysfunction should cause post-implantation complications, these experienced authors should have been expected to have mentioned it.

Discussion and conclusions

Although definitions and rates of post-prostatectomy incontinence may vary considerably, most recent urodynamic analyses of post-radical prostatectomy incontinence would suggest that sphincter damage is a significant contributing factor. A smaller number of urodynamic reports suggest that bladder dysfunction may also be present. It is important to distinguish between patients with incontinence following prostatectomy for cancer and benign disease, as the latter group may have more accompanying pre-operative bladder dysfunction. Reported experience with the artificial urinary sphincter would support the conclusion that treatment of sphincteric competence results in good management of post-radical prostatectomy incontinence. There are several possible ways in which the operating surgeon can imagine injuring the sphincter; it is less clear how the bladder itself would be injured.

Even though the reported incidence of bladder dysfunction after radical prostatectomy is limited to a few studies, its potential contribution to the overall problem should not be excluded. It is possible that post-prostatectomy sphincteric incompetence facilitates bladder dysfunction in three ways: (1) a weakened sphincter may be less likely to provide the necessary recruitment and reciprocal inhibition characteristic of the storage phase of the normal bladder; (2) urine distending an incompetent proximal urethra can provoke a feeling of impending urination and a bladder contraction; and (3) poor compliance may be evident in a chronically under-distended bladder.

Regardless of etiology, post-prostatectomy incontinence is a serious complication that, if sufficiently prevalent and uncontrolled, could lead to significant objection against surgical treatment of limited prostatic cancer, for the very group in whom cure is most likely to be achieved. For this reason, every effort should be made to determine the relative contributions of sphincteric and bladder damage to the etiology of this problem, and further refinements in anatomical understanding, surgical technique, accurate epidemiological reporting and further urodynamic testing of patients before and after surgery should be encouraged. Finally, improved outcome studies examining the consequences of incontinence and its true effect on quality of life must be undertaken if the problem is to be placed in a clinically useful and meaningful perspective.

References

1. Seaman, E. K., Jacobs, B. Z., Blaivas, J. G. and Kaplan, S. A. (1994). Persistence or recurrence of symptoms after transurethral resection of the prostate: a urodynamic assessment. *J. Urol.*, **152**, 935–7

2. Murphy, G. P., Mettlin, C., Mench, H., Winchester, D. P. and Davidson, A. M. (1993). National patterns of prostate cancer treatment by radical prostatectomy: results of a survey by the American College of Surgeons Commission on Cancer. *J. Urol.*, **152**, 1817–19

3. Fowler, F. J. Jr, Barry, M. J., Lu-Yao, G., Roman, A., Wasson, J. and Wennberg, J. E. (1993). Patient-reported complications and follow-up treatment after radical prostatectomy. The National Medicare Experience: 1988–1990 (updated June 1993). *Urology*, **42**, 622–9

4. Walsh, P. C. (1994). Editorial: the status of radical prostatectomy in the United States in 1993: where do we go from here. *J. Urol.*, **152**, 1816

5. Steiner, M. S., Morton, R. A. and Walsh, P. C. (1991). Impact of anatomical radical prostatectomy on urinary continence. *J. Urol.*, **145**, 512

6. Walsh, P. C., Partin, A. W. and Epstein, J. I. (1994). Cancer control and quality of life following anatomical radical retropubic prostatectomy: results at ten years. *J. Urol.*, **152**, 1831–6

7. Talcott, J. A., Richie, J. P. and Loughlin, K. A. (1993). Incontinence following radical prostatectomy: assessment by patient survey. *J. Urol.*, **149**, 234A

8. Geary, E. S., Dendinger, T. E., Freiha, F. S. and Stamey, T. A. (1995). Incontinence and vesical neck strictures following radical retropubic prostatectomy (Review). *Urology*, **45**, 1000–6

9. Skinner, E. C., Perez, M., Lieskovsky, G., Reynolds, B., Skinner, D. G. and Meterowitz, B. (1995). Quality of life following radical prostatectomy for carcinoma of the prostate. *J. Urol.*, **153**, 506A

10. Morten, J., Madsen, F. A., Rhodes, P. R. and Bruskewitz, R. C. (1995). Urinary incontinence in patients undergoing radical prostatectomy. *J. Urol.*, **153**, 506A

11. Fowler, F. J., Barry, M. J., Lu Yau, G., Roman, A., Wasson, J. and Wennberg, J. E. (1993). Patient-reported complications and follow-up treatment after radical prostatectomy. *Urology*, **42**, 622

12. Litweiler, S. E., Djavan, B., Richier, J. C., Schnitzer, B. and Roehrborn, C. G. (1995). Radical retropubic prostatectomy in a community practice setting: analysis of long-term outcomes, continence and potency rates, and retreatment rates. *J. Urol.*, **193**, 252A

13. Gosling, J. A., Dixon, J. S., Critchley, H. O. and Thompson, S. A. (1981). A comparative study of the human external sphincter and periurethral levator ani muscles. *Br. J. Urol.*, **53**, 35–41

14. Oelrich, T. M. (1980). The urethral sphincter muscle in the male. *Am. J. Anat.*, **158**, 229–46

15. de Leval, J., Chantraine, A. and Penders, L. (1984). [The striated sphincter of the urethra. 1: Recall of knowledge on the striated sphincter of the urethra] (French). *J. Urol.*, **90**, 439–54

16. Myers, R. P., Goellner, J. R. and Cahill, D. R. (1987). Prostate shape, external striated urethral sphincter and radical prostatectomy: the apical dissection. *J. Urol.*, **138**, 543–50

17. Myers, R. P. (1991). Male urethral sphincter anatomy and radical prostatectomy. *Urol. Clin. North Am.*, **18**, 211–25

18. Zvara, P., Carrier, S., Kour, N. W. and Tanagho, E. A. (1994). The detailed neuroanatomy of the human striated urethral sphincter (see comments). *Br. J. Urol.*, **74**, 182–7

19. Narayan, P., Konety, B., Aslam, K., Aboseif, S., Blumenfled, W. and Tanagho, E. (1995). Neuroanatomy of the external urethral sphincter: implications for urinary continence preservation during radical prostate surgery (see comments). *J. Urol.*, **153**, 337–41

20. Chao, R. and Mayo, M. E. (1995). Incontinence after radical prostatectomy: detrusor or sphincter causes (see comments). *J. Urol.*, **154**, 16–18

21. Prieto Chaparro, L., Jimenez Jimenez, F. J., Rodriguez de Bethencourt, F., Dehaini Dehaini, A., Hontoria Briso, J., Guil Cid, M., Cruces de Abia, F., Lera Fernandez, R., Salinas Casado, J. and Sanchez Chapado, M. (1994). [Radical prostatectomy: usefulness of selective electromyography of the periurethral sphincter in the assessment of urinary continence] (Spanish). *Arch. Espanoles Urol.*, **47**, 483–7

22. Hammerer, P., Schuler, J., Gonnerman, D. and Huland, H. (1993). Urodynamic parameters before and after radical prostatectomy. *J. Urol.*, **149**, 235A

23. Goluboff, E. T., Chang, D. T., Olsson, C. A. and Kaplan, S. A. (1995). Urodynamics and the etiology of post-prostatectomy urinary incontinence: the initial Columbia experience (see comments). *J. Urol.* **153**, 1034–7

24. Leach, G. E., Yip, C. M. and Donovan, B. J. (1987). Post-prostatectomy incontinence: the

influence of bladder dysfunction. *J. Urol.*, **138**, 574–8

25. Leach, G. E. (1995). Post-prostatectomy incontinence: the importance of bladder dysfunction [editorial; comment]. *J. Urol.*, **153**, 1038

26. Foote, J., Yun, S. K. and Leach, G. E. (1991). Post-prostatectomy incontinence: pathophysiology, evaluation and management. *Urol. Clin. North Am.*, **18**, 229

27. Aboseif, S. R., Konety, B., Schmidt, R. A., Goldfien, S. H., Tanagho, E. A. and Narayan, P. A. (1994). Preoperative urodynamic evaluation: does it predict the degree of urinary continence after radical retropubic prostatectomy? *Urol. Int.*, **53**, 68–73

28. Perez, L. M. and Webster, G. D. (1992). Successful outcome of artificial urinary sphincters in men with post-prostatectomy urinary incontinence despite adverse implantation features. *J. Urol.*, **148**, 1166–70

29. Fishman, I. J., Shabsigh, R. and Scott, F. B. (1989). Experience with the artificial urinary sphincter model AS800 in 148 patients. *J. Urol.*, **141**, 307–10

30. Malloy, T. R., Wein, A. J. and Carpiniello, V. L. (1989). Surgical success with AMS M800 GU sphincter for male incontinence. *Urology*, **33**, 274–6

31. Kil, P. J., De Vries, J. D., Van Kerrebroeck, P. E., Zwiers, W. and Debruyne, F. M. (1989). Factors determining the outcome following implantation of the AMS 800 artificial urinary sphincter. *Br. J. Urol.*, **64**, 586–9

32. Gundian, J. C., Barrett, D. M. and Parulkar, B. G. (1989). Mayo Clinic experience with use of the AMS800 artificial urinary sphincter for urinary incontinence following radical prostatectomy. *J. Urol.*, **142**, 1459–61

33. Furlow, W. L. and Barrett, D. M. (1985). Recurrent or persistent urinary incontinence in patients with the artificial urinary sphincter: diagnostic considerations and management. *J. Urol.*, **133**, 792–5

34. Barrett, D. M. and Furlow, W. L. (1983). Radical prostatectomy incontinence and the AS791 artificial urinary sphincter. *J. Urol.*, **129**, 528–30

35. Webster, G. D. and Sihelnik, S. A. (1984). Troubleshooting the malfunctioning Scott artificial urinary sphincter. *J. Urol.*, **131**, 269–72

36. Diokno, A. C., Sonda, L. P. and MacGregor, R. J. (1984). Long-term followup of the artificial urinary sphincter. *J. Urol.*, **131**, 1084–6

Trends in post-radical prostatectomy incontinence in Belgium and The Netherlands

11

J. L. H. R. Bosch

Urinary incontinence occurring after radical prostatectomy is a significant problem. The reported incidence of post-radical prostatectomy incontinence varies widely[1–4]. The main factors determining these reported percentages seem to be the definition of incontinence, the methodology used to determine the continence status of the patient, the duration of follow-up and the initial characteristics of the patient population.

The duration of follow-up is an important factor. The percentage of incontinent patients decreases dramatically in the first year of follow-up (Table 1). Immediately after removal of the stenting urethral catheter, more than 40–50% of the patients have serious difficulties with urinary control[2,3].

The tumor stage of the patient determines whether a nerve-sparing radical prostatectomy is feasible. Steiner and co-workers[1], describing the Johns Hopkins experience in 593 patients, have found no statistical differences in continence rates among patients with or without preservation of the neurovascular bundles.

The age of the patient may be another important factor. Patients over 70 years at the time of radical prostatectomy had a smaller chance of

Table 1 Evolution of post-radical prostatectomy incontinence in 188 patients. Experience at the Academic Hospital Rotterdam (data from reference 2)

	Incontinent
At removal of stenting catheter (3 weeks postoperatively)	107/188 (57%)
At 3-month follow-up	40/188 (21%)
At 1-year follow-up	24/170 (14%)

regaining continence in the Rotterdam series[2] (Table 2), although others have found that older patients regained continence less rapidly but eventually achieved continence rates comparable to those of younger patients[3].

The etiology of the problem is multifactorial. The major cause is impaired function of the external urethral sphincter, although detrusor instability and/or decreased compliance seems to be an additional major problem[5–7]. Conflicting data have been presented with regard to the percentage of patients with pure sphincteric weakness and detrusor instability with or without decreased compliance, or a combination of these features[5–7]. The reported percentage of post-radical prostatectomy incontinence patients with sphincteric weakness as the only cause has varied between 8 and 57%[5–7]. The percentage of those with sphincteric weakness

Table 2 Risk factors for incontinence in 188 radical prostatectomy patients. Experience at the Academic Hospital Rotterdam (data from reference 2)

	Statistics
Patient age (below 70 years vs. over 70 years)	$p = 0.02$
Anastomotic leakage	NS
Previous TURP	NS
Experience of surgeon	NS
Date (before 1987 vs. 1987; nerve-sparing)	$p = 0.02$
T stage (lower than T_3 vs. T_3 or higher)	NS
pT stage (lower than pT_3 versus pT_3 or higher)	NS

NS, not significant; TURP, transurethral resection of the prostate; T = clinical tumor stage; pT = pathological tumor stage in combination with other causes has varied between 39 and 52%[5–7]. All in all, sphincteric weakness is either the only cause or a major contributing cause in more than 80–85% of the patients. In the series of Leach and colleagues[5], 54 out of 102 patients incontinent after radical retropubic prostatectomy (53%), were treated by implantation of an artificial urinary sphincter.

In the National Medicare experience in the USA[4] it was found that 31% of patients 'wear pads, diapers or a penile clamp' after a radical prostatectomy (Table 3). In the series of Hautmann and associates[3] the percentage of patients using incontinence pads after more than 1 year of follow-up was 18.8%. In the Rotterdam series[2] this figure was 14.1% (Table 4). In the latter series 52% of the patients having to wear pads eventually underwent implantation of an artificial urinary sphincter. This is in agreement with the figure of 53% found by Leach and colleagues[5] in a series of 102 patients being incontinent after radical retropubic prostatectomy. On the basis of these figures one can

tentatively postulate that about half of the patients with post-radical prostatectomy incontinence severe enough to necessitate the use of protective pads are finally implanted with an artificial sphincter.

Data on the number of radical prostatectomies performed per year were obtained from the RIZIV (Rijksinstituut voor ziekte en invaliditeitsverzekering) for Belgium and from the SIG (Stichting informatiecentrum voor de gezondheidszorg) for The Netherlands. These numbers have increased significantly since 1987 (Figure 1). In Belgium 1294 radical prostatectomies were performed in 1993. In The Netherlands 433 radical prostatectomies were performed in 1994. The reason for the significant difference between these two countries is not clear. Data supplied by AMS Benelux show that the number of artificial sphincter implants in both countries increased along with the increase in the number of radical prostatectomies (Figure 2). The percentage of artificial sphincter implants that were inserted because of post-radical prostatectomy incontinence also increased in both countries (Figure 3). Between 1986 and 1995 the percentage of artificial sphincters implanted for post-radical prostatectomy incontinence increased from 19 to 59% in Belgium and from 14 to 42% in The Netherlands.

An artificial sphincter for post-radical prostatectomy incontinence is usually implanted

Table 3 Patient-reported incontinence after radical prostatectomy. The National Medicare experience in the USA (data from reference 4)

Report	%
'Some problem with wetness'	63
'Drip a few drops of urine every day'	47
'Wear pads, diapers or a penile clamp'	31
'Drip more than a few drops of urine *every* day'	23
'Had a surgical procedure to deal with incontinence'	6

Table 4 Severity of post-radical prostatectomy incontinence in patients with more than 1 year of follow-up. Experience at the Academic Hospital Rotterdam (data from reference 2)

	Proportion of patients
Grade 1 (two pads or less per day)	10/170 (5.9%)
Grade 2 (more than two pads per day)	14/170 (8.2%)
Grade 2, excluding patients incontinent prior to radical prostatectomy	11/170 (6.5%)
AMS 800 sphincter implants	11/170 (6.5%)

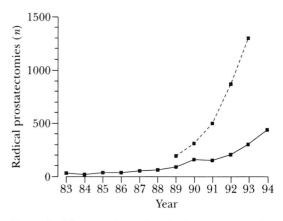

Figure 1 The number of radical prostatectomies per year in Belgium (dashed line) and The Netherlands (unbroken line)

96

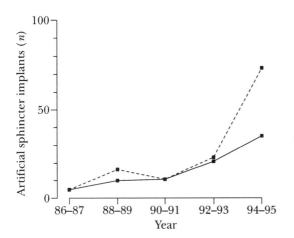

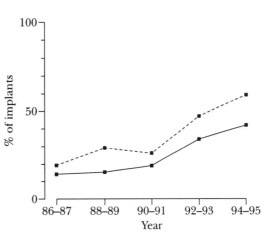

Figure 2 The number of artificial sphincter implants inserted because of post-radical prostatectomy incontinence in Belgium (dashed line) and The Netherlands (unbroken line)

Figure 3 Percentage of artificial sphincter implants inserted because of post-radical prostatectomy incontinence in Belgium (dashed line) and The Netherlands (unbroken line)

between 1 and 2 years after the radical prostatectomy. If the numbers of the radical prostatectomies are divided by the numbers of the sphincters implanted about 1 year later, the percentage of patients with incontinence severe enough to lead to implantation of an artificial sphincter can tentatively be calculated for both countries. For 1994–95 this figure is 4.7% for The Netherlands and 2.6% for Belgium. Based on previously published

results[2,5], these percentages should at least be doubled to come to the total percentage of men having to wear protective pads after the operation. The result of this calculation still gives very low incontinence rates. Because of the experience reported in the literature, it has to be assumed that these figures are far too low and that a significant rise in the number of implanted artificial sphincters can be expected in the near future.

References

1. Steiner, M. S., Morton, R. A. and Walsh, P. C. (1991). Impact of anatomical radical prostatectomy on urinary continence. *J. Urol.*, **145**, 512–15
2. Davidson, P. J. T., van den Ouden, D. and Schröder, F. H. (1996). Radical prostatectomy: prospective assessment of mortality and morbidity. *Eur. Urol.*, **29**, 168–73
3. Hautmann, R. E., Sauter, T. W. and Wenderoth, U. K. (1994). Radical retropubic prostatectomy: morbidity and urinary continence in 418 consecutive cases. *Urology*, **43** (Suppl. Febr.), 47–51
4. Fowler, F. J., Barry, M. J., Lu-Yao, G., Roman, A., Wasson, J. and Wennberg, J. E. (1993). Patient-reported complications and follow-up treatment after radical prostatectomy. The National Medicare experience: 1988–1990 (updated June 1993). *Urology*, **42**, 622–9
5. Leach, G. E., Trockman, B., Wong, A., Hamilton, J., Haab, F. and Zimmern, P. E. (1996). Post-prostatectomy incontinence: urodynamic findings and treatment outcomes. *J. Urol.*, **155**, 1256–9
6. Goluboff, E. T., Chang, D. T., Olsson, C. A. and Kaplan, S. A. (1995). Urodynamics and the etiology of post-prostatectomy urinary incontinence: the initial Columbia experience. *J. Urol.*, **153**, 1034–7
7. Chao, R. and Mayo, M. E. (1995). Incontinence after radical prostatectomy: detrusor or sphincter causes. *J. Urol.*, **154**, 16–18

Post-radical prostatectomy incontinence: treatment options and outcomes

12

F. Schreiter

Introduction

Radical prostatectomy is the therapy of choice for clinical localized prostate cancer. The postoperative incidence of incontinence varies from 0.5 to 40%[1,2]. This has a considerable psychosocial impact on the quality of life for these patients[3]. Geary and colleagues[4] provided more realistic data on their group of 450 patients, who underwent radical prostatectomy. Twelve months after radical prostatectomy, they found that 80% of the patients required no pads, 8% needed 1–2 pads, 7% needed 3–5 pads and 5% needed five pads or more. Only 2% were totally incontinent. In our own patients, we found 8.6% who required therapy for their postoperative incontinence

As regards the time for the return of continence, two-thirds of the patients became continent within 3 months, 20% within 6 months and 5% after 6 months.

There are many treatment options for postprostatectomy urinary incontinence, but there is no doubt that the implantation of an artificial sphincter (AS 800, American Medical Systems Inc.), which was developed and inaugurated in 1972 by Scott and associates[5,6] is the most reliable and most successful treatment in these patients.

Materials and methods

From 1974 to April 1996, 321 patients with postradical prostatectomy incontinence received an implantation of a bulbar artificial sphincter. The patient's ages ranged from 54 to 81 years, with a mean age of 65 years. From our own group of patients who underwent radical prostatectomy in our own institution, 34 (10.6%) were treated, and 287 (89.4%) came from other institutions. A total of 306 of them received the model AS 800 artificial sphincter, which has been available since 1983. The patients were followed from 1 month to 145 months, with an average of 64 months. All patients were checked neurourodynamically every 2 years, or immediately when problems occurred.

A total of 145/321 (45%) patients received previous anti-incontinence procedures: 33 (10.3%) had older models of the artificial sphincter, 93 had periurethral Teflon® or collagen injection (29%), and 19 (6%) had sling procedures (fascia and alloplastics). Three patients had a Rosen prosthesis and five patients a Kaufmann device. A total of 42 (13%) patients had a postoperative bladder neck contracture and had had a previous transurethral resection of the bladder neck. These were 15 patients (4.7%) who had a history of pelvic radiation before or after radical prostatectomy (Table 1).

Table 1 Previous anti-incontinence procedures used by 321 post-radical prostatectomy patients

	Patients	
	n	*%*
Artificial sphincters (older models)	33	10.3
Periurethral Teflon injections	42	13.1
Periurethral collagen injections	51	15.9
Sling procedures	19	6.0

All patients had a cuff implantation at the bulbous urethra, 56 of them a double cuff implantation simultaneously with, or secondary to, the sphincter implantation. A total of 314/321 were operated on with our own modified technique, which replaces the cuff at the very proximal bulbous urethra. A total of 287 (86.6%) of the patients received a pressure-regulating balloon in the range of 61–70 cmH₂O, 31 (9.7%) in the range of 51–60 cmH₂O, and only three (0.9%) in the range of 71–80 cmH₂O (Figure 1).

The implanted cuffs ranged from 4.5 to 6.0 cm in length: 98 (30.5%) received a cuff of 4.5 cm, 94 (29.3%) a cuff of 5.0 cm, 77 (24%) a cuff of 5.5 cm and 52 (16.2%) a cuff of 6.0 cm (Figure 2). All patients underwent deac-

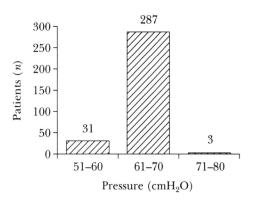

Figure 1 Ranges of pressure-regulating balloons used in 321 post-radical prostatectomy patients

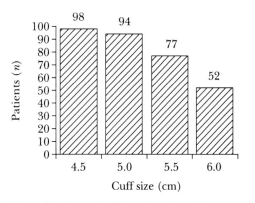

Figure 2 Sizes of cuffs implanted in 321 post-radical prostatectomy patients

tivation of the cuff for 4 to 6 weeks. Only a few difficult radiated cases underwent 3 months of deactivation.

Modified surgical technique

The bladder neck is the optimal location for the implantation of the cuff, which compresses the bladder neck in the intrapelvic cavity, the abdominal pressure transmission is optimal for the cuff and the whole device. During normal daily activities the compressive effect of the cuff occurs without loss of time, without fluid shift and immediately the abdominal pressure rises. Therefore, so stress incontinence or dribbling does not occur during coughing or heavy body activities. This is not the case in patients with bulbar cuff implantation. The cuff lies outside the pelvic cavity, so that the abdominal pressure will not be as effective as in cases with bladder neck implantation. A slide stress incontinence may occur, especially when the cuff is located at the distal part of the bulbous urethra. Additionally, the cuff at the distal part of the bulbous urethra lies in a position where the pressure during sitting will force fluid from the cuff to the pressure-regulation balloon. The empty cuff will then open the urethra and the patient leaks when he stands up.

The distal part of the bulbous urethra is of vulnerable cavernous tissue, involving a higher risk for tissue atrophy and erosion.

To exclude all these disadvantages of distal cuff implantation at the bulbous urethra, we changed our surgical technique in the following manner.

A midline perineal incision is made. The crura of the corpora cavernosa are exposed bilateral to the bulbocarvernous muscle (Figure 3).

The central tendon is dissected and the bulbous urethra is exposed up to the diaphragm of the pelvis (Figure 4).

Just below the bifurcation of the corpora cavernosa and above the membranous urethra, the diaphragm is split immediately below the posterior rim of the pubic bone (Figure 5). A right-angle clamp passes through the space between the pubic bone and behind the diaphragm (Figure 6). A cuff is pulled through, after the correct length of the cuff has been measured. The cuff is then closed deeply

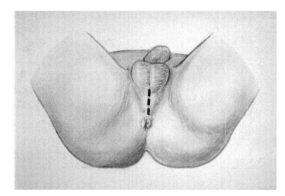

Figure 3 Midline perineal incision

around the proximal bulb of the urethra with all the surrounding and circular musculature (Figure 7). With suturing of the central tendon and reconstruction of the pelvic musculature, the cuff moves deeply to the pelvic floor and is located outside the compressing zone during sitting (Figure 8). Emptying of the cuff during sitting is therefore not possible (Figure 9).

A small incision is made in the lower abdominal wall. The peritoneum is opened and the pressure-regulating balloon implanted intraperitoneally. All the layers of the abdominal wall are closed. In the subcutaneous tissue and above the abdominal fascia of the oblique abdominal muscles, a pouch is bluntly prepared in the scrotum, between the tunica dartos and the tunica vaginalis (Figure 10).

The pump of the artificial sphincter is inserted into the pouch and fixed by means of a

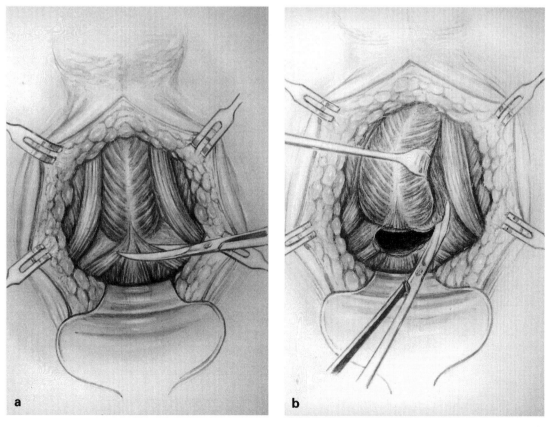

Figure 4 Dissection of the central tendon. (a) The cavernous muscle remains in place and is not dissected. (b) The bulbous and membranous urethra is dissected free up to the pelvic floor

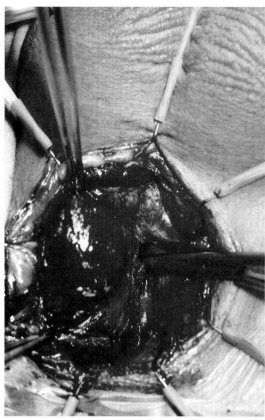

Figure 5 The ligamentum triangulare (diaphragm of the pelvis) is perforated just below the bifurcation of the corpora cavernosa. The pubic bone is contacted behind the ligamentum triangulare

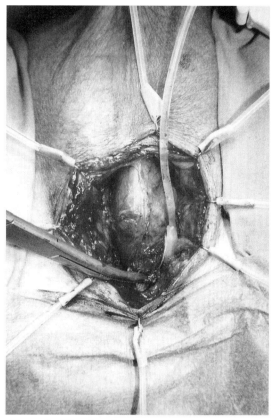

Figure 7 The closed cuff passes to the membranous urethra around the external sphincter musculature, its 'Natural place'

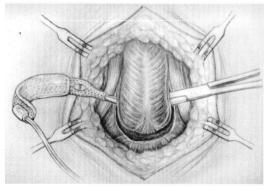

Figure 6 A right-angle clamp passes through the gap of the ligamentum triangulare and behind it. The cuff is pulled through

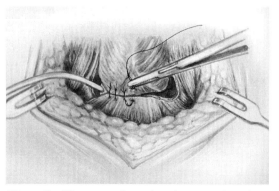

Figure 8 The central tendon is sutured and restored

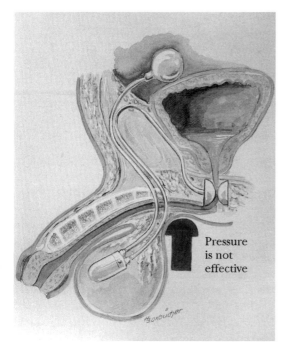

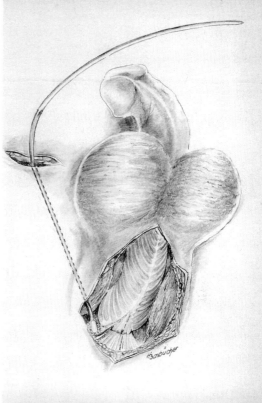

Pressure
is not
effective

Figure 9 With the cuff at the proximal position, just below the pelvic floor, it is out of the sitting pressure zone and in the region of the external sphincter. The cuff cannot be pressed empty during sitting and the patient remains dry

Figure 10 An inguinal incision is made and the cuff tube is passed through the subcutaneous tissue by means of a tubing passer. The pressure-regulating balloon is implanted intraperitoneally to prevent a fibrotic sheet forming around the balloon which may raise the pressure in the balloon and may lead to erosion

Babcock clamp until the end of the procedure. The pressure-regulating balloon is filled with a blood–isotone contrast medium dye or with physiological, saline solution in cases of allergic reactions to the dye.

The tube from the cuff is passed through the subcutaneous tissue into the abdominal subcutaneous tissue space and the tube connections are made by using a straight quick-connector to the balloon and a curved quick-connector from the pump to the cuff. Both wounds are closed without drainage.

Urinary diversion is created by means of a transurethral 8Fr. feeding tube. The device is deactivated for 4 to 6 weeks.

Table 2 Continence results in 306 post-radical prostatectomy patients

	No. pads	*No. patients*	*% patients*
Continent	≤ 1	257	84
Improved	2–3	19	6.2
Unsatisfied	≥ 4	17	5.6
Failed (device removed)		8	2.6

Results

Continence results are shown in Table 2: 257/306 (84%) of the patients who received the AS 800 device became continent, using at most one pad for their own safety; 19/306 (6.2%) were markedly improved, using 2–3 pads; 17 patients (5.6%) were unsatisfied, using four pads or more; eight patients (2.6%) were not improved and/or failed. In this group the total device or part of the device was removed.

Complications and revisions

Of the patients who were treated with the AS 800 artificial sphincter, 87/306 (28.5%) had 116 (38%) revisions; 219 (71.5%) did not require any revision (Table 3). Most of the revisions (69) were tissue related (22.5%); 47 revisions (15.5%) were device related (Table 4). The most frequent cause for tissue-related revisions was tissue atrophy beneath the cuff, leading to recurrence of incontinence (Table 5). There was no remarkable difference between the different cuff sizes. The time of revision for this reason was between 6 and 16 months. The mean interval was about 12 months. Eleven revisions (3.6%) were required because of urethral ero-

Table 3 Revision rate in 306 post-radical prostatectomy patients with the AS 800 artificial sphincter

No. patients	% patients	No. revisions
87	28.5	116
219	71.5	0

Table 4 Device-related complications in 87 patients out of 306 treated with the AS 800 artificial sphincter

	n	%
Cuff leak	31	10.1
Balloon leak	3	1.0
Connector leak	4	1.3
Pump malfunction	5	1.6
Tube kinking	4	1.3
Total	47	15.5

Table 5 Tissue-related complications in 87 patients out of 306 treated with the AS 800 artificial sphincter

	n	%
Infection	8	2.6
Cuff erosion	11	3.6
Tissue atrophy	46	15.0
Hematoma	4	1.3
Total	69	22.5

sion (nine) and scrotal pump erosion (two), due to subclinical infection with staphylococcus. Three of the cases with urethral erosion were in the radiation group. In eight patients (2.6%) the device had to be removed, due to infection on the plastic material. In six of these cases the device was reimplanted later on, with a successful reimplantation in four cases. Four patients (1.3%) developed a hematoma postoperatively that had to be drained in an open procedure.

Of the 47 (15.4%) patients who had to undergo revision because of device-related complications, 31 (10.1%) had a cuff leak, three (1.0%) had a balloon leak, four (1.3%) had a connector leak, five (1.6%) had a pump malfunction and four (1.3%) had tube kinking. Cuff leak was therefore the most common device-related reason for revision. This seems to be the weak point of the mechanical stability of the AS 800 and may be the typical late mechanical complication. In total, 237 sphincters (77.5%) required no revision and 259 patients (84.6%) suffered no mechanical failure.

Double cuff implantation

About 15% of the patients who had artificial sphincter implantation at the bulbous urethra did not become completely dry, due to incompetent closure pressure of the cuff. Urethral resistance is determined by the following relationships:

$$\text{Urethral resistance} = \text{balloon pressure} \times \text{compressing surface of the cuff}$$

There are two options to increase the urethral resistance: change the pressure-regulating balloon to the next higher level, or increase the compressing surface of the cuff. As the increase of the pressure to the urethra increases the risk of urethra erosion, it is advisable to increase the compressing surface of the cuff by using two cuffs, which are implanted side by side at the bulbous urethra (Figure 11).

We did this in 56 cases: 36 cases received the double cuff secondary to persisting or recurrent incontinence and 20 cases received a primary implantation of a double cuff, as we could not

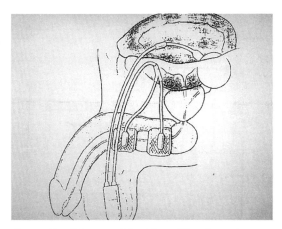

Figure 11   Schema of double-cuff implantation

Table 6   Improvement of continence with double cuff implantation in 306 patients

	No. patients	% patients
One cuff (at proximal bulbous urethra)	257	84.0
Double cuff	290	94.8

implant the single cuff to the proximal bulbous urethra because of previous urethral surgery in that region or previous radiation history. With the double cuff implantation we could increase the continence rate from 84 to 95% (Table 6). This phenomenon was first described by Britto and co-workers[7].

Discussion

Incontinence after radical prostatectomy is a most distressing complication[8]. There is a wide variation in the urological literature regarding postoperative incontinence after radical prostatectomy, ranging from 0.5 to 50%[1,2]. This variation may be in the definition of incontinence and the time of the evaluation of the patients. In the higher rates a great number of mild and also the severe cases are included, whereas in the lower rates only the severe cases are included. In our own patient group[8] only 8.6% of the patients who had a radical prostatectomy required therapy for postoperative incontinence.

In our study 321 patients were treated with an artificial sphincter (all models) at the bulbous urethra by a modified implantation technique[9]. As 95% of the patients became satisfactorily continent, the artificial sphincter is today the most reliable and most successful treatment of urinary incontinence after radical prostatectomy. Other treatment options, such as peri-

urethral Teflon and collagen injections as well as sling procedures, compressing procedures (Hauri procedure or Kaufman device) are not nearly as successful as the implantation of an artificial sphincter. Consequently, the artificial sphincter should be the therapy of choice for urinary incontinence after radical prostatectomy.

As in all prosthetic reconstructive surgery, revision surgery is the common necessity, and there are two problems that depend on the time after surgery. These are caused by the tissue reactions to the alloplastic material and by device-related difficulties, namely mechanical breakdowns.

A total of 116 (38%) revisions were carried out in 87 (28.5%) of 306 cases, which received the model AS 800. That means that 77.5% of the cases required no revision. Tissue atrophy and cuff leak were the main causes of revision. As there were no differences among the different cuff sizes, tissue atrophy represents the normal reaction of the tissue to the pressure, which is related to the level of the pressure-regulating balloon, which should be chosen to be as low as possible. The 61–70 cmH$_2$O balloon group may be the optimal range of pressure, as 86.5% of these patients became continent and the erosion rate remained low (3.6%). We also think that the site of cuff location plays an important role in prevention of urethral erosion. Around the proximal bulbous urethra, there is a protecting muscular layer. On the other hand, in the 6 o'clock position, the cuff penetrates the diaphragm pelvis so that this fascial part of the diaphragm acts as a protective sheath over the very vulnerable and thin corpus spongiosa urethra.

As the cuff is placed immediately beneath the membranous urethra, where the most effective abdominal pressure transmission can be registered by measuring the decending urethral pressure outside the pelvic floor, the continence rate is higher than in cases in which the cuff is placed at the distal part of the bulbous urethra. The advantage of our modified surgical technique is a higher continence rate and lower erosion rate. In patients with a history of radiation the cuff should not be placed at the proximal bulbus. The tissue may be damaged by radiation. In this case we prefer to place a double cuff at the distal part of the urethra, and have obtained quite good results.

The postoperative infection rate was 2.6%. This is a result of a number of precautions taken to prevent infection, such as the use of perioperative antibiotics, meticulous cleaning and disinfection of the genital skin area, careful surgical technique to prevent hematomas and the avoidance of wound drainage.

In conclusion, the results with the artificial sphincter used for treatment of urinary incontinence after radical prostatectomy are very encouraging, with an overall improvement of continence for 95% of patients. The revision rate is tolerable and patients' acceptance is overwhelming. Patients who had the experience of improvement of continence after becoming incontinent postoperatively always agreed to undergo a revision operation to improve their quality of life with a satisfactory working artificial sphincter.

References

1. Hodges, C. V. (1977). Vesicourethral anastomosis after radical prostatectomy: experience with the Jewett modification. *J. Urol.*, **118**, 209–10
2. Igel, T., Barrett, D. M., Segura, J. W., Benson, R. C. and Rife, C. C. (1987). Perioperative and postoperative complications from bilateral pelvic lymphadenectomy and radical retropubic prostatectomy. *J. Urol.*, **137**, 1189–91
3. Geary, E. S., Dendinger, T. E., Freiha, F. S. and Stamey, T. A. (1995). Incontinence and vesical neck strictures following radical retropubic prostatectomy. *Urology*, **45**, 1000–6
4. Fowler, F. J. Jr, Barry, M. J., Lu-Yao, G., Wasson, J., Roman, A. and Wennberg, J. (1995). Effect of radical prostatectomy for prostate cancer on patient quality of life: results from a Medicare survey. *Urology*, **45**, 1007–15
5. Scott, F. B., Bradley, W. E. and Timm, G. W. (1974). Treatment of urinary incontinence by an implantable prosthetic urinary sphincter. *J. Urol.*, **112**, 74
6. Gundian, J. C., Barrett, D. M. and Parulkar, B. G. (1989). Mayo clinic experience with use of the AMS 800 artificial urinary sphincter for urinary incontinence following radical prostatectomy. *J. Urol.*, **142**, 1459–61
7. Britto, C. G., Mulcahy, J. J., Mitchel, M. E. and Adams, M. C. (1993). Use of a double cuff AMS 800 artificial sphincter for severe stress incontinence. *J. Urol.*, **149**, 283–5
8. Heitz, M., Kluthe, A. E., Olianas, R. and Schreiter, F. J. (1996). Quality of life after radical prostatectomy: the problem of continence and potency. *Actuelle Urol.*, in press
9. Schreiter, F. (1985). Bulbar artificial sphincter. *Eur. Urol.*, **11**, 294–9

4

Endocrine Treatment of Locally Extensive and Metastatic Disease

Intermittent androgen suppression: rationale and clinical experience

13

M. Gleave, N. Bruchovsky, S. L. Goldenberg and P. Rennie

Background

No other treatment exists that equals or surpasses androgen ablation in controlling the growth of prostate cancer. Approximately 80% of prostate cancer patients achieve symptomatic and objective responses following androgen suppression, and serum prostate specific antigen (PSA) levels decrease in almost all patients. Surgical or medical castration results in a median progression-free survival of 12–33 months and a median overall survival of 23–37 months in patients with stage D_2 disease[1,2]. However, for reasons that remain unknown, the cell death process induced by androgen ablation by whatever means, fails to eliminate the entire malignant cell population[3]. Another limitation of conventional androgen ablation is that it increases the rate of progression of prostate cancer to an androgen-independent state[3], and after a variable period of time averaging 24 months, the tumor inevitably recurs with increasing serum PSA levels and is characterized by androgen- independent growth. Over the past 20 years, most efforts have focused on maximizing the degree of androgen suppression therapy by combining agents that inhibit or block both testicular and adrenal androgens. However, maximal androgen ablation increases treatment-related side-effects and expense, while prolonging time to androgen-independent progression by 3–6 months in most patients[2]. The paucity of information about cyclic hormonal therapy for breast and prostate malignancies can be attributed in part to the lack of suitable animal tumor models that regress predictably after castration and can be correctly termed hormone-dependent. Experimental animal and early clinical experience with intermittent androgen suppression suggests that quality of life is improved and progression to androgen independence may be delayed by using reversible androgen suppression and PSA level as the trigger point. Intermittent androgen suppression may offer a 'way out' of the immediate vs. delayed treatment controversy, by balancing the benefits of immediate androgen ablation with reduced treatment-related side-effects and expense.

Androgen dependence and independence

Androgen dependence is manifested by induction of apoptosis after androgen withdrawal in both normal and malignant tissues[4]. Androgen ablation has the double effect of triggering apoptosis and inhibiting DNA synthesis and cell proliferation. In the normal prostate, the cycle of androgen-induced cell growth and castration-induced apoptosis and regression can be continued through multiple cycles of androgen replacement and withdrawal. Data from animal studies and observations from the long-term follow-up of Chinese eunuchs demonstrate that normal prostatic epithelial cells undergo apoptotic regression and do not develop the ability to regenerate and grow in an androgen-depleted environment[5]. In contrast, progression to androgen independence nearly always occurs following androgen ablation therapy for patients with prostatic carcinoma. The inability of androgen withdrawal therapy to be curative may therefore result from pre-existing clones of androgen-independent cells in which the apoptotic process does not begin (clonal selection)[6,7], or from the up-regulation of androgen-repressed adaptive mechanisms capable of aborting the apoptotic process in subpopulations of cells (adaptation)[3,8].

Using the Dunning model, Isaacs and colleagues[6,7] emphasized the importance of genetic instability, which increases tumor heterogeneity by increasing the number of distinctly different clones of cells. Selective outgrowth of one or more androgen-resistant clones may occur after androgen ablation, resulting in androgen-independent progression. However, Dunning tumors are androgen sensitive and not androgen dependent, and apoptosis with tumor regression does not occur following castration. Intermittent androgen suppression may be harmful, because it would result in stimulation of androgen-sensitive cells when testosterone levels increase. Indeed, in an earlier study, Russo and associates[9] did not find intermittent androgen suppression to be superior to castration alone in the Dunning model. Maximal androgen ablation with the addition of cytotoxic agents that kill remaining androgen-independent cells appears to be the most effective therapy in this model[7].

In contrast, observations from the Shionogi and LNCaP tumor models suggest that progression to androgen independence is, in part, an adaptive response to androgen deprivation, which involves induction of a new resistant phenotype that develops from scattered cells throughout the tumor. The endpoint of androgen independence in the Shionogi model is loss of castration-induced apoptosis and *TRPM-2* gene expression[3,10], whereas the endpoint for progression in the LNCaP model is androgen-independent regulation of the PSA gene[11,12]. Androgen withdrawal in mice bearing Shionogi tumors precipitates apoptosis and tumor regression in a highly reproducible manner; however, despite complete remissions, castration fails to result in cure and androgen-independent progression invariably occurs within 60 days following castration[3,13]. Using an

in vivo limiting dilution assay to determine the proportions of androgen-dependent and androgen-independent tumorigenic stem cells in parent and recurrent tumors, Bruchovsky and co-workers[3] reported that the cells which survive androgen withdrawal may result from the ability of a small number of initially androgen-dependent stem cells to adapt to an androgen-depleted environment, possibly secondary to production of autocrine and paracrine growth factors, which may replace androgens as primary growth stimulatory factors[14].

LNCaP is an androgen-sensitive, PSA-secreting human prostate cancer cell line that is able to form tumors in male athymic mice under a variety of conditions[15], and provides accurate correlation between tumor volume and serum PSA levels *in vivo*[11]. Both androgens and tumor volume are important co-determinants of circulating PSA levels. Immediately after castration, serum PSA levels rapidly decrease by 80%, and they increase up to 20-fold following androgen supplementation; these changes in serum PSA occur without castration-induced tumor cell death or concomitant changes in tumor volume and reflect changes in androgen-regulated PSA gene expression. Despite decreasing by 80% after castration, LNCaP tumor cell mRNA PSA expression gradually returns to pre-castrate levels in the absence of testicular androgens beginning 4 weeks post-castration, heralding the onset of androgen- independent PSA gene regulation[16]. Further characterization of androgen-independent LNCaP cell lines produced a subline (C4-2) that metastasized to bone and, interestingly, the incidence of osseous metastases appeared higher in castrated than in intact male hosts, suggesting that continuous androgen suppression may facilitate development of androgen-independent osseous metastases[17,18].

The ability of benign or malignant prostate cells to undergo apoptosis and express PSA is acquired as a feature of differentiation of prostatic cells under the influence of androgens. In the absence of androgens, proliferating cells do not differentiate and cannot become pre-apoptotic again, which results in development of the androgen-independent phenotype and growth[3,4]. Progression to androgen independence is probably genetically programmed (up-regulation of androgen-repressed genes) but precipitated or directed by epigenetic factors (androgen ablation). In other words, androgen resistance may be a primary but quiescent property of some prostate cancer cells that is activated in response to androgen withdrawal. We hypothesize that if tumor cells which survive androgen withdrawal are forced into a normal pathway of differentiation by androgen replacement, then apoptotic potential might be restored and progression to androgen independence may be delayed. It follows that if androgens are replaced soon after regression of the tumor, it should be possible to bring about repeated cycles of androgen-stimulated growth, differentiation and androgen-withdrawal regression of the tumor.

Intermittent androgen suppression in animal models

Dunning R3327 rat prostatic adenocarcinoma

Treatment of the Dunning R3327 prostatic adenocarcinoma by cyclic therapy was studied by Trachtenberg[19] as a possible means of maintaining a population of hormonally dependent cells and preventing the emergence of an overwhelming number of hormonally independent cells. In his experiments, animals bearing the tumor were castrated and intermittently subjected to hormonal stimulation by means of indwelling silastic testosterone-filled implants. The growth of these tumors was compared to that of a castrate control group, a chronic implant group and an intact control group. No significant growth reduction with the intermittent stimulation group as compared to the implanted control or intact group was observed. It was concluded that intermittent hormonal therapy is inferior to early castration in preventing tumor growth.

The Dunning R3327 prostatic adenocarcinoma was also used by Russo and associates[9] to study the effects of intermittent diethylstilbestrol diphosphate (DES) administration. This work was prompted by an exploratory clinical trial by Klotz and co-workers[20] which examined the use of intermittent DES therapy in advanced symptomatic prostate cancer to diminish the morbidity of standard endocrine therapy. Treatment of animals bearing the Dunning R3327 tumor was started 60 days following implant and took the form of either intermittent high-dose DES or intermittent low-dose DES; in both cases the DES was administered in drinking water for 1 week, followed by 3 weeks off treatment. The growth of these tumors was compared to that of a castrate control group, and to two groups receiving either a low or a high dose of DES administered continuously in drinking water. The continuous low or high doses of DES as well as the intermittent treatments were shown to reduce serum testosterone to castrate levels during the week of hormone administration; furthermore, serum testosterone recovered to control levels after withdrawal of DES. All rats exposed to DES had a tumor volume at death smaller than that of control or castrate rats. Despite this, a significant survival advantage from the time of randomization was achieved only in the castrate or high-dose DES groups compared to the control group. Similarly, significant prolongation in tumor doubling time was achieved only in rats that had been castrated or had received high-dose DES. Although the intermittent regimen was successful in checking tumor volume, it did not yield a survival advantage and in this respect was inferior to castration.

The foregoing experiments on the Dunning R3327 prostatic adenocarcinoma draw attention to the importance of using cyclic androgen deprivation only for the treatment of androgen-dependent cancer. If the tumor lacks the androgen-dependent phenotype and does not undergo apoptotic regression when androgens are withdrawn, intermittent therapy is unlikely to be beneficial. Because the Dunning R3327 prostatic adenocarcinoma is androgen sensitive but not androgen dependent, the failure to demonstrate an improved outcome with intermittent hormone therapy is not an unexpected result.

Shionogi mouse carcinoma

The tumor best suited for studies on castration-induced cell death is the Shionogi carcinoma, a transplantable mouse mammary tumor that is androgen dependent and closely mimics the clinical course of prostate cancer in response to treatment. The parent Shionogi tumor grows only in male mice, regresses almost completely after castration and recurs with androgen-independent growth[3]. Because of its androgen-dependent behavior, the Shionogi tumor model is particularly useful in studying the mechanisms of androgen-independent progression, and the therapeutic approaches to delay or avert tumor progression. Intermittent androgen suppression of the parent Shionogi carcinoma has been carried out experimentally by transplanting the tumor into a succession of male mice, each of which was castrated when the estimated tumor weight was approximately 3 g. After the tumor regressed to 30% of the original weight, it was transplanted into the next non-castrated male. This cycle of transplantation and castration-induced apoptosis was successfully repeated four times before growth became androgen independent during the fifth cycle (see Figure 3)[10]. The mean time to androgen independence of 147 days compared to 51 days after one-time castration was in keeping with a retarding effect of cyclic therapy on tumor progression.

Some caution is required in the interpretation of these results, since the procedure of transplanting a regressing tumor from a castrated to a non-castrated animal temporarily may reduce the rate of cell division and give rise to an apparent delay in progression. In fact, a transplantation-related effect on doubling time during the early phase of tumor regeneration would be technically difficult to rule out; however, from the time the tumor becomes palpable (0.5 g), no differences in tumor doubling times are evident during successive cycles[10]. It seems more likely that the lag period between tumor regression and regeneration is determined by the number of stem cells in the regressing tumor at the time when androgen replacement begins. Although castration reduces the number of viable tumor cells by about 1 logarithm, the effect on stem cells is disproportionately greater, i.e. 2–3 logarithms. In addition to tumor growth, other markers of androgen-independent progression in this model include castration-induced apoptosis and *TRPM-2* gene expression. Both these intermediate markers of androgen dependence are maintained three times longer with intermittent androgen suppression compared to continuous therapy, paralleling and supporting the changes in tumor volume.

LNCaP human prostate tumor model

As in human prostate cancer, serum PSA levels in this model are regulated by androgen and are directly proportional to tumor volume[11]. After castration, serum and tumor-cell PSA levels decrease up to 80% and remain suppressed for 3–4 weeks before increasing again (Figure 1). With intermittent testosterone withdrawal and replacement in castrated mice bearing LNCaP tumors, a 3-fold delay in the development androgen-independent regulation of the *PSA* gene was observed[21]. Serum PSA levels remained below pre-castrate levels after 60 days in 75% of the intermittent androgen suppression group, but exceeded pre-castrate PSA levels after 28 days in 100% of the continuous androgen suppression group. By 15 weeks post-castration, PSA levels in the continuous androgen suppression group had increased 7.0-fold above pre-castrate levels, compared to only 1.9-fold in the intermittent androgen suppression therapy group (Figure 1). The success of intermittent androgen suppression in these animal models supports the concept that progression to androgen independence results from androgen-induced differentiation and/or down-regulation of androgen-repressed growth regulatory pathways.

Reversible androgen ablation therapy

With the introduction of antiandrogens such as cyproterone acetate and flutamide, and luteinizing hormone-releasing hormone agonists such as leuprolide acetate and goserelin acetate, new methods of androgen suppression have become available. These mimic the effects of orchidectomy by lowering the intranuclear concentration of dihydrotestosterone by 80% or more. Emphasis has been placed on the combined use of agents[2] with little attention given to their reversibility of action, the significance of which is far-reaching. The potential for a full recovery from therapy makes it possible to alternate a patient between periods of treatment and no-treatment. Furthermore, serial serum PSA measurements permit accurate monitoring of disease activity and serve as trigger points for stopping and re-starting therapy. When the patient is off-treatment, testicular function and serum testosterone levels return to normal slowly over a period of 8–14 weeks[10]. In response to this androgenic stimulus, atrophic cells are recruited into a normal pathway of differentiation, in which the risk of progression to androgen independence is reduced. With the

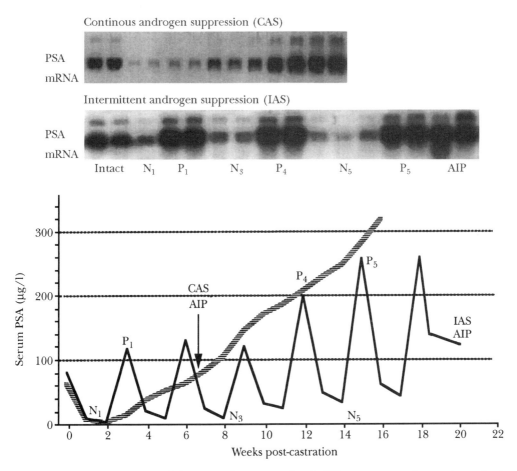

Figure 1 The LNCaP tumor model uses androgen-regulated *PSA* gene expression as its endpoint of progression to androgen-independence (AIP). Serum prostate specific antigen (PSA) (graph) and PSA mRNA (Northern analysis) levels increased above pre-castrate levels by 4 weeks post-castration with continuous androgen suppression (CAS), but remained androgen-regulated and suppressed 15 weeks post-castration with intermittent androgen suppression (IAS). By 15 weeks post-castration, PSA levels with CAS had increased 7.0-fold above pre-castrate levels, compared to only 1.9-fold in the IAS therapy group

associated movement through the division cycle, the cells become pre-apoptotic again, making it possible to repeat therapy.

Clinical observations

Reports of multiple regressions of hormone-dependent malignancy are rare in the clinical and scientific literature. Stoll[22] drew attention to the balance between inhibition and stimulation of the growth of breast cancer in an elderly woman who was treated intermittently with estrogen. Regression of the tumor occurred three times over a period of 5 years, after which an estrogen withdrawal response resulted in a fourth remission. Bruchovsky and co-workers[23] described the responses of pulmonary metastases of breast cancer in a female patient whose endocrine therapy consisted of a sequence of radiation ovariectomy, administration of androgen, discontinuation of androgen and adrenalectomy. Regressions followed each procedure and the tumor size was successfully held in check. Experiments conducted by Noble[24] focused on the effects of fractional hormone-replacement therapy on the progression of estrogen-dependent mammary tumors in male Nb rats. In animals whose tumors achieved a stationary growth pattern with a reduced dose of estrogen, no autonomous change was observed. Noble also conducted similar studies in Nb rats on an adenocarcinoma of the dorsal prostate, which grows only in estrogenized hosts[25]. Removal of estrogen from animals with growing tumors led to tumor regression; this was followed by progression and eventual re-growth of tumors that were autonomous. Replacement with lower doses of estrogen reduced the extent of regression and prevented autonomous change.

The intermittent regulation of serum testosterone levels for therapeutic purposes was first attempted with cyclic administration of estrogenic hormone[20]. Nineteen patients with advanced prostate cancer received DES until a clinical response was clearly demonstrated and then it was withheld until symptoms recurred. One additional patient was treated with flutamide, according to a similar schedule. The mean duration of initial therapy was 30 months (range 2–70 months). Subjective improvement was noted in all patients during the first 3 months of treatment. When therapy was stopped, 12 of 20 patients relapsed after a mean interval of 8 months (range 1–24 months) and all subsequently responded to re-administration of the drug. Therapy-induced impotence was reversed in nine of ten men within 3 months of the break in treatment. An improved quality of life was achieved, owing to the reduced intake of DES, and no adverse effects on survival were apparent.

In a more recent study, we reported preliminary results of intermittent androgen suppression in a group of 47 patients with prostate cancer, with a mean follow-up time of 125 weeks[26]. Sixty patients, 34 with clinically localized and 26 with metastatic disease, have now been treated (Table 1). The mean initial serum PSA level was 128 µg/l. Treatment was initiated with combined androgen blockade and continued for an average of 9 months. Because prognosis is poor in patients who do not achieve normal PSA levels after androgen ablation, only patients with PSA nadir levels below 4 µg/l are eligible for the intermittent androgen suppression protocol. Medication was then withheld until the serum PSA level increased to mean values between 10 and 20 µg/l. This cycle of treatment and no-treatment was repeated until

Table 1 Study group ($n = 60$)

Mean age: 67 years
Mean PSA level: 128 µg/l
Stages
  A_2: 2
  B_2: 1
  C: 31
    unRx: 14
    post-XRT: 12
    post-RRP: 5
  D_1: 10
  D_2: 16

PSA, prostate specific antigen; unRx, no treatment; post-XRT, ; post-RRP, after radical retropubic prostatectomy

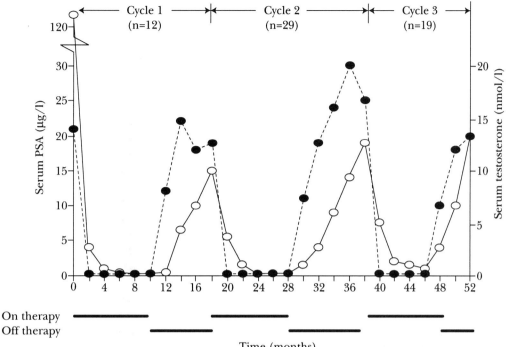

Figure 2 Composite results on 60 patients with prostate cancer treated with intermittent androgen suppression, of whom 12 are in their first cycle of treatment, 29 in their second cycle and 19 in their third or higher cycle. The mean serum level of prostate specific antigen (PSA) at the start of the first, second and third cycles was 128 µg/l, 14 µg/l and 17.3 µg/l, respectively. The first three cycles averaged 18, 18 and 15.5 months in length, respectively. Open circles, PSA; filled circles, testosterone

Table 2 Current cycle of intermittent androgen suppression (IAS) therapy for patients on IAS protocol

Current cycle	No. patients
1	12
2	29
3	11
4	6
5	2
Total	60

the regulation of the PSA level became androgen independent (Figure 2).

Twenty-nine men are currently in their second cycle and 19 are in their third or higher cycle (Table 2). The mean time to PSA nadir during the first three cycles was 5 months. The first two cycles averaged 18 months in length, with 45% of the time off therapy, and the third cycle averaged 15.5 months. The serum testosterone level returned to the normal range within 8 weeks (range 1–26 weeks) of stopping treatment. The off-treatment period in all cycles was associated with an improvement in sense of well-being, and the recovery of libido and potency in the men who reported normal or near-normal sexual function before the start of therapy.

Androgen-independent progression occurred in nine of 26 stage D patients and three of 34 with localized disease after a mean follow-up of 43 months. Of 16 stage D_2 patients, eight remain on the study, with stable disease. Eight patients have died, two from non-cancer-related illness, with median time to progression and overall survival of 26 and 38 months, respectively (Table 3).

Observations from this preliminary study suggest that intermittent androgen suppression

Table 3 Intermittent androgen suppression results in stage D patients. Numbers of patients are shown in parentheses

Stage	Median time on study (months)	Median time to progression (months)	Cycle
D$_2$ (16)			
alive and AD (8)	43	—	1 (1); 2 (3); 3 (3); 5 (1)
dead, from CaP (6)	45	26	2 (5); 5 (1)
dead, not from CaP (2)	38	38	2 (2)
D$_1$ (10)			
alive and AD (8)	40	—	1 (2); 2 (3); 3 (1); 4 (2)
alive and AI (2)	68	68	3 (1); 4 (1)

AD, androgen dependent; AI, androgen independent; CaP, cancer of the prostate

does not have a negative impact on time to progression or survival, both of which are similar to continuous combined therapy. However, phase III randomized studies are required for accurate assessment of the effects of intermittent treatment on these critical parameters. Intermittent androgen suppression does improve the quality of life by permitting recovery of libido and potency, increasing energy levels and enhancing sense of well-being during off-treatment periods (Table 4). The animal and preliminary clinical studies have helped identify groups of patients who are most likely to benefit from intermittent androgen suppression, to determine optimal duration of treatment, and to suggest trigger points on when to re-start therapy again. The therapeutic strategy and trigger points in each situation are guided by serum PSA levels.

Candidates for intermittent androgen suppression

In theory, this approach should be suitable for the long-term management of inoperable, incompletely excised, or locally recurrent prostate cancer, especially after local recurrences following external beam ionizing radiation. The standard regimen developed for stage D$_2$ prostate cancer (Figure 3) has been adapted for use in the treatment of men with initially localized prostate cancer, which has recurred after either irradiation or radical prostatectomy, as indicated by a rising serum PSA level and/or positive biopsy. Failure of serum PSA level

Table 4 Advantages of intermittent androgen suppression

Improved quality of life
recovery of libido and potency
greater sense of well-being
reduction in loss of bone mass
Reduced expense of treatment
Longer time to develop androgen resistance
Application to earlier stages of disease
Individualization allowed to a patient's particular medical and social preference
Innovative combination with other drugs

to nadir below 4 µg/l after 6 months of therapy is associated with a short duration of response to androgen ablation and a poor prognosis[27], and intermittent androgen suppression is not offered to these patients.

Length of treatment cycle

Conceptually, androgen ablation should be continued until maximal castration-induced apoptosis and tumor regression has been induced, but stopped before constitutive development of the androgen-independent phenotype. Premature termination of therapy would permit some cancer cells destined to undergo apoptosis to survive upon re-exposure to testosterone. After institution of androgen ablation therapy, serum PSA levels decrease rapidly and dramatically, due to cessation of androgen-regulated *PSA* gene expression and apoptosis[11]. In our group of patients treated with intermittent androgen suppression therapy, PSA nadir and

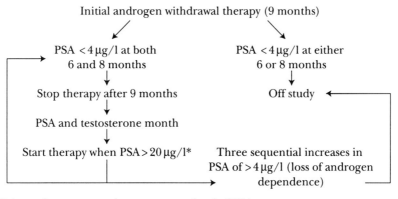

Initial androgen withdrawal therapy (9 months)

PSA < 4 μg/l at both
6 and 8 months

PSA < 4 μg/l at either
6 or 8 months

Stop therapy after 9 months

Off study

PSA and testosterone month

Start therapy when PSA > 20 μg/l*

Three sequential increases in
PSA of > 4 μg/l (loss of androgen
dependence)

* depends on stage and pre-treatment level of PSA

Figure 3 Schema of intermittent androgen suppression therapy for advanced prostate cancer

maximal soft tissue regression is not reached until 8 months in many patients with advanced stage C and D_2 disease[21]. Similarly, the duration of time necessary for PSA to reach its nadir in a group of patients with clinically confined disease after institution of neoadjuvant androgen withdrawal therapy is often longer than 6 months[28]. With the use of a lower limit of sensitivity of 0.2 μg/l, the PSA nadir was reached in only 34% after 3 months, 60% after 5 months, 70% after 6 months and 84% at 8 months. The serum PSA level was still decreasing at 8 months in 14%. The percentage of patients with a serum PSA nadir of ≤ 0.2 μg/l increased from 14% at 2 months, to 34% at 3 months, 56% at 5 months and 66% at 8 months. The initial rapid decrease in PSA results from cessation of androgen-regulated PSA synthesis and apoptosis, whereas the ongoing slower decline reflects decreasing tumor volume. On the basis of these observations, we now treat patients for 9 months prior to stopping therapy.

When to restart

The optimal time to reinstitute androgen ablation therapy remains undefined and empirical. Ideally, time off therapy should be long enough to permit normalization of libido and energy levels and testosterone-induced tumor cell differentiation. Until more information is obtained about PSA milestones from clinical trials

focusing on the subsets of patients indicated, the PSA thresholds and ceilings are regarded as tentative settings only. Trigger points are individualized and factors that are considered include pre-treatment PSA levels, stage, PSA velocity, presence of symptoms and tolerance of androgen ablation therapy. In general, in patients with metastatic disease and high pre-treatment PSA levels, therapy is re-started when the PSA level increases above 20 μg/l; in patients with locally recurrent disease and moderately elevated pre-treatment PSA levels, therapy is re-started when the PSA level increases above 4 μg/l, or earlier for post-radical prostatectomy recurrences.

Conclusions

In summary, both experimental and clinical evidence demonstrates that apoptosis and modulation of androgen-regulated gene expression can be induced multiple times with intermittent androgen suppression, and that maintenance of androgen dependence is likely to be due to androgen-induced differentiation and/or suppression of alternative growth stimulatory pathways. The first two treatment cycles in our ongoing phase II study averaged 18 months with 45% of the time off therapy, while the third cycle averaged 15 months with 33% of the time off therapy. The time to progression and survival of

16 stage D_2 patients was similar to the results expected with continuous therapy.

Available information about intermittent androgen blockade is still very limited and leaves several questions unanswered. The issue of survival is the most important and needs to be assessed in a randomized study of intermittent vs. continuous androgen deprivation. The possibility of expanding the use of intermittent therapy to earlier-stage disease should be examined in greater detail. Conceivably, the intermittent therapy option might become an alternative to radical prostatectomy or irradiation for the primary treatment of localized prostate cancer in men with life expectancies of less than 15 years. The prospect of improving the results of intermittent androgen suppression by increasing the length and number of cycles is attractive. Prolongation of the length of each 'off' treatment cycle may be possible with 5α-reductase inhibitors such as finasteride. Augmentation of intermittent therapy might be accomplished by the administration of cytotoxic drugs, differentiating agents, or gene therapies (e.g. antisense *BCL2*) at specific times during a cycle of treatment, when the modality of choice would have its maximum effect. Finally, it is clear that the concept of intermittent androgen suppression lends itself to other innovations, as in the example of long-term neoadjuvant therapy prior to radical prostatectomy or irradiation[28].

References

1. Bruchovsky, N. (1993). Androgens and anti-androgens. In Holland, J. F., Frei, E. III, Bast, R. C., Kufe, D. W., Morton, D. L. and Weichselbaum, R. R. (eds.) *Cancer Medicine*, 3rd edn, pp. 884–96. (Philadelphia: Lea & Febiger)
2. Denis, L. and Murphy, G. P. (1993). Overview of phase III trials on combined androgen treatment in patients with metastatic prostate cancer. *Cancer* (Suppl.) **72**, 3888–95
3. Bruchovsky, N., Rennie, P. S., Coldman, A. J., Goldenberg, S. L., To, M. and Lawson, D. (1990). Effects of androgen withdrawal on the stem cell composition of the Shionogi carcinoma. *Cancer Res.*, **50**, 2275–82
4. Bruchovsky, N., Brown, E. M., Coppin, C. M., Goldenberg, S. L., LeRiche, J. C., Murray, N. C. *et al.* (1987). The endocrinology and treatment of prostate tumour progression. In Coffey, D. S., Bruchovsky, N., Gardner, W. A. Jr, Resnick, M. I. and Karr, J. P. (eds.) *Current Concepts and Approaches to the Study of Prostate Cancer. Progress in Clinical and Biological Research*, pp. 348–87. (New York: Alan R. Liss)
5. Wu, C. P. and Gu, F. L. (1992). The prostate in eunuchs. *EORTC Genitourinary Group Monograph 10 – Urologic Oncology: Reconstructive Surgery, Organ Preservation, and Restoration of Function*, pp. 249–55. (New York: Wiley-Liss)
6. Isaacs, J. T., Wake, N., Coffey, D. S. and Sandberg, A. A. (1982). Genetic instability coupled to clonal selection as a mechanism for progression in prostatic cancer. *Cancer Res.*, **42**, 2353–61
7. Isaacs, J. T. (1984). The timing of androgen ablation therapy and/or chemotherapy in the treatment of prostatic cancer. *Prostate*, **51**, 1–17
8. van Weerden, W. M. (1991). Animal models in the study of progression of prostate and breast cancers to endocrine independency. In Berns, P. M. J. J., Romijn, J. C. and Schröder, F. H. (eds.) *Mechanisms of Progression to Hormone-Independent Growth of Breast and Prostate Cancer*, pp. 55–70. (Carnforth, UK: Parthenon Publishing)
9. Russo, P., Liguori, G., Heston, W. D. W., Huryk, R., Yang, C.-R., Fair, W. R., Whitmore, W. F. and Herr, H. W. (1987). Effects of intermittent diethylstilbestrol diphosphate administration on the R3327 rat prostatic carcinoma. *Cancer Res.*, **47**, 5967–70
10. Akakura, K., Bruchovsky, N., Goldenberg, S. L., Rennie, P. S., Buckley, A. R. and Sullivan, L. D. (1993). Effects of intermittent androgen suppression on androgen-dependent tumors: apoptosis and serum prostate specific antigen. *Cancer*, **71**, 2782–90
11. Gleave, M. E., Hsieh, J. T., Wu, H.-C., von Eschenbach, A. C. and Chung, L. W. K. (1992). Serum PSA levels in mice bearing human prostate LNCaP tumors are determined by tumor volume and endocrine and growth factors. *Cancer Res.*, **52**, 1598

12. Gleave, M. E., Bowden, M., Bruchovsky, N., Goldenberg, S. L. and Sullivan L. D. (1994). Predictors of time to androgen-independent progression in the LNCaP prostate tumor model (Abstr.). *J. Urol.*, **151**, 241

13. Rennie, P. S., Bruchovsky, N., Buttyan, R., Benson, M. and Cheng, H. (1988). Gene expression during the early phases of regression of the androgen-dependent Shionogi mouse mammary carcinoma. *Cancer Res.*, **48**, 6309–12

14. Sato, N., Watabe, Y., Suzuki, H. and Shimazaki, J. (1993). Progression of androgen-sensitive mouse tumor (Shionogi carcinoma 115) to androgen-insensitive tumor after long-term removal of testosterone. *Jpn. J. Cancer Res.*, **84**, 1300

15. Gleave, M. E., Hsieh, J. T., Gao, C. A., von Eschenbach, A. C. and Chung, L. W. K. (1991). Acceleration of human prostate cancer growth *in vivo* by factors produced by prostate and bone fibroblasts. *Cancer Res.*, **51**, 3753

16. Wu, H.-C., Hsieh, J. T., Gleave, M. E., von Eschenbach, A. C. and Chung, L. W. K. (1994). Derivation of androgen-independent human LNCaP prostate cancer sublines: role of bone stromal cells. *Int. J. Cancer*, **57**, 406

17. Hsieh, J. T., Wu, H.-C., Gleave, M. E. *et al.* (1993). Autocrine regulation of PSA gene expression in a human prostatic cancer (LNCaP) subline. *Cancer Res.*, **53**, 2852–7

18. Thalmann, G. N., Anezinis, P. E., Chang, S. H., Zhan, H. E., Kim, E. E., Hopwood, V. L., Pathak, S., von Eschenbach, A. C. and Chung, L. W. K. (1994). Androgen-independent cancer progression and bone metastasis in the LNCaP model of human prostate cancer. *Cancer Res.*, **54**, 2577

19. Trachtenberg, J. (1987). Experimental treatment of prostatic cancer by intermittent hormonal therapy. *J. Urol.*, **137**, 785–8

20. Klotz, L. H., Herr, H. W., Morse, M. J., Whitmore, W. F. Jr (1986). Intermittent endocrine therapy for advanced prostate cancer. *Cancer*, **58**, 2546–50

21. Sato, N., Gleave, M. E., Goldenberg, S. L., Bruchovsky, N., Rennie, P. and Sullivan, L. D. (1995). Intermittent androgen suppression delays time to androgen-independent progression in the LNCaP prostate tumor model. *J. Urol.*, **153**, 282A

22. Stoll, B. A. (1977). Palliation by castration or by hormone administration. In Stoll, B. A. (ed.) *Breast Cancer Management Early and Late*, pp. 133–46. (Chicago: Year Book Medical Publishers)

23. Bruchovsky, N., Rennie, P. S. and Van Doorn, E. (1978). Pathological growth of androgen-sensitive tissues resulting from latent actions of steroid hormones. *J. Toxicol. Environ. Health*, **4**, 391–408

24. Noble, R. L. (1977). Hormonal control of growth and progression in tumors of Nb rats and a theory of action. *Cancer Res.*, **37**, 82–94

25. Noble, R. L. (1977). Sex steroids as a cause of adenocarcinoma of the dorsal prostate in Nb rats, and their influence on the growth of transplants. *Oncology*, **34**, 138–41

26. Goldenberg, S. L., Bruchovsky, N., Gleave, M. E., Sullivan, L. D. and Akakura, K. (1995). Intermittent androgen suppression in the treatment of prostate cancer: a preliminary report. *Urology*, **45**, 839–45

27. Miller, J. I., Ahmann, F. R., Drach, G. W., Emerson, S. S. and Bottaccini, M. R. (1992). The clinical usefulness of serum prostate specific antigen after hormonal therapy of metastatic prostate cancer. *J. Urol.*, **147**, 956–61

28. Gleave, M. E., Goldenberg, S. L., Jones, E. C., Bruchovsky, N. and Sullivan, L. D. (1996). Maximal biochemical and pathological downstaging requires 8 months of neoadjuvant hormonal therapy prior to radical prostatectomy. *J. Urol.*, **155**, 213–19

Interactive Voting System

1 What do you believe is the predominant mechanism involved in progression to androgen independence after androgen ablation?

Response	Option
56%	Clonal selection and expansion of pre-existing AI cells.
36%	Adaptational changes in some cancer cells in response to androgen withdrawal.
1%	Stimulation by small amounts of residual adrenal androgens.
7%	Mutations in the androgen receptor.

Number of votes: 121

2   A 62-year-old male, sexually active and healthy, was treated 3 years ago with XRT for a T_{3B} moderately differentiated prostate cancer. His serum PSA level was 22 µg/l before treatment, decreased to a nadir of 0.8 µg/l, and has increased over the past year to 8.3 µg/l. DRE reveals a T_{3A} nodule at right base. Assuming his metastatic work-up is normal, what management would you recommend?

11%	Salvage prostatectomy with or without neoadjuvant hormone therapy.
30%	Delayed hormonal therapy until symptomatic or metastatic progression develops.
30%	Immediate continuous androgen ablation.
29%	Immediate intermittent androgen suppression.

Number of votes: 122

Clinical results of intermittent endocrine treatment in low-volume prostate cancer patients

14

U. W. Tunn

Permanent androgen withdrawal was introduced by Huggins and Hodges[1] more than 50 years ago as first-line treatment for advanced cancer of the prostate. It is still the 'gold standard' in therapy for cancer of the prostate. Despite a high initial response rate of 70–80% a relapse occurs in more than 50% of patients after an average time of 2 years. The median survival rate for metastatic disease of the prostate following treatment with complete androgen suppression is 36 months[2]. A meta-analysis of 22 randomized trials with 3283 deaths in 5710 patients has shown that maximum androgen blockade does not result in longer survival than conventional castration[3]. The reason might be that some of the malignant cell populations survive despite complete androgen ablation, and moreover they are able to proliferate in an androgen-free environment. This means that a population of androgen-dependent cells is transformed into a population of androgen-independent cells (Figure 1).

Permanent complete androgen deprivation (CAD) might even favor the androgen-independent progression. Bruchovsky and colleagues[4,5] showed in their experimental work that cyclic androgen withdrawal delayed time to tumor progression due to androgen independence. If this proves to be transferable to prostatic cancer it would mean a great improvement in therapeutic concepts.

A brief introduction follows to the theoretical basics of intermittent androgen deprivation (IAD) and the first clinical results.

Rationale of intermittent androgen deprivation

Basic knowledge about the positive effects of IAD in comparison to permanent androgen deprivation (PAD) was gathered by Bruchovsky and co-workers[4,5] in Vancouver; they used the Shionogi tumor as a model. The response of the initially androgen-dependent Shionogi carcinoma is similar in manner regarding proliferation, regression and progression to that of clinical prostatic cancer. Tumor proliferation occurs after transplantation of a defined number of tumor cells into intact male mice, after a set delay. Androgen withdrawal through castration leads to tumor regression and decrease of tumor volume by 90%. The relapse occurs after an average period of 50 days under the condition of permanent androgen deprivation. This

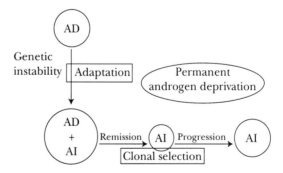

Figure 1 Schematic illustration of hypothetical adaptive and selective processes inducing androgen-withdrawal-independent tumor cell proliferation during permanent androgen deprivation. AD, androgen dependent; AI, androgen independent

secondary tumor progression is androgen independent. In the Shionogi model, a prolongation of the relapse-free interval was achieved with cyclic therapy in the form of cyclic androgen withdrawal.

After tumor regression and before secondary tumor proliferation, the tumor cells were reimplanted into the next generation of male mice. The tumor cells proliferated after the second transplantation, but regressed again in reaction to androgen withdrawal, produced by castration of the hosts.

Growth became androgen independent during only the fifth transplantation. The mean time to androgen independence achieved through IAD was 150 days compared with 50 days under PAD. The three-fold delay until androgen independence under cyclic androgen suppression with reduction in the number of tumor cells is the sum of latency time prior to tumor cell passage and tumor progression after testosterone replacement and regression after testosterone withdrawal. On the basis of this animal model Bruchovsky postulated that the transformation of surviving androgen-dependent to androgen-independent tumor cells is caused by the elimination of differentiated androgen-dependent stem cells in the primary tumor. Furthermore, there is evidence for the progression of the form of activation of previously androgen-repressed genes. Some of these possibly produce autocrine and paracrine growth factors that substitute for androgen and can stimulate the multitude of tumorigenic stem cells. This implies that replacement of androgens prior to secondary androgen-independent relapse could support the androgen-induced differentiation of the parent stem cell into a tumor cell population that is again androgen dependent, and again treatable by androgen withdrawal. The androgen-induced differentation of stem cells with recovery of apoptotic potential is thus the background for the cyclic IAD concept in the treatment of androgen-dependent tumors. The effect of IAD has been tested in LNCaP models[6]. A three-fold delay of the time interval until development of androgen independence with IAD was ob-

served. The success of intermittent therapy in this prostate tumor model supports the concept that permanent withdrawal of androgens leads to adaptive processes in the tumor cell and to an up-regulation of previously androgen-repressed growth regulatory pathways,

Clinical observations

The introduction of IAD for the treatment of prostate cancer can only be realised with reversible agents for the androgen deprivation such as luteinizing hormone releasing hormone (LHRH) agonists and antiandrogens, and a tumor marker able to monitor intervals of regression and progression is available. This is today the prostatic specific antigen (PSA). Prior to the introduction of PSA very few intermittent endocrine treatments of advanced prostatic cancer were used in clinical studies.

In 1980, Vahlensieck and Wegner[7] reported the intermittent use of estramustine phosphate in advanced prostatic cancer and failed to find a significant difference regarding clinical response[6,7]. Klotz and colleagues[8] used diethylstilbestrol in an intermittent regime in 19 patients with advanced cancer of the prostate. They reported an improved quality of life during the treatment-free interval which lasted an average of 8 months until relapse after the initial treatment of 30 months. With PSA as a marker to monitor progression and regression, IAD was used as a treatment in 47 patients with prostate cancer by Goldenberg and co-workers[9]. The clinical stage of the disease in these patients differed. There were 14 D_2, ten D_1, 19 C, two B_2 and two A_2 cases. The treatment consisted of complete androgen deprivation over at least 6 months until a serum PSA nadir was observed. Treatment was then withheld according to the increase of the PSA level. Treatment was restarted when the PSA level had increased to a mean value of 10–20 ng/ml (average 14 ng/ml). The first two treatment cycles (one cycle being the sum of treatment plus off-treatment time) lasted 73 and 75 weeks with a mean time off therapy of 30–33 weeks. During off-treatment time, a return to normal serum testosterone levels was observed after an average of 8 weeks. In seven out of 14 patients in clinical stage D₂, the mean time until androgen-independent relapse occurred was 128 weeks. The average cancer-specific survival time was 232 weeks. In all other patients the mean time to androgen-independent tumor progression in this non-randomized clinical study was 310 weeks.

Our own clinical observations

In our hospital, in a pilot study, patients with cancer of the prostate and a low tumor burden were initiated for IAD. We recruited patients with PSA progression after retropubic radical prostatectomy (RRP) and patients after transurethral resection of the prostate (TURP) with incidental cancer of the prostate (pT_1) who were unsuitable candidates for RRP. The mean time of PSA progression after RRP

was 14 months; the mean time for patients with pT_1 disease after TURP was 30 months. For this presentation we evaluated 25 patients with a mean follow-up duration of 30 months (12–50 months). Seventeen patients had a PSA progression after RRP and eight patients had incidental cancer of the prostate.

The study design is given in Figure 2. The mean pre-treatment PSA level was 5.1 ng/ml (4.2–9.0) in the RRP group and 9.3 (7.5–16.0) in the pT_1 group.

Androgen deprivation was achieved by complete androgen suppression with the use of LHRH agonists in combination with antiandrogens. In 20 patients leuprolide depot and in five patients buserelin depot was administered for medical castration by LHRH agonists. The duration of complete androgen suppression was 9 months. The primary parameter of this study was the time to androgen independence, i.e.

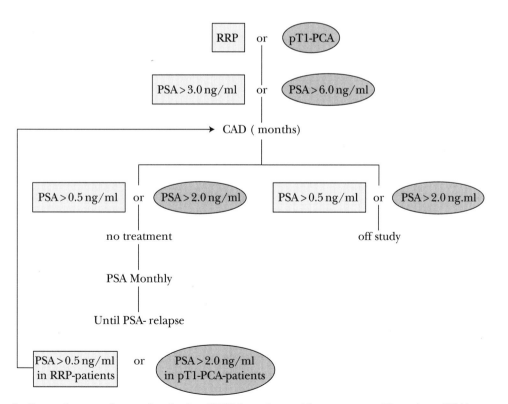

Figure 2 Intermittent androgen deprivation (IAD) in patients with prostate specific antigen (PSA) progression after radical retropubic prostatectomy (RRP) or incidental prostate cancer (pT₁-PCA)

123

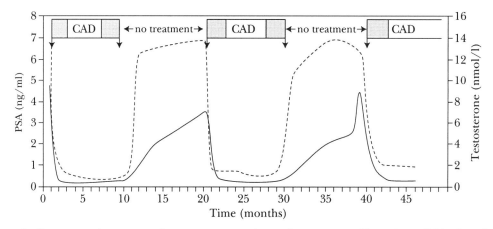

Figure 3 Representative course of serum concentrations of prostate specific antigen (PSA; dotted curve) and testosterone (unbroken curve) in a 59-year-old patient with PSA progression 15 months after radical retropubic prostatectomy and two cycles of intermittent androgen deprivation. CAD, complete androgen deprivation

PSA progression in spite of complete androgen deprivation. A representative course of the serum concentrations of PSA and testosterone is illustrated in Figure 3. During the 9 months of treatment, testosterone levels decreased to castrate levels. PSA levels dropped in the first and second cycles; a slower increase of the PSA levels was observed during off-treatment intervals in both cycles. Treatment was restarted when PSA levels reached the threshold of 3 ng/ml in RRP and 6 ng/ml in stage pT₁ patients with a repeated 9-month cycle of androgen deprivation. For these preliminary clinical results the data of 25 patients were available. The median time off treatment was 36 weeks (45% of the complete cycle). So far no patient has had androgen-independent tumor progression during the evaluated mean observation time of 30 months.

Conclusion

Permanent androgen suppression is the therapy of choice in the treatment of advanced prostate cancer. Intermittent androgen suppression, through reversible medical castration, results hypothetically in an androgen-induced differentiation of stem cells with recovery of the apoptotic potential. The cyclic changes of periods with and without androgen withdrawal should result in a slowing down of tumor progression and in an improvement in quality of life. The successful use of IAD is based on the concept of the cessation of development of a heterogeneous tumor cell population. In the initial pilot studies, IAD proved to be less successful in patients with high tumor burden than in patients with locally advanced prostatic cancer. In our own pilot study, patients with low tumor burden were successfully treated with IAD.

Until further studies have been completed, the therapeutic use of IAD should be treated as experimental in character. Only further prospective randomized phase III studies will be able to answer the question of whether the survival and quality of life of patients with cancer of the prostate can be considerably improved by using intermittent androgen suppression as a therapy of choice.

References

1. Huggins, C. and Hodges, C. V. (1941). Studies on prostate cancer. I. Effect of castration, estrogen, and androgen injection on serum phosphatases in metastatic carcinoma of the prostate. *Cancer Res.*, **1**, 293–7
2. Denis, L. and Murphy, G. P. (1993). Overview of phase III trials on combined androgen treatment in patients with metastatic prostate cancer. *Cancer,* **72** (Suppl.), 3888–95
3. Prostate Cancer Trialists' Collaborative Group (1995). Maximum androgen blockade in advanced prostate cancer: an overview of 22 randomized trials with 3283 deaths in 5710 patients. *Lancet,* **346**, 265–9
4. Akakura, K., Bruchovsky, N., Goldenberg, S. L., Rennie, P. S., Buckley, A. R. and Sullivan, L. D. (1993). Effects of intermittent androgen suppression on androgen-dependent tumors: apoptosis and serum prostate specific antigen. *Cancer,* **71**, 2782–90
5. Bruchovsky, N., Rennie, P. S., Goldman, A. J., Goldenberg, S. L., To, M. and Lawson, D. (1990). Effects of androgen withdrawal on the stem cell composition of the Shionogi carcinoma. *Cancer Res.*, **50**, 2275–82
6. Gleave, M. E., Hsieh, J. T., Wu, H.-C., von-Eschenbach, A. C. and Chung, L. W. (1992). Serum PSA levels in mice bearing human prostate LNCaP tumours are determined by tumour volume and endocrine and growth factors. *Cancer Res.*, **52**, 1598–605
7. Vahlensieck, W. and Wegner, G. (1980). Continuous versus intermittent oral therapy with estramustine phosphate (Estracyt). *Scand. J. Urol. Nephrol.* (Suppl.), **55**, 147–9
8. Klotz, L. H., Herr, H. W., Morse, M. J. and Withmore, W. F. Jr (1986). Intermittent endocrine therapy for advanced prostate cancer. *Cancer,* **58**, 2546–50
9. Goldenberg, S. L., Bruchowsky, N., Gleave, M. E., Sullivan, L. D. and Akadura, K. (1995). Intermittent androgen suppression in the treatment of prostate cancer: a preliminary report. *Urology,* **45**, 839–44

Interactive Voting System

1   Restart of androgen deprivation in IAD therapy should be done:

Response	*Option*
11%	When PSA nadir is reached.
1%	When normal testosterone levels are achieved.
0%	When the patient becomes symptomatic.
84%	When PSA levels increase above an individual pathological cut-off value.
4%	After 9 months.

Number of votes: 134

2   Intermittent androgen deprivation therapy:

1%	Is a routine approach in the treatment of advanced prostate cancer.
1%	Is a routine approach in the treatment of localized prostate cancer.
87%	Should be offered only as part of prospective trials.
4%	Offers improved quality of life in phase III trials.
7%	Is appropriate for patients with failure of serum PSA to decrease to normal range after initiating androgen withdrawal.

Number of votes: 133

PSA and other serum markers as prognostic factors of response duration and patient survival in metastatic prostate carcinoma

15

R. A. Janknegt

Introduction

The initial results of hormonal therapy in metastatic prostate cancer seem to be very favorable. Symptomatic improvement is seen in 70–80% and the biochemical improvement for prostate specific antigen (PSA), alkaline phosphatase (ALP) and prostate acid phosphatase (PAP) is 99%[1]. However, it is well known that the overall results are not as encouraging. First of all, the improvement lasts for a limited period of time and it shows a high variation in individual patients. In large groups, it does not seem to make much difference whether there is improvement in the biochemical factors and whether castration or maximum androgen blockade are used. In recent publication by Dalesio and colleagues[2], who performed a meta-analysis of 25 trials, it was shown that the 5-year survival was 22.8% for castration and 26.2% for maximum androgen blockade. There was a difference of 3.5% with a 95% confidence interval of 0–7%. This study did not show a significant difference, or additional benefit of maximum androgen blockade over castration.

It is our opinion that studies on the various levels of biochemical improvements should be performed. Riedl and co-workers[3] examined a group of 50 patients with stage C and D prostate carcinoma for PSA levels after orchidectomy. An elevated PSA was initially found in 98% of all patients, the PSA level had decreased in 99% after 3–6 months. However, there was a large difference in the mean remission of three

groups. In group 1, the PSA level was < 1 ng/ml after 45.9 months; in group 2, the PSA level was 1–10 ng/ml after 16.7 months; and in group 3, the PSA level was > 10 ng/ml after 12.5 months. This small study demonstrates that it is important to assess the amount of decrease in the level of PSA.

The relationship between PSA doubling time and DNA ploidy was also studied[4]. Diploid tumors had the longest PSA doubling time and non-ploid tumors a short PSA doubling time. PSA doubling time also seems to be a strong predictor of prognosis. The patients with the shortest PSA doubling time apparently required more aggressive combined treatment, again showing the value of assessing the individual variations of PSA level.

ALP flare after orchidectomy was studied in a recent series of 112 patients undergoing castration[5]. The initial ALP level was already shown to be a very important predictor of progression. An ALP level of ≥ 2 times normal was a very negative predictor. The study of the level of ALP within 28 days after the orchidectomy showed four groups:

(1) Group 1: there was no increase and the median time to survival was average;

(2) Group 2: there was an increase of < 1.5 times the initial value;

(3) Group 3: there was an increase of 1.5–2 times the initial value; and

(4) Group 4: there was an increase of > 2 times the initial value.

All showed an increasing negative predictive factor for progression.

In stage D_2 untreated prostate cancer, we performed a long-term double-blind placebo-controlled multicenter randomized study comparing orchidectomy plus nilutamide (Anandron) vs. orchidectomy plus placebo. We have published the favorable effect of maximal androgen blockade in terms of progression-free survival[6]. In all evaluable patients ($n = 202$) we showed that the median time for maximal androgen blockade was 21.2 months vs. orchidectomy plus placebo ($n = 208$) of over 14.7 months (Figure 1). The p-value was 0.0036. We retrospectively studied the PSA variations after 3 months, the ALP levels at baseline and the PAP levels at 3 months.

Aim of the study

Our aim was to define a subgroup of patients who might derive more benefit from hormonal therapy: either complete or partial hormone deprivation.

Materials and methods

A large multi-center double-blind placebo-controlled study was performed mainly in Europe, but we also had patient entry from centers in the United States, Canada, South Africa and South America. In this study, castration by orchidectomy plus nilutamide was compared with orchidectomy plus placebo[6]. Nilutamide was given at a daily dose of 300 mg for 1 month and 150 mg daily thereafter. All patients had stage D_2 carcinoma of the prostate with bone metastasis, as documented by either radioisotope bone scan and X-ray or computerized tomography (CT) scan. The three serum markers were obtained before treatment and at months 1, 3, 6 and every 6 months thereafter as long as the patient remained in the study. Blood tests for PSA were performed in a central laboratory (CERBA, France).

Values of > 2.5 ng/ml were considered abnormal by this assay. Progression was assessed according to the criteria described by the National Prostate Cancer Project. PAP and ALP levels were assayed by the laboratories of each participating centre. The reference was the ratio to the upper limit of the normal range for each individual laboratory.

We performed two steps of analysis: (1) regardless of treatment; and (2) with regard to treatment groups.

Regardless of treatment   We explored PSA, PAP and ALP alone on continuous variable or multivariate analysis of the prognostic value of these three markers. The multivariate analysis was restricted to the levels of the markers at baseline, month 1 and month 3. With the information obtained later, this point was of less clinical interest.

With regard to treatment groups   Patients were classified into prognostic groups based upon these data. The association between markers and outcome (time to progression and survival) was analyzed by means of the Cox proportional hazards model. The Cox regression proportional hazards model and Wald χ^2 statistics were used for the association between markers and endpoints. Kaplan–Meier estimates for progression-free survival rates, and logrank tests for between-group comparison, were used.

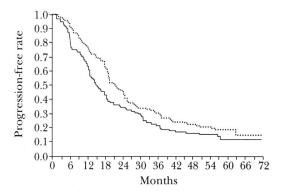

Figure 1 Progression-free survival in evaluable patients. Dotted line, nilutamide ($n = 202$), median 21.2 months; continuous line, placebo ($n = 208$), median 14.7 months; $p = 0.0036$

Results

A total of 457 patients were enrolled, of whom 423 were eligible for efficacy analysis. Only seven patients (1.7%) had a normal PSA level at baseline; normal ALP level at baseline was seen in 139 (33%) patients; and the PAP level was normal at baseline in 20%. The median follow-up was 52–78 months. Endpoints were time to objective progression, time to death by cancer, or time to death by any cause.

Stepwise regression removed PAP measurement, so all further studies evaluated only PSA and ALP.

Prognostic value of measurement of baseline ALP level

In those patients with an ALP level of ≤ 2 times normal ($n = 245$), we found a median time to progression-free survival in all evaluable patients of 23.2 months. The progression-free survival with an ALP level of > 2 times normal ($n = 173$) was 12.5 months ($p < 0.0001$) (Figure 2). The overall survival in evaluable patients with an ALP level of ≤ 2 times normal ($n = 245$) was a median of 33.2 months and with an ALP level of > 2 times normal ($n = 173$) was 19.0 months ($p = 0.0001$).

Prognostic value of PSA measurement at month 3

The progression-free survival of month 3 PSA measurement for PSA level below the normal value ($n = 121$) was 24.1 months median time and for PSA level above the normal value ($n = 151$) it was 17.3 months ($p = 0.0001$) (Figure 3). The overall survival in all evaluable patients for PSA level below or at the normal value ($n = 121$) was 37.0 months median time, and for PSA level above the normal value ($n = 151$) it was 24.3 months ($p = 0.0001$).

Prognostic value of month 3 PSA measurement in patients with baseline ALP level of ≤ 2 times normal

In those patients who had a favorable decrease of month 3 PSA level to below the nadir in comparison with baseline ALP level, the results were even more favorable. The progression-free survival for PSA level below the nadir ($n = 80$) was a median of 36.2 months, and for PSA level above the nadir ($n = 76$), it was 18.3 months.

In an assessment of the combined prognostic factors for median time to progression, only the combination with baseline ALP level of < 2 times normal was favorable for month 3 PSA measurement. In all patients with a baseline ALP level

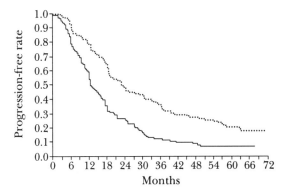

Figure 2 Progression-free survival in evaluable patients, showing the prognostic value of measurement of baseline alkaline phosphatase (ALP) level. Dotted line, ALP ≤ 2 times normal ($n = 245$), median 23.2 months; continuous line, ALP > 2 times normal ($n = 173$), median 12.5 months; $p < 0.0001$

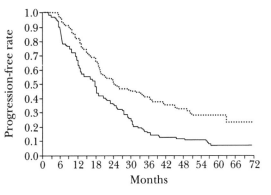

Figure 3 Progression-free survival in evaluable patients, showing the prognostic value of month 3 measurement of prostate specific antigen (PSA) level. Dotted line, PSA level at or below the normal value ($n = 121$), median 24.1 months; continuous line, PSA level above the normal value ($n = 151$), median 17.3 months; $p < 0.0001$

Table 1 Median time to progression (months) for patients have determinations of both baseline levels of alkaline phosphatase (ALP) and month 3 levels of prostate specific antigen (PSA)

| Baseline ALP | Month 3 PSA | | Total patients | p-Value |
	≤ Nadir	> Nadir		
≤ 2 times normal	34.0 (n = 79)	18.2 (n = 75)	154	0.0011
> 2 times normal	15.6 (n = 37)	15.9 (n = 74)	111	0.3014

of > 2 times normal, there was no difference of month 3 PSA level, either normalizing to below the normal value or remaining above the normal value (Table 1).

With regard to treatment group

When looking at the rate of PSA normalization at month 3, we found that maximum androgen blockade (orchidectomy plus nilutamide; $n = 137$) had 59% normalization vs. 29% in orchidectomy plus placebo ($n = 135$). Even more favorable was the outcome with the combined prognostic factors that showed PSA normalization at month 3 in those patients who had a baseline ALP level of ≤ 2 times normal. The maximum androgen blockage group ($n = 84$) showed a normalization of 66% vs. 35% with orchidectomy plus placebo ($n = 72$) (Figure 4).

Discussion

Instead of looking at the overall survival of the entire group, it now seems clear that there is a wide variation of response and that the prognosis can be predicted by individual serum markers such as baseline ALP level and month 3 PSA measurement. The combination of the two markers shows the most favorable results in patients starting with a lower than normal value ALP level and a month 3 PSA level below the normal value.

Irrespective of the treatment groups, we showed that the PSA level soon after initiation of hormonal therapy is strongly correlated with the three long-term endpoints. We also found that the PSA level itself is a better predictor than its decrease from baseline in general.

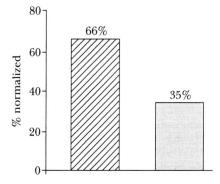

Figure 4 Rate of normalization of prostate specific antigen level at month 3 for patients with an alkaline phosphatase level of ≤ 2 times normal. Hatched bar, orchidectomy plus nilutamide ($n = 84$); shaded bar, orchidectomy plus placebo ($n = 72$)

Combining baseline ALP value and month 3 PSA level brings early reliable information on patient outcome.

Nilutamide combined with castration significantly increased the rate of early PSA normalizations: overall 59% vs. 29% and, in patients with ALP level < 2 times normal, 66% vs. 35%.

It might be speculated that in the future these markers could open the possibility of individual cascade therapy. In **step 1**, monotherapy with an antiandrogen might be started in those patients who are still sexually active. If the baseline ALP level was < 2 times normal and the PSA level decreased to the normal value, the patient could remain on this therapy under control of the PSA assessment on a monthly basis. During this time, the quality of life of this patient could be relatively good.

As soon as there is a PSA rise of > 2.5 times normal, **step 2** might be introduced, namely, maximum androgen blockade. If the PSA level then decreases again to the normal value, the patient would be left under this therapy until a further rise of the PSA level. **Step 3** would be addition of chemotherapy (for example estramustin).

New studies that assess these variations of serum markers, perhaps also including the free/total ratio of PSA, may increase our understanding of the various heterogeneous groups of prostate cancer and also derive more benefit for special subgroups of patients.

References

1. Smith, J. A. Jr, Lange, P. H., Janknegt, R. A., Abbou, C. C. and De Gery, A. (1996). Serum markers as a predictor of response duration and patient survival after hormonal therapy for metastatic carcinoma of the prostate. *J. Urol.*, in press
2. Prostate Cancer Trialists' Collaborative Group (1995). Maximum androgen blockade in advanced prostate cancer: an overview of 22 randomised trials with 3283 deaths in 5710 patients. *Lancet*, **346**, 265–9
3. Riedl, C. R., Huebner, W. A., Mossig, H., Ogris, E. and Pflueger, H. (1995). Prognostic value of prostate-specific antigen minimum after orchidectomy in patients with stage C and D prostatic carcinoma. *Br. J. Urol.*, **76**, 34–40
4. Pollack, A., Zagars, G. K., El-Naggar, A. K. and Terry, N. H. (1994). Relationship of tumor DNA-ploidy to serum prostate-specific antigen doubling time after radiotherapy for prostate cancer. *Urology*, **44**, 711–18
5. Pelger, R. C. M., Lycklama à Nijeholt, G. A. B., Zwinderman, A. H., Papapoulos, S. E. *et al.* (1995). The flare in serum alkaline phosphatase activity after orchiectomy: a valuable negative prognostic index in metastatic prostate cancer (Abstr. 739). *J. Urol.*, **153**, 412A
6. Janknegt, R. A., Abbou, C. C., Bartoletti, R., Bernstein-Hahn, L., Bracken, B., Brisset, J. M., Calais, da Silva, F., Chisholm, G., Crawford, E. D., Debruyne, F. M. J., Dijkman, G. D., Frick, J., Goedhals, L., Knönagel, H. and Venner, P. M. (1993). Orchiectomy and nilutamide or placebo as treatment of metastatic prostatic cancer in a multinational double-blind randomized trial. *J. Urol.*, **149**, 77–83

Interactive Voting System

1 In metastatic prostate carcinoma the mean survival for hormonal therapy is 25 months in most studies. If your patient on M.A.B. has a favorable nadir in 3 months, would you think this leads to average improvement of progression by 50% and survival by 50%?

Response	*Option*
42%	Yes.
58%	No.

Number of votes: 95

2 Would you change your treatment strategy?

28%	Yes.
72%	No.

Number of votes: 111

Hot flushes under endocrine treatment and their management   16

E. Varenhorst and M. Hammar

Introduction

Hot flushes are accepted as a characteristic symptom of the menopause in women and are a consequence of decreasing estrogen levels. Flushing in men after bilateral orchidectomy or administration of gonadotropin releasing hormone (GnRH) analogs suggests that testicular failure may also be associated with disturbed regulation of vasomotion.

In 1896 Cabot reported 'uncomfortable flushes of heat' in males castrated for treatment of benign enlargement of the prostate[1]. In 1941 Huggins and co-workers[2] described, probably for the first time, hot flushes after orchidectomy for carcinoma of the prostate. 'Hot flushes, beginning 2 to 6 weeks postoperatively were associated with profuse perspiration, often occurring at night, forcing the patient to throw off the bed covers'[2]. Since then there has been little in the literature concerning hot flushes in patients treated for prostate cancer. Later reports appearing after the introduction of GnRH analogs in the therapy of prostate cancer, however, emphasize that the majority of men who have undergone androgen deprivation therapy suffer from hot flushes and episodic sweating that often interfere with their quality of life[3–6].

Characteristics of hot flushes in males – an objective phenomenon

Hot flushing is difficult to study, because of the rapidity of the physiological response and because people who claim they flush frequently may not always do so in the laboratory. Ginsburg and O'Reilly[7] first objectively investigated the thermovascular reaction during a hot flush in a man treated with orchidectomy for carcinoma of the prostate. Circulatory studies performed during an attack showed a pronounced increase in hand blood flow that coincided with the onset of symptoms. An increase also occurred in forearm blood flow and in pulse rate. These results were later confirmed in another investigation[8]. Among 66 males suffering from hot flushes after orchidectomy, 13 men with the highest frequency were selected for a study concerning the temporal correlation between the subjective symptoms and the physiological changes during the hot flushes[8]. Measurements of cutaneous blood flow and sweating were performed continuously for an average of 3 h. During this time, nine out of 13 patients experienced a total of 23 attacks of hot flushing. Sweating was recorded with an evaporimeter and cutaneous blood flow with a laser Doppler flow meter. Eight patients had at least one flush with an increase in water evaporation. One man with only a single attack showed no increase in water evaporation but a pronounced increase in cutaneous blood flow. Eight patients had at least one attack with an increase in blood flow to more than 150% of the basal value. One patient with six attacks showed no detectable increase in blood flow but a moderate increase in water evaporation.

All patients experienced a sensation of warmth, often spreading from the chest to the rest of the body, followed by sweating mostly from the forehead, chest and back but, interestingly enough, not involving the palms and soles, areas having pronounced emotional sweating.

Only four of 13 patients showed a faint flush, but in most cases nothing obvious could be seen. The duration of each attack varied from 30 s to 5 min with a mean of 2.5 min. Synchronously with the patients' experience of a hot flush, a marked increase in the rate of water evaporation was seen in 68% of the attacks, probably reflecting activation of sweat glands.

Provoking factors for the hot flushes and feelings afterwards

In many cases hot flushes come on without premonitory symptoms, with no obvious relation to external factors. In an evaluation by questionnaire of 30 patients who reported hot flushes during androgen deprivation therapy, 15 stated that there were no provoking factors for the flushes. In the other patients flushes were provoked by heat, physical activity, stress, hot drinks, alcohol or salt-rich meals. In another group of patients who flushed, 34% said that anxiety was a precipitating cause[9]. McCallum and Reading[10] studied ten men suffering from hot flushes after orchidectomy or GnRH analog treatment regarding provoking factors and concluded that the flushes were induced by thermogenic stimuli. They found that in men who reduced the temperature of their hot drinks and the amount of night clothing they wore, the frequency of flushing was halved.

After the flushing, 60% of the patients denied any further symptoms, but the remaining had unpleasant sensations such as fatigue, headache and a globus sensation in the throat; one man described a metallic taste in the mouth[9].

Prevalence of hot flushes

The hot flushes begin within a period of a few days to 12 months after castration[5]. In a study of 90 orchidectomized patients flushes in most cases started within 4 weeks, but in 10% they appeared after 3 months[6]. In clinical trials with GnRH analogs the prevalence of hot flushes increased from 25% within 6 weeks to 53% after 6 weeks or 31% within 12 weeks to 51% in 12–48 weeks while on treatment[11,12].

In an evaluation by questionnaire of 90 consecutive orchidectomized patients, 66 (73%) had hot flushes[8]. The prevalence and frequency per day of flushing correlates well with another report, which collected data by questionnaire[5]. In different studies, the prevalence of hot flushes in patients who underwent surgical or medical castration varied from 43 to 77% (Table 1).

Pattern with time and severity of hot flushes

There are few long-term reports in the literature. Charig and Rundle[5] followed 50 men for 6

Table 1 Prevalence of hot flushes in patients with carcinoma of the prostate treated with surgical or medical (GnRH analogs) castration

Reference	Treatment	Prevalence of hot flushes (%)
Huggins et al. (1941)[2]	orchidectomy	43
Varenhorst et al. (1983)[6]	orchidectomy	73
Smith (1984)[3]	leuprolide	77
Parmar et al. (1987)[4]	triptorelin	76
Charig and Rundle (1989)[5]	orchidectomy	76
Peeling (1989)[13]	goserelin	63
	orchidectomy	58
De Voogt et al. (1990)[11]	buserelin	53
Kaisary et al. (1991)[14]	goserelin	63
Falkson et al. (1991)[15]	buserelin	69
Tyrrell et al. (1991)[16]	goserelin	64
Atala et al. (1992)[17]	orchidectomy	54
Dijkman et al. (1995)[12]	goserelin	54

months to 4 years. Of 38 patients, 19 (50%) had ceased flushing after 2 years.

In an attempt to establish whether the hot flushes persist for 5 years or more, 77 men were evaluated by a questionnaire 5–11 years after the start of treatment for advanced carcinoma of the prostate[9]. Hot flushes after orchidectomy or GnRH analog treatment still occurred in almost half of the patients after more than 5 years.

The use of logbooks with daily recording of the number and intensity of hot flushes is sometimes employed to monitor the attacks[8,18,19]. In this way the number of hot flushes recorded in 66 of 90 patients over 24 h was 1–3 in 44%, 4–10 in 47% and > 10 in 9%, 2–48 months after orchidectomy (mean 14 months)[8]. Fifty per cent were not troubled by the flushes, 23% were slightly inconvenienced and 27% were greatly distressed[8]. The intensity of the attacks as experienced by the patients corresponded closely with the recorded nature of the flushing by other workers[5]. However, no patient was classified as being untroubled by the flushes[5]. Since there seems to be a high correlation between the two recorded variables (frequency per 24 h and intensity), the number of hot flushes per 24 h might be sufficient for monitoring hot flushes[19].

Pathogenesis of hot flushes

It is not known why some patients have hot flushes and some do not. It has been speculated that those without flushes may have a higher level, although within the castration range, of non-testicular androgens circulating after castration, which by itself or after conversion to an estrogen prevents vasomotor symptoms[5].

The precise etiology of the hot flush is still unknown. Lability in the thermoregulatory center appears to be the cause. Changes in hypothalamic neurotransmitter activity such as β-endorphin or norepinephrine, which in turn stabilize the thermoregulatory center, have been suggested[20]. It is possible that changed hormonal levels result in sensitization of peripheral and central neurons, making them more susceptible to neural input.

There is a temporal correlation between elevated luteinizing hormone concentrations caused by a GnRH pulse and the hot flushes. β-Endorphin inhibits the release of GnRH and may also influence the thermoregulatory center, which is located in the hypothalamus. Sex steroids stimulate the release of endogenous β-endorphins which may explain the beneficial effects of estrogens on hot flushes[21]. Neuropeptide Y, widely distributed in the central or peripheral nervous system, is considered to be a possible transmitter or modulator of sympathetic activity[22].

Another neuropeptide of possible importance is calcitonin gene-related peptide (CGRP). This is a potent vasodilator produced in the central as well as the peripheral nervous system and may be involved in the mechanisms behind flushing. Recently it has been shown that the release of CGRP at the spinal cord level is modulated by endogenous opioids. The systemic infusion of CGRP also induced a flush in the face, neck, upper arm and upper trunk. After successful treatment of perimenopausal hot flushes in women by acupuncture, the excretion of CGRP in urine decreased[19]. A study in men concerning changes in the level of this peptide in relation to hot flushes after castration is in progress.

Management of hot flushes

The treatment remains essentially empirical.

Estrogens

It has long been known that estrogens reduce the severity and frequency of hot flushes. As early as 1941 Huggins and co-workers[2] mitigated hot flushes for many weeks by oral or subcutaneous administration of 1 mg of stilbestrol daily for 5 days, but the matter subsequently fell into oblivion. Nearly 3 decades later, treatment with 3 mg/day of diethylstilbestrol (DES) was reported to be effective in the treatment of post-orchidectomy hot flushes in one man[23]. DES at a dose of 0.33 mg daily likewise improved troublesome post-orchidectomy hot flushes in nine of 12 patients. Five men, however, experienced gynecomastia or breast soreness[24].

A double-blind, placebo-controlled cross-over trial confirmed that the treatment of hot flushes can be effectively managed with a low dose of DES (1 mg daily). Fourteen patients demonstrated a 100% response. Twelve of the 14 patients (86%) treated with DES had complete resolution of hot flushes and two patients (14%) demonstrated a significant reduction in the frequency, duration and severity of hot flushes[17].

Medroxyprogesterone acetate and megestrol acetate

In a small pilot study the progestational agent medroxyprogesterone acetate, 5 mg twice daily, was tried and appeared to be an effective agent for controlling the flushes[5]. In a formal randomized double-blind cross-over trial, megestrol acetate, another progestational agent, was tested in 66 men. A dose of 20 mg twice daily was well tolerated and substantially decreased the frequency of hot flushes after bilateral orchidectomy or during treatment with a GnRH analog[25].

Cyproterone acetate

Cyproterone acetate (CPA), a steroid with progestational as well as antiandrogenic properties, has been used in the treatment of hot flushes for many years. The usefulness of CPA in hot flushes was proved in a double-blind placebo-controlled cross-over trial at a dosage of 100 mg orally taken three times per day. Compared to placebo, CPA caused the number of hot flushes to decrease significantly. For the first 3 weeks of the study, eight patients received CPA and four patients received placebo. Five of the 12 patients complained of lassitude while on CPA. In one patient the dosage had to be reduced to 100 mg daily. This dosage completely suppressed the hot flushes[26]. A dose–response study confirmed this observation and showed that a dose of 50–100 mg daily seemed to be as effective as 300 mg daily[27].

Similarly in an open trial with CPA at a dosage of 100 mg daily, the occurrence of hot flushes was suppressed in 21 of 22 patients[28].

In a much larger placebo-controlled double-blind study including 273 patients who had hot flushes or outbreaks of sweat after orchidectomy, 150 mg CPA per day was given. In the CPA group both phenomena were significantly reduced. After 6 months hot flushes were experienced by 33% of patients receiving CPA and 60% in the placebo group; 24% of CPA-treated patients had outbreaks of sweating compared to 47% of placebo-treated patients[29].

Non-endocrine treatment has also been used in men with hot flushes, but with limited success.

Clonidine

Clonidine is a central α-adrenergic agonist, which has been tried as a treatment for hot flushes. In a pilot study in seven patients with frequent and bothersome hot flushes after bilateral orchidectomy, it was suggested that a 0.1 mg per day, transdermal clonidine patch weekly could control hot flushes in men[30]. Contrary to these findings, elimination of hot flushes was rare in 14 patients receiving 1 mg oral clonidine daily. Only five patients had a partial response and eight had no change[31]. Similar findings were noted when a clonidine patch was used. Three of seven patients had a partial response and four were unchanged[31]. Despite these promising pilot studies a randomized double-blind cross-over trial on 17 men suffering from hot flushes who had undergone medical or surgical castration demonstrated that clonidine did *not* significantly decrease the frequency and severity of hot flushes[18].

Phenobarbital plus ergotamine

Some palliative effect was seen in an open study in 21 patients who received a combination of phenobarbital plus ergotamine, 1 tablet twice daily. One patient had a complete response, nine had a partial response and 11 reported no change[31].

Endocrine vs. non-endocrine drugs

In a comparison of non-endocrine treatment (phenobarbital plus ergotamine or clonidine) to endocrine treatment with DES or megesterol acetate, endocrine treatment provided the best therapeutic response. Sixteen patients self-titrated the dose of DES to the lowest amount that could eliminate or improve the hot flushes and often took as little as 0.25 mg daily. The complete response rate with DES was statistically superior to that achieved with combined phenobarbital plus ergotamine or clonidine. Most patients had, however, at least some degree of tender gynecomastia even at these low DES doses. Megesterol acetate (20 mg twice daily) was used in 11 patients. A complete response was noted in seven patients, a partial response in two and no change in one. As with DES, the complete response rate with megesterol acetate was statistically superior to that achieved with combined phenobarbital plus ergotamine or clonidine[31].

Non-pharmacological therapies

These have yet not been studied in men with hot flushes, but acupuncture was found to reduce the number of hot flushes significantly among postmenopausal women[19]. The explanation may be the influence of acupuncture on hypothalamic β-endorphins.

Conclusion

In summary, the most accepted treatment modalities of advanced carcinoma of the prostate are bilateral orchidectomy or GnRH analogs. Apart from impotence the onset of hot flushes is the most frequently reported side effect. In many patients these symptoms are mild. However, up to 50% of men experience significant discomfort, which affects their quality of life and can persist for more than 5 years[9]. It is not understood why some men do not flush. Hot flushes come on without premonitory symptoms or are precipitated by emotional upset, hot drinks, meals or a warm environment. The precise pathophysiology of hot flushes is not well understood. The latest theories postulate an involvement of endogenous opioids and vasodilating neuropeptides.

Treatment, then, remains essentially empirical. Several non-hormonal and hormonal drugs have been proposed for treatment of hot flushes in men who have undergone androgen deprivation therapy, but only DES, cyproterone acetate and megestrol acetate, in double-blind placebo-controlled trials, have been shown to be effective in ameliorating post-castration hot flushes (Table 2).

The similarity of the vasomotor symptoms in men and women suggests the same causal mechanism. Accordingly, similar treatments could work in males and females.

Table 2 Placebo-controlled double-blind trials evaluating the prevention of hot flushes in patients with carcinoma of the prostate treated with surgical or medical castration

Reference	Drug dosage	Patients (n)	Results
Eaton and McGuire (1983)[26]	CPA 300 mg daily, orally	12	significant reduction of the frequency of HF
Krämer *et al.* (1992)[29]	CPA 150 mg daily, orally	273	significant reduction of the severity and frequency of HF
Atala *et al.* (1992)[17]	DES 1 mg daily, orally	14	significant reduction of the severity and frequency of HF
Loprinzi *et al.* (1994)[18]	clonidine transdermally, equivalent to daily oral dose of 0.1 mg	77	no significant reduction of the severity and frequency of HF
Loprinzi *et al.* (1994)[25]	megestrol acetate 40 mg daily, orally	66	significant reduction of the severity and frequenty of HF

CPA, cyproterone acetate; DES, diethylstilbestrol; HF, hot flushes

Today the treatment of choice for women suffering from hot flushes is without doubt estrogen replacement, which could be delivered orally or via a transdermal patch, which circumvents the enhanced hepatic actions of the hormone[32,33]. The transdermal administration could probably avoid the risk of increased cardiovascular morbidity, when estrogens are given in men. To our knowledge clinical experience with transdermal estrogen treat-ment in men with hot flushes is so far limited. To evaluate this promising possibility, a double-blind placebo-controlled randomized trial to assess the efficacy and toxicity of transcutaneous estrogen in men suffering from post-castration hot flushes should be conducted.

Complete understanding of the pathogenesis of the hot flush is, however, a prerequisite of causal therapy.

References

1. Cabot, A. T. (1896). The question of castration for enlarged prostate. *Ann. Surg.*, **24**, 265–309
2. Huggins, C., Stevens, R. C. and Hodges, C. V. (1941). Studies on prostatic cancer. II. The effects of castration of advanced carcinoma of prostate gland. *Arch. Surg.*, **43**, 209–23
3. Smith, J. A. (1984). Androgen suppression by a gonadotropin releasing hormone analogue in patients with metastatic carcinoma of the prostate. *J. Urol.*, **131**, 1110–12
4. Parmar, H., Edwards, L. and Philips, R. H. (1987). Orchiectomy versus long-acting D-Trp-6-LHRH in advanced prostatic cancer. *Br. J. Urol.*, **59**, 248–54
5. Charig, C. R. and Rundle, J. S. (1989). Long-term side effect of orchiectomy in treatment of prostatic carcinoma. *Urology*, **33**, 175–8
6. Varenhorst, E., Frödin, T. and Ålund, G. (1983). Climacteric flushing in a man (Letter). *Br. Med. J.*, **287**, 838–9
7. Ginsburg, J. and O'Reilly, O. (1983). Climacteric flushing in a man. *Br. Med. J.*, **287**, 262
8. Frödin, T., Ålund, G. and Varenhorst, E. (1985). Measurement of skin blood-flow and water evaporation as a means of objectively assessing hot flushes after orchidectomy in patients with carcinoma of the prostate. *Prostate*, **7**, 203–8
9. Karling, P., Hammar, M. and Varenhorst, E. (1994). Prevalence and duration of hot flushes after surgical or medical castration in men with prostatic carcinoma. *J. Urol.*, **152**, 1170–3
10. McCallum, K. A. and Reading, C. (1989). Hot flushes are induced by thermogenic stimuli. *Br. J. Urol.*, **64**, 507–10
11. De Voogt, H. J., Klijn, J. G. M., Studer, U., Schröder, F., Sylvester, R., De Pauw, M. and Members of the EORTC-Gu Group (1990). Orchidectomy versus buserelin in combination with cyproterone acetate, for 2 weeks or continuously, in the treatment of metastatic prostatic cancer. Preliminary results of EORTC-trial 30843. *J. Steroid. Biochem. Molec. Biol*, **36.**, 965–9
12. Dijkman, G. A., Debruyne, F. M. J., Fernandez del Moral, P., Plasman, J. W. M. H., Hoekfakker, J. W., Idema, J. G. and Sykes, M. (1995). A randomised trial comparing the safety and efficacy of the Zoladex 10.8-mg Depot, administered every 12 weeks, to that of the Zoladex 3.6-mg Depot, administered every 4 weeks, in patients with advanced prostate cancer. *Eur. Urol.*, **27**, 43–6
13. Peeling, W. B. (1989). Phase III studies to compare goserelin (Zoladex) with orchidectomy and with diethylstilboestrol in treatment of prostatic carcinoma. *Urology*, **33** (Suppl.) 45–52
14. Kaisary, A. V., Tyrell, C. J., Peeling, W. B. and Griffiths, K. (1991). Comparison of LHRH analogue (Zoladex) with orchiectomy in patients with metastatic prostatic carcinoma. *Br. J. Urol.*, **67**, 502–8
15. Falkson, C. I., Falkson, G. and Falkson, H. C. (1991). Long term follow-up of patients with advanced prostatic cancer treated with nasal buserelin. *Ann. Oncol.*, **2**, 303–4
16. Tyrrell, C. J., Altwein, J. E., Klippel, F., Varenhorst, E., Lunglmayr, G., Boccardo, F., Holdawy, I. M., Haefliger, J.-M., Jordaan, J. P. and Sotarauta, M. for the International Prostate Cancer Study Group (1991). A multicenter randomized trial comparing the luteinizing hormone-releasing hormone analogue goserelin acetate alone and with flutamide in the treatment of advanced prostate cancer. *J. Urol.*, **146**, 1221–6
17. Atala, A., Amin, M. and Harty, J. I. (1992). Diethylstilbestrol in treatment of postorchiectomy vasomotor symptoms and its relationship with

serum follicle-stimulating hormone, luteinizing hormone, and testosterone. *Urology*, **39**, 108–10

18. Loprinzi, C. L., Goldberg, R. M., O'Fallon, J. R., Quella, S. K., Miser, A. W., Mynderse, L. A., Brown, L. D., Tschetter, L. K., Wilwerding, M. B., Dose, A. M. and Oesterling, J. E. (1994). Transdermal clonidine for ameliorating postorchiectomy hot flushes. *J. Urol.*, **151**, 634–6

19. Wyon, Y., Lindgren, R., Lundeberg, T. and Hammar, M. (1995). Effects of acupuncture on climacteric vasomotor symptoms, quality of life, and urinary excretion of neuropeptides among postmenopausal women. *Menopause*, **2**, 3–12

20. Olson, G. A., Olson, R. D. and Kastin, A. J. (1991). Endogenous opiates: 1990. *Peptides*, **12**, 1407–32

21. Shoupe, D. and Lobo, R. (1987). Endogenous opioids in the menopause. In Speroff, L. and Lobo, R. (eds.) *Role of Opioid Peptides in Reproductive Endocrinology. Seminars in Reproductive Endocrinology*, Vol. 5, No. 2, pp. 199–206. (New York: Thieme Medical Publishers)

22. Tatemoto, K., Carlquist, M. and Mutt, V. (1992). Neuropeptide Y – a novel brain peptide with structural similarities to peptide YY and pancreatic polypeptide. *Nature (London)*, **296**, 659–60

23. Steinfeld, A. D. and Reinhardt, C. (1980). Male climacteric after orchiectomy in patient with prostate cancer. *Urology*, **16**, 620–2

24. Miller, J. I. and Ahmann, F. R. (1992). Treatment of castration-induced menopausal symptoms with low dose diethylstilbestrol in men with advanced prostate cancer. *Urology*, **40**, 499–502

25. Loprinzi, C. L., Michalak, J. C., Quella, S. K., O'Fallon, J. R., Hatfield, A. K., Nelimark, R. A., Dose, A. M., Fischer, T., Johnson, C., Klati, N. E., Bate, W. W., Respond, R. M. and Oesterling, J. E.

(1994). Megestrol acetate for the prevention of hot flushes. *N. Engl. J. Med.*, **331**, 347–52

26. Eaton, A. C. and McGuire, N. (1983). Cyproterone acetate in treatment of postorchidectomy hot flushes. Double-blind cross-over trial. *Lancet*, **10**, 1336–7

27. Jansen, J. E. (1990). Prevention of hot flushes with cyproterone acetate (CPA). In Murphy, G., Khoury, S., Chatelain, C. and Denis, L. (eds.) *Recent Advances in Urological Cancers – Diagnosis and Treatment*, pp. 70–1. (Paris)

28. Ålund, G. and Knönagel, H. (1989). Therapie der Hitzewallungen nach Hormonentzug wegen Prostatakarzinom. *Z. urol. poster* 2, 114

29. Krämer, P., Andrzejak-Nolten, N., Kallischnigg, G. and Heumann, F. (1992). Prevention of hot flushes with CPA in the hormonal treatment of prostatic cancer. Results of a placebo-controlled double-blind trial. In Murphy, G., Khoury, S., Chatelain, C. and Denis, L. (eds.) Third International Symposium on *Recent Advances in Urological Cancer Diagnosis and Treatment*, pp. 111–15. (Paris: SCI, Zeneca Pharmaceuticals)

30. Para, R. O. and Gregory, J. G. (1990). Treatment of post-orchiectomy hot flushes with transdermal administration of clonidine. *J. Urol.*, **143**, 753–4

31. Smith, J. A. (1994). A prospective comparison of treatments for symptomatic hot flushes following endocrine therapy for carcinoma of the prostate. *J. Urol.*, **152**, 132–4

32. Steingold, K. A., Laufer, L., Chetkowski, R. J., DeFazio, J. D., Matt, D. W., Meldrum, D. R. and Judd, H. L. (1985). Treatment of hot flushes with transdermal estradiol administration. *J. Clin. Endocrinol. Metab.*, **61**, 627–32

33. Judd, H. (1987). Efficacy of transdermal estradiol. *Obstet. Gynecol.*, **156**, 1326–31

Interactive Voting System

1   Have you ever seen flushing in a patient?

Response	Option
46%	Yes.
54%	No.

Number of votes: 106

2   How do you treat hot flushing in your patients who have had castration for carcinoma of the prostate?

12%   Estrogen.
70%   Cyproterone acetate.
 6%   Medroxyprogesterone or megestrol acetate.
 1%   Clonidine.
11%   Non-pharmacological treatment.

Number of votes: 127

Antiandrogens as monotherapy for metastatic prostate cancer: a preliminary report on EORTC protocol 30892

17

F. H. Schröder, P. Whelan, K. H. Kurth, R. Sylvester, M. de Pauw and members of the EORTC Genitourinary Group

Castration, the use of luteinizing hormone releasing hormone (LHRH) agonists and antiandrogen monotherapy remain options in the treatment of human prostate cancer. Total androgen blockade cannot be considered to be the 'gold standard' for various reasons, but mainly because of marginal advantages in effectiveness[1] and the very high costs. Two types of antiandrogens are available for monotherapy, steroidal antiandrogens of the cyproterone acetate (CPA) type and non-steroidal antiandrogens (pure antiandrogens) of the flutamide, nilutamide and bacalutamide type. Potential advantages of the use of antiandrogens are the quick achievement of a maximal effect, the reversibility of the antiandrogenic effect, the oral application and the potential preservation of libido and potency with the use of non-steroidal antiandrogens.

CPA has been compared in randomized studies to standard forms of treatment such as estradiol undecylate[2,3], to diethylstilbestrol (DES) 3 mg/day[4], and more recently to Zoladex® and 3 mg of DES[5]. The last, in preliminary reporting, does not show differences in response rates and time to treatment failure, but shows an advantage of control treatments (Zoladex and DES) above CPA. There is, however, an imbalance of numbers of patients, with only 35 being evaluable in the CPA arm. On the basis of earlier studies, CPA is considered to be equally effective as standard treatment with 3 mg of DES. The results of randomized studies

comparing 50 mg and 100 mg/day of bacalutamide to castration are available[6]. They show a significant advantage of castration with respect to time to progression and other endpoints. Another study comparing Casodex 150 mg/day to castration has not yet been finally evaluated[7]. Data given in this monograph reveal no significant difference in favor of castration with relation to time to progression, disease-specific and overall survival in metastatic patients; the data on M0 patients are insufficiently mature (*see* Chapter 18, pp. 147–155). Flutamide and nilutamide have not been studied in large randomized studies with sufficient power to reject a hypothesis of 'no difference'.

No randomized comparative study is available so far to evaluate the effectiveness and potential side effects of a pure antiandrogen in comparison to a steroidal antiandrogen. In 1989 the EORTC Genitourinary Group designed such a protocol. The features of this study are summarized in Table 1. Flutamide and CPA at standard dosages were compared in a randomized fashion in previously untreated patients with painless, metastatic prostate cancer, with good-risk prognostic factors. In order to qualify for the study, patients had to have at least two of the three favorable prognostic factors: performance status WHO 0, a normal alkaline phosphatase level and less than T4 classification of the primary tumor. Patients with painful metastases and/or T4 disease were excluded. Patients with a history of myocardial infarctions who presented with active coronary disease were not eligible. The protocol was activated in September 1990 and closed on 1st April 1996. It recruited 308 patients. The objectives of the study were to compare overall death rates and those related to prostate cancer in each treatment group, to compare time to progression in each treatment group, to assess potency and side effects in the two treatment arms and to evaluate the 1987 TNM classification. This last goal of the study was dropped later on. The study was conducted in a large number of centers, indicated in Table 2. A sample size of 280 patients with 96 deaths on each arm was considered sufficient to detect a difference of 50% in median survival. A total of 280 patients were considered to be sufficient to detect a difference of about 15% in the incidence of side effects and impotence.

Results

In this paper preliminary results related to side effects and sexual performance are presented as they were evaluated immediately after closure of the protocol on 1 April 1996. Reasons for going off study are indicated in Table 3. Nine patients were ineligible; this number may be incomplete at this time. Clearly, the relatively small proportion of patients who died or progressed so far shows that this trial is still immature and not ready for a final evaluation of the major endpoints.

Prognostic factors at entry

Most prognostic factors were equally distributed between the two treatment arms. This concerned the non-prostate cancer-related as

Table 1 EORTC 30892: Flutamide vs. cyproterone acetate in metastatic, painless, good-risk prostate cancer (April 1996)

Treatment	Flutamide 250 mg three times per day vs. cyproterone acetate 100 mg three times per day
Good risk	No painful metastases and presence of two of the three factors: (1) Performance status WHO = 0 (2) Normal alkaline phosphatase level (3) Classification < T4
Activation	September 1990
Closure	1 April 1996
Number of patients	308 randomized
Study coordinator	F. H. Schröder

Table 2 EORTC 30892: participating institutions (March 1996)

St James, Leeds	UCL St Luc, Brussels	Hosp. Mutua, Terrassa
AMC, Amsterdam	Hosp. Civils, Strasbourg	CHR, Besançon
Erasmus, Rotterdam	Pr. Royal, Hull	Radiumhosp., Oslo
St Maarten, Kortrijk	CH, Auxerre	Univ., Debrecen
Bordet, Brussels	OLVG, Amsterdam	CHU, Toulouse
AZ VU, Amsterdam	Den Bosch Medicentrum	UZ, Gent
Univ., Palermo	Kaizer Franz Univ., Graz	Hosp. Distrital, De Xira
Ramaz., Carpi	St Elisabeth, Tilburg	AZ VUB, Brussels
Middelheim, Antwerp	Do Desterro, Amadora	Hosp. N. S. Del Pino, Las Palmas
Marmara, Istanbul	Zuiderz., Rotterdam	Dokuze Eylul, Izmir
St Radboud, Nijmegen	Kromeriz, Chech Rep.	Lierse Ziekenh., Lier
Inselspital, Bern	Santa Maria, Lisbon	Ufficio S & P, Rome
Gen. Inf., Pontefract	Med. Radiol. C., Obninsk	UZ UIA, Antwerp

well as the prostate cancer-related factors, WHO performance status, chronic disease, previous myocardial infarction, previous cerebrovascular accidents, a history of thromboembolism, the T category, grade and ureteric obstruction. A previous transurethral resection (TUR) was carried out more frequently in the CPA arm as a result of more frequent prostatic obstruction in this group of patients. The elevation of prostate specific antigen (PSA) values was also equally distributed between the two treatment arms at entry. The PSA level was evaluated by multiples of the normal value.

Progression and survival

Progression and survival rates with a median follow-up time of 2.2 years are immature and cannot yet be considered.

Side effects

Side effects are summarized in Table 4. In the flutamide and CPA arms, 130 and 134 patients,

respectively, were evaluable for side effects. Only side effects that showed significant differences between the treatment arms are listed in detail. Painful gynecomastia was the most frequent side effect, followed by diarrhea, nausea and deterioration of liver function. All these side effects were more frequent on the flutamide arm. Myocardial infarction and cerebrovascular accident did not show differences; other thromboembolic events were more frequent on the CPA arm. Other side effects that did not differ between treatment arms are not listed. Cardiovascular deaths, which might be related to side effects, were seen in six cases (4.6%) in the flutamide arm and in seven cases (5.2%) in the CPA arm.

Toxicity requiring discontinuation of treatment

Serious toxicity requiring discontinuation of treatment is listed in Table 5. Discontinuation of treatment was more frequent on the flu-

Table 3 EORTC 30892: reasons for going off study (308 patients)

	Flutamide		CPA		
	n	%	n	%	Total (n)
Progression	51	54.3	43	45.7	94
Death	51	52.6	46	47.4	97
Loss to follow-up	3	27.3	8	72.7	11
Toxicity	19	73.1	7	26.9	26
Others	1	33.4	2	66.6	3
Ineligible	5	55.6	4	44.4	9

CPA, cyproterone acetate

Table 4 EORTC 30892: side effects (March 1996)

	Flutamide (n = 130)		CPA (n = 134)		
	n	%	n	%	p-Value
Painful gynecomastia	59	45.4	10	7.5	0.001
Diarrhea	30	23.1	13	9.7	0.000
Nausea	25	19.2	8	6.0	0.002
Liver function deterioration	13	10.0	6	4.5	0.045
Thrombosis, embolus	0		6	4.5	0.011

CPA, cyproterone acetate
Other side effects not differing between treatment arms: myocardial infarction, cerebrovascular accident, gynecomastia not painful, hot flushes, dizziness, others

tamide arm. Liver toxicity and gastrointestinal toxicity, mostly diarrhea and nausea, were the most common reasons. Thromboembolic events led to discontinuation of treatment in one patient on the CPA arm. Other side effects not detailed were dizziness and an unknown reason on the flutamide arm, diabetes mellitus, dyspnea and tiredness and an unknown reason on the CPA arm.

Potency and sexual performance
One of the potential advantages of the use of a pure antiandrogen is preservation of libido, potency and sexual performance. In this protocol these parameters were evaluated by the following five questions:

(1) Did you notice an erect penis sometimes during the night or when waking up (last 3 months)?

(2) Do you consider yourself sexually active in some way?

(3) Do you have an erection with sexual excitement?

(4) Do you reach an orgasm during sexual activity?

(5) Do you ejaculate with sexual activity?

Questions 3 to 5 were supposed to be asked only if question 2 was answered positively. The investigators were, however, not consistent in following this rule.

Table 6 gives an inventory of the answers to these questions according to treatment arm at entry. It is evident that there is an equal distribution of positive answers over both treatment arms. The most remarkable finding was that only about one-quarter of the patients were sexually active at entry; positive answers to the other questions were obtained in 21–38% of cases.

Table 7 summarizes the positive answers given during follow-up. Answers were only evaluated in those patients who answered 'yes' to the respective question at entry. A positive answer was scored only in those patients who consistently answered 'yes' to either question. Only question 1 (spontaneous erections at night or when waking up) showed a significant difference between flutamide and CPA in favor

Table 5 EORTC 30892: toxicity requiring discontinuation of treatment (March 1996)

	Flutamide (*n* = 130)	*CPA* (*n* = 134)
Liver toxicity	8	2
Gastrointestinal	7	1
Gynecomastia + pain	2	—
Venous thrombosis	—	1
Others	2	3
Total	19 (14.6%)	7 (5.2%)

CPA, cyproterone acetate

Table 6 EORTC 30892: potency at entry (March 1996)

	Flutamide (*n* = 148)		*CPA* (*n* = 150)		
	n	*%*	*n*	*%*	*p-Value*
(1) Morning erections	49	33.1	57	38.0	NS
(2) Sexually active	34	23.0	38	25.3	NS
(3) Erections with sexual excitement	37	25.0	35	23.3	NS
(4) Orgasm	34	23.0	36	24.0	NS
(5) Ejaculation	33	22.3	32	21.3	NS

CPA, cyproterone acetate; NS, not significant
Questions 3–5 only to be asked if answer to question 2 was 'yes'

Table 7 EORTC 30892: potency in follow-up (March 1996)

		Flutamide		CPA		
		n	%	n	%	p-Value
(1)	Morning erections	15	30.6	7	12.5	0.005
(2)	Sexually active	11	32.4	7	18.4	NS
(3)	Erections with sexual excitement	14	37.8	18	51.4	NS
(4)	Orgasm	15	44.1	13	36.1	NS
(5)	Ejaculation	13	39.4	10	31.3	NS

CPA, cyproterone acetate; NS, not significant
Answers were only evaluated in those who answered 'yes' to the respective question at entry; 'no' was scored if 'no' was stated at least once

of flutamide. Sexual activity was less frequent in patients using CPA; the difference, however, was not significant. The answers to the remaining questions were positive in remarkably similar proportions of previously sexually active men. No significant differences of sexual behavior on the flutamide and the CPA arms were found with questions 3–5. A time-dependent analysis of both treatments on potency is pending.

Discussion and conclusions

In conclusion, it must be said that many of the available data are still preliminary. This is especially true for progression and death rates; less than half of the patients have progressed or died. PSA progression has not yet been conclusively evaluated. Toxicity is clearly more pronounced with flutamide. However, toxicity was acceptable to most patients in both arms.

Serious toxicity was also seen more frequently on flutamide; 19 patients in this arm had to be taken off the study for toxicity, as opposed to seven in the CPA arm.

As far as potency and sexual behavior are concerned, this study has produced interesting and relevant data. Only 25–30% of patients were sexually active and potent at entry. Of those who have given positive answers to the potency-related questions, again only about one-third has remained so on both arms. Surprisingly, no significant differences were seen with respect to the two treatment arms except for a significantly more frequent occurrence of spontaneous erections at night or in the early morning hours.

The present data suggest that CPA is a less toxic drug in monotherapy of metastatic prostate cancer. Obviously, data on effectiveness will be crucial for a more comparative determination of the role of both drugs in this study.

References

1. Prostate Cancer Trialists' Collaborative Group (1995). Maximum androgen blockade in advanced prostate cancer: an overview of 22 randomised trials with 3283 deaths in 5710 patients. *Lancet*, **346**, 265–9
2. Jacobi, G. H., Altwein, J. E., Kurth, K. H., Basting, R. and Hohenfellner, R. (1980). Treatment of advanced prostatic cancer with parenteral cyproterone acetate: a phase III randomised trial. *Br. J. Urol.*, **52**, 208–15
3. Neumann, F. and Jacobi, G. H. (1982). Antiandrogens in tumour therapy. *Clin. Oncol.*, **1**, 41–64
4. Pavone-Macaluso, M., de Voogt, H. J., Viggiano, G., Barasolo, E., Lardennois, B., de Pauw, M. and Sylvester, R. (1986). Comparison of diethylstilbestrol, cyproterone acetate and medroxyprogesterone acetate in the treatment of advanced prostatic cancer: final analysis of a randomized phase III trial of the European Organization for

Research on Treatment of Cancer Urological Group. *J. Urol.*, **136**, 624–31

5. Osborne, D. R., Moffat, L. E. F., Kaisary, A., Rees, D. L. P. and Weaver, J. P. (1990). A comparison of Zoladex, cyproterone acetate and stilboestrol in the treatment of patients with advanced prostatic carcinoma. In Murphy, G., Khoury, S., Chatelain, C. and Denis, L. (eds.) *Recent Advances in Urological Cancers – Diagnosis and Treatment*, pp. 53–5. (New York: Alan R. Liss)

6. Bales, G. T. and Chodak, G. W. (1996). A controlled trial of bicalutamide versus castration in patients with advanced prostate cancer. *Urology*, **47** (Suppl. 1A), 38–43

7. Blackledge, G. P. (1996). High-dose bicalutamide monotherapy for the treatment of prostate cancer. *Urology*, **47** (Suppl. 1A), 44–7

Interactive Voting System

1   Maintenance of libido and potency justify the use of flutamide monotherapy in spite of side-effects.

Response	Option
25%	Yes.
66%	No.
9%	No opinion.

Number of votes: 114

2   If maximal anti-androgen blockade is not preferred, cyproterone acetate can be considered for monotherapy based on effectiveness and side-effects.

78%	Yes.
11%	No.
11%	No opinion.

Number of votes: 118

Endocrine therapy: goals and limitations 18

P. Iversen

Introduction

In the 16th century, Andreas Vesalius and Ambroise Paré were among the first to describe the anatomy of the prostate. Two hundred years later, observations reported by John Hunter strongly indicated the importance of intact testes for normal prostatic growth and function. However, two more centuries passed, before Charles Huggins' discoveries in the 1940s led to the introduction of androgen deprivation as a therapeutic modality in prostate cancer. Today, more than 50 years later, endocrine manipulation remains the corner stone in the management of advanced cancer of the prostate.

The treatment is effective. Following androgen ablation, 70–80% of treated patients with metastatic disease will experience symptomatic relief, i.e. reduced bone pain, increased performance status and a general improvement with increased sense of well-being. In the majority, an objective response can be demonstrated.

Unfortunately, the use of androgen deprivation in patients with prostate cancer has limitations. Most importantly, endocrine treatment as used today is considered palliative in nature, and relapse of the malignancy occurs if the patient survives competing causes of death. The median survival in metastatic patients from initiation of androgen deprivation is in the order of 2–2.5 years.

Also, although mild compared to many other forms of anticancer therapy, side effects and toxicity associated with endocrine manipulation are common. With loss of sexual function as the most obvious, a number of side effects, some of which are poorly defined, such as fatigue, depression and lack of energy, result in reduced quality of life.

Bilateral orchidectomy or orally administered estrogen were the treatments of choice for many years. During the last two decades a number of new pharmacological agents for androgen deprivation have been introduced. Although more therapeutic options have led to greater patient compliance, the optimal use of endocrine therapy in patients with cancer of the prostate is far from being a settled issue. Timing of therapy is still controversial, and new (and some revived) derived concepts such as endocrine therapy in very early cancer and even chemoprophylaxis are issues of debate and subjects of clinical trials. Also being investigated are non-steroidal antiandrogen monotherapy, combined androgen blockade, intermittent androgen suppression and neoadjuvant and adjuvant therapy.

Parallel to the current limitations of androgen deprivation, the goals for improved endocrine manipulation are two-fold: first, improved anticancer efficacy in terms of increased rate and duration of response as well as prolongation of survival; and second, minimal toxicity and improved quality of life.

In this paper, some of the new modalities and concepts in endocrine manipulation of prostate cancer are discussed.

Pharmacological castration: LHRH agonists

Bilateral orchidectomy removes the primary source of circulating androgen, and the castrate range of testosterone in serum is reached within 24 h. While orchidectomy is still considered the 'gold standard' treatment, the primary drawback is the psychological impact; also the need for, and waiting time for, surgical intervention contributed to the enthusiasm when a pharmacological alternative was introduced.

Many studies have found treatment with luteinizing hormone releasing hormone (LHRH) agonists to be comparable to surgical castration with regard to efficacy. Like the endogenous LHRH, synthetic agonists stimulate the pituitary to release luteinizing hormone (LH). However, continuous stimulation by potent synthetic agonists with longer half-life than the endogenous LHRH results in downregulation of pituitary LHRH receptors and a paradoxical suppression of circulating levels of LH and sex steroids. The castrate range of testosterone is generally reached within 2 weeks and maintained for the duration of therapy[1]. The initial stimulatory effect of LHRH agonists occurring during the first week of treatment is associated with objective and subjective signs, referred to as the 'flare phenomenon'. Antiandrogens or estrogens given during this initial period of LHRH agonist therapy counteract the flare. Recently, synthetic and potent LHRH antagonists have been introduced[2]. These agents cause an immediate inhibition of the release of LH, follicle stimulating hormone (FSH) and sex steroids. Whether LHRH antagonists have clinical potential either alone or in combination with LHRH agonists awaits further research.

LHRH agonists are polypeptides and cannot be administered orally. Depot preparations for monthly injections are most commonly used: 2- or even 3-monthly depots are currently being introduced[3].

Estrogens revisited

The antigonadotropic effect of estrogens has been used in the treatment of prostate cancer since Huggins' discoveries. Both experimental and clinical evidence suggest that estrogen therapy may be superior to castration in terms of efficacy, perhaps because of a direct effect on the tumor[4,5]. However, apart from adverse feminizing effects, an unacceptable cardiovascular toxicity[4-6] has brought the use of oral estrogens into disrepute. The dose-dependent cardiovascular side effects seem to be caused by an altered production of coagulation factors: increased factors VII and X and decreased antithrombin III[7] as a result of a 'first-pass' effect of portal blood with high estrogen concentration following oral intake. However, recent studies have shown that parenterally administered estrogens do not entail an increased risk of thrombosis or cardiovascular disease[8].

There is therefore a renewed interest in the use of estrogens. A multicenter study (SPCG 5) conducted by the Scandinavian Prostatic Cancer Group, comparing polyestradiol phosphate (Estradurin®) 240 mg intramuscularly every 4 weeks (every 2 weeks for the first 2 months) with total androgen blockade has recently completed recruitment of more than 900 planned patients. No comparative data on major endpoints are yet available.

Antiandrogens

Antiandrogens are defined as substances that compete with testosterone and dihydrotestosterone (DHT) for the androgen receptor and thereby inhibit the action of androgens on their target site. Antiandrogens are administered orally and can be divided into two groups[9]: steroid and non-steroid antiandrogens.

Steroid antiandrogens

Steroid antiandrogens, e.g. cyproterone acetate (CPA), have a dual mechanism of action: they compete for the androgen receptors but also possess progesterone-like antigonadotropic activity, leading to a decreased secretion of LH and FSH with a consequent decline in testosterone production and loss of sexual function. CPA is effective in preventing flare in conjunction with LHRH agonist treatment and can be used to suppress hot flushes following orchidectomy or LHRH agonist treatment.

Non-steroid or pure antiandrogens

These interact with the androgen receptor and block the intracellular effects of testosterone and DHT. Flutamide, nilutamide and bicalutamide belong to this group of antiandrogens. The negative feedback of androgens at the hypothalamic level is also blocked, resulting in reflex increments of LH, testosterone and DHT levels.

Treatment with non-steroid antiandrogens does not lead to obligatory loss of sexual function. This has obvious implications for quality of life, especially in younger patients with a strong desire to preserve potency. However, the marked rise in serum testosterone level is disturbing, because it may 'overcome' the blockade of androgen receptors by the antiandrogen.

Clinically, non-steroid antiandrogens have been used in long-term combination with either surgical or medical castration, as well as antiflare therapy when treatment is initiated with LHRH agonists. Bicalutamide (Casodex®) in monotherapy has been compared with castration in large international trials. A daily dose of 50 mg was found to be inferior to castration in terms of progression-free and overall survival, thus nourishing the fear that the androgen blockade with antiandrogen monotherapy may be insufficient[10].

Higher doses of bicalutamide in monotherapy have been investigated. In two European studies more than 1400 patients with locally advanced or metastatic prostate cancer were randomized between surgical/pharmacological castration and bicalutamide 150 mg daily. Although bicalutamide at this dosage is inferior to castration in patients with metastatic disease, it seems to be at least as effective in patients with only locally advanced prostate cancer[11]. However, the data in the latter group of patients are preliminary, and further follow-up is necessary before valid conclusions can be drawn.

What could be the explanation for this possible interaction between treatment and tumor burden? The same interaction is believed to exist when antiandrogens are used in combination with castration, and is dealt with further below.

Although antiandrogens are often used in combination with castration in combined androgen blockade, another combination has lately attracted attention. 5α-Reductase inhibitors do not seem to have a role as monotherapy in prostate cancer; however, they may be of value in combination with non-steroidal antiandrogens. In principle, the combination is rational. While the former inhibits the formation of the most active androgen, DHT, the latter blocks the androgen receptors. Further, the combination holds the possibility of maintained sexual function and low toxicity. Preliminary studies are encouraging and larger comparative studies are under way[12].

Antiandrogen withdrawal response

First described as a flutamide withdrawal response[13], the phenomenon has currently been extended to an antiandrogen withdrawal response[14,15]. Most probably caused by an androgen receptor mutation, the withdrawal response may be observed in 30–60% of prostate cancer patients after discontinuation of the antiandrogen at the time of progression. The phenomenon has predominantly been reported in patients to whom the antiandrogen is administered as a component of combined androgen blockade. Not only has a decline in prostate specific antigen (PSA) been observed, but other objective signs of tumor regression and symptomatic responses have also been reported. What is not clear at present is whether the withdrawal response reflects a serious drawback per se in the use of antiandrogens or whether the phenomenon, when exploited correctly, represents an extra possibility for improving progression-free and overall survival. The withdrawal response has served to emphasize the fact that we are far from fully understanding the mechanisms involved in the development of 'hormone-refractory' cancer of the prostate.

Combined androgen blockade

Whether the combination of castration (surgical or pharmacological) and an antiandrogen is superior to castration alone has been the issue of much debate since Labrie and colleagues advocated the clinical importance of adrenal androgens and introduced the principle of total or combined androgen blockade based on theoretical considerations and experimental observations[16].

The first clinical series of Labrie and colleagues was essentially uncontrolled, and several trials, randomizing thousands of patients, were initiated to test the hypothesis. The designs of the studies have varied: three different antiandrogens have been used, two non-steroidal and one steroidal: flutamide, nilutamide and CPA. Various LHRH agonists or bilateral orchidectomy have been used for castration in one or both arms. Few studies were double-blinded, and most studies have various methodological flaws or shortcomings, the most common of which is lack of statistical power to detect a meaningful difference in survival.

Both the flare phenomenon associated with LHRH agonist monotherapy and the antiandrogen withdrawal response add to the controversy surrounding combined androgen blockade. None of the concepts were sufficiently well known when most of the trials were protocolled, and it is not clear to what extent these phenomena have contributed to observed differences between treatment arms and individual studies.

No consensus abut the value of combined androgen blockade in the treatment of prostate cancer appears from the published reports. However, when the results of the individual studies are reviewed, the following cautious conclusions may be drawn: the remarkable difference in favor of combined androgen blockade first reported by Labrie and co-workers has not been confirmed. Only two studies[17,18] have shown a clear statistically significant survival advantage for combined androgen blockade. Some studies have demonstrated a significantly improved progression-free survival

in treated patients. More studies have found some evidence of improved objective or subjective response (fall in PSA/prostatic acid phosphatase; relief of symptoms). Whenever a difference in parameters of anti-cancer efficacy has been reported, it has always been to the advantage of combined androgen blockade. Where benefits from combined androgen blockade have been demonstrated or suggested, the antiandrogen used has been a non-steroidal antiandrogen (flutamide or nilutamide). Finally, in all studies addressing the issue, a clear tendency towards more adverse effects, although generally not severe, has been observed among patients treated with combined androgen blockade.

An overview, or meta-analysis, of 25 trials initiated before December 1989 has recently been published[19]. In the analysis, where only overall survival was analyzed, individual patient data were obtained from 22 of the trials, totalling 5710 patients with advanced prostate cancer (87% M_1) of whom 3283 had died (57%). The median follow-up was 40 months.

Overall, mortality was 56.3% in the combined androgen blockade group compared with 58.4% among patients treated with castration alone. The 5-year survival estimates were 26.2% and 22.8%, respectively. These differences, although in favor of combined androgen blockade and corresponding to a 6.4% reduction in the annual odds of death, are not statistically significant. Although differences in favor of combined androgen blockade were only found in studies using non-steroidal antiandrogens, exclusion of the studies employing CPA did not make the gain in survival statistically significant.

Therefore, the meta-analysis did not demonstrate combined androgen blockade to be superior to castration in terms of survival, and one can conclude that if combined androgen blockade entails a gain in survival, it is unlikely to be large.

However, the meta-analysis has been criticized. First of all, potential benefits such as symptom relief and length of symptom-free survival were not evaluated. Also, a lack of knowledge about prognostic factors makes a comparison between treatments, as well as analysis of subgroups, impossible[20]. Trial maturity heterogeneity, and how this affects the statistical power of the meta-analysis for reaching a negative ('no difference') conclusion, has also been questioned[21].

The Southwest Oncology Group embarked on a new study in 1989, INT 0105, investigating the addition of flutamide vs. placebo to surgical castration. Inclusion of almost 1400 patients is complete, and the first results are eagerly expected in 1996. Hopefully, this large study will provide us with a more precise understanding of the value and indications for combined androgen blockade.

Minimal disease

In the two studies, EORTC 30853[17] and INT 0036[18], the benefit of combined androgen blockade was particularly evident in patients with good performance status and minimal disease, according to the definition by Crawford and co-workers[18]. Even though the reported differences in progression-free and overall survival are considerable (median survival improved 19 months for this subgroup in INT 0036), numbers are few, and the differences have not been validated statistically. Is the benefit of combined androgen blockade limited to this particular subgroup of patients, and did these two studies include a larger percentage of such patients? In the EORTC 30853, published hazard ratios for different prognostic groups of patients strongly indicate that the gain in survival disappeared in patients with poor performance and severe disease[17]. Published survival curves from the INT 0036 point in the same direction, although a difference in favor of combined androgen blockade seems to persist, also in patients with severe disease and poor performance status[18].

No other studies have published data on the subgroup of patients with minimal disease. However, in the study by the Danish Prostatic Cancer Group, we have identified 34 and 38 patients in the orchiectomy and LHRH agonist plus flutamide treatment arms, respectively fulfilling the criteria. No difference in progression-free and overall survival was found. Further, if metastatic patients with a low tumor burden should benefit particularly from combined androgen blockade, it is tempting and logical to extrapolate that to patients with only locally advanced prostate cancer. In the study by Tyrrell and associates[22], 246 patients with locally advanced prostate cancer were randomized between combined androgen blockade and goserelin acetate alone. No difference in objective response and overall survival could be demonstrated. However, median survival had not been reached at the time of analysis.

Interestingly, the hypothesis that combined androgen blockade is of special benefit to patients with minimal disease is to some extent supported by the meta-analysis[19]. No difference in mortality was observed at all during the first 2 years, but thereafter a difference appeared in favor of combined androgen blockade. Since patients with minimal disease typically will not contribute to cancer mortality before 2 years, this finding may concur with the hypothesis. Longer follow-up of existing studies as well as new studies specifically addressing this issue are warranted. The maturing INT 0105 stratified between minimal and severe disease at inclusion, and large numbers of patients of the first category were recruited.

What could be the explanation for this possible interaction between treatment and tumor burden? As mentioned earlier, the same kind of interaction is suspected in preliminary data from trials comparing the novel non-steroidal antiandrogen bicalutamide in monotherapy with castration. Considering the competitive action of antiandrogens, is the efficacy of antiandrogens correlated to the numbers of androgen receptors in prostatic tumor tissue (i.e. the tumor burden)? And does the addition of antiandrogen in combined androgen blockade make a difference only when the numbers of receptors are limited? Another contributing explanation could be that secretion of adrenal androgens declines not only with age, but also in patients with advanced illness[23].

Timing of treatment

The indication for androgen deprivation in management of prostate cancer is clear and nearly absolute in patients with spinal compression, ureteral obstruction and/or painful osseous metastases. Otherwise, no clear consensus exists on when to start hormonal therapy.

Conceptually, endocrine therapy is palliative and therefore should be administered with quality of life as a high priority. Furthermore, not enough exact knowledge exists about the optimal timing. Should such therapy be immediate, i.e. instituted as soon as prostate cancer is diagnosed and it is clear that the patient is beyond curative reach, or may it just as well be deferred until symptoms appear?

In the 1960s a large number of patients with advanced prostate cancer were randomized in the VACURG study[24] to immediate endocrine therapy vs. placebo followed by deferred endocrine treatment when they became symptomatic. No difference in survival was demonstrated. With today's standards, the study had several methodological and analytic flaws, and a later re-analysis actually found younger patients with poorly differentiated tumors to gain from immediate endocrine therapy[25]. Nonetheless, for many years the study formed the scientific basis for withholding endocrine therapy until symptoms appeared, thus avoiding adverse effects and loss of sexual function as long as possible.

However, a number of developments have renewed the interest for immediate or at lest early endocrine therapy: in many countries more patients are diagnosed with early disease; the appearance of new and well-tolerated treatment modalities such as LHRH agonists and non-steroid antiandrogens has increased patient compliance; interest in multimodal therapy has grown; and the introduction of PSA has enabled better monitoring to be carried out of the disease process.

There is no doubt that immediate/early endocrine therapy may satisfy a psychological need in some patients for therapeutic action instead of expectancy only. However, there are questions that should be answered before immediate endocrine therapy is advocated in general.

Will immediate endocrine therapy prolong the time to progression, and if so, does this translate into longer survival? Several uncontrolled and non-randomized studies have indicated a longer progression-free and overall survival associated with immediate endocrine therapy[26]. Large randomized trials are underway both in Europe and in the USA. Preliminary data[27] strongly indicate a longer progression-free survival in prostate cancer patients with stages N+, MO, but a longer overall survival has not yet been proven to result from immediate endocrine therapy.

If immediate therapy carries a clear advantage over deferred therapy, a logical consequence would be to investigate the effect of early endocrine therapy in early, organ-confined cancer of the prostate, e.g. in patients not suited for, or rejecting, surgery, realizing that such treatment would have to be given for many years. Several co-operative groups have initiated such ambitious studies.

Will immediate endocrine therapy, by reducing the tumor burden or sensitizing tumor cells, enhance the effect of other therapies, e.g. surgery, irradiation, chemotherapy or other systemic treatment? The concept of neo-adjuvant endocrine therapy was introduced as early as 1944 but has recently gained new momentum with the employment of reversible forms of androgen deprivation. While the ultimate goal for this concept must be improved prospects for cure with longer progression-free and overall survival, more immediate aims of neo-adjuvant endocrine therapy, usually given for 3 months before surgery or radiation in patients with localized or locally advanced cancer of the prostate, are to reduce the tumor burden, i.e. 'downsize', and possibly 'downstage' (stage reduction) and 'downgrade' the cancer. Subsequent surgery may be facilitated, and in case of radiotherapy tumor cell kill may be enhanced and adverse effects minimized, due to reduced target volume.

Several uncontrolled and non-randomized studies have suggested that neo-adjuvant therapy may induce stage reduction, and in some cases downgrading or even disappearance of the malignancy have been described. The first prospective, randomized studies have been published[28,29], and more are under way. At present, a cautious conclusion based on available evidence is that neo-adjuvant endocrine therapy does indeed downsize by 35–50% and, more important, the rate of positive margins is lowered by approximately 50%. Furthermore, the degree of PSA suppression after 3 months of endocrine therapy seems to hold important prognostic information about whether or not the cancer is organ confined. On the other hand, downstaging of clinical T$_3$ as well as downgrading have not been convincingly demonstrated. Time to PSA increase as well as clinical progression and survival remain the most important endpoints, for which we have to wait several years.

Will immediate endocrine therapy identify patients not responding to, or failing, androgen deprivation, earlier than with deferred therapy? If so, will the patients' better general condition result in improved results of an often toxic second-line therapy? Cytotoxic chemotherapy has traditionally been administered in later stages of disease, when patients are generally weakened, and therefore the true effectiveness of such treatment is difficult to ascertain. If the hormonal refractory patients were identified at an earlier point in the course of disease they may well be able to tolerate more intensive chemotherapy with the possibility of improved response rates. The introduction of PSA testing has meant that progression following initial endocrine therapy can be demonstrated much earlier than before, since a rise in PSA level precedes both symptomatic and other objective signs of progression, typically by 6 months. Several trials with a wide range of second-line therapeutic modalities are ongoing or being planned in patients with such early 'PSA progression'.

Intermittent androgen suppression

Intermittent therapy adds further to the controversy surrounding timing of endocrine treatment. The cell death process induced by androgen withdrawal is incomplete and surviving tumor cells progress to an androgen-independent state. Bruchovsky and associates[30] found evidence that this progression is a consequence of a lack of androgen-induced differentiation of stem cells in the primary tumor, with resultant loss of apoptotic potential; new growth factors substituting for androgens and stimulating tumor growth may also be generated. Therefore, if androgen stimulation of the surviving stem cells were resumed in a cyclic form, this could allow the tumor to repopulate with androgen-sensitive cells, with recovery of apoptotic potential and hence the possibility of re-treatment by androgen withdrawal[9,31]. Potential benefits of this intermittent therapy might include prolongation of the androgen-dependent state of the tumor, and perhaps a better quality of life, with recovery of libido and potency. While the principle has been tried before in treatment of advanced prostate cancer, the use of PSA to monitor the cancer has formed the basis for a revived enthusiasm. Studies employing this principle are under way.

Chemoprevention

Chemoprevention may be considered as the extreme use of early endocrine manipulation. Androgens play an important role in the development and progression of prostate cancer. DHT is the most powerful androgen in men and is synthesized from testosterone through the action of the enzyme 5α-reductase in the prostatic cell. 5α-Reductase inhibitors competitively inhibit this enzyme and are capable of reducing prostate volume and serum PSA level. The observations of the absence of prostate cancer in prepubertally castrated men, in men with 5α-reductase deficiency and in men with androgen-insensitive syndrome have given rise to the hypothesis that a suppression of DHT with a 5α-reductase inhibitor prior to the development of clinically evident cancer may decrease the incidence of prostate cancer. A large chemopreventive study, prompted by the United States National Cancer Institute, with planned inclusion of 18 000 healthy males 55 to 70 years of age, randomizing between a 5α-reductase inhibitor (5 mg finasteride) or placebo, is at present recruiting in the USA.

Concluding remarks

Exciting progress is being made in basic cancer research, and there is hope that this will result in major breakthroughs in the management of prostate cancer in the not-so-distant future. As a urologist, I have in this discussion focused upon clinical aspects. It is apparent that continued clinical research is necessary. In the final phases of such research there is no alternative to the controlled randomized trial, and experience from the last decade has stressed the importance of sufficient statistical power in such studies. To provide such power and be able to give valid answers to important questions, collaboration in large-scale multicenter and even multinational trials is mandatory.

References

1. Conn, P. M. and Crowley, W. F. Jr (1991). Gonadotrophin-releasing hormone and its analogues. *N. Engl. J. Med.*, **324**, 93–103
2. Pinski, J., Yano, T., Miller, G. and Schally, A. V. (1992). Blockade of the LH response induced by the agonist D-Trp-6-LHRH in rats by a highly potent LH-RH antagonist SB-75. *Prostate*, **20**, 213–24
3. Dijkman, G. A., Debruyne, F. M. J., Fernandez del Moral, P., Plasman, J. W. M. H., Hoefakker, J. W., Idema, J. G. and Sykes, M. (1995). A randomised trial comparing the safety and efficacy of the Zoladex 10.8-mg Depot, administered every 12 weeks, to that of the Zoladex 3.6-mg Depot, administered every 4 weeks, in patients with advanced prostate cancer. *Eur. Urol.*, **27**, 43–6
4. Byar, D. P. (1973). The Veterans Administration Cooperative Urological Research Group's studies of cancer of the prostate. *Cancer*, **32**, 1126–30
5. Cox, R. L. and Crawford, E. D. (1995). Estrogens in the treatment of prostate cancer. *J. Urol.*, **154**, 1991–8
6. Johansson, J.-E., Andersson, S.-O., Holmberg, L. and Bergström, R. (1991). Primary orchiectomy versus estrogen therapy in advanced prostatic cancer – a randomised study: results after 7 to 10 years of followup. *J. Urol.*, **145**, 519–23
7. Henriksson, P., Blombäck, M., Bratt, G., Edhag, O. and Eriksson, A. (1986). Activators and inhibitors of coagulation and fibrinolysis in patients with prostatic cancer treated with oestrogen or orchidectomy. *Thrombosis Res.*, **44**, 783–91
8. Stege, R. and Sander, S. (1993). Endocrine treatment of prostatic cancer. A renaissance for parenteral estrogen. *Tidsskr. Nor. Laegeforen*, **113**, 833–5
9. Bruchovsky, N. (1993). Androgens and anti-androgens. In Holland, J. F., Frei, E. III, Bast, R. C., Kufe, D. W., Morton, D. L. and Weichselbaum, R. R. (eds.) *Cancer Medicine*, 3rd edn, pp. 884–96. (Philadelphia: Lea & Febiger)
10. Iversen, P (1994). Update of monotherapy trials with the new anti-androgen, Casodex (ICI 176,334). *Eur. Urol.*, **26** (Suppl. 1), 5–9
11. Iversen, P. (1995). European randomized trials (1453 patients) of bicalutamide (Casodex) versus castration in the treatment of advanced prostate cancer. Presented at the Symposium *Bicalutamide (Casodex) – Its Potential in Management of Prostate Cancer*, July, Boston, USA
12. Fleshner, N. E. and Trachtenberg, J. (1993). Treatment of advanced prostate cancer with the combination of finasteride plus flutamide: early results. *Eur. Urol.*, **24** (Suppl. 2), 106–12
13. Scher, H. I. and Kelly, W. K. (1993). Flutamide withdrawal syndrome: its impact on clinical trials in hormone-refractory prostate cancer. *J. Clin. Oncol.*, **11**, 1566–71
14. Small, E. J. and Carroll, P. R. (1994). Prostate-specific antigen decline after Casodex withdrawal: evidence for an antiandrogen withdrawal syndrome. *Urology*, **43**, 408–10
15. Dawson, N. A. and McLeod, D. G. (1995). Dramatic prostate specific antigen decrease in response to discontinuation of megestrol acetate in advanced prostate cancer: expansion of the

antiandrogen withdrawal syndrome. *J. Urol.*, **153**, 1946–7

16. Labrie, F., Dupont, A. and Belanger, A. (1985). Complete androgen blockade for the treatment of prostatic cancer. In DeVita, V. T., Hellman, S. and Rosenberg, S. A. (eds.). *Important Advances in Oncology*, pp. 193–217. (Philadephia: J. B. Lippincott)

17. Denis, L. J., Whelan, P., Carneiro de Moura, J. L., Newling, D., Bono, A., Depauw, M., Sylvester, R. and the EORTC GU-Group (1993). Goserelin acetate and flutamide versus bilateral orchiectomy: a phase III EORTC trial (30853). *Urology*, **42**, 119–30

18. Crawford, E. D., Eisenberger, M. A., McLeod, D. G., Spaulding, J. T., Benson, R., Dorr, F. A. *et al.* (1989). A controlled trial of Leuprolide with and without Flutamide in prostatic carcinoma. *N. Engl. J. Med.*, **321**, 419–24

19. Prostate Cancer Trialists' Collaborative Group (1995). Maximum androgen blockade in advanced prostate cancer: an overview of 22 randomised trials with 3283 deaths in 5710 patients. *Lancet.*, **346**, 265–9

20. Denis, L. (1996). Endocrine treatment – should it be total (maximal) blockade? In Peeling, W. B. (ed.) *Questions and Uncertainties about Prostate Cancer*, pp. 246–54. (Oxford: Blackwell Science)

21. Blumenstein B. A. (1995). Overview analysis issues using combined androgen deprivation overview analysis as an example. *Urol. Oncol.*, **1**, 95–100

22. Tyrrell, C. J., Altwein, J. E., Klippel, F., Varenhorst, E., Lunglmayr, G., Boccardo, F. *et al.* (1991). A multicenter randomized trial comparing the luteinizing hormone-releasing hormone analogue goserelin acetate alone and with flutamide in the treatment of advanced prostate cancer. *J. Urol.*, **146**, 1321–6

23. Parker, L. N. (1989). *Adrenal Androgens in Clinical Medicine*, Chapter 25. (New York: Academic Press; Harcourt, Brace, Johanovich)

24. Byar, D. P. (1973). The Veterans Administration Cooperative Urological Research Group's studies of cancer of the prostate. *Cancer*, **32**, 1126–30

25. Sarosdy, M. F. (1990). Do we have a rational treatment plan for stage D-1 carcinoma of the prostate? *World J. Urol.*, **8**, 27–33

26. Kozlowski, J. M., Ellis, W. J. and Grayhack, J. T. (1991). Advanced prostatic carcinoma. Early versus late endocrine therapy. *Urol. Clin. North Am.*, **18**, 15–24

27. van den Ouden, D., Tribukait, B., Blom, J. H. M., Fossa, S. D., Kurth, K. H. ten Kate, F. J. W., Heiden, T., Wang, N. and Schroder, F. H. (1993). Deoxyribonucleic acid ploidy of core biopsies and metastatic lymph nodes of prostate cancer patients: impact on time to progression. *J. Urol.*, **150**, 400–6

28. Soloway, M. S., Sharifi, R., Wajsman, Z., McLeod, D., Wood, D. P., Puras-Baez, A. and the Lupron Depot Neoadjuvant Prostate Cancer Study Group (1995). Randomized prospective study comparing radical prostatectomy alone versus radical prostatectomy preceded by androgen blockade in clinical stage B2 (T2b,NxM0) prostate cancer. *J. Urol.*, **154**, 424–8

29. van Poppel, H., de Ridder, D., Elgamal, A. A., van de Voorde, W., Werbrouck, P., Ackaert, K., Oyen, R., Pittomvils, G., Baert, L. and the Members of the Belgian Uro-Oncological Study Group (1995). Neoadjuvant hormonal therapy before radical prostatectomy decreases the number of positive surgical margins in stage T2 prostate cancer: interim results of a prospective randomized trial. *J. Urol.*, **154**, 429–34

30. Bruchovsky, N., Rennie, P. S., Coldman, A. J., Goldenberg, S. L., To, M. and Lawson, D. (1990). Effects of androgen withdrawal on the stem cell composition of the Shionogi carcinoma. *Cancer Res.*, **50**, 2275–82

31. Akakura, K., Bruchovsky, N., Goldenberg, S. L., Rennie, P. S., Buckley, A. R. and Sullivan, L. D. (1993). Effects of intermittent androgen suppression on androgen-dependent tumors: apoptosis and serum prostate-specific antigen. *Cancer*, **71**, 2782–90

5

Early Detection of Prostate Cancer

Rationale for trials of screening for prostate cancer 19

F. E. Alexander

Introduction

Screening for the early detection of cancer is an important method of disease control alongside primary prevention and improved clinical management. Prospects for primary prevention of prostate cancer are limited and the majority of cases presenting symptomatically are already unsuitable for curative therapy. Available data provide hope that screening may reduce mortality, but it is also possible that the net effect of screening may be harmful. The rationale for randomized controlled trials to resolve this issue is discussed below, within a framework provided by relevant points of the World Health Organization criteria[1] for screening:

(1) The disease is an important public health problem.

(2) Screening tests are available and are safe, acceptable and valid.

(3) An early stage of the disease is recognized and the subsequent natural history is known.

(4) Effective therapy is available for early disease, and treatment given while still asymptomatic improves the prognosis.

Prostate cancer as a public health problem

Prostate cancer is the second most common form of male cancer in many countries[2]; in the United States it has now overtaken lung cancer in terms of incidence, but remains second as cause of death[3]. Prostate cancer afflicts elderly men and, in consequence, absolute numbers and crude rates are extremely sensitive to the age structure of the population. Increases in life expectancy have been substantial in developed countries and are now predicted for the rest of the world, as the epidemiological transition occurs[4]. When this is combined with the baby-boom of 1945–55 it will lead to an accelerating future rise in numbers of both cases and deaths, *even if age-specific rates remain stable*[5]. Prostate cancer is undoubtedly a major public health problem.

Screening tests for prostate cancer

Three screening tests for the early detection of prostate cancer are available: digital rectal examination (DRE), transrectal ultrasound examination (TRUS) and prostate specific antigen (PSA) measurement. The last is now accepted as forming the basis of screening for prostate cancer, although opinions differ as to the desirability of including other modalities. These tests are all simple, safe and acceptable to men screened, but acceptance rates of invitations to screening can be disappointingly low[6,7]. Blood tests are widely acceptable[8], so that detection of prostate cancer in the population may be maximized by use of PSA testing alone, although omission of DRE will certainly lead to some missed cancers in men screened[9]. The further requirement for screening tests is validity: that they provide accurate information about the potential presence or absence of disease (Table 1).

Table 1 Validity of screening tests

	True state of nature	
	Diseased	*Healthy*
Test result		
+ve	a	b
−ve	c	d
Sensitivity	a/(a + c) × 100	
Specificity	d/(b + d) × 100	

Sensitivity of the tests

Quantification of sensitivity and specificity of screening tests (as opposed to diagnostic tests) is hampered by ignorance of the current true state of nature for men who test negative (i.e. c + d in Table 1). Most estimates for the prostate cancer tests have been derived by using a combination of tests to provide the benchmark classification. This, in effect, measures relative sensitivity; results for PSA are in the range 57–79%[10].

There are clear disadvantages to this approach; in particular, the 'healthy' group may include an unknown number of men with prostate cancer destined to be fatal, and, conversely, the prostate cancer group may include another unknown number whose disease would never have become symptomatic. Two alternative approaches are possible.

Firstly, sensitivity can be considered in terms of its ability to detect the cancers that would actually arise in the population. The proportional incidence of interval cancers[11] is:

$$(1 - I/R) \times 100$$

where I is the rate of interval cancers (i.e. cancers arising symptomatically between screens) and R the underlying incidence rate in the absence of screening. This deals with the sensitivity of a screening program rather than just the test; few data are available, except for the Quebec program in which annual PSA screening has 100% sensitivity according to this criterion[9]. This may not be sufficient for prostate cancer, since over half of all cases have extended beyond the gland when symptoms arise[12]. However, the Quebec program has also

succeeded in eliminating stage D and drastically reducing stage C cancers in the population of screened men (apart from cases detected at first screening).

The most recent approach involves retrospective evaluation of stored serum from cohorts of men whose subsequent experience of prostate cancer morbidity and mortality is known. Results from three studies[13-15] have been reported, with 767 cases of prostate cancer and 2339 controls who were free of prostate cancer at the end of the follow-up period. The studies consistently showed that over 72% of cases of prostate cancer arising symptomatically within the 3–4 following serum collection years had abnormal baseline PSA levels. These roughly corresponded to the conventional 4 mg/ml of the monoclonal Hybritech assay, but only one of the studies[15] used this assay, and these authors used 4 times the normal median (age- and center adjusted) rather than an absolute threshold. Two studies reported low probabilities of detecting cases that would arise more than 5 years after serum collection[14,15], although the third[13] found that PSA begins to increase rapidly (doubling times of 4.3 years as opposed to the control 24.9 years) 13 years before symptomatic presentation of stage B–D tumors. These studies provide firm evidence that PSA has high sensitivity, in the sense that regular screening (at 3–4 year intervals) will detect most tumors before they become symptomatic but, unfortunately, they failed to demonstrate that these cases would have been suitable for curative therapy at the time of detection[16].

Modifications of the PSA test are being evaluated, but we can conclude that PSA shows sufficient promise of having good sensitivity to justify screening trials, although not for recommendation of screening as public health policy.

Specificity of the tests and the problem of overdiagnosis

The problems due to ignorance of the 'true state of nature' have already been alluded to; not only is this knowledge unavailable for men screened negative (at least initially), but it is not clear whether, if detected, an invasive carcinoma that would *not* have grown fast enough to cause morbidity during the lifetime of the host should be a 'true' rather than 'false' positive. This is the problem of overdiagnosis.

With a PSA threshold for further investigation of 4 ng/ml, the specificity of PSA used alone is around 88%; this is acceptable, but somewhat less than ideal, and means that 12% of men without evidence of prostate cancer may be recalled for further tests, possibly including sextant prostate biopsies.

There are two different but tenable interpretations of overdiagnosis. The first is that screening diagnoses prostate cancers that are clinically unimportant. Stamey and colleagues[17] classified tumors of < 0.5 ml as clinically unimportant, and others have added that the tumor must have no part with Gleason score 4 or 5[18]. According to these criteria the majority of screen-detected cases (90% or more) are clinically important and there is little overdiagnosis[9,19,20].

The second, more stringent, definition considers that overdiagnosis occurs whenever a cancer is diagnosed that would never have become clinically overt or never have been fatal. Approaches to estimation of the potential for overdiagnosis in this sense include analyses of stored serum and examination of cumulative incidence rates in screened men. The proportions of the controls in the prospective studies who have normal PSA levels are, superficially at least, very encouraging (88%[13], 91%[14] and 94%[15]). Further inspection, however, leads to the conclusion that if prostate cancer had been diagnosed in 4% of controls with abnormal PSA levels, then screening could lead to the diagnosis (and treatment) in four of each 1000 men screened who would not have experienced any clinical symptoms during the next 10 years. The number of men overtreated in this sense is similar to reasonable estimates of prostate cancer deaths prevented[21].

The best available estimates of detection rates at second or later screens are 0.8% for annual screens[9]; from this figure, the cumulative incidence for men screened from age 55 to 69 years can be estimated at 12–14% (depending on the prevalence screen detection rate at age 55 years, for which good data are not available). If this is compared with the current North American estimate of 10% lifetime incidence, there is little problem of overdiagnosis[9]. However, incidence rates for prostate cancer are unreliable indicators of disease burden[5,22], and a more conservative approach considers prostate cancer mortality (or incidence rates in countries with lower incidence : mortality ratios). Since, at age 55, a US male has a risk of dying from prostate cancer of around 3%[23], 10% of men screened regularly from age 55 will have a prostate cancer detected that would not have proved fatal. Incidence rates from Denmark (which has the same prostate cancer mortality as other Nordic countries, but much lower reported incidence[22]) suggest that at age 55 men may have 'underlying' risk of prostate cancer to age 70 of no more than 6%, which may then be doubled by screening.

These data highlight the need to approach screening cautiously, since overdiagnosis in the second sense is a real possibility. At present, in the absence of reliable estimates of mortality benefit, it is not possible to know how much overdiagnosis is acceptable[24].

Early stage and natural history of prostate cancer

Disease confined to the prostate gland (T_1, T_2) is the recognized early stage. The Wilson and Junger criteria[1] also require that the natural history should be understood, but this is at present far from the case for prostate cancer. There is evidence of latent foci of prostate cancer in substantial proportions of middle-aged (30%) and elderly (50%) men at autopsy[25], figures confirmed from examination of tissues removed during surgery for benign prostate and bladder disease. It is generally believed that, given sufficient time, these lesions all have the capacity to progress, but this is not certain and of largely academic relevance. Progression is undoubtedly often slow, with typical median times to progression of 13.5 years for T_{1A}, 4.75 years for T_{1B}[26] and 6 years for T_2 taken together[27] having been reported. Few patients live long enough to die of prostate cancer; in large series of untreated patients with T_1 or T_2 disease, the mortality rate after 10 years of follow-up was below 10%[28], but longer follow-up may alter this[29]. Tumor volume, degree of differentiation and time influence the probability of progression, but cannot explain the differences between cases, and, at present, it is not possible at the time of detection to identify with certainty those whose disease is potentially lethal though still curable.

Effective therapy

Three therapies are available for localized prostate cancer: radical prostatectomy, radical radiotherapy and watchful waiting (therapy deferred until evidence of progression emerges). These are discussed elsewhere, but a number of points are relevant here. Firstly, they are all effective therapies for early prostate cancer[30]. Secondly, there is at present no proof that active therapy reduces prostate cancer mortality; evidence from randomized controlled trials is awaited, but if it fails to emerge then this will be an important argument against prostate cancer screening. Thirdly, the frequencies of serious side effects of the active therapies is of a magnitude that cannot be ignored[31]. These include operative mortality (1–2%), incontinence (up to 25%) and impotence (up to 30%) and, in consequence, screening may have major harmful effects on quality of life and possibly also on length of life.

Some authors have suggested that screening, even in trials, should await conclusive results from trials of therapy. However, there are two critical counter-arguments: firstly, screening trials may not be possible in future, since unscreened control groups cannot be recruited; secondly, the optimum therapy for screen-detected disease need not be the same as that for symptomatic confined disease[32].

Potential advantages and disadvantages of screening

Personal

The potential advantages are easy to see: death from prostate cancer may be avoided and so, also, may morbidity from advanced prostate cancer. In addition those screened negative will perceive themselves to be reassured that they are free of cancer. On the other hand, there are clear potential disadvantages: in particular, receiving treatment for prostate cancer that might never have caused any morbidity or mortality and the side effects of that treatment. For those who choose to remain untreated, there is unnecessary anxiety and the effects of being labelled as a cancer patient.

At present there is inadequate scientific knowledge to quantify these or determine the direction of the net effect, but it is clear that most benefits are long-term, while adverse consequences are immediate. It follows that screening is clearly unsuitable for men with reduced life expectancy.

Community

Advantages include reduction in prostate cancer deaths and the need to provide care for advanced cases. The main disadvantages are the costs of screening and further diagnostic investigations and the cost of therapy both for prostate cancer and for the side effects of primary therapy. Once again scientific guidance is lacking, but the financial costs of prostate cancer to national health services are likely to be increased by screening[31].

Expert opinion

The American Cancer Society recommends annual screening by PSA and DRE for all men over 50 years[33]. At the opposite extreme, some scientists consider that the chance of net harm to men screened is such that screening, even with randomized trials, contravenes the Helsinki declaration[34]. The US Preventative

Health Task Force does not recommend routine screening for prostate cancer by either DRE or PSA and this view is shared by many other experts[7,24,35].

It is clear that, while many individual clinicians and scientists have deeply held convictions for and against screening for prostate cancer, the current general consensus position is one of agnosticism and equipoise.

Rationale for randomized controlled trials

The foregoing discussion has demonstrated an urgent need to determine whether population screening for prostate cancer can achieve its primary objective of reducing mortality from this disease. Evaluation of screening, whilst superficially straightforward, is susceptible to three important biases: selection bias, lead time bias and length-biased sampling. Selection bias occurs if mortality from prostate cancer is compared in men who have and have not been screened, but it was the men themselves who chose whether or not to be screened. There are many differences between people who would choose to receive screening if it were available and those who would decline it, some known and others unknown, and it is entirely possible that factors such as underlying rate of prostate cancer, stage at presentation, concurrent morbidity and post-therapy survival would differ between the two groups.

Lead time bias (Figure 1) arises when survival time is compared in screened and unscreened men, with time measured from date of diagnosis. As a result of the earlier diagnosis of the screen-detected cases, their survival time will then be longer, even if the date of death is unchanged. Length-biased sampling is also illustrated in Figure 1. The 'sojourn time' during which a tumor remains detectable but pre-clinical will be longer for some tumors than others; those tumors that have longer sojourn times will be more likely to be screen-detected (since the chance of one or more screens occurring during the sojourn time is greater). Therefore, in any comparison of screen-detected

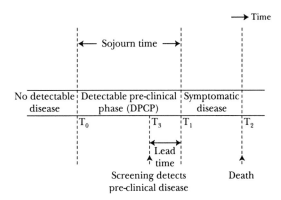

Figure 1 The progression of chronic disease

tumors with other tumors, the two groups will differ not just by their method of detection but also by their mean sojourn time. It is likely that tumors with long sojourn times will be less aggressive, so that this bias, like lead-time bias, can be expected to favor screening.

The only scientifically acceptable way of evaluating screening for early detection of prostate cancer (and other cancers) is to use a randomized controlled trial. The essential features are that a defined population is randomized, one (the study) arm is offered screening while the other is a control group. The follow-up period begins with the date of randomization. Prostate cancer mortality in the whole of the study arm during the follow-up period is compared with that in the control arm. Within this basic framework there are two important alternatives: the trial population may be a defined geographical population (Figure 2) or a volunteer group (Figure 3). There are ethical and scientific advantages for both designs and they adopt, respectively, the single-consent or the usual-consent design. Either will yield a reliable answer to the basic question, provided that the numbers are large enough to ensure adequate statistical power. For this answer to be of clinical relevance, follow-up periods in excess of 10 years are essential.

Either of these designs will also provide a framework for subsidiary studies, which will provide reliable estimates of the proportion of cases detected by screening, the extent of any

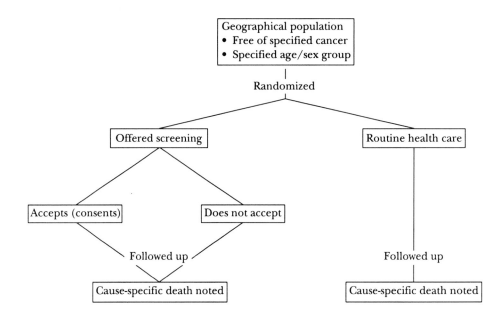

Figure 2   The classical design of screening trials

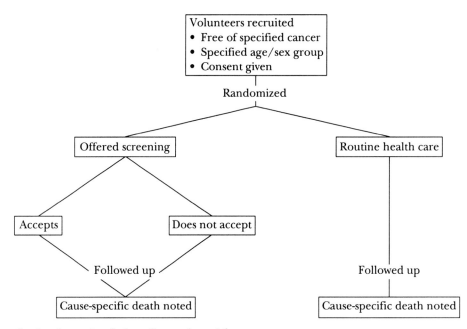

Figure 3   An alternative design of screening trials

overdiagnosis, the cost-effectiveness of screening and its relation to other methods of prostate cancer control and the impact of screening on the quality of life of those screened and those diagnosed. The conclusion will permit informed comparisons of the advantages and disadvantages of screening and of screening for prostate cancer with other health care.

Adami and colleagues[34] have argued that randomized controlled trials of screening are unethical, since it has not been demonstrated to their satisfaction that the possibility of net harm to the men screened is low. Their arguments are both important and persuasive; in particular they emphasize the need for the provision of clear and honest information to men offered screening, so that each man may make his own informed decision about whether to accept screening. Each will attach his own weights to the possible harms and benefits in order to reach this decision. If this is done, then, in a situation of equipoise in the medical community, the conduct of trials of screening are not unethical. Conversely, they are essential to provide firm conclusions, since the present data are consistent with both considerable benefit and serious harm; in addition, if screening is not effective, then it is an enormous waste of scarce health care resources.

References

1. Wilson, J. M. G. and Junger, G. (1968). *Principles and Practice of Screening for Disease*, Public Health Paper no 34. (Geneva: WHO)
2. Parkin, D. M., Muir, C. S., Whelan, Y. T. *et al.* (1992). *Cancer Incidence in Five Continents.* (Lyon: WHO, IARC)
3. Pisani, P., Parkin, D. M. and Ferlay, J. (1993). Implications for prevention and projections of future burdens. *Int. J. Cancer*, **55**, 891–903
4. World Bank (1993). *World Development Report.* (Washington, DC: World Bank)
5. Alexander, F. E. and Boyle, P. (1995). The rise in prostate cancer: myth or reality? In Garraway, M. (ed.) *Epidemiology of Prostate Disease.* (Berlin: Springer)
6. Schroder, F. H., Damhuis, R. A. M., Kirkels, W. J. *et al.* (1996). European randomised study of screening for prostate cancer. *Int. J. Cancer*, **65**, 145–51
7. Denis, L. J. (1995). Prostate Cancer Screening and Prevention: Realities and Hopes. *Urology*, **46**, SS55–61
8. Smith, W. C. S., Turnstall-Pedoe, H., Crombie, I. K. and Tavendale, R. (1989). Concomitants of excess coronary deaths – major risk factor and lifestyle findings from 10359 men and women in the Scottish Heart Health Study. *Scot. Med. J.*, **34**, 550–5
9. Labrie, F., Bernand, C., Leonello, C. *et al.* (1996). Diagnosis of advanced or noncurable prostate cancer can be practically eliminated by prostate-specific antigen. *Urology*, **47**, 212–16
10. Cupp, M. R. and Oesterling, J. E. (1993). Prostate-specific antigen, digital rectal examination, and transrectal ultrasonography: their roles in diagnosing early prostate cancer. *Mayo Clin. Proc.*, **68**, 297–306
11. Day, N. E., Williams, D. R. R. and Khaw, K. T. (1989). Breast cancer screening programs: the development of a monitoring and evaluation system. *Br. J. Cancer*, **59**, 954–8
12. Mettlin, C., Jones, G. W. and Murphy, G. P. (1993). Trends in prostate care in the United States, 1974–1990: observations from the patient care evaluation studies of the American College of Surgeons Commission on Cancer. *CA Cancer J. Clin.*, **48**, 83–91
13. Whittemore, A. S., Chitra, L. and Friedman, G. D. (1995). Prostate-specific antigen as predictor of prostate cancer in black men and white men. *J. Natl. Cancer Inst.*, **87**, 354–60
14. Gann, P. H., Hennekens, C. H. and Stampfer, M. J. (1995). A prospective evaluation of plasma prostate specific antigen for detection of prostatic cancer. *J. Am. Med. Assoc.*, **273**, 289–94
15. Parkes, C., Wald, N. J., Murphy, P. *et al.* (1995). Prospective observational study to assess value of prostate cancer. *Br. Med. J.*, **311**, 1340–3
16. Neal, D. E. and Hamdy, F. C. (1996). Prospective observational study to assess value of prostate specific antigen as screening test for prostate cancer. *Br. Med. J.*, **312**, 709
17. Stamey, T. A., Freika, F. S., McNeal, J. E. *et al.* (1993). Localised prostate cancer. Relationship of tumor volume to clinical significance for treatment of prostate cancer. *Cancer*, **91**, 933–8
18. Ohori, M., Wheeler, T. M., Dunn, J. K., Stamny, T. A. and Scardino, P. T. (1994). The pathological features and prognosis of prostate cancers detectable with current tests. *J. Urol.*, **152**, 1714–20
19. Brendler, C. B. (1995). Characteristics of prostate cancers found with early detection regimes. *Urology*, **46**, SS71–6

20. Miles, B. J. (1995). Impact of Therapy on Adenocarcinoma. In Garraway, M. (ed.) *Epidemiology of Prostate Disease*, pp. 239–47 (Berlin: Springer)

21. Fulton, M. (1995). Screening for prostate cancer: background. In *Epidemiology of Prostate Disease*, pp. 248–55 (Berlin: Springer)

22. Tretli, S., Engeland, A., Haldorsen, T., *et al.* (1996). Prostate Cancer – Look to Denmark. *J. Natl. Instit. Cancer*, **88** (2), 128

23. Scardino, P. T., Weaver, R. and Hudson, M. A. (1992). Early detection of prostate cancer. *Hum. Pathol.*, **23**, 211–22

24. Schroder, F. H. (1995). Screening, early detection and treatment of prostate cancer – a European view. *Urology*, **46**, SS62–70

25. Breslow, N., Chan, C. W., Dhom, G., *et al.* (1977). Latent carcinoma of prostate at autopsy in seven areas. *Int. J. Cancer*, **20**, 680–5

26. Lowe, B. A. and Listrom, M. B. (1988). Incidental carcinoma of the prostate: an analysis of the predictors of progression. *J. Urol.*, **140**, 1340–4

27. Whitmore, W. F., Warner, J. A. and Thompson, I. M. (1990). Expectant management of localized prostatic cancer. *Cancer*, **67**, 1091–6

28. Johansson, J. E. (1995). Natural history in untreated prostate cancer. In Garraway, M. (ed.) *Epidemiology of Prostate Disease*, pp. 225–38 (Berlin: Springer)

29. Aus, G. (1994). Prostate cancer mortality and morbidity after non-curative therapy with aspects on diagnosis and treatment. *Scand. J. Urol. Nephrol.* (Suppl.), **67**, 1–41

30. National Cancer Institute (NCI) (1988). Consensus development conference on the management of localised prostate cancer. *NCI Monogr.*, **7**,

31. Kramer, B. S., Brown, M. L., Prorok, P. C., Potosky, A. L. and Gohagen, J. K. (1993). Prostate cancer screening: what we know and what we need to know. *Ann. Intern. Med.*, **119**, 914–23

32. Parkes, C., Murray, P., Wald, N. J., George, L. and Watt, H. C. (1996). Authors reply (letter) *Br. Med. J.*, **312**, 709–10

33. Mettlin, C., Jones, G., Averette, H., Gusberg, S. B. and Murphy, G. P. (1993). Defining and updating the American Cancer Society guidelines for the cancer related check-up: prostate and endometrial cancers. *CA Cancer J. Clin.*, **43**, 42–6

34. Adami, H. O., Barron, J. A. and Rotham, K. J. (1994). Ethics of prostate cancer screening trials. *Lancet*, **343**, 958–60

35. Denis, L. J., Murphy, G. P. and Schröder, F. H. (1995). Report for the consensus workshop on screening and global strategy for prostate cancer. *Cancer*, **75**, 1187–207

The European Randomized Study of Screening for Prostate Cancer (ERSPC): international co-operation and preliminary data

20

A. Auvinen, F. Calais da Silva, L. J. Denis, J. Hugosson and F. H. Schröder, on behalf of the Scientific Committee ERSPC and all other associates of the study

Introduction

After a series of pilot studies were conducted, the European Randomized Study of Screening for Prostate Cancer (ERSPC) was initiated in 1994. International co-operation has been established within the International Prostate Screening Trial Evaluation Group (IPSTEG) to establish a prospective evaluation plan of all ongoing randomized screening studies[1,2]. The purpose of this overview is to describe the organization of the ERSPC and the international co-operation that has been established, and to review the progress made so far. The ERSPC has participated in an effort to reach consensus on essential screening-related issues[3].

Goal and features of the ERSPC

The main aim of the ERSPC is to establish or to disprove the effect of active screening on prostate cancer mortality. In addition, based on the overall mortality within the study and prostate cancer mortality, life-years gained by screening and early treatment will be calculated. Quality of life evaluation will allow calculation of the quality-adjusted life years (QUALYs). Furthermore, the evaluation of the screening tests and the optimal use in the general population is an early goal of the study. Eventually, a complete cost-effectiveness analysis will be carried out. Interim endpoints such as prostate cancer morbidity, progression rates, stage distribution at diagnosis, etc. will be evaluated according to a preset plan. Side studies are encouraged, but have to be presented and approved within the study group. The goals of the ERSPC are summarized in Table 1.

A number of common features have been agreed upon. A few exceptions have been made and will lead to appropriate adjustments in the final evaluation phase. The age range at the time of first recruitment is 55–70 years. Some centers use different upper-range limits. Re-screening after 4 years or sooner is a minimal requirement for all participants. All study centers use the same test for prostate specific antigen (PSA), the Hybritech Tandem E or R assays. Biopsy indications are minimally a PSA level of 4.0 ng/ml or more, and/or an abnormal rectal examination and/or transrectal ultrasonography. Cancer cases found will be treated unless treatment is not indicated. Treatment policies within the screening arm are as much as possible in agreement with regional policies. Watchful waiting is one option. Watchful waiting is, however, not identical with no treatment. Treatment may

Table 1 Goals of the ERSPC

To establish or disprove an effect of active screening on prostate cancer mortality
To predict life years gained and to calculate the cost of screening policies
To study quality of life
To evaluate the efficiency of the screening tests
To carry out side-studies

be initiated whenever signs of progression occur. There is full agreement on the major endpoint of the trial: prostate cancer mortality. Table 2 gives an indication of common features of the ERSPC, but it is far from complete.

Sample size

All sample size calculations established so far in the United States, Canada and Europe assume that a prostate cancer mortality reduction of at least 20% should be achieved. Obviously, quality of life evaluation will be a decisive factor in the evaluation of the ongoing randomized screening studies. Table 3 shows a summary of several sample size calculations, some of which are used in ongoing studies. Obviously, prostate cancer diagnosed and cured at a very young age (50–55 years) would give a very long added lifespan. On the other hand, prostate cancer is rare in these young age groups. Their inclusion leads to a very important increase in sample size. It is mainly for this reason that the lower age limit of 55 years is used within the ERSPC. The upper age limit is very disputable. There is an agreement around the world that radical prostatectomy should be limited to men aged 70 or slightly

older, who are biologically younger than their true age would suggest. On the other hand, radiotherapy is applied to older age groups, certainly up to age 75. Most centers have decided to accept the ERSPC policy of using age 70 as a cut-off for screening.

The sample size within the ERSPC is determined by the choice of age 55–70. At least 122 218 men will have to be included to be able to show a prostate cancer mortality reduction of 20% with a statistical power of 90% based on Dutch mortality rates and 1 : 1 randomization.

Contamination of the control arm by use of the screening test is an important factor, which influences sample size in an exponential fashion. Contamination is to be evaluated. In the Rotterdam study at the time of initiation within the last 4 years prior to entry 8% of the men had undergone a PSA test. Upfront contamination increased to 11% in 1995. During the study period sample size may have to be adjusted according to such findings.

Recruitment and participants

To achieve the main goal of the ERSPC – to show or rule out an effect on prostate cancer mortality of early detection and treatment – a minimum of 122 000 men will have to be recruited. This number may have to be increased, depending on the possible increased use of the screening test in the control group. Table 4 gives an indication of the potential contributions of the individual centers and the number of men randomized to the study so far. Obviously, there is still a long way to go. However, the total number of more than 30 000 men randomized

Table 2 ERSPC: Common features

Age range 55–70 years, general population
Re-screening after 4 years or less
Same PSA test
Biopsy with PSA $\geq$ 4.0 ng/ml, abnormal DRE and/or TRUS
Treatment policy
Endpoints, 10-year follow-up

PSA, prostate specific antigen; DRE, digital rectal examination; TRUS, transrectal ultrasonography

Table 3 Sample size considerations: randomized screening studies for prostate cancer (PC)

Age (years)	PC mortality reduction (%)	Power (%)	Sample size/arm
50–64	20	90	145.425*
55–64	20	90	75.555*
55–70	20	90	61.1009[†]
55–74	20	90	49.140[†]
60–74	20	90	37.000*

*Prorok and colleagues[9]; [†]de Koning[10]

Table 4 European Randomized Study of Screening for Prostate Cancer (ERSPC): participants

Center	Start date	No. on study	No. expected
Antwerp	1.4.95	1685	20 000
Göteborg	1.1.95	15 570	32 000*
Portugal	1994	1318	5000
Finland	1.5.96	—	75 000*
Rotterdam	1.6.94	11 600	40 000
Total		30 173	172 000

*Randomization control/screening ± 2 : 1

is encouraging. Two centers have elected to randomize more men to the control group than to the screening group. In Göteborg 5190 men have been screened; with 2 : 1 randomization the sample recruited so far amounts to 15 570 men. Separate statistical considerations have been made concerning the protocols running in Göteborg, Sweden and Helsinki/Tampere, Finland.

Co-operation at an international level and at the scale necessary to run this study requires firm commitments from all parties. Such co-operation has been established within the Scientific Committee of the ERSPC, the group that is responsible for the conduct of the study. Each center delegates two members to this Committee. Co-operative agreement besides the common features already mentioned above includes an agreement on rules for participation, on a minimal data set necessary for common evaluation of the national studies and on a common Committee structure and quality control procedures. All centers agree on a final common evaluation with respect to the main endpoint. Within this structure national differences are reviewed and can be accepted.

The minimal data set, which is also agreed upon by international partners such as the representatives of the Prostate Lung Ovary and Colon Study of the National Cancer Institute of the USA (PLCO) and a Canadian project that is seeking funding at this time, will be published shortly[4]. The minimal data set includes baseline information on each participant, the date of entry, follow-up information relating to the results of screening, follow-up concerning cancer cases including staging, grading and treatment, process evaluation (evaluation of

contamination), recommendations for a quality of life evaluation and many other features, some of which are summarized in Table 5.

The Committee structure of the ERSPC includes a Data Monitoring Committee, the Scientific Committee, which actually runs the study, the Quality Control Committee, an Epidemiology Committee, national Causes of Death Committees with international co-ordination, a PSA Committee and a Pathology Committee, which is still in the process of being set up. The Data Monitoring Committee is an external Committee that supervises the ERSPC. The Committee has established stopping rules and has the right to advise discontinuation of the study in case a significant difference with regard to the major endpoint is reached or in the case of ethically unacceptable events or complications. The final evaluation of the ERSPC will be delegated to a data center, which is still to be determined. The Quality Control Committee has the important task of supervising the internal consistency of data as well as the adherence to the mutually agreed features of the protocol and the minimal data set. The Causes of Death Committee is in the process of establishing an operational definition of prostate cancer death. It will subsequently have the task of supervising the proper assignment of causes of death. The PSA Committee is in the process of setting up a quality control between the centers involved and hopefully will eventually come up with standardization measures concerning the PSA assay.

International co-operation is supported by grants from Europe Against Cancer and the National Cancer Institute of the USA.

Progress reports by center

The five centers indicated in Table 4 are full participants of the ERSPC. Although Finland had a late start, for various reasons, the study group has successfully completed a pilot study[4]. Candidate centers include Padua (Italy), Florence (Italy), Brussels (Belgium) and Edinburgh/Newcastle (UK). Tables 6–9 give an indication of progress made by centers.

Table 5 Co-operative agreement: minimal data set

Baseline information (age, date, etc.)
Follow-up (alive, dead, cause of death, etc.)
Screening information (screen results, failures, complications)
Prostate cancer follow-up (pathology, tumor node metastasis, treatment)
Process evaluation (contamination)
Quality of life evaluation

After Auvinen and colleagues[1]

In Antwerp, three pilot studies had been concluded by 1993[5]. The main study started in April 1995. Up to March 1996, 1685 men were randomized. The detection rate amounted to 2.7% (Table 6). Not all randomized men have as yet been screened.

The study in Göteborg, Sweden will be subject to a separate report in this volume. After a pilot phase the protocol started on 1 January 1995. In December 1994, 32 414 men were randomized. In Sweden an informed consent is not necessary in the control group. Of the 10 000 randomly assigned to the screening group, 5190 agreed (52.0%). The study group uses a pre-screen with PSA measurement. Men with a PSA value of < 3.0 ng/ml are excluded from further evaluation. On the other hand, everyone who has a PSA level above 3.0 will undergo a biopsy. There is re-screening of the screened population after 2 years. To date, 5190 men were screened for PSA level, 460 underwent a biopsy and 94 cancers were found, amounting to a detection rate of 2.4%. A total of 4.9 biopsies were necessary to find one cancer. About 12% of the population undergoes a biopsy. A total of 48% of men were treated by radical prostatectomy, 22% by other forms of treatment, mainly radiotherapy and 30% were managed by active watchful waiting (Table 7).

In Portugal, after a short pilot phase, recruitment started during the year 1994. Participants are recruited from the patient registries of general practitioners. The number of men invited is for this reason not known. By October 1995, 1557 were randomized; 769 were screened. There was a biopsy indication in 117 (15.2%); 13 cancers (1.7%) were detected; 7.6 biopsies were necessary to find one cancer. The results may reflect the lower incidence of prostate cancer in the Mediterranian area (Table 8).

The results of the Rotterdam study section, which has been ongoing since June 1994, are summarized in Table 9. At the time of writing this article, 11 600 patients have been randomized. This number falls slightly short of the goal of including 200 men per week. Otherwise,

Table 6 Progress by center: Antwerp, April 1995–March 1996

Invited	4681
Randomized	1685 (36.0%)
Screened (so far)	641
Biopsied	69 (10.8%)
Cancers	17
Detection rate	17/641 (2.7%)

Table 7 Progress by center: Göteborg, February 1996

Start date: 1 January 1995	
Cut-off: March 1996	
Age 50–65, randomization control : screen = 2 : 1	
Biopsy: PSA ≥ 3.0 ng/ml; re-screen: 2 years	
Sample	32 414
Invited to screen	10 000
PSA measured (agreed)	5190 (52%)
Evaluated	3890 (75%)
Biopsies	460 (11.8%)
Cancers	94
Detection rate	94/3890 (2.4%)
Treatment: radical 48%, others 22%, watchful waiting 30%	

Table 8 Progress by center: Portugal, October 1995

Start: 1994 (pilot phase), March	
Recruitment from registries of general practitioners	
Invited	?
Randomized	1557
Screened	769
Biopsy indication	117 (15.2%)
Cancers (detection rate)	13 (1.7%)
Biopsies/prostate cancer	7.6

Table 9 Progress by center: Rotterdam

Main study: June 1994–June 1995	
Invited	13 940
Randomized	6155 (44%)
Screened	2518
Biopsied	529 (21%)
Cancers (detection rate)	103 (4.1%)
Biopsies/prostate cancer	5.1
Randomized by March 1996: 11 600	

this part of the study is running according to protocol. The results of five Rotterdam pilot studies have been published[6].

Evaluation of the screening tests

Since Rotterdam is the first center that was able to recruit patients on a large scale, this group has taken on the task of evaluating the available screening tests in the study population, which is assumed to be as close as possible to the general population. During the initial phase, PSA testing, digital rectal examination (DRE) and transrectal ultrasonography (TRUS) were applied to all participants randomized to the screening group. Results of this evaluation and of a simulation of different screening strategies have recently been reported[7,8]. In this series, biopsies were carried out in all men with a PSA level of ≥ 4.0 ng/ml, as well as in those with a positive DRE and/or TRUS. In addition, an evaluation of the free/total PSA ratio, of PSA density and of age-specific reference ranges was included. Table 10 shows a summary of some of the results. Clearly, an improvement of specificity (reduction of biopsies) can be achieved with all strategies evaluated. PSA density in this respect seems to be the most effective. However, the trade-off that always exists between sensitivity and specificity needs to be considered. With both, the use of PSA density or free/total ratio combined with rectal examination, $11 \pm 3.8\%$ of the cancers would have been missed. In this respect, the best balance seems to be achieved with a PSA pre-screen. A total of 68% of all men were shown to have a PSA level below 2.0 ng/ml. If these are excluded from rectal examination and transrectal ultrasonography, 30% fewer biopsies will be carried out and $6 \pm 2.9\%$ cancers will be missed. The biopsy rate per cancer would be 3.4, an important improvement with respect to the 4.6 biopsies to detect one cancer with the application of PSA, DRE and TRUS to the whole population. A more definitive evaluation of the whole study population is ongoing.

The PSA pre-screen with a cut-off value of 2.0 ng/ml will be applied within the Finnish study and to a planned Canadian study. Within the Swedish protocol a PSA cut-off level of 3.0 ng/ml is used. Decisions as to the alteration of the screening regimen in Rotterdam, Antwerp and Portugal are still pending. Unfortunately, the present evaluation has the limitation that no PSA-driven biopsies are done with PSA values below 4.0 ng/ml. Such studies are presently carried out elsewhere.

Discussion and conclusions

A multi-center randomized screening study of prostate cancer is feasible in Europe. The study should contribute to resolve the controversy around early diagnosis and treatment of prostate cancer. Although the ongoing investigations are very expensive, the cost of uncontrolled screening as it is developing in the United States at this time would be much higher. The results of this study should enable health care policy makers to take important decisions concerning the use of early detection measures and recommendations concerning early treatment of this disease. Quality of life studies form an essential part of this endeavor,

Table 10 Biopsy indications and simulated results – 1726 men, 308 biopsies, 67 cancers. Standard errors are shown in parentheses

Biopsy indication	Reduction in biopsies (%)	Loss of prostate cancer (%)	Biopsies/cancer
PSA ≥ 4 ng/ml, DRE, TRUS	—	—	4.6
PSA ≥ 4 ng/ml, DRE	17 (2.1)	3 (2.1)	3.9
PSA, age, DRE	37 (2.8)	12 (4.0)	3.3
PSA ≥ 4 ng/ml, PSAD, DRE	39 (2.8)	11 (3.8)	3.2
PSA ≥ 4 ng/ml, F/T, DRE	37 (2.8)	11 (3.8)	3.3
PSA pre-screen > 2.0 ng/ml			
PSA ≥ 4 ng/ml, DRE, TRUS	30 (2.6)	6 (2.9)	3.4

After Bangma and colleagues[8]
PSA, prostate specific antigen; DRE, digital rectal examination; TRUS, transrectal ultrasonography; PSAD, PSA density; F/T, free/total

and may be decisive in the end, especially in a situation where small differences between the screening and the control arms may be encountered.

Acknowledgements

The trialists and different study groups are grateful for financial support by many ideal and financial sponsors. Among these are: Europe Against Cancer, the National Cancer Institute (USA) and Hybritech Inc. Local sponsors are: The Flemisch Cancer League, the Finnish Cancer Society, Wallac Oy, the Dutch Cancer Society (KWF), the Dutch Prevention Fund, Hel Singin Sanomat Centenary Fund (Finland), Pirkanmaa Cancer Society (Finland) and Finnish Culture Foundation (Finland). The acknowledgements from Portugal are: Administração Regional de Saúde de Lisboa e Vale do Tejo, Administração Regional de Saúde do Norte, Administração Regional de Saúde do Centro and Administração Regional de Saúde da Região Autónoma da Madeira.

References

1. Auvinen, A., Rietbergen, J. B. W., Denis, L. J., Schröder, F. H. and Prorok, P. C. (1996). Prospective evaluation plan for randomized trials of prostate cancer screening. *J. Med. Screening*, in press
2. Reynolds, T. (1993). Prostate cancer experts debate screening, treatment at workshop. *J. Nat. Cancer Inst.*, **85**, 1104–6
3. Denis, L. J., Murphy, G. P. and Schröder, F. H. (1995). Report of the consensus workshop on screening and global strategy for prostate cancer. *Cancer*, **75**, 1187–207
4. Auvinen, A., Tammela, T., Stenman, U.-H. *et al.* (1996). Screening for prostate cancer using serum prostate specific antigen: a randomized, population-based pilot study in Finland. *Br. J. Cancer*, in press
5. Schröder, F. H., Denis, L. J., Kirkels, W. J., de Koning, H. J. and Standaert, B. (1995). European randomized study of screening for prostate cancer, progress report of Antwerp and Rotterdam pilot studies. *Cancer*, **76**, 129–34
6. Schröder, F. H., Damhuis, R. A. M., Kirkels, W. J., de Koning, H. J., Kranse, R., Nijs, H. G. T. and Blijenberg, B. G. (1996). European randomized study of screening for prostate cancer – the Rotterdam pilot studies. *Int. J. Cancer*, **65**, 145–51
7. Bangma, C. H., Kranse, R., Blijenberg, B. G. and Schröder, F. H. (1995). The value of screening tests in the detection of prostate cancer. Part I: Results of a retrospective evaluation of 1726 men. *Urology*, **46**, 773–8
8. Bangma, C. H., Kranse, R., Blijenberg, B. G. and Schröder, F. H. (1995). The value of screening tests in the detection of prostate cancer. Part II: Retrospective analysis of free/total prostate-specific analysis ratio, age-specific reference ranges, and PSA density. *Urology*, **46**, 779–84
9. Prorok, P. C., Connor, R. and Baker, S. G. (1990). Statistical considerations in cancer screening programs. *Urol. Clin. North Am.*, **17**, 699–708
10. de Koning, H. (1993). *Protocol ERSPC*. (Rotterdam: ERSPC)

Interactive Voting System

1   Screening for prostate cancer:

Response	Option
12%	Should be recommended to all elderly men.
11%	Should not be used in asymptomatic men.
77%	Should be evaluated in a randomized study.

Number of votes: 107

Characteristics of prostate cancers detected in a population-based screening study (ERSPC data, Rotterdam region)

21

J. B. W. Rietbergen, W. J. Kirkels, R. Kranse and F. H. Schröder

Introduction

Over the last decades it became clear that prostate cancer is a serious health problem in elderly men. In The Netherlands it is the second leading cause of male cancer deaths. In 1991, 4915 cases were detected and 2222 deaths from cancer of the prostate were recorded in a male population of 7.5 million[1]. The incidence rates show an important increase from the age of 50 (Table 1). In the European community the overall prostate cancer incidence was 54.9 per 100 000. The lifetime risk in this group of men is approximately 4%, the age-corrected mortality due to prostate cancer was 22.6 per 100 000, or a lifetime mortality of 1.2%[2].

Prostate cancer develops within the prostate and may even spread outside the prostate with no signs or symptoms for many years. Generally the clinically diagnosed cancer has already spread outside the prostate, usually into the bones, before the first diagnosis is made. Roughly half of the patients who are diagnosed with prostate cancer present with locally advanced and/or metastatic disease[3]. In the Rotterdam region the clinical stage distribution with local invasion or metastases was responsible for 37% of all diagnosed prostate cancers in the year 1993 (Table 2). The prognosis of patients with metastatic prostate cancer is poor. Cure is impossible and median survival is in the range of 18–30 months in spite of endocrine treatment[4].

The most promising way to control prostate cancer and to reduce mortality seems to be through early detection and treatment. Screening of the male population in the high-risk age group, however, is still controversial. This controversy arises from the fear of overdiagnosis and subsequent overtreatment. The discrepancy between incidence and mortality with screening suggests overdiagnosis in the range of 2 to 3 times mortality[5]. This is still limited, since autopsy and cystoprostatectomy studies have shown that approximately 30% of all men who

Table 2 Stage distribution of prostate cancer found in 1993 in the Rotterdam region before the start of the screening study. Unpublished results 1993, I.K.R.

	T_x	T_1	T_2	Advanced disease T_3	T_4	$T-$
Metastases	M_0	M_0	M_0	M_0	M_0	M_1
Percentage	4	11	48	10	5	22

Table 1 Age-specific prostate cancer incidence and mortality rates. From reference 1

Age (years)	40–44	45–49	50–54	55–59	60–64	65–69	70–74	75–79	80–84	85+	Total
Incidence	5	15	64	186	418	793	1107	1073	741	513	4915
Mortality	—	5	14	30	110	210	356	484	488	525	2222

come to necropsy harbor latent prostate cancer[6]. Kabalin and associates[7] found a 38% incidence in cystoprostatectomy specimens obtained from men with normal digital rectal examinations who underwent operation for a pathological condition of the bladder. These tumors, however, are different from those detected clinically. Their volumes are smaller (mean 0.11 ml, range 0.01–1.10 ml), they are often well differentiated and usually confined to the prostate. Only 10–15% of screen-detected cancers have the features of autopsy cancers[8,9]. In several European countries randomized screening studies are conducted with prostate cancer mortality as the major endpoint, in order to find a possible solution to the present controversy[10]. The features of detected cancers within the ERSPC section Rotterdam are presented.

Methods

Patient population

Between July 1994 and January 1996, 8668 men between 55 and 74 years of age responded to a letter of invitation, sent by our department, to enter the European Randomised Study of Screening for Prostate Cancer (section Rotterdam). The only exclusion criterion for entry into the study was a previous diagnosis of prostate cancer. Written informed consent was obtained from all study subjects. Those who responded were randomized into either the screening arm or the control arm. The 4324 men in the control arm were not tested.

Of the 4344 men in the screening arm 3963 underwent a serum prostate specific antigen (PSA) determination, digital rectal examination and transrectal ultrasonography. An abnormality by any of the three diagnostic tests prompted a sextant prostate biopsy.

Techniques

All men underwent determination of serum PSA concentration (Hybritech Tandem-E PSA im-munoenzymetric assay); blood samples were drawn before the other tests were performed. The cut-off level of the PSA test was set at 4.0 ng/ml; any value greater than 3.9 ng/ml was considered to be elevated. At the time of screening the members of the screening team were not aware of the PSA results. Digital rectal examination was performed by a resident urologist or an ultrasound technician. Nodularity, induration and asymmetry of the prostate were considered to be abnormal.

Biplanar transrectal ultrasonography was performed by a resident urologist or an X-ray technician using a Bruel & Kjaer® model 1846 mainframe and a 7-MHz endorectal transducer with the subject in the left lateral decubitus position. The sonographic criteria for prostate cancer described by Lee and co-workers[11] were used. All prostate biopsies were performed by a resident urologist under ultrasound guidance, using a MAGNAN pro-mag® 2.2 biopsy gun and an 18-gauge Bard® biopsy needle. If the biopsy indication was an elevated PSA level or an abnormal digital rectal examination, sextant biopsies were performed. In case of a hypoechoic lesion, the lesion was sampled in addition to the sextant biopsy. All subjects received antimicrobial prophylaxis.

The pathological findings from sextant and ultrasound-guided biopsies were the reference test for determining the presence or absence of prostate cancer.

Results

Population

The mean age of the screened men in this population was 64.2 years (range 55–75); the median age was 64 years. Of the 4344 subjects in the screening group, 3963 underwent all screening tests. In 1050 (26.5%) subjects there was an indication for biopsy. In 69 cases the biopsy was not performed for various reasons; 42 men refused a biopsy and will be rescreened after 1 year, 24 men could not be biopsied for medical reasons and three biopsies are pending.

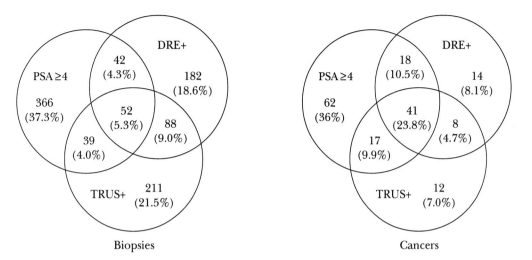

Biopsies   Cancers

Figure 1 Number of biopsies specified per screening test or combination of tests (total 980); and number of cancers detected, specified per screening test or combination of tests (total 172). Each circle represents a screening test. The overlapping fields represent combinations of the tests. PSA ≥ 4, prostate specific antigen level of ≥ 4 ng/ml; DRE+, suspicious digital rectal examination findings; TRUS+, suspicious transrectal ultrasonography findings

Cancer detection

A total of 981 biopsies were performed. (In the evaluation, one biopsy is missing, because the outcome of the digital rectal examination is unknown). One hundred and seventy-two prostate cancers were diagnosed, resulting in an overall detection rate of 4.3%. The performance of the various screening tests expressed in number of biopsies and number of cancers found is detailed in two Venn diagrams (Figure 1). A total of 499 men had PSA levels of ≥ 4 ng/ml; in this group 138 (80.2%) cancers were found. A total of 481 men had PSA levels of < 4 ng/ml and 34 (19.8%) cancers were found. Table 3 shows the clinical stage distribution of all cancers at the moment of screening.

Biopsy rates

Figure 2 shows the number of biopsies performed for each cancer detected, specified per screening test or combination of tests. At PSA levels of ≥ 4 ng/ml, 3.6 biopsies were performed to find one cancer. At PSA levels of < 4 ng/ml, 14.2 biopsies were required to detect one cancer.

Table 3 Clinical stage (cT) distribution at screening, expressed as percentages

	T_{1C}	T_{2A}	$T2B$	T_{2C}	T_{3A}	T_{3B}	T_{3C}	T_{4A}	T_{4B}
cT	36.7	42.2	7.2	4.8	6.6	1.8	0.6	0	0

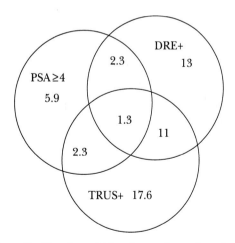

Figure 2 Number of biopsies performed to detect one prostate cancer. PSA ≥ 4, prostate specific antigen level of ≥ 4 ng/ml; DRE+, suspicious digital rectal examination findings; TRUS+, suspicious transrectal ultrasonography findings

Cancer treatment

All patients were informed about the various treatment options. Information about the treatment of 143 patients is available: radical prostatectomy was chosen for the treatment in 73 patients. Fifty-five men received radiotherapy. Watchful waiting was chosen by 12 patients. In three patients metastases were found. These patients have received endocrine treatment.

Radical prostatectomy specimens

As stated before, 73 radical prostatectomies were performed. The clinical stage distribution and the pathological stage distribution are detailed in Table 4. Table 5 illustrates the fact that the clinical stage of the tumor is generally underestimated at the moment of screening compared with the pathological stage.

The grade distribution of the radical prostatectomy specimens is detailed in Table 6 in relation to the pathological tumor stage. In Table 7 the grade of the biopsy specimen is shown vs. the grade of the radical prostatectomy specimen. In two biopsy specimens it was impossible to determine the grade; both these radical prostatectomy specimens were grade 1.

In 24 (33%) of the radical prostatectomy specimens, one or more surgical margins were not free of tumor. This concerned the apex margin in 15 cases. The lateral margin was positive in 13 prostatectomies and the bladder neck in two.

Table 4 The clinical stage (cT) distribution at screening vs. the pathological stage (pT) distribution of all 73 radical prostatectomies, expressed as percentages

	T_{1C}	T2A	T2B	T2C	T3A	T3B	T3C	T4A	T4B
cT	39.7	43.8	8.2	6.8	1.4	0	0	0	0
pT	—	22.2	4.2	36.1	16.7	5.6	5.6	8.3	1.4

Table 5 Clinical stage (cT) vs. pathological stage (pT) of the radical prostatectomy specimen

	pT_2	pT_3	pT_4
cT_1	18	9	1
cT_2	27	10	6
cT_3	0	1	0
cT_4	0	0	0

Table 6 The pathological grade (pG) distribution vs. the pathological stage (pT) distribution in the radical prostatectomy specimens expressed as percentages

	pG_1 (44.9%)	pG_2 (40.6%)	pG_3 (14.5%)
pT_2	35	26.5	3
pT_3	9	10	6
pT_4	1.5	3	6

Table 7 The biopsy grade distribution (cG) vs. the grade in the radical prostatectomy specimen (pG) in 71 radical prostatectomies, expressed as percentages

	pG_1	pG_2	pG_3	Total
cG_1	35	18	4	57
cG_2	10	23	9	42
cG_3	0	0	1	1
Total	45	41	14	100

Discussion

Concern has been raised that screening for prostate cancer, although it increases the rate of cancer detection, may identify tumors of little biological significance that pose no threat to a patient's life. If we take autopsy studies and cystoprostatectomy studies into consideration, detection rates up to 30% are theoretically possible, but undesirable. Essential for screening for prostate cancer is the diagnosis of those cancers that are a possible threat to the host within his life expectancy. The autopsy cancers evidently have not been such a threat. On the other hand, very small tumors (stage A or T_{1A}) that were well differentiated have been shown to be potentially dangerous[12] in patients with a life expectancy of 15 years or more.

The performance of the screening tests in the ERSPC Rotterdam region is depicted in three Venn diagrams. At PSA levels of ≥ 4 ng/ml, 3.6 biopsies had to be performed to diagnose one cancer. In this PSA range 80.2% of all cancers were detected. Digital rectal examination and transrectal ultrasonography do have additional value in this PSA range. If both or either of these examinations were positive, the number of biopsies needed to find one prostate cancer was reduced. At PSA levels of < 4 ng/ml, 19.8% of cancers were detected and 14.2 biopsies were performed to detect one cancer. These cancers were detected through digital rectal examination and/or transrectal ultrasonography. From these data we can conclude that digital rectal examination and transrectal ultrasound examination do have additional value, but that the PSA level seems to be the strongest predictor for prostate cancer. The tumors that were found through PSA testing only formed a substantial part of all tumors found; 37% of the detected cancers were classified as T_{1C}.

The clinical stage distribution at the moment of screening shows that most tumors are locally confined when palpable or visible with ultrasound. This can also be seen in the evaluation of the radical prostatectomy specimens; 62.5% of all tumors were locally confined (stage T_2). There is an impressive number of moderate to high grade lesions; 55% of the radical prostatectomy specimens showed MD Anderson grade 2 and 3. The cancers that are locally confined are generally well (grade 1) or moderately (grade 2) differentiated. The locally advanced tumors are often grade 3. The grade of the tumor is often underestimated in the biopsy specimen. In Table 7 the grades of the biopsy specimens and the radical prostatectomy specimens are depicted. Nine out of ten grade 3 radical prostatectomy specimens were undergraded at biopsy. This underestimation trend is also seen in the clinical vs. pathological stage distribution of the radical prostatectomy specimens (Tables 4 and 5).

Metastases were found in only three patients. One had clinical stage T_{1C} and a well-differentiated cancer in the biopsy specimen. The other two had locally advanced disease (T_{3B} and T_{3C}) and grade 3 lesions in the biopsy specimen.

The tumors that were diagnosed in the pre-PSA era were generally locally advanced and/or metastases were present[3]. The results from this study demonstrate that metastases were present in only three cases (1.7%) vs. 22% in the Rotterdam region in 1993. This was before the screening study started, but after the introduction of PSA testing, which may have had its effect on the stage distribution at the time of diagnosis. The first signs are favorable in that most tumors are locally confined. The answer to the question of whether diagnosis and treatment of these early tumors have a significant impact on prostate cancer mortality will have to come from large randomized screening studies.

References

1. Visser, O., Coebergh, J. W. W. and Schouten, L. J. (1995). Incidence of cancer in the Netherlands 1992. *Fourth Report of The Netherlands Cancer Registry* (Utrecht)
2. Jensen, O., Esteve, J., Möller, H. and Renard, H. (1990). Cancer in the European community and its member states. *Eur. J. Cancer*, **26**, 1167–256
3. Mettlin, C., Natarajan, M. and Murphy, G. P. (1989). Recent patterns of care of prostate cancer patients in the United States: results from the survey of the American College of Surgeons Commission on Cancer. *Int. Adv. Surg. Oncol.*, **5**, 277–321
4. Crawford, E. D., Eisenberger, M. A. and McLeod, D. G. (1989). A controlled trial of leuprolide with and without flutamide in prostatic carcinoma. *N. Engl. J. Med.*, **321**, 419–24
5. Schröder, F. H. (1995). Screening, early detection and treatment of prostate cancer: a European view. *Urology*, **46**, 62–70
6. Franks, L. M. (1954). Latent carcinoma of the prostate. *J. Path. Bact.*, **68**, 603–16
7. Kabalin, J. N., McNeal, J. E., Price, H. M., Freiha, F. S. and Stamey, T. A. (1989). Unsuspected adenocarcinoma of the prostate in patients undergoing cystoprostatectomy for other causes:

incidence, histology and morphometric observations. *J. Urol.*, **141**, 1091–4

8. Ohori, M., Wheeler, I. M., Dunn, J. K., Stamey, T. A. and Scardino, P. T. (1994). The pathological features and prognosis of prostate cancers detectable with current diagnostic tests. *J. Urol.*, **152**, 1714–20

9. Epstein, J. I., Walsh, P. C., Carmichael, M. and Brendler, C. B. (1994). Pathologic and clinical findings to predict tumor extent of nonpalpable (stage T1c) prostate cancer. *J. Am. Med. Assoc.*, **271**, 368–74

10. Schröder, F. H., Denis, L. J., Kirkels, W. J., de Koning, H. J. and Standaert, B. (1995). European randomised study of screening for prostate cancer (progress report of Antwerp and Rotterdam pilot studies). *Cancer*, **76**, 129–34

11. Lee, F., Gray, J. M., McCleary, R. D., Meadows, T. R., Kumansaka, G. H., Borlaza, G. S., Straub, W. H., Lee, F. Jr, Solomon, M. H. and McHugh, T. A. (1985). Transrectal ultrasound in the diagnosis of prostate cancer: location, echogenicity, histopathology and staging. *Prostate*, **7**, 117–29

12. Blute, M. L., Zincke, H. and Farrow, G. M. (1986). Long-term follow-up of young patients with stage A adenocarcinoma of the prostate. *J. Urol.*, **136**, 840–3

European randomized study for prostate cancer: results of PSA-related screening in Göteborg

22

J. Hugosson

Introduction

Screening for prostate cancer is still an unresolved and controversial question. In the USA, early detection and curative treatment has been recommended by several organizations. In Europe, the attitude among many urologists is more sceptical to such a concept. Most European urologists believe that there are still many issues to be evaluated before screening may be recommended in the general population.

Introduction of prostate specific antigen (PSA) measurement, transrectal ultrasound and transrectal core biopsies of the prostate have markedly changed the prospects of early detection. How these different techniques may best be combined into a screening program is, however, not fully evaluated. The most common combination of screening has been the combination of digital rectal examination (DRE) and serum PSA measurement with a cut-off value of 4 ng/ml. However, some have proposed only the measurement of serum PSA as a screening test[1]. The cut-off value for PSA screening has been discussed and some have proposed lower values for younger men[2].

Apart from the requirement of an efficient screening tool, screening demands the existence of an effective therapy before it can be recommended. Even if results after radical prostatectomy are excellent with up to 15 years of follow-up, we still lack proof that this is not an effect of selection, since conservative treatment of early prostate cancer may also result in a low mortality from prostate cancer, at least within 10 years after diagnosis[3,4]. However, although prostate cancer usually develops extremely slowly, it has at the same time a high malignant potential, in that it may spread outside the prostate at an early stage. Tumors larger than $4 cm^3$ are seldom cured by radical prostatectomy, whereas tumors smaller than $1.5 cm^3$ have a much more favorable prognosis[5]. It thus seems that there is a 'window' with early cancer that may be suitable for curative treatment[5].

Two problems exist. The first is the question of how often these small tumors progress, or in other words what is the risk for overtreatment if all these tumors are treated? Secondly, most of these early cancers do not give rise to any symptoms. When a tumor gives rise to symptoms, it is usually too large to be suitable for treatment with curative intent. This means that if we want to treat early prostate cancers we probably have to look for them.

Screening by PSA measurement may detect these unsymptomatic tumors suitable for curative treatment[1,6]. One problem with PSA, however, is its low specificity for slightly increased values, i.e. values in the range of 4–10 ng/ml[7]. This low specificity is particularly problematic in a screening situation, since most tumors detected have a PSA value within this range. Only one out of five men with PSA levels between 4 and 10 ng/ml turns out to have cancer[8]. This means that a lot of men are worried and receive investigations with biopsies of the prostate unnecessarily. One way to increase the specificity of PSA has been the introduction of measuring free vs. complex-bound PSA[9]. The PSA leak in prostate cancer seems to be complex-bound, whereas the PSA increase in patients with benign prostatic hyperplasia (BPH) is mainly free PSA[9]. The present study was initiated to investigate whether measurement of free vs. complex-bound PSA may increase the specificity for prostate cancer in a screening situation. The Göteborg study has also joined the European Randomized Study of Screening for Prostate Cancer (ERSPC) with the aim of studying whether screening for prostate cancer may decrease the mortality from prostate cancer.

Patients and methods

Patients

The base of the screening population was formed from men living in the city of Göteborg (440 000 inhabitants) and born between 1 January 1930 and 31 December 1944 ($n = 22 471$). Fifty-four men with known prostate cancer were excluded. Of the remainder, 10 000 were randomized to active screening and the 32 417 constituted a control group. Men in the screening group were invited to have their PSA level assayed. A blood sample was drawn and serum was frozen at −70 °C within 3 h.

PSA method

All sera were stored at −70 °C for at most 2 weeks until analysis. Both free and total PSA were measured (Wallac Oy, Finland).

Screening algorithm

Men with a total PSA level of 3 ng/ml or more were further invited to an examination by a urologist. This examination included DRE, transrectal ultrasound scanning and sextant biopsies. Men with PSA levels of less than 3 ng/ml were informed by letter and no further investigations were done. The DRE and transrectal ultrasound examinations were carried out with the subjects in a left-sided position, and palpable abnormalities were characterized according to

the criteria of UICC 92. Transrectal ultrasound examinations were performed with Brüel and Kjaer 3535 ultrasound equipment, with a 7-MHz biplane probe, model 8551, attached (Brüel and Kjaer Medical A/S, Naerum, Denmark). Hypoechoic lesions were registered and the total volume of the prostate was calculated according to the volume formula of the prostate was calculated according to the volume formula of the ellipsoid (width × height × length × $\pi/6$). Ultrasound-guided transrectal sextant biopsies were taken with 1.2-mm tru-cut needles (Colibri Medical, Helsingborg, Sweden) mounted in a spring-loaded biopsy gun (Bard Ltd) and directed as described by Stamey[10].

Results

The study started in January 1995, and in March 1996 all 10 000 men had been invited at least once. To date 53% ($n = 5267$) of the men have accepted the invitation and had their PSA level assayed. The distribution of PSA levels is very skew, with 50% of men with values of < 1 ng/ml and 11.8% ($n = 622$) with values exceeding 3 ng/ml (Figure 1a). The distribution of free PSA was also very skew, with 70% having values of < 0.4 and 96% having values of < 1 ng/ml (Figure 1b). The ratio of free/total PSA followed a more uniform distribution. In the total population 82% had values exceeding 18% (Figure 1c). Of those with elevated values of PSA, 418 have so far been further examined, with complete results available. Sextant biopsies were carried out in 380, other types of biopsies in 29 (mean 3.6 biopsies) and no biopsies in nine (five refused, two had acute prostatitis and there were other reasons in two). Of those biopsied, 85 (21%) were found to have cancer and 324 had benign biopsies. The characteristics of these two groups are given in Table 1. The relationship between positive and negative biopsies at various PSA levels is given in Table 2. Of those with cancer, none had bone metastasis and only two had lymph node metastasis. The distribution of Gleason grade and number of positive cores is presented in Table 3. The distribution of free and the ratio of free/total PSA

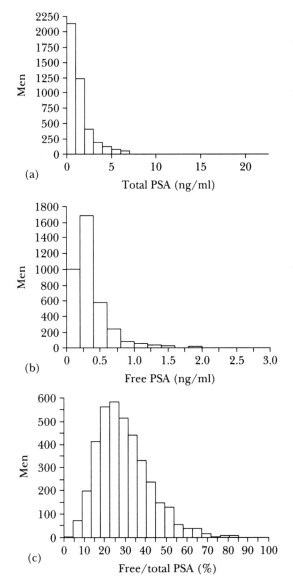

(a)

(b)

(c)

Figure 1 Distribution among men aged 50–65 years of (a) total prostate specific antigen (PSA), (b) free PSA and (c) ratio of free/total PSA

is presented in Figures 2 and 3. If the ratio of free/total PSA with a cut-off at 18% had been used in those with PSA levels in the interval of 3–10 ng/ml, an increase in positive predictive value from 16% to 36% would have been gained. Only five cancers with PSA levels of 3–10 ng/ml had a ratio exceeding 18%. The characteristics of these five cancers are presented in Table 4.

Discussion

The optimal treatment for early prostate cancer is not established. However, it seems that all prostate cancers pass through a curable stage, at which, with modern techniques, they may easily be diagnosed. How many of these cancers will eventually end up as lethal is also not established, but ongoing randomized studies may give us this information. As prostate cancer is one of the most rapidly increasing causes of death in the Western world, and is also a disease associated with much suffering, better management resulting in better survival is urgently needed. As no treatment today or in the near future seems able to reduce mortality for advanced disease, the strategies have focused on early diagnosis. Introduction of PSA testing has given us the tool for early diagnosis, but as a single screening instrument, its specificity is very low. A higher specificity would have several advantages: sampling for PSA testing is easy and cheap and associated with almost no complications, whereas further investigations with DRE, transrectal ultrasound and biopsies are rather complicated and expensive investigations, with a risk for complications such as hemorrhage and infection. Infections after prostate biopsy may become serious, and even lethal cases have been described. A low specificity will also give rise to much anxiety in many men with only benign conditions. How men perceive the message that they have an increased PSA level and how they react in the meantime to further investigations and even afterwards is so far only marginally studied.

In this study, with a cut-off level at 3 ng/ml, as many as 12% of men aged 50–65 had increased values, but only one out of five of these with increased PSA levels turned out to have cancer. The PSA distribution in our study was similar to that found by Kane and co-workers[11]. The cancer detection rate in the present study was 2.3%, somewhat lower than that found in other studies. The higher detection rate found, for example, in the study of Labrie and associates[8] may be due to the higher age at invitation in that study. Even higher detection rates have

Table 1 Comparison between those with benign and malignant biopsies

	Benign (n = 324)	Cancer (n = 85)	p-Value
PSA (ng/ml)	5.6	12.4	$p < 0.001$
PSA density (ng/ml/cm^3)	0.15	0.43	$p < 0.0001$
Prostate volume (cm^3)	40.7	31.1	$p < 0.01$
Age (years)	59.7	60.7	NS
Normal DRE (%)	82	62	$p < 0.05$
Normal TRUS (%)	60	29	$p < 0.01$

PSA, prostate specific antigen; PSAD, prostate specific antigen density; DRE, digital rectal examination; TRUS, transrectal ultrasound examination

Table 2 Relationship between positive and negative biopsies and distribution of detected cancers at different prostate specific antigen (PSA) intervals

PSA interval (ng/ml)	No. of men with positive biopsies	No. of men with negative biopsies	Positive predictive value (%)	No. with focal cancer	No. cancers with ratio* > 18%
3–4	19	141	12	6	4
4–7	26	142	16.7	5	1
7–10	11	26	29.7	1	0
10–20	17	13	57	0	0
20–30	5	1	83	0	0
30–40	6	1	86	0	0
> 40	1	0	100		0

*Ratio of free/total PSA

Table 3 Distribution of T-stage, Gleason grade and number of positive biopsies in 85 patients with screening-detected cancer

T-stage	Patients n	Patients %	Gleason grade	Patients n	Patients %	No. of positive cores	Patients n	Patients %
T$_{1C}$	48	58	3	13	15	1	22	26
T$_{2A}$	20	24	4	29	34	2	17	20
T$_{2B}$	8	10	5	19	23	3	23	27
T$_{2C}$	2	2	6	15	18	4	8	9
T$_{3A}$	2	2	7	5	6	5	1	1
T$_{3B}$	2	2	8	1	1	6	14	16
T$_{3C}$	0		9	1	1			
T$_4$	1	1	10	0				
T$_X$	2	2	G$_X$	2	2			

been found in studies that have not been population based, for example in the study of Cooner and colleagues[12], but persons attending that study were invited by advertising.

Cancers detected in the present study were in general early-stage prostate cancers, none detected to date had distant metastasis and only two had positive lymph glands. Of 85 detected cancers, 73 (86%) had PSA values of < 20 ng/ml, 56 (66%) had values of < 10 ng/ml and 19 (22%) had values of 3–4 ng/ml. This is

in sharp contrast to the situation without screening, in which only a minority are diagnosed with localized disease. The specificity for prostate cancer increased with increasing PSA level. However, in the region of 3–10 ng/ml, in which most localized cancers are diagnosed, the positive predictive value was only 15%. In programs with repeated screening most cancers are probably diagnosed within this interval[8]. The low positive predictive value in this interval may be enhanced considerably by using the ratio of

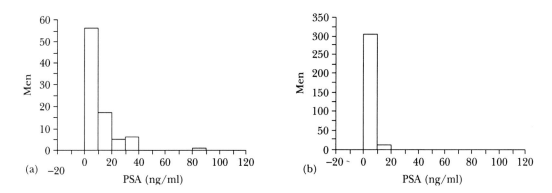

Figure 2 Distribution of prostate specific antigen (PSA) levels among men aged 50–65 years with total serum PSA levels of > 3 ng/ml. (a) Those with findings of cancer at biopsy; (b) those with benign biopsies

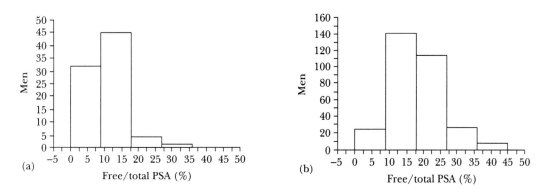

Figure 3 Distribution of the ratio of free/total prostate specific antigen (PSA) among men aged 50–65 years with total serum PSA levels of > 3 ng/ml. (a) Those with findings of cancer at biopsy; (b) those with benign biopsies

Table 4 Characteristics of five patients with cancer in biopsies and a ratio of free/total prostate specific antigen (PSA) of > 18%

Patient	Total PSA (ng/ml)	Ratio free/total PSA (%)	T-stage	Prostate volume (cm³)	No. of positive biopsies	Treatment
1	3.07	20.8	T_{1C}	42	2 (G1)	Watchful waiting
2	3.16	21.2	T_{1C}	55	1 (G1)	Watchful waiting
3	4.17	22.3	T_{1C}	49.9	1 (G1)	Watchful waiting
4	3.35	25.8	T_{1C}	51	1 (G1)	Watchful waiting
5	3.96	35.9	T_{1C}	74.5	3 (G1)	Watchful waiting

G, Gleason grade

free/total PSA. If men with a ratio exceeding 18% had been withdrawn, we would have spared 37% of the men in this interval further examination (Table 5). Five cancers detected in this study had a ratio exceeding 18%, four of these had focal high-grade cancers and none of these four were recommended to have curative treatment. The fifth patient had a large BPH (volume 74 cm³), but also had a small Gleason grade 6 cancer in the peripheral zone.

In conclusion, it seems that population-based PSA screening detects mainly clinically localized

Table 5 Detection rate (%) and positive predictive value (PPV) at four different combinations of prostate specific antigen (PSA) and the ratio of free/total PSA

	Biopsied		PPV (%)	Cancer detected	
	n	%		n	%
PSA > 3 ng/ml	428	11.3	19	82	2.16
PSA > 3 ng/ml + ratio	270	7.1	29	77	2.03
PSA > 4 ng/ml	252	6.6	25	64	1.68
PSA > 4 ng/ml + ratio	174	4.6	36	63	1.66

prostate cancer, which in most instances is suitable for curative treatment. As the long-term results of treating these tumors seems promising[3] at least the first criteria for possible positive long-term effects of screening are fulfilled. By further evaluating the use of free/total PSA evaluation, we may in the future find a more selective screening tool better suited for mass screening than is PSA testing alone.

References

1. Brawer, M. K., Chetner, M. P., Beatie, J., Buener, D. M., Vessella, R. L. and Lange, P. H. (1992). Screening for prostatic carcinoma with prostate specific antigen. *J. Urol.*, **147**, 841–5
2. Oesterling, J. F., Jacobsen, S. J., Chute, C. G., Guess, H. A., Girman, C. J., Panser, L. A. and Lieber, M. M. (1993). Serum prostate-specific antigen in a community-based population of healthy men: establishment of age-specific reference ranges. *J. Am. Med. Assoc.*, **270**, 860–4
3. Zincke, H., Oestering, J. E., Blute, M. L., Bergstrahl, E. J., Myers, R. P. and Barrett, M. (1994). Long-term (15 years) results after radical prostatectomy for clinically localized (stage T$_{2c}$ or lower) prostate cancer. *J. Urol.*, **152**, 1850–7
4. Johansson, J.-F., Adami, H.-O., Andersson, S.-O., Bergström, R., Holmberg, L. and Krusemo, U. B. (1992). High 10-year survival rate in patients with early, untreated prostatic cancer. *J. Am. Med. Assoc.*, **267**, 2191–5
5. Babaian, R. J., Troncoso, P., Steelhammer, L. C., Lloreta-Trull, J. and Ramirez, E. I. (1995). Tumour volume and prostate specific antigen: implications for early detection and defining a window of curability. *J. Urol.*, **154**, 1808–12
6. Catalona, W. J., Smith, D. S., Ratliff, T. L. and Basler, J. W. (1993). Detection of organ-confined prostate cancer is increased through prostate-specific antigen-based screening. *J. Am. Med. Assoc.*, **25**, 948–54
7. Luderer, A. A., Chen, Y.-T., Soriano, T. F., Kramp, W. J., Carlson, G., Cuny, C., Sharp, T., Smith, W., Petteway, J., Brawer, M. K. and Thiel, R. (1995). Measurement of the proportion of free to total prostate-specific antigen improves diagnostic performance of prostate-specific antigen in the diagnostic gray zone of total prostate-specific antigen. *Urology*, **46**, 187–94
8. Labrie, F., Candas, B., Cusan, L., Gomez, J.-L., Diamond, P., Suburu, R. and Lemay, M. (1996). Diagnosis of advanced or noncurable prostate cancer can be practically eliminated by prostate-specific antigen. *Urology*, **47**, 1–7
9. Christensson, A., Björk, T., Nilsson, O., Dahlen, U., Matikainen, M. T., Cockett, A. T., Abrahamsson, P. A. and Lilja, H. (1993). Serum prostate-specific antigen complexed to alfa 1-antichymotrypsin as an indicator of prostate cancer. *J. Urol.*, **150**, 100–5
10. Stamey, T. A., Kabaln, J. N. and McNeil, J. E. (1989). Prostate specific antigen in the diagnosis and treatment of adenocarcinoma of the prostate II radical prostatectomy treated patients. *J. Urol.*, **141**, 1076–81
11. Kane, R. A., Littrup, R. J., Babaian, R., Drago, J. R., Lee, F., Chesley, A., Murphy, G. P. and Mettlin, C. (1992). Prostate-specific antigen levels in 1695 men without evidence of prostate cancer. *Cancer*, **69**, 1201–7
12. Cooner, W. H., Mosley, B. R., Rutherford, C. L., Beard, J. H., Pond, H. S., Terry, W. J., Igel, T. C. and Kidd, D. D. (1990). Prostate cancer detection in a clinical urological practical by ultrasonography, digital rectal examination and prostate specific antigen. *J. Urol.*, **143**, 1146–52

6

PSA and the Early Detection of Prostate Cancer

PSA and the natural course of prostate cancer

23

H. B. Carter and J. D. Pearson

Introduction

The natural course of prostate cancer has been considered by some investigators to be poorly defined. There is increased interest in the natural course of prostate cancer because routine testing of prostate specific antigen (PSA) has resulted in the earlier diagnosis of prostate cancer, and greater numbers of these men are choosing surgical treatment due to improvements in surgical technique. This has led to controversy regarding the need for early detection and aggressive treatment of localized prostatic cancer – a controversy that is based on differences of opinion regarding the natural course of the disease.

The dilemma – on a population level – is due to the long, protracted course of most prostate cancers, and the fact that the majority of men are diagnosed with the disease at a time when there is a limited number of remaining years of life. For the clinician and policy maker, who are both interested in providing optimum care while minimizing harm, understanding the natural course of prostate cancer has never been more important.

The natural course of prostate cancer has important implications with respect to prostate cancer screening, since screening is unlikely to be beneficial in reducing prostate cancer deaths, if (1) most early, localized cancers that are detectable will never progress; and (2) most aggressive cancers are already advanced when detection is possible. Alternatively, screening may reduce prostate cancer mortality, if (1) most early, localized cancers that are detectable eventually progress; and (2) biologically aggressive cancers have a window of opportunity during which detection and cure is possible. Longitudinal PSA data evaluated over decades before the diagnosis of prostate cancer support the concept of inexorable progression for most detectable prostate cancers that are contained, and a phase during which even the most biologically aggressive cancers can be detected at a time when cure is possible.

Prostate specific antigen, digital rectal examination and prostate cancer

Data from autopsy and radical prostatectomy series have demonstrated the following important findings with respect to PSA, digital rectal examination (DRE) and prostate cancer. First, in the setting of PSA elevations, most prostate cancers – more than 80% – are significant in terms of size, grade and pathological extent[1,2]. Epstein and associates[1,3] evaluated the pathological features of PSA-detected prostate cancers using tumor size, grade and pathological stage as surrogates for biological aggressiveness. They discovered that PSA-detected cancers (stage T_{1C}) more closely resembled DRE-detected cancers (stage B or T_2), than the smallest cancers detected by transurethral prostate resection (stage A_1 or T_{1A}), which are often managed expectantly. Other investigators have demonstrated the similarity between PSA- and DRE-detected prostate cancers in terms of size and grade[4-6].

Second, the PSA level is directly related to the volume of cancer present[7]. Numerous studies have shown that for groups of men with prostate cancer, the serum PSA level correlates directly with advancing clinical and pathologic stage[7-9].

Third, in the pre-PSA era, most cancers were discovered at an advanced stage by DRE when progression was likely, even with treatment. When DRE has been used alone to detect prostate cancer, organ-confined disease has been found in less than 50% of men undergoing surgery[10-12]. Furthermore, 75% of 366 men in the Physicians Health Study who were diagnosed with prostate cancer in an era when DRE was the primary diagnostic method available ultimately died of prostatic cancer[13]. Since the cancers detected in the pre-PSA era were most often advanced, significant cancers, evaluation of the course of PSA – with the use of frozen sera – in men who were diagnosed in the pre-PSA era can provide information with respect to the natural course of the disease, with PSA used as a surrogate for cancer progression.

The Baltimore Longitudinal Study of Aging

The Baltimore Longitudinal Study of Aging (BLSA) is an ongoing, long-term, prospective aging study of the National Institute of Aging (Bethesda, MD), which has as its goal the study of the processes of aging in humans[14]. Since the BLSA was established in 1958, more than 1500 men with an average of almost seven visits and 16 years of follow-up have participated in the study. At present, there are approximately 600 active male subjects enrolled in the BLSA. Participants are community-dwelling volunteers who return every 2 years for several days of evaluations; during return visits serum samples are stored for current and future studies. Participants are predominantly white and well educated. Previous analysis of this population of men[15] revealed the age-specific prevalence of prostate disease to be similar to that in the white male population[16].

Longitudinal PSA data

Data from the BLSA has allowed evaluation of the course of serum PSA – from frozen sera – for up to 2 decades before the diagnosis of prostate cancer was made in men at a time when PSA was not used for diagnosis. Thus, the data provide a longitudinal assessment of the natural course of prostate cancer among men who were diagnosed at a time when the majority of detected cancers were already advanced.

The demographic data for the BLSA study groups is shown in Table 1. Controls ($n = 254$) are subjects in the BLSA with no history of medical or surgical treatment of prostate disease. Subjects with benign prostatic hyperplasia (BPH cases; $n = 38$) all had surgical treatment for BPH, and histological confirmation of a benign diagnosis. Cancer cases ($n = 52$) all had histological confirmation of the diagnosis of prostate cancer. The cancer cases are divided into aggressive and non-aggressive, based on the presence or absence of a Gleason histological score of 7 or greater, or clinical evidence of metastatic disease – criteria that have proven predictive value in terms of prognosis. No information regarding Gleason score, or presence or absence of metastatic disease, was available for 12 men who were classified as indeterminate. All

Table 1 Study groups

	Control cases	BPH cases	Non-aggressive cancers	Aggressive cancers	Indeterminate cancers
n	254	38	23	17	12
Median age at diagnosis (years)	69	72	70	75	76
Median follow-up (years)	18	17	17	19	20
Median number of repeat PSA tests	6	5	5	7	5
Median PSA level at visit nearest diagnosis (ng/ml)	1.5	2.5	5.8	14.9	5.6

BPH, benign prostatic hyperplasia; for definitions of study groups see text subjects were over the age of 55 and had at least three serial PSA measurements made on frozen serum samples (Hybritech Tandem-R). Median values for age at diagnosis, years of follow-up, number of repeat PSA tests and the PSA level closest to diagnosis are also shown in Table 1 for the study groups. Data regarding clinical stage and Gleason histological score for the 52 cancers are presented in Table 2.

A mixed-effects longitudinal regression analysis was used to evaluate all longitudinal PSA data[17]. Time of diagnosis was defined for cancer cases as the date of diagnosis of cancer; for BPH cases as the date of simple prostatectomy; and for controls as the date of exclusion of prostate disease. The changes in average PSA levels (95% confidence limits) over time for control subjects, BPH cases and all cancer cases are presented in Figure 1. Average PSA levels over time in men without a diagnosis of prostate cancer demonstrate a slow progressive linear rise. This rise in PSA level has been shown to correspond, among BPH cases, to autopsy data on the doubling time of BPH in aging men[18]. On a

Table 2 Stage and grade of cancer cases ($n = 52$)

	Non-aggressive ($n = 23$)	Aggressive ($n = 17$)	Indeterminate ($n = 12$)
Evidence of metastasis			
M_0	15	4	—
M+	—	11	—
Unknown	8	2	12
Gleason score			
2–4	6	—	—
5–6	15	3	—
7–10	—	14	—
Unknown	2	—	12

For definitions of non-aggressive, aggressive and indeterminate cancers see text; M_0, no clinical evidence of metastasis; M+, clinical evidence of metastasis

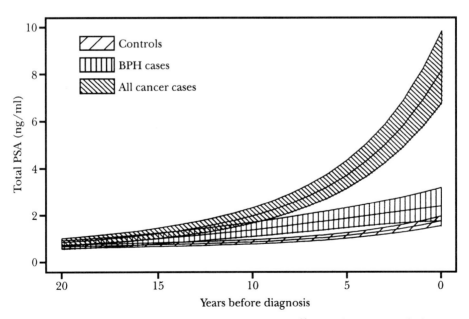

Figure 1 Average prostate specific antigen (PSA) levels and 95% confidence intervals for control cases ($n = 254$), benign prostatic hyperplasia cases (BPH; $n = 38$), and cancer cases ($n = 52$) as a function of years before diagnosis or exclusion of prostate disease

population level, men with prostate cancer demonstrate exponential PSA increases, in contrast to the linear increases in men without prostate cancer. The average PSA levels over time for all men with prostate cancer overlap PSA levels for men without prostate cancer until approximately 7–10 years before diagnosis, at which time the PSA levels for cancer cases become exponential. The exponential rise in PSA occurs at a total PSA level of around 2.0 ng/ml. Using a cut-off level of 4.0 ng/ml as an indicator for the presence of prostate cancer would provide an average lead time for diagnosis of approximately 3–4 years in the BLSA population.

Average PSA levels over time for aggressive and non-aggressive cancers are shown in Figure 2, together with PSA levels in men without prostate cancer for comparison. The curves representing aggressive and non-aggressive cancers overlap until approximately 5–7 years before diagnosis. This suggests that aggressive and non-aggressive cancers are similar early in the natural course of the disease, and that

aggressive cancers may evolve over time from a non-aggressive counterpart. These data also suggest that the non-aggressive cancers may have been diagnosed 5–7 years earlier than the aggressive cancers.

On a population level within the BLSA, prostate cancers exhibit PSA progression that is consistent with the slow but inexorable clinical progression of disease. The finding that average PSA levels for cancer cases become exponential approximately 7 years before diagnosis (Figure 1) is consistent with data from Whittemore and co-workers[19], who suggested that incidental prostate cancers take approximately 7 years to present clinically, based on the relationship between age-specific low-grade tumor volume and clinical incidence rates. In the BLSA population of cancer cases, the median PSA doubling times for aggressive and non-aggressive cancers are around 2–3 years[20], consistent with other investigators' estimates[21,22]. Assuming that PSA doubling times reflect tumor growth – on a population level – it would take approximately three tumor doublings (or 6–9 years) for a small

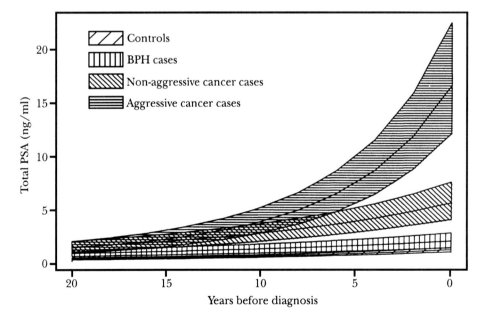

Figure 2 Average prostate specific antigen (PSA) levels and 95% confidence intervals for control cases (n = 254), benign prostatic hyperplasia cases (BPH; n = 38), non-aggressive cancers (n = 23) and aggressive cancers (n = 17) as a function of years before diagnosis or exclusion of prostate disease. For definition of non-aggressive and aggressive cancers, see text

tumor $(0.5 \, cm^3)$ to reach the average size $(4.0 \, cm^3)$ of most T$_2$ tumors[23]. Since most prostate cancers are still localized at lower PSA levels in the 4–5 ng/ml range, one can see from Figure 2 that, on average, it would take more than 10 years to reach a PSA level consistent with metastatic disease in the 20 ng/ml range. Thus, based on longitudinal PSA data it would appear that prostate cancers slowly progress over time, and that even among the most aggressive cancers a window of opportunity exists when diagnosis is possible before the development of advanced disease. These long-term longitudinal PSA data are consistent with the clinical studies of men with localized – moderately to poorly differentiated – prostate cancers who have been treated expectantly or ineffectively, and those men with localized high-grade cancers who have undergone surgical treatment.

Longitudinal clinical data

More than 80% of the cancers detected with DRE and PSA testing are moderately to poorly differentiated prostate cancers. A number of studies provide information regarding the natural course of these tumors. Aus and colleagues[24] studied a large population of unselected men with prostate cancer who were managed expectantly and who all eventually died of the disease or from other causes. Fifty-three per cent of 284 men with clinically confined, moderately to poorly differentiated prostate cancers eventually died of prostate cancer, and not of other causes. A meta-analysis of expectant management series[25] revealed that metastatic rates at 10 years for men with clinically localized moderately to poorly differentiated cancers who did not die of other causes was 42–74% – an optimistic calculation, since androgen ablation was used at the time of progression, delaying the onset of metastases. Finally, Fuks and associates[26] evaluated 403 men with negative pelvic lymph node dissection who underwent ^{125}I implants. Ten-year metastatic rates of 50–70% were found for those men with moderately to poorly differentiated localized cancers – consistent with expectant manage-ment studies. Therefore, longitudinal PSA data and the clinical studies of men treated expectantly or ineffectively support the concept that the natural course of prostate cancer is one of inexorable progression for most localized moderately to poorly differentiated cancers. These are the cancers that are most often detected with routine DRE and PSA testing.

Follow-up of men with poorly differentiated prostate cancers that are detected early in the natural course of the disease, and treated effectively, suggests that a window of opportunity exists for detection and cure of even the most biologically aggressive prostate cancers. Partin and colleagues[27] demonstrated a 45% likelihood of having an undetectable PSA level in men with specimen-confined, poorly differentiated prostate cancer 5 years after radical prostatectomy. Ohori and co-workers[28] demonstrated no difference in the probability of residual disease (PSA recurrence) in men undergoing radical prostatectomy who had organ-confined prostate cancer, regardless of tumor grade. Therefore, longitudinal PSA data are consistent with the clinical studies evaluating men with poorly differentiated prostate cancer that is detected early, and treated effectively. These data suggest that a window of opportunity exists for detection and cure of even the most biologically aggressive cancers.

Summary

The natural course of most clinically localized prostate cancers is slow, but inexorable, progression of disease. This concept is supported by (1) longitudinal PSA data that reveal gradual PSA progression in the majority of clinically detectable localized prostate cancers; and (2) long-term follow-up of men with localized, moderately to poorly differentiated cancers that are managed expectantly or ineffectively. Furthermore, it would appear that there is a window of opportunity for detection at a time when cure is possible even for biologically aggressive cancers – a concept supported by (1) longitudinal PSA data that demonstrate a similar PSA progression for aggressive and non-aggressive cancers early in the natural course of the disease; and (2)

long-term follow-up of men with poorly differentiated cancers detected early and treated effectively with radical prostatectomy.

References

1. Epstein, J. I., Walsh, P. C., Carmichael, M. and Brendler, C. B. (1994). Pathologic and clinical findings to predict tumor extent of non-palpable (stage T1c) prostate cancer. *J. Am. Med. Assoc.*, **271**, 368–74

2. Brawn, P. N., Speights, V. O., Kuhl, D., Riggs, M., Spiekerman, A. M., McCord, R. G., Coffield, K. S., Stewart, D. T. and Lind, M. L. (1991). Prostate-specific antigen levels from completely sectioned, clinically benign, whole prostates. *Cancer*, **68**, 1592–9

3. Epstein, J. I., Walsh, P. C. and Brendler, C. B. (1994). Radical prostatectomy for impalpable prostate cancer: the Johns Hopkins experience with tumors found on transurethral resection (Stages T1a and T1b) and on needle biopsy (Stage T1c). *J. Urol.*, **152**, 1721–9

4. Stormont, T. J., Farrow, G. M., Myers, M. L., Blute, M. L., Zincke, H., Wilson, T. M. and Oesterling, J. E. (1993). Clinical stage B0 or T1c prostate cancer: nonpalpable disease identified by elevated serum prostate-specific antigen concentration. *Urology*, **41**, 3–8

5. Skaletsky, R., Koch, M. O., Eckstein, C. W., Bicknell, S. L., Gray, G. F. Jr and Smith, J. A. Jr (1994). Tumor volume and stage in carcinoma of the prostate detected by elevations in prostate specific antigen. *J. Urol.*, **152**, 129–31

6. Ohori, M., Wheeler, T. M. and Scardino, P. T. (1994). The new American joint committee on cancer and international union against cancer TNM classification of prostate cancer: clinicopathologic correlations. *Cancer*, **73**, 104–14

7. Stamey, T. A., Yang, N., Hay, A. R., McNeal, J. E., Freiha, F. S. and Redwine, E. (1987). Prostate-specific antigen as a serum marker for adenocarcinoma of the prostate. *N. Engl. J. Med.*, **317**, 909–16

8. Oesterling, J. E., Chan, D. W., Epstein, J. I., Kimball, A. W., Bruzek, D. J., Rock, R. C., Brendler, C. B. and Walsh, P. C. (1988). Prostate specific antigen in the preoperative and postoperative evaluation of localized prostatic cancer treated with radical prostatectomy. *J. Urol.*, **139**, 766–72

9. Partin, A. W., Carter, H. B., Chan, D. W., Epstein, J. I., Oesterling, J. E., Rock, R. C., Weber, J. P. and Walsh, P. C. (1990). Prostate specific antigen in the staging of localized prostate cancer: influence of tumor differentiation, tumor volume and benign hyperplasia. *J. Urol.*, **143**, 747–52

10. Thompson, I. M., Rounder, J. B., Teague, J. L., Peek, M. and Spence, C. R. (1987). Impact of routine screening for adenocarcinoma of the prostate on stage distribution. *J. Urol.*, **137**, 424–6

11. Mueller, E. J., Crain, T. W., Thompson, I. A. and Rodriguez, F. R. (1988). An evaluation of serial digital rectal examinations in screening for prostate cancer. *J. Urol.*, **140**, 1445–7

12. Chodak, G. W., Keller, P. and Schoenberg, H. W. (1989). Assessment of screening for prostate cancer using the digital rectal examination. *J. Urol.*, **141**, 1136–8

13. Gann, P. H., Hennekens, C. H. and Stampfer, M. J. (1995). A prospective evaluation of plasma prostate-specific antigen for detection of prostatic cancer. *J. Am. Med. Assoc.*, **273**, 289–94

14. Shock, N. W., Greulich, R. C., Andres, R., Arenberg, D., Costa, P. T. Jr, Lakatta, E. G. and Tobin, J. D. (1984). *Normal Human Aging: The Baltimore Longitudinal Study of Aging*, NIH publication 84-2450. (Washington, DC: US GPO)

15. Arrighi, H. M., Guess, H. A., Metter, E. J. and Fozard, J. L. (1990). Symptoms and signs of prostatism as risk factors for prostatectomy. *Prostate*, **16**, 253–61

16. National Institutes of Health (1988). *1987 Annual Cancer Statistics Review*, NIH publication 88-2789. (Washington, DC: National Institutes of Health)

17. Lindstrom, M. J. and Bates, D. M. (1988). Newton–Raphson and EM algorithms for linear mixed-effects models for repeated-measures data. *J. Am. Stat. Assoc.*, **83**, 1014–22

18. Carter, H. B., Morrell, C. H., Jay, D., Pearson, J. D., Plato, C. C., Metter, E. J., Chan, D. W., Fozard, J. L. and Walsh, P. C. (1992). Estimation of prostatic growth using serial prostate specific antigen measurements in men with and without prostate disease. *Cancer Res.*, **52**, 3323–8

19. Whittemore, A. S., Keller, J. B. and Betensky, R. (1991). Low-grade, latent prostate cancer volume: predictor of clinical cancer incidence? *J. Natl. Cancer Inst.*, **83**, 1231–5

20. Pearson, J. D. and Carter, H. B. (1994). Natural history of changes in prostate-specific antigen in early-stage prostate cancer. *J. Urol.*, **152**, 1743–8

21. Stamey, T. A. and Kabalin, J. N. (1989). Prostate-specific antigen in the diagnosis and treatment of adenocarcinoma of the prostate. I: untreated patients. *J. Urol.*, **141**, 1070–5

22. Schmid, H. P., McNeal, J. E. and Stamey, T. A. (1993). Observations on the doubling time of prostate cancer: the use of serial prostate-specific antigen in patients with untreated disease as a measure of increasing cancer volume. *Cancer*, **71**, 2031–40

23. Partin, A. W., Epstein, J. I., Cho, K. R., Gittelsohn, M. A. and Walsh, P. C. (1989). Morphometric measurement of tumor volume and per cent of gland involvement as predictors of pathological stage in clinical stage B prostate cancer. *J. Urol.*, **141**, 341–5

24. Aus, G., Hugosson, J. and Norlen, L. (1995). Long-term survival and mortality in prostate cancer treated with noncurative intent. *J. Urol.*, **154**, 460–5

25. Chodak, G. W., Thisted, R. A., Gerber, G. S., Johansson, J.-E., Adolfsson, J., Jones, G. W., Chisholm, C. B. E., Moskovitz, B., Livne, P. M. and Warner, J. (1994). Results of conservative management of clinically localized prostate cancer. *N. Engl. J. Med.*, **330**, 242–8

26. Fuks, Z., Leibel, S. A., Wallner, K. E., Begg, C. B., Fair, W. R., Anderson, L. L., Hilaris, B. S. and Whitmore, W. F. (1991). The effect of local control on metastatic dissemination in carcinoma of the prostate: long-term results in patients treated with ^{125}I-implantation. *Int. J. Radiat. Oncol. Biol. Phys.*, **21**, 537–47

27. Partin, A. W., Lee, B. R., Carmichael, M., Walsh, P. C. and Epstein, J. I. (1994). Radical prostatectomy for high grade disease: a reevaluation. *J. Urol.*, **151**, 1583–6

28. Ohori, M., Goad, J. R., Wheeler, T. M., Eastmen, J. A., Thompson, T. C. and Scardino, P. T. (1994). Can radical prostatectomy alter the progression of poorly differentiated prostate cancer? *J. Urol.*, **152**, 1843–9

Interactive Voting System

1   The natural history of most detectable early cancers is:

Response	Option
3%	To remain quiescent.
88%	Slowly to progress.
6%	Rapidly to progress.
3%	None of the above.

Number of votes: 91

2   Available data suggest that high-grade biologically aggressive cancers:

27%	Have a poor prognosis regardless of stage.
1%	Are advanced from inception.
72%	Can be detected early in their natural history and treated effectively.
0%	None of the above.

Number of votes: 115

Free and total PSA: background information and rationale for use

24

H. Lilja

Prostate specific antigen (PSA) is a serine protease occurring at very high concentration in the seminal fluid (about 0.2 mg/ml) mainly in the catalytically active form. The catalytically active single-chain fraction constitutes approximately 70% of the seminal fluid PSA, whereas about 30% of PSA lacks catalytic activity, e.g. due to the internal peptide bond hydrolysis between Lys_{145} and Lys_{146}. This internal peptide bond cleavage generates a free, non-complexed, inactive two-chain form of PSA, but internal peptide bond cleavages at other positions have also been demonstrated to exist. In addition, up to 5% of PSA in the seminal fluid is inactive, due to complex formation with the protein C inhibitor (PCI). This is a 55-kDa, mainly seminal-vesicle-derived serine protease inhibitor that has a mechanism of action similar to that of α_1-antichymotrypsin (ACT).

The structure of the glandular ductal system in the prostate promotes the secretion of very high concentrations of PSA into the seminal fluid, and efficiently prevents exit of PSA into the different extracellular compartments. This may mainly be attributed to the function of the basement membranes in the acini, a basal cell layer, and stromal cells which normally prevent the escape of PSA into the blood at concentrations higher than 4 ng/ml, a level of PSA in the serum that roughly corresponds to 10^{-6} of the concentration of PSA in the seminal fluid. Moreover, it might be vitally important to control the proteolytic activity of PSA carefully, if the protein exits into compartments other than the glandular ducts in the prostate. The biosynthesis of PSA therefore generates an inactive PSA-precursor that stepwise is processed post-translationally to generate the catalytically active form of PSA. Upon escape of the catalytically active form of PSA, there is a very large molar excess of extracellular protease inhibitors such as ACT and α_2-macroglobulin (AMG) present in the extracellular fluids. ACT and AMG are two of the major, mainly liver-derived protease inhibitors occurring at approximately 3–7 μmol/l concentrations which corresponds to approximately 10^4–10^5-fold excess to the normal serum concentration of PSA, i.e. a PSA concentration of 3 ng/ml corresponds to a molar concentration of approximately 0.1 nmol/l. The formation of covalently stabilized equimolar complexes of approximately 90–kDa between PSA and ACT requires the presence of the catalytically active form of PSA, but the rate at which ACT irreversibly inactivates PSA is not very high. Still, about 75–80% of the PSA activity may be inhibited in 10 min *in vitro* at only ten-fold molar excess of ACT. Therefore, it may be considered unlikely that any significant amounts of catalytically active PSA may remain unreacted with ACT at the very large molar excess of ACT in the interstitial fluids. Furthermore, the reaction of PSA with ACT is less rapid than the *in vitro* inactivation of PSA by AMG, which may be present at somewhat lower concentration than ACT in the interstitial fluids. However, no antigenic epitopes on the PSA molecule remain exposed when PSA has been complexed to AMG, unless denaturing conditions are used to change the native conformation of this complex drastically. Therefore, most immunoassays fail to recognize the PSA–AMG complexes under non-denaturing conditions, and the concentrations of PSA–AMG complexes in the extracellular fluids remain unknown. In contrast, only one major PSA epitope is shielded upon the complex formation with ACT. This epitope may be used for very specific detection of the free, non-complexed form of PSA, also in the presence of a large excess of PSA–ACT complexes, i.e. sensitive and specific free-PSA detection with a cross-reactivity of less than 0.2% from PSA–ACT complexes. However, there are several independent antigenic epitopes on the PSA molecule that remain exposed when PSA has complexed to ACT and that can interact with different anti-PSA monoclonal antibodies. This makes it possible to construct immunoassays that may detect both the free, non-complexed form of PSA and the PSA–ACT complexes uniformly in an equimolar fashion (i.e. equimolar detection of total PSA concentrations in serum).

PSA has extensive structural similarity with the glandular kallikreins, in particular the human prostatic glandular kallikrein-1 (hGK-1 or hK$_2$) that has 80% identity in primary structure to PSA. We used recombinant production of hK$_2$ and PSA in both pro- and eukaryotic cells to study the immunological cross-reactivity of PSA and hK$_2$. Our studies have demonstrated that only seven out of 23 monoclonal anti-PSA immunoglobulin (Ig)Gs (monoclonal antibodies) cross-reacted with PSA, whereas 16 monoclonal antibodies defined epitopes unique to PSA, despite the extensive similarity of the two proteins. These data have now also been used to design an immunofluorometric assay for detection of hK$_2$ (detection limit 0.1 ng/ml) with low cross-reactivity to recombinant PSA (less than

0.7%), and evaluations of the putative clinical significance of these measurements have now been initiated.

PSA complexed to ACT is the major form of PSA in serum, and *in vitro* the rate at which this covalently formed 90-kDa complex dissociates has been shown to be remarkably low. A free, non-complexed form of PSA is less abundant in the serum, but the free form in serum is unlikely to manifest enzyme activity, as there is such a large molar excess of ACT and AMG available to react with any catalytically active PSA present in the serum. The proportion of PSA–ACT complexes to total PSA (i.e. free and complexed PSA) is significantly higher in cancer of the prostate than in benign prostatic hyperplasia (BPH), but analysis of the ratio is free PSA to total PSA, which is significantly lower in prostate cancer than in BPH, appears to be a more efficient means to discriminate subjects with BPH alone from those with prostate cancer. We have developed a dual-label immunoassay for the simultaneous measurement of the ratio of free PSA to total PSA, which significantly increases the ROC area under the curve compared to measurements of only total PSA concentrations in serum. However, it is not yet understood why a larger proportion of PSA is complexed to ACT in prostate cancer than in BPH, although it could be speculated that it may relate to local production of ACT and PSA in malignant prostate tissue, as demonstrated by immunocytochemical and *in situ* hybridization techniques.

Interactive Voting System

1   Is it likely that any of the molecular forms of PSA in the serum manifests enzymatic activity?

Response	*Option*
60%	Yes.
40%	No.

Number of votes: 72

2   Which of the following aspects will be most important in the clinical utility of the measurements of free and total PSA?

   8%   To increase the sensitivity in the analysis of total PSA concentrations in serum.
   50%   To increase the specificity in the analysis of total PSA in serum.
   42%   To increase both the sensitivity and the specificity in the analysis of total PSA.

Number of votes: 103

The ratio of free to total PSA level: clinical implications

25

M. K. Brawer

Prostate specific antigen (PSA) has revolutionized out approach to diagnosis, staging and monitoring of patients who are suspected of, or who currently carry the diagnosis of, prostatic carcinoma. Its role in early detection and screening is entrenched in the literature and indeed has resulted in the recommendation of the American Cancer Society[1] and the American Urological Association[2] for serum PSA determination in conjunction with a carefully performed digital rectal examination in men seeking a prostate cancer check-up. Moreover, the use of PSA in early detection has resulted in a substantial increase in the incidence of prostate carcinoma[3,4], and there is an increasing number of carcinomas detected at a stage amenable to extirpative surgery or radiation[5–7]. Finally the majority of men with carcinoma identified because of elevation of the PSA level have clinically significant carcinoma, as evidenced by histological grade, pathological stage and tumor volume[8–13].

Despite the impressive yield of PSA testing in a diagnostic setting with resulting positive predictive values[5,14–23] (Table 1), there has been considerable effort to improve the performance of PSA measurement. This stems from two salient observations: approximately two out of three men with a PSA level of > 4.0 ng/ml (the usual cut-off level for recommendation for biopsy) have negative initial biopsy[5,15,16,21,24,25], and approximately 20–25% of men will be shown to have carcinoma with a serum PSA level of < 4.0 ng/ml[5,15,16,21,24,26].

Several attempts at manipulating the PSA test to improve its performance have been made. In general, efforts have been directed at enhancing the specificity, owing to the fact that false-positive results carry with them considerable cost. Not only are there economic costs, owing to the fact that an elevated PSA level requires follow-up studies (usually ultrasound and biopsy), but in addition, the emotional cost from the burden of human anxiety is immeasurable when a man is told that he has an abnormal PSA finding.

It must be kept in mind that any attempt at enhancing the specificity will result in diminu-

Table 1 Positive predictive value for PSA level of > 4.0 ng/ml

Authors	Year	Population	No. of biopsies	Positive predictive value (%)
Babaian and Camps[18]	1991	mixed	67	31.3
Bazinet et al.[19]	1994	referral	565	37.0
Brawer and Lange[17]	1989	referral	188	54.2
Brawer et al.[16]	1992	screening	105	30.5
Catalona et al.[15]	1991	screening	112	33.0
Catalona et al.[5]	1993	screening	1325	37.1
Catalona et al.[14]	1994	screening	686	31.5
Cooner et al.[20]	1988	referral	96	51.2
Cooner et al.[21]	1990	referral	436	35.0
Mettlin et al.[22]	1991	screening	70	41.4
Rommel et al.[23]	1994	referral	2020	41.0

tion in the sensitivity. Figure 1 demonstrates the yield of ultrasound-guided biopsy with various PSA cut-off levels[1,16,27]. As is readily apparent, an increase in specificity associated with a higher PSA cut-off level results in a diminution in test sensitivity.

Among the efforts at enhancing PSA performance have been tests of PSA density, PSA velocity, age-specific PSA value and measurement of the ratio of the free to total PSA[27]. PSA density, the quotient derived from the serum PSA level divided by the volume in the prostate, was first promulgated by Benson and associates[28]. In actuality, Babaian and co-workers[29] were the first to demonstrate the correlation of serum PSA level and prostate volume. Benson and colleagues theorized that by normalizing the prostate volume, any spurious elevation of PSA level emanating from hyperplastic cells would be reduced. Indeed, they were they able to demonstrate considerable stratification of those men with and without prostate cancer by utilizing this modality[28,30]. Others reported similar increased cancer yield[19,23,31,32]. We[33], as well as Mettlin and co-workers[24], were unable to reproduce these findings. Sampling consideration may explain the discrepancy. All the reports that showed enhancement in the ability to detect carcinoma with PSA density revealed that the prostates were considerably smaller in those glands with cancer than in those without[19,23,31,32]. In contrast, in our study and that of Mettlin and associates, the prostates

with cancer were the same size or slightly larger[24,27,33].

Another attempt at enhancing the performance of PSA testing has been the concept of PSA velocity. This assumes that the PSA increases over time are greater in those men with cancer than in those without. Carter and colleagues[34] were the first to promulgate this concept. They demonstrated significant prediction of cancer if the PSA level increased by 0.75 ng/ml/year. Others have also found PSA velocity useful in predicting carcinoma[35,36]. We were unable to recapitulate these findings with short-term interval and PSA determinations[37], but these findings have been substantiated by Carter and associates[38]. One possible explanation for the discrepancy in the literature is the considerable biological variation of PSA level, which has been reported ranging from 10 to 50%[39–42].

The recognition that PSA level increases in all men with advancing age resulted in Oesterling and colleagues[43] as well as Dalkin and associates[44] recommending age-specific cut-off values for PSA. Utilizing different cut-off values for differing age groups has resulted in increased sensitivity in younger men and increased specificity in older men. Other investigations, however, have failed to demonstrate substantial improvement in the accuracy of PSA by utilizing age-specific cut-off levels, owing to a decreased detection of carcinoma in the older man, in whom the prevalence is, of course, greater[24,45,46].

It also would appear that while some investigators have demonstrated an improvement of PSA testing, utilizing manipulation such as PSA density, PSA velocity and age-specific cut-off levels, other studies have refuted these results. Several prospective evaluations of these efforts are currently under way.

Probably the most encouraging development in enhancing the performance of PSA testing involves measuring the different constituents of PSA in the systemic circulation. Two Scandinavian research groups[47,48] independently observed that PSA exists in at least three distinct forms in the systemic circulation. The free form of PSA, which is not complexed to other protein

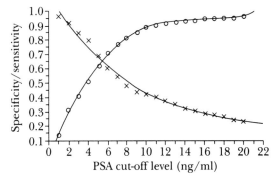

Figure 1 Sensitivity (crosses) and specificity (circles) relative to various PSA cut-off levels

moieties, is similar to the form of PSA found in the ejaculate.

The largest component of PSA in the systemic circulation appears to be complexed α_1-antichymotrypsin (ACT). A third form is complexed to α_2-macroglobulin (AMG). It is thought, as shown in Figure 2[49], that the free form of PSA has five prostate epitopes available for reactionable antibodies. It appears that ACT sterically hinders three of the epitopes. AMG causes blocking of all the recognized epitopes. This form of PSA is not identified by conventional immunoassays.

In 1991 Stenman and associates[50] demonstrated that the ratio of free to total PSA was greater in men without carcinoma than in men with prostate carcinoma. Investigating 67 patients with prostate cancer and 30 men with clinical evidence of benign prostatic hyperplasia (BPH), along with healthy male and female controls, these authors demonstrated that they could separate those men with cancer from those without, on the basis of the ratio of free to complexed (ACT) PSA. In a subsequent investigation, of 120 patients with cancer and 144 with BPH, Christensson and associates[51] again observed a significant decrease in the proportion of free PSA in patients with cancer. The median ratio of free to total PSA in untreated prostate cancer was 0.16 and in BPH patients 0.28. Utilizing the free-to-total PSA cut-off level of 0.18, these authors reported a 71% sensitivity and 95% specificity in men with a total PSA range from 4.0 to 20.8 ng/ml.

Tables 2 and 3 demonstrate the performance of the ratio of free to total PSA in several large series[52]. Luderer and associates[53] (Figures 3 and 4) reported the utility of the ratio of free total PSA in men with a total PSA level between 4.0 and 10.0 ng/ml. Whereas the ratio offers no enhanced prediction of carcinoma over the entire PSA range, in this important interval these authors noted an increased specificity from 37 to 52% with a minimal reduction of sensitivity from 93 to 87% as compared to measurement of total PSA alone. Utilizing a free-to-total PSA cut-off value of 0.25 or less, these authors noted that 31% of unnecessary biopsies could be prevented without missing any men with cancer.

Catalona and colleagues[54] evaluated 63 patients with BPH and 50 men with carcinoma. They divided the patients with cancer into those

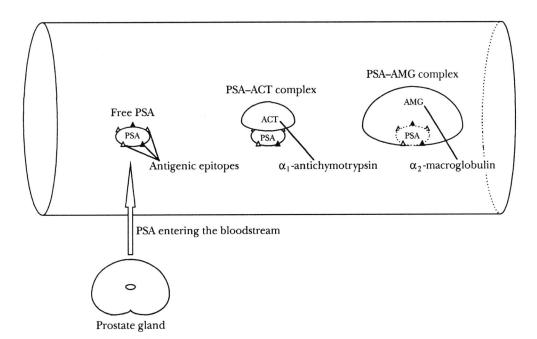

Figure 2 Major molecular forms of prostate specific antigen (PSA)

Table 2 Measurement of free PSA in the recent literature. Standard deviations given in parentheses

Authors	Histology	n	Median total PSA	Median % free PSA
Lauderer et al.[53]	benign	62	4.89 (4.12)	21 (13)
		64	1.07 (0.81)	23 (14)
		55	9.60 (15.18)	13 (6)
Catalona et al.[54]	benign	63	6.0 (1.4)	18.8 (6.8)
	CAP (GL. > 40)	30	6.6 (1.5)	15.9 (3.9)
	CAP (GL. > 40)	20	5.3 (1.3)	9.2 (3.3)
Bangma et al.[55]	benign	1659	1.2	28
	CAP	67	7.6	12
Prestigiacomo et al.[56]*	benign	48	8.9[†] (3.2)	16.5 (6.22)
	CAP	51	10.0[†] (6.3)	8.9 (5.5)
Prestigiacomo et al.[56]†	benign	47	8.9[†] (7.2)	15.5 (8.1)
	CAP	50	10.0[†] (6.3)	9.1 (5.8)
Petteway et al.[52]‡	benign	166	4.9 (7.9)	18.5 (11.8)
	CAP	47	10.7 (46.3)	13.3 (6.7)
Petteway et al.[52]**	benign	166	4.9 (7.9)	21.1 (16.4)
	CAP	47	10.7 (46.3)	14.5 (9.2)

CAP, cancer of the prostate; GL. > 40, prostate gland volume > 40 cm^3; *Delfia; † mean; ‡ Hybritech; ** Dianon

Table 3 Performance of free total PSA measurement by various assays, reported in the recent literature

Authors	Assay	CAP	Benign	Cut-off Level	Sensitivity (%)	Specificity (%)
Bangma et al.[55]	Delfia	33	140	28	91	19
		33	140	17	71	68
Bangma et al.[55]*		22	81	19	91	49
		22	81	14	82	74
Petteway et al.[52]	Hybritech	47	166	38	100	6
				25	96	24
				22	90	37
Petteway et al.[52]	Dianon	47	166	50	100	7
				31	94	26
				30	92	30
Petteway et al.[52]†	Hybritech			22	100	33
		12	69	21	92	42
	Dianon	12	69	30	100	17
				22	92	32
Catalona et al.[54]	Hybritech	50	63	30	90	38
Catalona et al.[54]‡		30	63	21	90	38
Catalona et al.[54]**		20	67	14	90	76
Luderer et al.[53]	Dianon	55	62	25	98	34
				15	87	71
				10	53	89
Luderer et al.[53]†	Dianon	25	32	25	100	31
				15	72	75
				10	24	88
Prestigiacomo et al.[56]	Delfia	51	48	15	95	56
	Hybritech	50	47	14	90	64

CAP, cancer of the prostate; cut-off levels for volume of prostate:* < 50 cm^3; ‡ > 40 cm^3; ** < 40 cm^3; † PSA 4.0–10.0 ng/ml

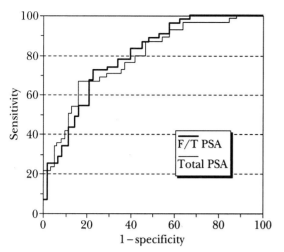

Figure 3 Receiver-operating characteristic curve analysis comparing total PSA and the ratio of free/total (F/T) PSA over the total range

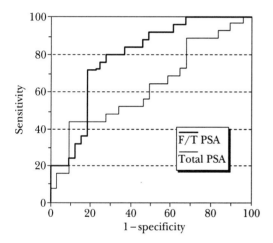

Figure 4 Receiver-operating characteristic curve analysis comparing total PSA and the ratio of free/total (F/T) PSA over the range 4.0–10.0 ng/ml

with prostate size of less than 40 cm³ to maintain a 90% sensitivity in men with cancer, and for glands less than 40 cm³ a cut-off value of 0.137 was required. To afford the same sensitivity in men with larger prostates, a cut-off value of the free-to-total ratio of 0.205 was used. The specificity for all cancers utilizing these cut-off levels was 38.1% in those with a gland less than 40 cm³, with 76.2% sensitivity. Furthermore, Catalona and co-workers showed significant enhance-

ment in specificity over testing of total PSA in men who had normal digital rectal examinations. Similar enhancement in PSA performance has been observed by Bangma and associates[55] based on their impressive screening population, as well as by the Stanford group[56].

It would thus appear that the free-to-total PSA ratio offers a significant advantage in the diagnostic gray zone of a PSA level between 4.0 and 10.0 ng/ml. Several concerns remain, before widespread application of free-to-total PSA can be recommended. First and foremost is the recognition that unless very high cut-off ratios are selected, there will be some compromise in the cancer detection rate (decreased sensitivity). Urologists will have to determine how many cancers they are willing to miss to afford a significant reduction in unnecessary biopsies. After this is decided, the optimum cut-off ratio can be selected. Another concern is the fact that owing to differences between manufacturers in the free as well as the total PSA measurement, some effort at standardization will be required, or different cut-off levels will be necessary for each manufacturer. Utilizing the quotient of free to total PSA will potentially increase the assay variability between manufacturers. We and others have reported considerable bias, for example, between the Abbott total PSA assay and that achieved on the same patient serum with the Hybritech assay[57]. It does appear in this regard that the Ciba Corning PSA assay and the Hybritech assay offer comparable results for the measurement of total PSA[57]. Such data have not been reported for different manufacturers' free PSA assay.

Finally, even without change in the recommendation for biopsy in a man with a PSA level > 4.0, as a result of the free PSA measurement, there will be considerable application for this ratio. One certain application is to help determine which men who have undergone prostate biopsy with negative results should have repeat biopsy. Standard methods, including measurement of serum PSA level, do not appear to enhance our predictability in this regard[58]. Another important application for the use of the free-to-total PSA ratio would be in men with a total PSA level of < 4.0. Certainly this constitutes the majority of patients undergoing testing with PSA, and if indeed they have another indication for biopsy, such as an abnormality on digital rectal examination, this may help predict who will have carcinoma.

In conclusion, it appears that the ratio of the free to total PSA level offers the most significant enhancement in the predictability of PSA level for carcinoma to be found on the biopsy. Certainly, with future refinements, as additional data become apparent, the optimum role of this modality will be realized.

References

1. Mettlin, C., Jones, G., Averette, H. Gusberg, S. B. and Murphy, G. P. (1993). Defining and updating the ACS guidelines for the cancer related check-up: prostate and endometrial cancer. *CA Cancer J. Clin.*, **43**, 42–6
2. AUA (1992). *American Urological Association Policy Statement: Early Detection of Prostate Cancer and Use of Transrectal Ultrasound.* (Baltimore: American Urological Association)
3. Scher, H. I. and Fossa, S. (1995). Prostate cancer in the era of prostate-specific antigen. *Curr. Opin. Oncol.*, **7**, 281
4. Potosky, A. L., Miller, B. A., Albertsen, P. C. and Kramer, B. S. (1995). The role of increasing detection in the rising incidence of prostate cancer. *J. Am. Med. Assoc.*, **273**, 548
5. Catalona, W. J., Smith, D. S., Ratliff, T. L. and Basler, J. W. (1993). Detection of organ-confined prostate cancer is increased through PSA-based screening. *J. Am. Med. Assoc.*, **270**, 948–54
6. Jacobsen, S. J., Katusic, S. K., Bergstralh, E. J., Oesterling, J. E., Ohrt, D., Klee, G. G. *et al.* (1995). Incidence of prostate cancer diagnosis in the eras before and after serum prostate-specific antigen testing. *J. Am. Med. Assoc.*, 274, 1445
7. Slawin, K. M., Ohori, M., Dillioglugil, O. and Scardino, P. T. (1995). Screening for prostate cancer: an analysis of the early experience. *CA Cancer J. Clin.*, **45**, 134–47
8. Dugan, J. A., Bostwick, D. G., Myers, R. P., Qian, J., Bergstralh, E. J. and Oesterling, J. E. (1996). The definition and pre-operative prediction of clinically insignificant prostate cancer. *J. Am. Med. Assoc.*, **275**, 288
9. Ohori, M., Wheeler, T. M., Dunn, J. K., Stamey, T. A. and Scardino, P. T. (1994). Pathological features and prognosis of prostate cancer detectable with current diagnostic tests. *J. Urol.*, **152**, 1714–20
10. Blackwell, K. L., Bostwick, D. G., Myers, R. P., Zinke, H. and Oesterling, J. E. (1994). Combining prostate-specific antigen with cancer and gland volume to predict more reliably pathological stage: the influence of prostate-specific antigen cancer density. *J. Urol.*, **151**, 1565
11. Stamey, T. A., Freiha, F. S., McNeal, J. E., Redwine, E. A., Whittemore, A. S. and Schmid, H. P. (1993). Localized prostate cancer: relationship of tumor volume to clinical significance for the treatment of prostate cancer. *Cancer*, **71**, 993
12. Schmid, H. P., McNeal, J. E. and Stamey, T. A. (1993). Observations on the doubling time of prostate cancer: the use of serial prostate specific antigen in patients with untreated disease as a measure of increasing cancer volume. *Cancer*, **71**, 2031–40
13. D'Amico, A. V. and Hanks, G. E. (1993). Linear regressive analysis using prostate-specific antigen doubling time for predicting tumor biology and clinical outcome in prostate cancer. *Cancer*, **72**, 2638
14. Catalona, W. J., Richie, J. P., Ahmann, F. R., Hudson, M. A., Scardino, P. T., Flanigan, R. C. *et al.* (1994). Comparison of DRE and serum PSA in the early detection of prostate cancer: results of a multicenter clinical trial of 6,630 men. *J. Urol.*, **151**, 1283–90
15. Catalona, W. J., Smith, D. S., Ratcliff, T. L., Dodds, K. M., Coplen, D. E., Yuan, J. J. J. *et al.* (1991). Measurement of prostate-specific antigen in serum as a screening test for prostate cancer. *N. Engl. J. Med.*, **324**, 1156–61
16. Brawer, M. K., Chetner, M. P., Beatie, J., Buchner, D. M., Vessella, R. L. and Lange, P. H. (1992). Screening for prostatic carcinoma with PSA. *J. Urol.*, **147**, 841–5
17. Brawer, M. K. and Lange, P. H. (1989). PSA in the screening, staging and follow up of early-stage prostate cancer: a review of recent developments. *World J. Urol.*, **7**, 7–11
18. Babaian, R. J. and Camps, J. L. (1991). The role of PSA as part of the diagnostic triad and as a guide when to perform a biopsy. *Cancer*, **68**, 2060–3
19. Bazinet, M., Meshref, A. W., Trudel, C., Aronson, S., Peloguin, F., Nachabe, M. *et al.* (1994).

Prospective evaluation of prostate specific antigen density and systematic biopsies for early detection of prostatic carcinoma. *Urology*, **43**, 44–51

20. Cooner, W. H., Mosley, B. R. and Rutherford, C. L. Jr (1988). Clinical application of transrectal ultrasonography and prostate specific antigen in the search for prostate cancer. *J. Urol.*, **139**, 758–61

21. Cooner, W. H., Mosley, R. B. C. L., Rutherford, J., Beard, J. H., Pond, H. S., Terry, W. J. *et al.* (1990). Prostate cancer detection in a clinical urological practice by ultrasonography, digital rectal examination and prostate specific antigen. *J. Urol.*, **143**, 1146–52

22. Mettlin, C., Lee, F., Drago, J. and Murphy, G. P. (1991). The American Cancer Society National Prostate Cancer Detection Project: findings on the detection of early prostate cancer in 2425 men. *Cancer*, **67**, 2949–58

23. Rommel, F. M., Augusta, V. E., Breslin, J. A., Huffnagle, H. W., Pohl, C. E., Sieber, P. R., *et al.* (1994). The use of PSA and PSAD in the diagnosis of prostate cancer in a community based urology practice. *J. Urol.*, **151**, 88–93

24. Mettlin, C., Littrup, P. J., Kane, R. A., Murphy, G. P., Lee, F., Chesley, A. *et al.* (1994). Relative sensitivity and specificity of serum PSA level compared with age-referenced PSA, PSA density and PSA change. *Cancer*, **74**, 1615–20

25. Crawford, E. D. and DeAntoni, E. P. (1993). PSA as a screening test for prostate cancer. *Urol. Clin. North Am.*, **20**, 637

26. Ellis, W. J., Chetner, M., Preston, S. and Brawer, M. K. (1994). Diagnosis of prostatic carcinoma: the yield of serum PSA, DRE and TRUS. *J. Urol.*, **152**, 1520–5

27. Brawer, M. K. (1995). How to use PSA in the early detection or screening for prostatic carcinoma. *CA Cancer J. Clin.*, **45**, 148–64

28. Benson, M. C., Whang, I. S., Pantuck, A., Ring, K., Kaplan, S. A., Olsson, C. A. *et al.* (1992). Prostate specific antigen density: a means of distinguishing benign prostatic hypertrophy and prostate cancer. *J. Urol.*, **147**, 815–16

29. Babaian, R. J., Fritsche, H. A. and Evans, R. B. (1990). PSA and prostate gland volume: correlation and clinical application. *J. Clin. Lab.*, **4**, 135–7

30. Benson, M. C., Whang, I. S., Olsson, C. A., McMahon, D. J. and Cooner, W. H. (1992). The use of prostate-specific antigen density to enhance the predictive value of intermediate levels of serum prostate-specific antigen. *J. Urol.*, **147**, 817–21

31. Seaman, E., Whang, M., Olsson, C. A., Katz, A., Cooner, W. H. and Benson, M. C. (1993). PSA density (PSAD), role in patient evaluation and management. *Urol. Clin. North Am.*, **20**, 653

32. Ohori, M., Dunn, J. K. and Scardino, P. T. (1995). Is prostate-specific antigen density more useful than prostate-specific antigen levels in the diagnosis of prostate cancer. *Urology*, **46**, 666

33. Brawer, M. K., Aramburu, E. A. G., Chen, G. L., Preston, S. D. and Ellis, W. J. (1993). The inability of PSA index to enhance the predictive value of PSA in the diagnosis of prostatic carcinoma. *J. Urol.*, **150**, 369–73

34. Carter, H., Morrell, C. H., Pearson, J. D., Brant, L. J., Plato, C. C., Metter, E. J. *et al.* (1992). Estimation of prostatic growth using serial prostate-specific antigen measurements in men with and without prostate disease. *Cancer Res.*, **52**, 3323–8

35. Smith, D. S. and Catalona, W. J. (1994). Rate of change in serum prostate specific-antigen levels as a method for prostate cancer detection. *J. Urol.*, **152**, 1163

36. Littrup, P. J., Kane, R. A., Mettlin, C. J., Murphy, G. P., Lee, F., Toi, A. *et al.* (1994). Cost-effective prostate cancer detection: reduction of low-yield biopsies. *Cancer*, **74**, 3146–58

37. Porter, J. R., Hayward, R. and Brawer, M. K. (1994). The significance of short-term PSA change in men undergoing ultrasound guided prostate biopsy. *J. Urol.*, **151** (Suppl.), 293 A

38. Carter, H. B., Pearson, J. D., Chan, D. W., Guess, H. A. and Walsh, P. C. (1995). Prostate-specific antigen variability in men without prostate cancer: effect of sampling interval on prostate-specific antigen velocity. *Urology*, **45**, 591

39. Dejter, S. W., Jr, Martin, J. S., McPherson, R. A. and Lynch, J. H. (1988). Daily variability in human serum PSA and prostatic acid phosphatase: a comparative evaluation. *Urology*, **32**, 288

40. Glenski, W. J., Klee, G. G., Bergstralh, E. J. and Oesterling, J. E. (1992). Prostate-specific antigen establishment of the reference range for the clinically normal prostate gland and the effect of digital rectal examination, ejaculation, and time on serum concentrations. *Prostate*, **21**, 99

41. Riehmann, M., Rhodes, P. R., Cook, T. D., Grose, G. S. and Bruskewitz, R. C. (1993). Analysis of variation in prostate-specific antigen values. *Urology*, **42**, 390

42. Lanz, K. J., Wener, M. H., Brawer, M. K., Strobel, S. A., Smith, K. M. and Parson, R. E. (1996). Biological variation in serum PSA level. *J. Urol.*, **155** (Suppl.), 696

43. Oesterling, J. E., Jacobsen, S. J., Chute, C. G., Guess, H. A., Girman, C. J., Panser, L. A. *et al.* (1993). Serum PSA in a community-based popu-

lation of healthy men. *J. Am. Med. Assoc.*, **270**, 860–4

44. Dalkin, B. L., Ahmann, F. R. and Kopp, J. B. (1993). PSA levels in men older than 50 years without clinical evidence of prostatic carcinoma. *J. Urol.*, **150**, 1837–9

45. El-Galley, R. E. S., Petros, J. A., Sanders, W. H., *et al.* (1995). Normal range prostate-specific antigen versus age-specific prostate-specific antigen in screening prostate adenocarcinoma. *Urology*, **46**, 200

46. Petteway, J. and Brawer, M. K. (1995). Age specific vs. 4.0 ng/ml as a PSA cutoff in the screening population: impact on cancer detection. *J. Urol.*, **153** (Suppl.), **465A**

47. Christensson, A., Laurell, C. B. and Lilja, H. (1990). Enzymatic activity of prostate-specific antigen and its reaction with extracellular serine proteinase inhibitors. *Eur. J. Biochem.*, **194**, 755

48. Lilja, H., Christensson, A., Dahlen, U., Matkainen, M. T., Nilsson, O., Pettersson, K. *et al.* (1991). PSA in human serum occurs predominantly in complex with alpha-1 antichymotrypsin. *Clin. Chem.*, **37**, 1618–25

49. Nixon, R. G. and Brawer, M. K. (1996). Refinements in serum prostate-specific antigen testing for the diagnosis of prostate cancer. In Kirby, R. and O'Leary, M. P. (eds.) *Recent Advances in Urology.* (London: Churchill Livingstone) in press

50. Stenman, U., Leinonen, J., Alfthan, H., Rannikko, S., Tuhkanen, K. and Althan, O. (1991). A complex between PSA and α_1-antichymotrypsin is the major form of PSA in serum of patients with prostatic cancer: assay of the complex improves clinical sensitivity for cancer. *Cancer Res.*, **51**, 222

51. Christensson, A., Bjork, T., Nilsson, O., Dahlen, U., Matikainen, M., Cockett, A. *et al.* (1993). Serum prostate-specific antigen complexed to alpha 1-antichymotrypsin as an indicator of prostate cancer. *J. Urol.*, **150**, 100–5

52. Petteway, J. C., Brawer, M. K. and Meyer, G. E. (1996). Comparison of two investigative assays for the free form of PSA. *J. Urol.*, **155**, 371A

53. Luderer, A. A., Chen, Y., Thiel, R., Sariano, T., Kramp, B., Carlson, G. *et al.* (1995). Measurement of the proportion of free to total PSA improves diagnostic performance of PSA in the diagnostic gray zone of total PSA. *Urology*, **46**, 187–94

54. Catalona, W. J., Smith, D. S., Wolfert, R. L., Wang, T. J., Rittenhouse, H. G., Ratliff, T. L. *et al.* (1995). Evaluation of percentage of free serum prostate-specific antigen to improve specificity of prostate cancer screening. *J. Am. Med. Assoc.*, **274**, 1214–20

55. Bangma, C. H., Kranse, R., Blijenberg, B. G. and Schroder, F. H. (1995). The value of screening tests in the detection of prostate cancer. Part I: results of a retrospective evaluation of 1726 men. *Urology*, **46**, 773–8

56. Prestigiacomo, A. F., Lilja, H., Pettersson, K., Wolfert, R. L. and Stamey, T. A. (1996). A comparison of the 'free' fraction of serum prostate specific antigen (PSA) in men with benign and cancerous prostates: the 'best case' scenario. *J. Urol.*, in press

57. Brawer, M. K., Daum, P., Petteway, J. C. and Wener, M. H. (1995). Assay variability in serum PSA determination. *Prostate*, **26**, 1–6

58. Ellis, W. J. and Brawer, M. K. (1995). Repeat prostate needle biopsy: who needs it? *J. Urol.*, **153**, 1496–8

Interactive Voting System

1 Do you use free/total PSA ratios in determining whom to biopsy?

Response	Option
15%	Yes.
81%	No.
4%	Sometimes.

Number of votes: 100

2 To reduce the number of benign biopsies I perform, I would be willing to miss:

22%	0%.
55%	5%.
19%	10%.
4%	15%.

Number of votes: 88

Utility of total serum PSA, free/total PSA ratio, age-specific reference ranges and PSA density: Rotterdam experience (ERSPC)

26

Introduction

Screening for prostate carcinoma has been performed from 1994 onwards in the Rotterdam area as part of the European Randomized Study of Screening for Prostate Carcinoma (ERSPC), to study the usefulness of early detection in the general population.

The screening protocol of the ERSPC differs in at least two important aspects from various other screening programs around the world. Firstly, the study is randomized for various reasons explained elsewhere[1]. Secondly, all participants randomized for screening undergo phlebotomy for determination of serum levels of prostate specific antigen (PSA) (Hybritech Tandem E), digital rectal examination (DRE)

and transrectal ultrasonography (TRUS). These screening tests are performed independently by a team of experienced urological residents and a specially schooled radiological laboratory technician. The screening protocol is described in Figure 1.

In screening for prostate cancer, selection of candidates for prostate biopsy is complicated by the fact that all screening modalities lack sufficient specificity. This results in a high ratio between the number of biopsies (Bx) and the number of detected carcinomas (PC). In most screening studies, about five biopsies are needed to detect one carcinoma[2-6]. This number seems to be acceptable with

Identification of men age 55–74 from the population registry
|
Informed consent
|
Randomization (screening versus control)
|
PSA + DRE + TRUS (only in screening group)
|
Biopsy (if suspicious DRE or TRUS, or PSA >4.0 ng/ml)
|
Treatment of cancer cases (radical prostatectomy, radiotherapy, endocrine therapy, watchful waiting)
|
Re-screening after 4 and 8 years, re-evaluation of suspicious cases after 1 year (if biopsy was negative)
|
Follow-up (10 years)

Figure 1 Basic protocol of the Rotterdam site of the ERSPC

207

regard to screening ethics and pragmatic considerations.

The reciprocal relationship between sensitivity and specificity is well illustrated in the distribution of PSA values among participants with and without a carcinoma of the prostate (Figure 2). From that figure the question: 'What is the best cut-off level for PSA as an indication for prostate biopsy?' is impossible to answer. As the nature of the early detected cancers is not ultimately known, and the result of their therapy can be compared only after several years to the symptomatic cancers which present in the randomized control group, the best strategy at the moment is to detect all cancers in the population, and to study their course. As all three screening modalities are applied in the ERSPC, that protocol offers relatively the best possibilities to detect as many cancers as possible, and to evaluate the screening modalities at lower serum PSA levels. Still, even that protocol results in a detection rate of 4% in the Dutch population, whereas literature studies suggest a much higher prevalence of prostate cancer found with autopsy.

In order to reduce the ratio between biopsies and detected carcinomas (Bx/PC), several additional parameters have been analyzed, such as prostate volume and age[2,5]. In these studies the main importance of reducing the Bx/PC ratio is based on cost-effectiveness, and minimizing the disturbing psychological effects of biopsies on the participants. The result of diminishing the Bx/PC ratio contributes to a certain reduction of the cancer detection rate by the reduction of the number of negative biopsies. The effect of the application of the various additional parameters has been illustrated in the literature. However, knowledge concerning the nature of those cancers lost to detection is limited, and is merely confined to grade and stage. At the moment, there are three parameters directly correlated with serum PSA level, which correct for the volume of the prostate, age and the percentage of PSA that is complexed to serum proteins. These concepts have resulted in the definition of PSA density (PSAD)[7], the age-specific reference ranges[8] and the free to total PSA ratio (F/T ratio)[9].

These three additional parameters have not yet been studied prospectively. Retrospective analysis of all three parameters simultaneously in 1726 subsequent participants was performed at the Rotterdam site of the ERSPC[10]. Optimal determination of their value would have been accomplished in a study in which all men would undergo prostate biopsy in order to evaluate the histological status of their prostates. In most screening protocols the application of TRUS volumetry is restricted to those selected for

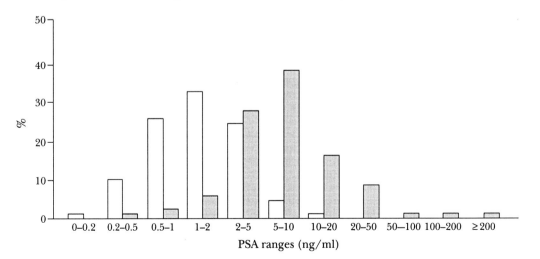

Figure 2 Distribution of detected carcinomas according to PSA range (logarithmic). Plain, no cancer; shaded, cancer

biopsy by DRE and a PSA value of 4.0 ng/ml or more. In the ERSPC, however, the PSAD, age-related reference values and F/T ratio were determined in 1726 subsequent participants regardless of PSA, DRE or diagnostic TRUS results.

As all men with a PSA value of 4.0 ng/ml or more were biopsied, two groups were created with different indications for biopsy: those men biopsied with an abnormal TRUS or DRE result and a PSA value of less than 4.0 ng/ml, and those men biopsied regardless of DRE and TRUS results with a PSA value of 4.0 ng/ml or more. This is reflected in the relative incidence of carcinomas for various PSA groups (Figure 2), due to the biopsy rate which was 8.4% in the first, and 100% in the second group. It might lead to the idea that the prevalence of carcinomas below a PSA value of 4.0 ng/ml is low and hopefully unimportant, and that only palpable carcinomas might be of interest due to their size. To be detected, initially smaller tumors have to appear by rescreening due to a rise in PSA level, or palpability. However, in the ERSPC study, it has been observed that cancers removed in men with a PSA level of 4.0 ng/ml or less may be clinically important with regard to their pathological stage and grade (J. B. W. Rietbergen, this symposium). It is clear that the results of analysis of the three PSA-correcting parameters has to be different between both groups, as the methods of detection and therefore most probably the nature of the detected tumors is different. Still, the main interest of the scientific community lies in the study of the 'gray' area of the PSA range between 4.0 and 10.0 ng/ml, where PSA values of benign and malignant participants overlap most.

In the study group of 1726 participants, 308 men underwent prostate biopsies. By means of backwards deletion logistic regression analysis, the information given by total serum PSA, free PSA, DRE, TRUS, total prostate volume, volume of the prostatic inner zone and age was used to find a predictor that specifies the chance of a positive biopsy result as a function of the variables most relevant to this end. All variables with insignificant Wald statistics were deleted[11]. Table 1 shows the result of the first step of this procedure, in which the serum PSA and DRE results were the most important predictors, followed by free PSA and inner zone volume. Age and TRUS appeared to be insignificant[12].

To determine the value of PSAD, age-specific reference ranges and the F/T ratio, a simulated case selection for biopsy was performed. For PSAD a cut-off value of 0.12^2 was used (step-section planimetric volumetry); for the F/T ratio a cut-off value of 0.20 was used (ProStatus F/T, Wallac); age-specific reference ranges were calculated from this population[12]. The results of the simulation study are illustrated in Table 2. Also, the distribution of organ-confined (pathological stage T2 or less) and extended carcinomas (pathological stage T3 and more) according to the histological results of 38 out of 67 men, who underwent radical prostatectomy and

Table 1 Results of logistic regression analysis of independent parameters for predicting a positive biopsy in 308 men, prostate specific antigen (PSA) range 0–200 ng/ml

Variable	B	SE	Wald	Significance
Log PSA	5.84	0.98	35.12	0.00
Log Free PSA	−2.32	1.15	4.03	0.04
DRE	−0.93	0.24	14.97	0.00
Volume (Total)	−0.01	0.01	0.58	0.44
Volume (Inner)	−0.03	0.02	3.71	0.05
Age	0.04	0.04	1.06	0.30
TRUS	−0.18	0.22	0.63	0.42

B, predictor for a positive biopsy; SE, standard error of the predictor; Wald, statistic = square of the ratio of the predictor to its standard error; Significance, significance of Wald statistic, threshold 0.05; DRE, digital rectal examination; TRUS, transrectal ultrasonography

Table 2 Simulated case selection for biopsy of 1726 men by various combinations of parameters, and distribution of organ-confined and extended carcinomas of the subgroup after radical prostatectomy

Biopsy (Bx) indication	Number (Bx/PC)	Reduction in Bx		PC missed		Bx/PC	Number con/ext
		%	SE	%	SE		
PSA ≥ 4, or DRE, or TRUS	308/67					4.6	22/16
PSA ≥ 4, or DRE	255/65	17	2.1	2	2.1	3.9	20/16
PSAD, or DRE	212/60	28	2.4	11	3.8	3.6	19/16
PSA–age, or DRE	195/59	37	2.8	12	4.0	3.3	19/14
PSA ≥ 4 and PSAD, or DRE	188/60	39	2.8	11	3.8	3.2	17/16
PSA ≥ 4 and F/T, or DRE	196/60	37	2.8	11	3.8	3.3	17/16

PC, prostate carcinoma; PSA ≥ 4, PSA level is 4.0 ng/ml or more; PSA–age, total serum PSA larger than age-specific reference range; PSAD, PSA density 0.12 ng/ml/cm^3 or more; F/T, free/total PSA ratio of 0.20 or less; DRE, abnormal DRE result; TRUS, ultrasonic lesion detected by TRUS; con/ext, number of organ-confined and extended PC after radical prostatectomy; SE, standard error; Bx/PC, ratio between number of biopsies and detected prostate cancer cancers

were selected/detected by the combination of parameters, is given.

It can be seen that the combination of an abnormal DRE and a F/T ratio of 0.20 or less in the PSA range above 4.0 ng/ml selects participants for biopsy with a high sensitivity combined with a low Bx/PC ratio (this is a high specificity). The combination of DRE and PSAD in the intermediate PSA range detects statistically as many cancers as the combination of F/T ratio with DRE, but application of the F/T ratio has the advantage that its determination is reproducible, and easy to perform in the same serum sample as is used for the total PSA assay. The equimolar ProStatus F/T assay combines the determination of total serum PSA level and the F/T ratio automatically. All cancers lost for detection by application of these regimes appeared to be confined to the prostate (five out of 22 pathological confined cancers). In contrast, selection by age-specific reference ranges would even have missed some extended carcinomas. It has to be shown in due time whether it is likely that the 'undetected' confined cancers would have been detected in a following screening round. The nature of these cancers is at present under investigation: their tumor volumes and grade distribution are being determined by histological step-section.

In the simulation study, a F/T ratio cut-off value of 0.20 was used according to earlier population-derived data[12]. Other cut-off values would have induced different values of sensitivity and specificity. To compare the F/T ratio for any value of cut-off to the most important predictors (PSA and DRE), receiver operating characteristic (ROC) curves were constructed, in which each point of the curve fits a combination of sensitivity with its specificity[13]. ROC curves illustrate the characteristics of a test (or combination of tests), and the discriminatory potential of various tests can be compared by their area under the curve.

For the intermediate PSA range between 4.0 and 10.0 ng/ml a separate study was recently completed. Out of 991 men from the Rotterdam site of the ERSCP who all underwent sextant biopsies as indicated by the protocol, 441 men were assessed within the PSA range between 4.0 and 10.0 ng/ml, according to the ProStatus F/T assay. This assay is correlated well with the Hybritech Tandem-E assay, which is used in the ERSCP study (correlation coefficient $r = 1.0$; ProStatus = 1.06; Tandem E -0.45[12]. Figure 3 shows the ROC curves for PSA, the combination of PSA and DRE, and that of the F/T ratio. It can be appreciated that both the last are significantly better predictors of a positive biopsy than PSA alone. The difference between both combinations is not significant (defined by a difference in the area under the curve of at least two standard errors).

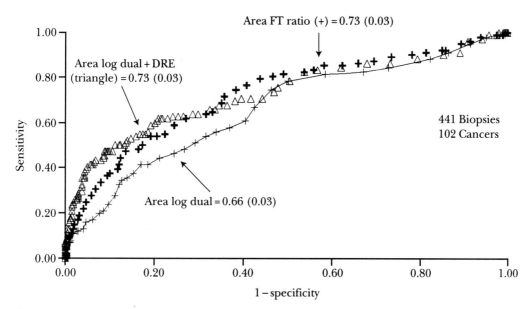

Figure 3 The relative effectiveness of diagnostics illustrated in ROC curves of 441 men in the PSA range between 4.0 and 10.0 ng/ml (standard error of the areas = 0.03); dual = total PSA

In conclusion, selected application of the F/T ratio in the intermediate PSA range appears to be an intriguing parameter to reduce the number of biopsies in a screening population. In the Rotterdam site of the ERSPC 8% of the participants had a PSA value in the intermediate range, in which the application of a F/T ratio of less than 0.20 as an indicator for biopsy would induce a reduction of 37% of biopsies, and a loss of locally confined cancers of 11% in the whole screening population. This percentage of undetected cancers, however, seems to be considerable.

Acknowledgements

These studies have been supported by grants from 'Europe against Cancer', the Dutch Cancer Society (KWF), and the Prevention Fund of the Netherlands, as well as by an educational grant of Wallac Oy, Finland.

References

1. Schröder, F. H. and Boyle, P. (1993). Screening for prostate cancer – necessity or nonsense. *Eur. J. Cancer*, **29A**, 656–61
2. Mettlin, C., Lee, F., Drago, J. and Murphy, G. P. (1991). The American Cancer Society National Prostate Cancer Detection Project, findings on the detection of early prostate cancer in 2425 men. *Cancer*, **67**, 2949–58
3. Brawer, M. K., Chetner, M. P., Beatie, J., Buchner, D. M., Vesella, R. L. and Lange, P. H. (1992). Screening for prostatic carcinoma with prostate specific antigen. *J. Urol.*, **147**, 841–5
4. Labrie, F., Dupont, A., Suburu, R., Cusan, L., Tremblay, M., Gomez, J.-L. and Emond, J. (1992). Serum prostate specific antigen as pre-screening test for prostate cancer. *J. Urol.*, **147**, 846–52
5. Catalona, W. J., Richie, J. P., Ahmann, F. R., Hudson, M. A., Scardino, P. T., Flanigan, R. C., deKernion, J. B., Ratliff, T. L., Kavoussi, L. R.,

Dalkin, B. L., Waters, W. B., MacFarlane, M. T. and Southwick, P. C. (1994). Comparison of digital rectal examination and serum prostate specific antigen in early detection of prostate cancer: results of multicenter clinical trial of 6630 men. *J. Urol.*, **151**, 1283–90

6. Schröder, F. H., Denis, L. J., Kirkels, W., De Koning, H. J. and Standaert, B. (1995). European randomized study of screening for prostate cancer, progress report of Antwerp and Rotterdam pilot studies. *Cancer*, **76**, 129–34

7. Benson, M. C., Whang, I. S., Pantuck, A., Ring, K., Kaplan, S. A., Olsson, C. A. and Cooner, W. H. (1992). The use of prostate specific antigen density to enhance the predictive value of intermediate levels of serum prostate specific antigen. *J. Urol.*, **147**, 817–21

8. Oesterling, J. E., Jacobsen, S. J. and Cooner, W. H. (1995). Use of age-specific reference ranges for serum prostate specific antigen in men 60 years old or older. *J. Urol.*, **153**, 1160–3

9. Stenman, U., Leinonen, J., Alfthan, H., Rannikko, S., Tuhkanen, K. and Alfthan, O. (1991). A complex between prostate-specific antigen and alpha 1-antichymotrypsin is the major form of prostate-specific antigen in serum of patients with prostatic cancer: assay of the complex improves clinical sensitivity for cancer. *Cancer Res.*, **51**, 222–6

10. Bangma, C. H., Kranse, R., Blijenberg, B. G. and Schröder, F. H. (1995). The value of screening tests in the detection of prostate cancer. 2. A simulation of the role of the F/T ratio, age specific reference ranges, and PSA density. *Urology*, **46**, 779–84

11. Norusis, M. J. (1990). *SPSS/PC+ Advanced Statistics 4.0*, (Chicago: SPSS)

12. Bangma, C. H., Kranse, R., Blijenberg, B. G. and Schröder, F. H. (1995). The value of screening tests in the detection of prostate cancer. 1. Results of a retrospective evaluation of 1726 men. *Urology*, **46**, 773–8

Interactive Voting System

1   Do you consider the F/T ratio suitable as a screening parameter for all screening participants?

Response	*Option*
25%	Yes.
75%	No.

Number of votes: 72

2   What would you say to screening of your own prostate?

38%	Yes.
23%	No.
39%	Cheese.

Number of votes: 76

3   What would be your favorite screening modality?

21%	PSA total.
5%	DRE.
33%	F/T ratio.
39%	PSA total.
2%	PSAD.

Number of votes: 82

4.   Screening for prostate cancer:

11%	Should be recommended to all elderly men.
17%	Should not be used in asymptomatic men.
72%	Should be evaluated in a randomized study.

Number of votes: 29

7

Management of Locally Confined Prostate Cancer

Can progression of prostate cancer be predicted by pre-treatment parameters?

27

H. B. Carter and A. W. Partin

After the diagnosis of adenocarcinoma of the prostate has been histologically confirmed, an accurate assessment of the stage – or extent – of the disease is necessary for a rational recommendation of therapy. The extent of disease correlates directly with prognosis in men with newly diagnosed prostate cancer. Treatment directed at eradication of the primary tumor is not likely to affect prognosis when the disease is no longer confined, because adjuvant therapy capable of eradicating extra-prostatic disease is unavailable. Thus, an assessment of disease extent – or progression – is a pivotal step when counselling the patient with newly diagnosed prostate cancer regarding the options of curative vs. palliative treatment. Studies evaluating the pathological extent of prostate cancer after removal of the prostate suggest that the use of clinical stage, tumor grade and prostate specific antigen (PSA) level – when used in combination – optimize the pre-treatment prediction of progression.

In the PSA era, the majority of prostate cancers detected are clinically localized (T_1–T_2) to the prostate gland. Catalona and colleagues[1] found that, with serial PSA screening, 97% of detected cancers were clinically localized to the prostate, and that of these 83% had PSA levels of 4–10 ng/ml. Thus, in comparison to the pre-PSA era when most cancers were detected at an advanced stage of disease by digital rectal examination (DRE)[2–4], the addition of routine PSA testing has resulted in the detection of prostate cancer earlier in the natural course of the disease. For these men, pre-treatment determination of progression provides valuable information regarding the probability of success of curative treatment. Table 1 lists some of the

Table 1 Pre-treatment parameters for prediction of progression

Digital rectal examination (T stage)
Prostate biopsy
  tumor grade
  tumor volume
  seminal vesicle involvement
  perineural invasion
Tumor markers
  prostate specific antigen
  prostatic acid phosphatase
Imaging
  transrectal ultrasound
  computed tomography/magnetic resonance
   imaging

pre-treatment parameters of importance with respect to prediction of progression in men with prostate cancer. In this article, the pre-treatment parameters that are readily available to the practicing urologist are discussed.

Local extent of disease (T stage)

Determination of the local extent of disease – primarily by DRE – is referred to as the T stage. Table 2 provides a comparison between clinical and pathological stages from radical prostatectomy series[5–9]. Because DRE is subjective, both understaging and overstaging are found when the pathological extent of disease is correlated with pre-treatment DRE findings.

Earlier studies involving small groups of men, in whom extraprostatic disease spread had been expected by DRE – and who subsequently underwent radical prostatectomy – confirmed the clinical impression in only 25% of the cases[10,11]. Histological evaluation of surgical specimens after radical prostatectomy for presumed organ-confined disease demonstrates a significant degree of understaging by DRE[12].

Determination of the sensitivity and specificity of DRE in determining the organ-confined status was evaluated in a large series[7] in which all DREs and radical prostatectomies were performed by one urologist, with pathological evaluations completed by a single pathologist. Within this series of 565 men, in whom the DRE suggested organ-confined disease (T_2), 52% actually had organ-confined disease, 31% had capsular penetration and the remaining 17% exhibited either seminal vesicle or lymph node involvement. Within the same series, of the 36 men in whom extraprostatic disease was suspected by DRE (T_{3A}), 19% were organ-confined, 36% had capsular penetration and 45% had involvement of either the seminal vesicles or the lymph nodes. This represents a sensitivity of 52% and a specificity of 81% for prediction of organ-confined disease by DRE alone. Thus, DRE is a more reliable predictor of progression when the findings on DRE suggest the presence of advanced disease. DRE alone is an unreliable method of predicting progression when the findings on DRE suggest localized prostate cancer.

Prostate biopsy data

Gleason histological grade

The most commonly used histological grading system for prostate cancer is the Gleason system[13,14], which has been shown to correlate directly with the pathological extent of disease. Table 3 shows the distribution of Gleason scores determined on pre-treatment prostate biopsy, as a function of final pathological stage for 703 men who underwent surgery for clinically localized prostate cancer[7]. The importance of histological grading is supported by multi-variate analyses[6,7,15–20] of prognostic criteria for men with clinically localized disease that demonstrates Gleason sum (or grade) as a strong predictor of disease extent. Epstein and colleagues[6,15,16,19,20] have suggested that all new prognostic indicators should be compared with

Table 2 Comparison of clinical and pathological stages in radical prostatectomy series. Data from references 5–9

Clinical stage	Patients (n)	Pathological stage: organ confined	
		n	%
T_{1A}	93	88	94
T_{1B}	288	196	68
T_{1C}	299	161	54
T_2	3837	1779	46
T_{3A}	36	7	19

Table 3 Distribution of Gleason score by pathological stage in 703 men with clinically localized prostate cancer. Adapted from reference 7

Gleason score	Patients		Organ-confined disease		Established capsular penetration		Positive seminal vesicles		Positive lymph nodes*	
	n	%	n	%	n	%	n	%	n	%
2–4	64	9	49	77	12	19	2	3	1	1
5	168	24	116	69	43	26	3	2	6	4
6	303	43	173	57	89	30	16	5	25	8
7	130	19	39	30	50	38	15	12	26	20
8–10	38	5	5	13	9	24	8	21	16	42
Total	703	100	382	54	203	29	44	6	74	11

*Includes patients who did not undergo radical retropubic prostatectomy because of positive lymph nodes at pelvic lymph node dissection

the Gleason sum (grade), and provide statistically independent predictive information before being considered to be clinically useful.

Volume of cancer

The volume of cancer present within the prostate, as determined by step-sectioning of a radical prostatectomy specimen, has been shown to correlate with disease extent and progression. McNeal and co-workers[21] found that when the tumor volume exceeded 12.0 cm^3, locally advanced or metastatic disease was almost always present; whereas when the tumor volume was less than 4.0 cm^3, the tumor was almost always confined and associated with a good prognosis. Therefore, accurate pre-treatment knowledge of tumor volume would be desirable information that could help in predicting the probability of treatment success. Numerous studies have evaluated needle biopsy criteria as a predictor of prostate cancer volume to aid in prediction of tumor extent[22-24]. The various needle biopsy criteria evaluated include the percentage of cancer present, percentage of biopsy cores involved with cancer, length of cancer (millimeters) within the biopsy, and number of biopsy cores involved with cancer. Direct correlations exist between the amount of cancer present in the needle biopsy and the actual volume of prostate cancer present in the operative specimen. However, there is great variation between the biopsy findings and the actual volume of cancer present. Cupp and associates[22] found that, for 46 men with stage T$_{1C}$ disease and 84 men with stage T$_2$ disease, the volume of cancer for a given percentage of cancer in the biopsy specimen had significant variability (standard error 6.1 cm^3). Therefore, the prediction of cancer volume and disease progression would appear to be limited when based on the amount of cancer within the pre-treatment needle biopsy.

Seminal vesicle biopsy

The finding of seminal vesicle invasion on pathological evaluation after radical prostatec-tomy is associated with a low probability of total eradication of tumor, and a high probability of distant failure[12,17,25]. Pre-treatment biopsy of the seminal vesicles has been recommended by some investigators as a means to improve staging before recommending treatment options[26-28]. Terris and colleagues[26] suggested the use of pre-treatment seminal vesicle biopsies in selected individuals based on the results of DRE, transrectal ultrasound and serum PSA measurement. Among 67 men who underwent radical prostatectomy for clinically localized prostate cancer, Vallancien and co-workers[27] found that seminal vesicle biopsy detected 61% of those men with seminal vesicle invasion with no false-positive biopsies. They recommended seminal vesicle biopsy in all men with localized prostate cancer and a PSA level of more than 10.0 ng/ml – since no men with a PSA level of less than 10.0 ng/ml had positive seminal vesicle biopsies. Stone and colleagues[28] found that clinical stage, tumor grade and PSA level correlated directly with the probability of seminal vesicle invasion. They recommended seminal vesicle biopsy for all men with a Gleason score of more than 4, PSA level of more than 10.0 ng/ml, or a clinical stage of T$_{2B}$ or greater. Given the presence of these criteria, the probability of seminal vesicle invasion was around 20%. However, with selection of those men who are most likely to benefit from a curative approach, contemporary radical prostatectomy series demonstrate a prevalence of seminal vesicle invasion of less than 10% without routine seminal vesicle biopsy[5,17]. Seminal vesicle biopsy, to rule out progression before treatment, is most likely to be beneficial if men with bulky, higher grade tumors are considered to be candidates for radical prostatectomy. In this setting, pre-treatment seminal vesicle biopsy may provide additional information that would be helpful in recommending the most appropriate treatment option.

Perineural invasion

Branches of the neurovascular bundle enter the prostate on the posterolateral surface. Prostatic cancer most frequently penetrates the capsule of the prostate through perineural space invasion[29]. This accounts for the finding that in non-transition zone cancers, capsular penetration occurs posterolaterally in 50% of cases[30]. Bastacky and co-workers[31], evaluated the finding of perineural invasion on needle biopsy as a predictor of capsular penetration among 302 men with stage T_2 prostate cancer who underwent radical prostatectomy. Perineural invasion was seen in 20% of pre-treatment needle biopsies. As a marker of capsular penetration, perineural invasion had a sensitivity of 27% and a specificity of 96%. Therefore, the absence of perineural invasion on pre-treatment biopsy does not exclude the presence of capsular penetration. However, the finding of perineural invasion on pre-treatment biopsy is associated with the finding of capsular penetration after removal of the prostate in over 90% of cases. This finding on pre-treatment biopsy provides useful information in guiding the surgeon with respect to the necessity for wider excision to prevent positive margins.

Serum tumor markers

Two prostatic tumor markers – serum prostatic acid phosphatase (PAP) and serum prostate specific antigen (PSA) – have been used as indicators of disease extent in prostate cancer. The lower sensitivity of PAP compared to PSA in the prediction of advanced disease, and the close correlation between PSA and extent of disease, has led some experts to question the need for measurement of PAP in men with newly diagnosed prostate cancer.

Prostatic acid phosphatase

Prior to the availability of PSA, PAP was the most often utilized serum marker for the staging of prostate cancer. The isoenzymes detected by assays that measure PAP are not found exclusively in the prostate. Therefore, although PAP activity is 1000-fold greater in the prostate than in any other tissue, PAP is not prostate-specific,

because detectable levels are noted even after removal of all prostate tissue.

In terms of prostate cancer staging, PAP elevations are directly related to the extent (stage) of disease[32]. Radioimmunoassays (RIA) for measurement of PAP are more sensitive, but less specific, than enzymatic assays as a marker of advanced disease. The enzymatic assay using thymolphthalein monophosphate as a substrate for hydrolysis of PAP (Roy enzymatic assay) is a specific assay for the presence of advanced disease in the absence of other diseases that cause acid phosphatase elevations. Numerous studies have documented the close relationship between advanced disease and enzymatic elevations of PAP[33–35]. Abnormal PAP values (Roy enzymatic assay) and values in the upper half of the normal range suggest a high likelihood (> 80%) of extraprostatic disease[34,35]. However, a normal enzymatic PAP level is not highly predictive for the absence of extraprostatic disease.

In the PSA era, use of PAP in staging has a limited role, due to the closer relationship between PSA and disease extent[36]. PAP rarely adds additional information in those men who are considered to have clinically localized prostate cancer based on the results of DRE, PSA and Gleason grade[37].

Prostate specific antigen

Numerous studies have shown that for groups of men with prostate cancer, the serum PSA level correlates directly with advancing clinical and pathological stage[7,36,38,39]. However, in most cases, the PSA level alone does not provide accurate staging information for the individual patient, because of overlap in PSA levels between stages. PSA is directly related to the volume of cancer present[36], but other variables influence the overall PSA level. The preoperative interpretation of serum PSA level as it relates to tumor extent is confounded by both the volume of benign prostatic hyperplasia (BPH) tissue present and the tumor grade; both of which influence serum PSA levels in men with prostatic cancer[40].

The contribution of BPH to overall serum PSA level has been estimated to be 0.3 ng/ml per gram of BPH tissue[36] with the use of the Yang Pros-Check polyclonal immunoassay (Bellevue, WA). The Yang polyclonal (Bellevue, WA) and Tandem monoclonal assays (Hybritech, San Diego, CA) are not equivalent, but in general the Yang assay gives values 1.4 to 1.9 times higher than the Tandem assay[41]. This conversion would yield an estimated 0.15 ng/ml of PSA per gram of BPH tissue with the use of the monoclonal assay – the PSA density cut-off level that is most often used to distinguish between BPH and cancer. An accurate assessment of the BPH contribution to the overall serum PSA level is not possible for a given individual, because (1) the epithelial component of BPH is the source of PSA; (2) there is a variable amount of epithelium and stroma within BPH tissue; and (3) no non-invasive methods are available for distinguishing between epithelium and stroma within BPH tissue.

Partin and co-workers[40] have shown that men with disease of a more advanced stage have tumors of higher grade and higher volume, and that produce less PSA per gram of tumor. The heterogeneity of prostate cancer with respect to tumor grade prevents an accurate assessment of the affect of grade on overall serum PSA level before treatment.

The confounding variables of BPH and tumor grade result in the overlap of serum PSA levels between stages, which hinders the prediction of final pathological stage with the use of PSA alone for most patients. As general guidelines, the majority of men (70–80%) with PSA values of < 4.0 ng/ml have pathologically organ-confined disease; more than 50% of men with PSA levels of > 10 ng/ml already have established capsular penetration; most men (75%) with serum PSA levels of > 50 ng/ml have positive pelvic lymph nodes[7,40]. However, approximately 60% of men with clinically localized prostate cancer have serum PSA levels between 4.0 and 50.0 ng/ml[40]; this is a large group of men for whom PSA is of limited use for preoperative staging when used alone. Table 4 shows the relationship between serum PSA level and pathological stage in a recently published radical prostatectomy series[7].

PSA density

One method of accounting for the BPH contribution to PSA is to adjust the PSA level for the ultrasound-determined prostate volume (PSA density or PSAD). Seaman and colleagues[42] studied the role of PSAD in predicting the probability of total eradication of tumor with radical prostatectomy. In 107 men with clinically localized prostate cancer, they defined success after radical prostatectomy as local excision of all tumor with negative margins, seminal vesicles and lymph nodes, and an undetectable PSA level. Men with a PSAD of 0.35 or lower had a 90% chance of success, whereas men with a PSAD of 0.35 or greater had a 66% chance of failure. Thus, PSAD correlates with tumor extent and in the study by Seaman and associates[42] was more predictive of surgical success than was the Gleason score used alone. However, no single value of PSAD, when used alone, can be used to identify those men who will or will not benefit from a curative treatment approach. PSAD was not an independent predictor of response for prostate cancer treated by conformal radiotherapy[43].

Table 4 Pathological stage as a function of preoperative prostate specific antigen (PSA) level. Data from reference 7

PSA level (ng/ml)	Patients (n)	Organ-confined disease		Non-organ-confined disease	
		n	%	n	%
0.0–4.0	284	211	75	73	25
4.0–10.0	246	131	53	115	47
> 10.0	173	50	28	123	72

Radiographic imaging

Radiographic imaging rarely adds additional information regarding the local extent of disease over that gained with DRE. Transrectal ultrasound (TRUS) is an insensitive method for detecting local extension of tumor that is not suspected by DRE[44]. Pelvic imaging with computed tomography (CT) or magnetic resonance imaging (MRI) for detection of local extension of disease or the presence of lymph node metastases, is not routinely useful, because of low sensitivity[44–46]. Pelvic imaging for lymph node assessment may be warranted in men at higher risk of metastases when suspected by locally advanced disease on DRE, marked PSA elevations (> 20 ng/ml) or the presence of poorly differentiated cancer on needle biopsy. Wolf and colleagues[46] suggested on the basis of decision analysis that the probability of lymph node metastases would need to be > 30% for pelvic imaging to be cost effective. Individuals at high risk for pelvic lymph node disease can be identified by means of probability tables (see below). The majority of men found to have prostate cancer with PSA testing and DRE, excluding those with poorly differentiated tumors, will not benefit from pelvic imaging.

Combined use of clinical data to predict progression of prostate cancer

When used alone, the prognostic value of any clinical criteria used to predict tumor extent is

Table 5 Multivariate logistic regression analysis for prediction of pathological stage with organ-confined disease by means of prostate specific antigen (PSA) level, Gleason score and clinical stage (TNM). Adapted from reference 51

Gleason score	Clinical stage						
	T_{1A}	T_{1B}	T_{1C}	T_{2A}	T_{2B}	T_{2C}	T_{3A}
PSA level 0.0–4.0 ng/ml							
2–4	100	85	92	88	76	82	—
5	100	78	81	81	67	73	—
6	100	68	69	72	54	60	42
7	—	54	55	61	41	46	—
8–10	—	—	—	48	31	—	—
PSA level 4.1–10.0 ng/ml							
2–4	100	78	82	83	67	71	—
5	100	70	71	73	56	64	43
6	100	53	59	62	44	48	33
7	100	39	43	51	32	37	26
8–10	—	32	31	39	22	25	12
PSA level 10.1–20.0 ng/ml							
2–4	100	—	—	61	52	—	—
5	100	49	55	58	43	37	26
6	—	36	41	44	28	37	19
7	—	24	24	36	19	24	14
8–10	—	11	—	29	14	15	9
PSA level > 20 ng/ml							
2–4	—	—	33	20	7	—	—
5	—	—	24	32	—	3	—
6	—	—	22	14	1	4	5
7	—	—	7	18	4	5	3
8–10	—	—	3	3	—	2	2

limited for the individual patient with prostate cancer. The staging accuracy for prostate cancer can be significantly enhanced by combining the parameters of local disease extent (T stage), serum PSA level and Gleason grade from the prostate biopsy specimen[7,47-50]. Probability tables, based on the parameters of preoperative clinical stage, serum PSA level and Gleason sum, have been constructed from the values of large numbers of men who have undergone radical prostatectomy with precise determination of the pathological stage. In Tables 5 and 6, numbers within the nomogram represent the percentage probability of having a given final pathological stage based on logistic regression analyses for all three variables combined; dashes represent data categories in which insufficient data existed to calculate a probability. This information is useful in counselling men with newly diagnosed prostate cancer with respect to treatment alternatives and probability of complete eradication of tumor. As examples, a man with a serum PSA level of 3.0 ng/ml who has a clinical stage T_{2A} cancer with a Gleason score of 5 has an 81% chance of having organ-confined disease; whereas a man with a serum PSA level of 15 ng/ml who has a clinical stage T_{1C} cancer and a Gleason score of 7 would only have a 24% chance of having organ-confined disease.

Summary

A number of clinical parameters are available to the clinician for the prediction of prostate

Table 6 Multivariate logistic regression analysis for prediction of pathological stage with lymph node status by means of prostate specific antigen (PSA) level, Gleason score and clinical stage (TNM). Adapted from reference 51

Gleason score	Clinical stage						
	T_{1A}	T_{1B}	T_{1C}	T_{2A}	T_{2B}	T_{2C}	T_{3A}
PSA level 0.0–4.0 ng/ml							
2–4	0	2	< 1	1	2	4	—
5	0	4	1	2	4	8	—
6	0	8	2	3	9	17	15
7	—	15	2	7	18	31	—
8–10	—	—	—	13	32	—	—
PSA level 4.1–10.0 ng/ml							
2–4	0	2	1	1	2	5	—
5	0	4	1	2	5	10	8
6	0	9	2	4	11	19	16
7	0	18	3	8	20	34	28
8–10	—	30	5	15	35	53	50
PSA level 10.1–20.0 ng/ml							
2–4	0	—	—	1	3	—	—
5	0	5	3	2	6	13	11
6	—	11	4	5	13	22	20
7	—	21	7	9	24	39	35
8–10	—	41	—	17	40	59	54
PSA level > 20 ng/ml							
2–4	—	—	6	2	7	—	—
5	—	—	9	3	—	29	—
6	—	—	8	9	18	53	31
7	—	—	24	11	44	62	55
8–10	—	—	41	35	76	73	65

cancer progression. No single parameter when used alone provides accurate information regarding the probability of progression. One approach to improve prediction of the extent of prostate cancer in a man with clinically localized disease is to combine the readily available parameters of local disease extent (T stage) determined by DRE, Gleason histological score from pre-treatment prostate biopsy and

pre-treatment serum PSA level prior to biopsy. This approach allows one to estimate the probability of disease progression and to help patients choose the most reasonable treatment option. In the future, more accurate molecular markers may be available that will help avoid unnecessary treatment for those men who will not benefit from attempts at local eradication of a tumor.

References

1. Catalona, W. J., Smith, D. S., Ratliff, T. L. and Basler, J. W. (1993). Detection of organ-confined prostate cancer is increased through prostate-specific antigen based screening. *J. Am. Med. Assoc.*, **270**, 948–54

2. Thompson, I. M., Rounder, J. B., Teague, J. L., Peek, M. and Spence, C. R. (1987). Impact of routine screening for adenocarcinoma of the prostate on stage distribution. *J. Urol.*, **137**, 424–6

3. Mueller, E. J., Crain, T. W., Thompson, I. A. and Rodriguez, F. R. (1988). An evaluation of serial digital rectal examinations in screening for prostate cancer. *J. Urol.*, **140**, 1445–7

4. Chodak, G. W., Keller, P. and Schoenberg, H. W. (1989). Assessment of screening for prostate cancer using the digital rectal examination. *J. Urol.*, **141**, 1136–8

5. Catalona, W. J. and Bigg, S. W. (1990). Nerve-sparing radical prostatectomy: evaluation of results after 250 patients. *J. Urol.*, **143**, 538–44

6. Epstein, J. I., Walsh, P. C. and Brendler, C. B. (1994). Radical prostatectomy for impalpable prostate cancer: the Johns Hopkins experience with tumors found on transurethral resection (Stages T$_{1a}$ and T$_{1b}$) and on needle biopsy (Stage T$_{1c}$). *J. Urol.*, **152**, 1721–9

7. Partin, A. W., Yoo, J. K., Carter, H. B., Pearson, J. D., Chan, D. W., Epstein, J. I. and Walsh, P. C. (1993). The use of prostate-specific antigen, clinical stage and Gleason score to predict pathological stage in men with localized prostate cancer. *J. Urol.*, **150**, 110–14

8. Paulson, D. F. (1994). Impact of radical prostatectomy in the management of clinically localized disease. *J. Urol.*, **152**, 1826–30

9. Zincke, H., Oesterling, J. E., Blute, M. L., Bergstralh, E. J., Myers, R. P. and Barrett, D. M. (1994). Long-term (15 years) results after radical prostatectomy for clinically localized (stage T$_{2c}$ or lower) prostate cancer. *J. Urol.*, **152**, 1850–7

10. Turner, R. D. and Belt, E. A. (1957). A study of 229 consecutive cases of total perineal prostatectomy for cancer of the prostate. *J. Urol.*, **77**, 62–77

11. Byar, D. P., Mostofi, F. K. and the Veterans Administration Cooperative Urological Research Group (1972). Carcinoma of the prostate: prognostic evaluation of certain pathological features in 208 radical prostatectomies examined by step-section technique. *Cancer*, **30**, 5–13

12. Walsh, P. C. and Jewett, H. J. (1980). Radical surgery for prostatic cancer. *Cancer* (Suppl.), **45**, 1906–11

13. Gleason, D. F. (1966). Classification of prostatic carcinoma. *Cancer Chemother. Rep.*, **50**, 125–8

14. Gleason, D. F. and the VACURG (1977). Histological grading and clinical staging of prostatic carcinoma. In Tannenbaum, M. (ed.) *Urologic Pathology: The Prostate*, pp. 171–97. (Philadelphia: Lea and Febiger)

15. Epstein, J. I., Pizov, G. and Walsh, P. C. (1993). Correlation of pathologic findings with progression after radical retropubic prostatectomy. *Cancer*, **71**, 3582–93

16. Epstein, J. I., CarMichael, M. J., Pizov, G. and Walsh, P. C. (1993). Influence of capsular penetration on progression following radical prostatectomy: a study of 196 cases with long-term follow-up. *J. Urol.*, **150**, 135–41

17. Partin, A. W., Pound, C. R., Clemens, J. Q., Epstein, J. I. and Walsh, P. C. (1993). Prostate-specific antigen after anatomic radical prostatectomy: the Johns Hopkins experience after ten years. *Urol. Clin. North Am.*, **20**, 713–25

18. Partin, A. W., Piantadosi, S., Sanda, M. G., Epstein, J. I., Marshall, F. F., Mohler, J. L., Brendler, C. B., Walsh, P. C. and Simons, J. W. (1995). Selection of men at high risk for disease recurrence for experimental adjuvant therapy

following radical prostatectomy. *Urology*, **45**, 831–8

19. Epstein, J. I., Walsh, P. C., CarMichael, M. and Brendler, C. B. (1994). Pathologic and clinical findings to predict tumor extent of non-palpable (stage T_{1c}) prostate cancer. *J. Am. Med. Assoc.*, **271**, 368–74

20. Epstein, J. I., CarMichael, M. and Partin, A. W. (1995). OA-519 (fatty acid synthase) as an independent predictor of pathologic stage in adenocarcinoma of the prostate. *Urology*, **45**, 81–6

21. McNeal, J. E., Villers, A., Redwine, E. A., Freiha, F. S. and Stamey, T. A. (1990). Capsular penetration in prostate cancer: significance for natural history and treatment. *Am. J. Surg. Pathol.*, **14**, 240–7

22. Cupp, M. R., Bostwick, D. G., Myers, R. P. and Oesterling, J. E. (1995). Volume of prostate cancer in biopsy specimen cannot reliably predict quantity of cancer in radical prostatectomy specimen on individual basis. *J. Urol.*, **153**, 1543–8

23. Dietrick, D. D., McNeal, J. E. and Stamey, T. A. (1995). Core cancer length in ultrasound-guided systematic sextant biopsies: a preoperative evaluation of prostate cancer volume. *Urology*, **45**, 987–92

24. Loch, T., McNeal, J. E. and Stamey, T. A. (1995). Interpretation of bilateral positive biopsies in prostate cancer. *J. Urol.*, **154**, 1078–83

25. Catalona, W. J. and Smith, D. J. (1994). Five-year tumor recurrence rates after anatomic radical retropubic prostatectomy for prostate cancer. *J. Urol.*, **152**, 1837–42

26. Terris, M. K., McNeal, J. E., Freiha, F. S. and Stamey, T. A. (1993). Efficacy of transrectal ultrasound-guided seminal vesicle biopsies in the detection of seminal vesicle invasion by prostate cancer. *J. Urol.*, **149**, 1035–9

27. Vallancien, G., Bochereau, G., Wetzel, O., Bretheau, D., Prapotnich, D. and Bougaran, J. (1994). Influence of preoperative positive seminal vesicle biopsy on the staging of prostatic cancer. *J. Urol.*, **152**, 1152–6

28. Stone, N. N., Stock, R. G. and Unger, P. (1995). Indications for seminal vesicle biopsy and laparoscopic pelvic lymph node dissection in men with localized carcinoma of the prostate. *J. Urol.*, **154**, 1392–6

29. Villers, A., McNeal, J. E., Rewine, E. A., Freiha, F. S. and Stamey, T. A. (1989). The role of perineural space invasion in the local spread of prostatic adenocarcinoma. *J. Urol.*, **142**, 763–8

30. Villers, A. (1994). Extracapsular tumor extension in prostatic cancer. In Stamey, T. A. (ed.) *Monographs in Urology*, pp. 61–77. (Montverde, FL: Medical Directions Publishing Co. Inc.)

31. Bastacky, S. I., Walsh, P. C. and Epstein, J. I. (1993). Relationship between perineural tumor invasion on needle biopsy and radical prostatectomy capsular penetration in clinical stage B adenocarcinoma of the prostate. *Am. J. Surg. Pathol.*, **17**, 336–41

32. Heller, J. E. (1987). Prostatic acid phosphatase: its current clinical status. *J. Urol.*, **137**, 1091–103

33. Whitesel, J. A., Donohue, R. E., Mani, J. H., Mohr, S., Scanavino, D. J., Augspurger, R. R., Biber, R. J., Fauver, H. E., Wettlaufer, J. N. and Pfister, R. R. (1984). Acid phosphatase: its influence on the management of carcinoma of the prostate. *J. Urol.*, **131**, 70–2

34. Bahnson, R. R. and Catalona, W. J. (1987). Adverse implications of acid phosphatase levels in the upper range of normal. *J. Urol.*, **137**, 427–30

35. Oesterling, J. E., Brendler, C. B., Epstein, J. I., Kimball, A. W. and Walsh, P. C. (1987). Correlation of clinical stage, serum prostatic acid phosphatase and preoperative Gleason grade with final pathological stage in 275 patients with clinically localized adenocarcinoma of the prostate. *J. Urol.*, **138**, 92–8

36. Stamey, T. A., Yang, N., Hay, A. R., McNeal, J. E., Freiha, F. S. and Redwine, E. (1987). Prostate-specific antigen as a serum marker for adenocarcinoma of the prostate. *N. Engl. J. Med.*, **317**, 909–16

37. Burnett, A. L., Chan, D. W., Brendler, C. B. and Walsh, P. C. (1992). The value of serum enzymatic acid phosphatase in the staging of localized prostate cancer. *J. Urol.*, **148**, 1832–4

38. Oesterling, J. E., Chan, D. W., Epstein, J. I., Kimball, A. W., Bruzek, D. J., Rock, R. C., Brendler, C. B. and Walsh, P. C. (1988). Prostate specific antigen in the preoperative and postoperative evaluation of localized prostatic cancer treated with radical prostatectomy. *J. Urol.*, **139**, 766–72

39. Hudson, M. A., Bahnson, R. R. and Catalona, W. J. (1989). Clinical use of prostate-specific antigen in patients with prostate cancer. *J. Urol.*, **142**, 1011–17

40. Partin, A. W., Carter, H. B., Chan, D. W., Epstein, J. I., Oesterling, J. E., Rock, R. C., Weber, J. P. and Walsh, P. C. (1990). Prostate specific antigen in the staging of localized prostate cancer: influence of tumor differentiation, tumor volume and benign hyperplasia. *J. Urol.*, **143**, 747–52

41. Graves, H. C. B., Wehner, N. and Stamey, T. A. (1990). Comparison of a polyclonal and monoclonal immunoassay for PSA: need for an international antigen standard. *J. Urol.*, **144**, 1516–22

42. Seaman, E. K., Whang, I. S., Cooner, W., Olsson, C. A. and Benson, M. C. (1994). Predictive value

of prostate-specific antigen density for the presence of micrometastatic carcinoma of the prostate. *Urology*, **43**, 645–8

43. Corn, B. W., Hanks, G. E., Lee, W. R., Bonin, S. R., Hudes, G. and Schultheiss, T. (1995). Prostate specific antigen density is not independent predictor of response for prostate cancer treated by conformal radiotherapy. *J. Urol.*, **153**, 1855–9

44. Rifkin, M. D., Zerhouni, E. A., Gatsonis, C. A., Quint, L. E., Paushter, D. M., Epstein, J. I., Hamper, U., Walsh, P. C. and McNeil, B. J. (1990). Comparison of magnetic resonance imaging and ultrasonography in staging early prostate cancer. Results of a multi-institutional cooperative trial. *N. Engl. J. Med.*, **323**, 621–6

45. Tempany, C. M., Zhou, X., Zerhouni, E. A., Rifkin, M. D., Quint, L. E., Piccoli, C. W., Ellis, J. H. and McNeil, B. J. (1994). Staging of prostate cancer: results of Radiology Diagnostic Oncology Group project comparison of three MR imaging techniques. *Radiology*, **192**, 47–54

46. Wolf, J. S. Jr, Cher, M., Dall'era, M., Presti, J. C. Jr, Hricak, H. and Carroll, P. R. (1995). The use and accuracy of cross-sectional imaging and fine needle aspiration cytology for detection of pelvic lymph node metastases before radical prostatectomy. *J. Urol.*, **153**, 993–9

47. Kleer, E., Larson-Keller, J. J., Zinke, H. and Oesterling, J. E. (1993). Ability of pre-operative serum prostate-specific antigen value to predict pathologic stage and DNA ploidy. *Urology*, **41**, 207–16

48. Kleer, E. and Oesterling, J. E. (1993). Prostate-specific antigen and staging of localized prostate cancer. *Urol. Clin. North Am.*, **20**, 675–704

49. Humphry, P. A., Walther, P. J., Currin, S. M. and Vollmer, R. T. (1991). Histologic grade, DNA ploidy, and intraglandular tumor extent as indicators of tumor progression of clinical stage B prostate carcinoma. *Am. J. Surg. Pathol.*, **15**, 1165–70

50. Bluestein, D. L., Bostwick, D. G., Bergstralh, E. J. and Oesterling, J. E. (1994). Eliminating the need for bilateral pelvic lymphadenectomy in select patients with prostate cancer. *J. Urol.*, **151**, 1315–20

51. Partin, A. W. and Carter, H. B. (1994). Prostate specific antigen: use in clinical practice. In *Campbell's Urology*, 6th edn, update 10. (Philadelphia: W. B. Saunders)

Interactive Voting System

1 In most men with newly diagnosed prostate cancer, PSA level alone is not an accurate marker of progression, because:

Response	Option
8%	PSA levels overlap between stages.
2%	PSA is not related to cancer volume.
10%	Other factors in addition to tumor volume influence PSA levels.
80%	Both 1 and 3 are correct.

Number of votes: 105

2 The best pre-treatment assessment of progression in men with prostate cancer is made by:

2%	Calculation of tumor volume from needle biopsies.
0%	PSA level.
0%	Seminal vesicle biopsy.
98%	Combination of T-stage, Gleason score and PSA level.

Number of votes: 110

Molecular alterations associated with prostate cancer development

28

Y. Tamimi, M. J. G. Bussemakers and J. A. Schalken

Introduction

Prostate cancer, the malignancy with the highest incidence in the Western male population, is characterized by the fact that at clinical presentation, the majority of patients have disease extended beyond the prostate, i.e. capsular penetration and/or established locoregional or distant metastases. For prostate cancer the clinical consequences of established metastatic disease are profound, since no curative therapy is available. Systemic palliative methods, based on androgen ablation, are usually successful, but of limited duration. The outgrowth of androgen-insensitive cells is inevitable and will eventually result in the patient's death.

Patients with localized tumors can be cured by radical prostatectomy. A considerable proportion of these patients, however, will show clinical progression to metastatic disease. Obviously, identification of these patients at risk is of great importance. Moreover, it is likely that the number of patients with small localized tumors will steadily increase as a consequence of incidental and/or systematic screening of the male population older than 50 years. In this group three categories are present which, as yet, cannot be discriminated: (1) the patients with small tumors that do not need any treatment; (2) those who should undergo a radical prostatectomy but have a low risk for clinical progression; and (3) the high-risk patients with tumors that are likely to progress to metastatic disease.

At this time, no accepted method is available to make this distinction, which makes systematic screening programs at least questionable. Therefore, methods for prediction of the meta-static potential of tumor cells are urgently needed. Many research laboratories are using molecular approaches to this problem. These approaches are all based on the question of whether molecular differences at the DNA, RNA or protein level can be identified that can serve as progression markers for malignant prostatic disease. Here, an overview is given of results obtained by the use of molecular approaches to the identification of markers for prostate cancer development.

Molecular changes in prostate cancer

Tumor progression is associated with phenotypic changes, which are determined by the pattern of protein expression. Aberrant protein expression patterns that mark the progression, however, often find their origin in genomic alterations. Therefore, studies on the involvement of specific genetic changes, such as chromosomal abnormalities, can serve as a lead to identify genes that are implicated in the onset and progression of cancer. The molecular biology of human cancer has seen explosive progress in the last decade. Several cancer susceptibility genes have been identified and have provided a basis for the understanding of the relationship between inherited malignancies and sporadic forms of common human cancers. However, despite the high prevalence of prostate cancer, little is known with regard to the molecular pathogenesis of this disease. Several studies have focused on chromosomal loss, which might indicate areas of the genome that harbor important tumor suppressor genes.

Genetic changes

Until a few years ago, the genetic changes leading to the development and progression of prostate cancer were poorly characterized. Classical cytogenetic studies are difficult to carry out in prostate cancer, due to the low mitotic index of prostatic tissue and to the preferential growth of non-malignant cells in tissue culture. Nonetheless, the involvement of some specific chromosomal changes has been identified: loss of chromosomes 1, 2, 5, 11 and Y, trisomy of chromosomes 7, 14, 20 and 22 and structural changes involving chromosomal segments 2p, 7q and 10q were the most common changes reported[1]. Of these, deletions of 7q and 10q were found in late-stage cancer. These findings, however, are all based on small numbers of patients. A less complicated technique that overcomes the previously mentioned problems with prostatic tissue is allelotyping. Using DNA probes that recognize restriction fragment length polymorphisms (RFLPs), one can identify deletions of parts of a chromosome. Allelic loss studies have been instrumental in the identification of putative tumor suppressor gene loci in a variety of cancers, for instance the frequent deletion of the long arm of chromosome 17 in colon cancer was revealed, leading to the identification of p53 as a potential tumor suppressor gene[2]. Several allelotype analyses have been performed for prostate cancer: Carter and collaborators[3] examined 'loss of heterozygosity' by means of RFLP analysis in 28 prostate cancer specimens (most of them organ-confined, stage B lesions), using probes for 7q and 10q (until then reported as most frequently showing loss) as well as probes for chromosomes documented to harbor tumor suppressor genes. They reported frequent loss of 10q and 16q. Kunimi and colleagues[4] studied ten primary tumors and eight metastatic lesions and found, besides loss of chromosomes 10 and 16, also frequent loss of chromosome 8. Bergerheim and colleagues[5] extended this study in 18 prostate cancer specimens and demonstrated that the highest frequency of allelic loss was restricted to the short arm of chromosome 8. Frequent allelic loss of chromosome 8p has since then been confirmed by several other studies[6–8] and research is ongoing to identify and characterize the putative tumor suppressor gene, located on chromosome 8p, which is involved in prostate cancer development. Interestingly, chromosome 8p is also frequently lost in colorectal cancer (45%), non-small cell lung cancer (50%), hepatocellular carcinoma (45%) and bladder cancer (25%). Future studies will have to reveal whether the same gene is affected in these cancers.

Whereas on 8p and 10q as yet no candidate tumor suppressor genes are mapped, an invasion suppressor gene, i.e. E-cadherin, is located on 16q22. Clearly, the relevant suppressor genes are candidates for use as molecular markers of prostate cancer development and progression.

Differential gene expression

Another way to identify candidates for such analyses that are not directly implicated in molecular genetic alterations, such as mutational activation or inactivation, is to identify genes that are differentially expressed. Differential and subtraction hybridization analyses provide a direct approach for identification of genes that are expressed at different levels in the tissues studied, being based on comparison of a 'steady state' mRNA population. Differential or subtraction hybridization offers several possibilities: one can screen for genes that are up-regulated (e.g. genes that are overexpressed as a result of, for instance, gene amplification or oncogene activation) as well as for genes that are down-regulated (e.g. genes that are no longer expressed, due to allelic loss, or transcriptional down-regulation/inactivation). Furthermore, the reagents that become available, i.e. cDNA clones, are easy to characterize by DNA sequence analysis and can be tested for usefulness in the diagnosis by Northern blot analysis or RNA *in situ* hybridization. Differential and subtraction hybridization have been successfully applied, to identify genes differentially expressed when comparing normal to malignant tissue. For prostate cancer, differential hybridization was used to study general changes in gene expression. In our laboratory, we identified a number of cDNAs overexpressed in metastasizing rat prostatic cancers[9–11]. One of those clones was shown to be identical to high mobility group (HMG) protein I(Y)[10]. HMG-I(Y) is a small non-histon nuclear protein implicated in transcription and replication processes. Its overexpression in dedifferentiated, fast-proliferating cells was reported earlier. The value of HMG-I(Y) as a progression marker was further investigated by means of RNA *in situ* hybridization[12]. This was done on paraffin-embedded tissue, thus enabling retrospective evaluation of the value of this marker. In the first evaluation it appeared that in human prostate cancers also, HMG-I(Y) was overexpressed in high-grade lesions and was associated with the presence of metastases[12].

Recently, the technique of differential display was developed and has proven to be a powerful tool to identify and clone differentially expressed genes[13]. Differential display analysis has some major advantages over traditional differential or subtraction hybridization, in that (1) it allows simultaneous comparison of multiple RNA samples; (2) both up- and down-regulated expression of genes can be studied in one experiment; (3) it is less time-consuming; and (4) only small amounts of RNA are required for this technique, allowing the use of sometimes rare and/or small human specimens. Differential display analysis is likely to reveal several new genes that are up- or down-regulated in prostate cancer development.

Recently, it has been shown that, in addition to deletions, mutations and chromosomal translocations, alterations in DNA methylation can also affect gene expression. Hypermethylation of CpG islands (areas of the genome rich in the sequence CpG, associated with the 5′ regulatory regions of genes) has been associated with gene inactivation. Lee and colleagues[14] studied the methylation of the regulatory sequences at the locus of the glutathione S-transferase gene-pi (GSTP1 – the protein encoded by this gene can catalyze the detoxification of electrophilic carcinogens by conjugation with reduced glutathione) and found that hypermethylation occurred in 20 of 20 human prostatic tumors, but not in normal prostatic tissue or in benign hyperplasia of the prostate (BPH). A striking decrease of GSTP1 expression was found to accompany human prostate carcinogenesis. This group further analyzed 91 prostatic carcinomas by staining with an anti-GSTP1 antibody and they were unable to show GSTP1 expression in 88 of these cancer specimens, suggesting that (hyper)methylation of GSTP1 regulatory sequences leading to decreased GSTP1 expression may be one of the most common genetic alterations yet described for prostate cancer.

Oncogenes and tumor suppressor gene involvement in prostate cancer

For prostate cancer, studies have been carried out on typical tumor suppressor genes, such as the tumor suppressor genes p53 and Rb and the oncogene *ras*, which are frequently affected in other solid tumors. With regard to the p53 gene, the frequency of mutations in primary prostate cancer is low in comparison with other common cancers. However, preliminary data from a number of laboratories suggest that bone metastatic deposits of prostate cancer may frequently exhibit mutant p53. This suggests that p53 mutations are 'late events' in the progression of prostate cancer[15,16]. Obviously, more studies are required to establish the role of p53 in (the progression of) this disease.

For Rb, mutations have been found in a subset of prostatic adenocarcinomas, but also here, more studies are required. Concerning a role for *ras* gene mutations in prostate cancer, the data obtained in American patients show that activation of the *ras* oncogenes via point mutations is not a common event in either the initiation or the progression of prostatic neoplasia[17]. In contrast to this, two reports on *ras* gene mutations in Japanese patients with prostate cancer showed a significant occurrence of *ras* mutations in both latent and clinically manifest disease[18,19]. This raises the question of whether significant differences exist in the genetic events associated with the development of prostate cancer in American vs. Japanese men.

Prostate cancer susceptibility genes

More recently it has become clear that, as in breast cancer, a subset of prostate cancer has a familial background. Therefore, linkage studies have been initiated in prostate cancer families in order to characterize the loci harboring the susceptibility genes involved in hereditary forms of this common disease. From initial studies it has been reported[20] that the gene responsible for this predisposition may account for 9% of the total cases of prostate cancer observed and for 45% of the cases observed in men under 55 years of age.

It is anticipated that these studies will provide critical information regarding the genetic mechanisms involved not only in hereditary prostate cancer but also in the more common sporadic disease.

Molecular prognostic factors

Despite the tremendous increase in our knowledge of the molecular basis of prostate cancer, relatively few reports are available on the value of these findings for molecular diagnostics.

E-cadherin/α-catenin immunohistochemistry

One of the best-studied candidates is E-cadherin. This molecule mediates Ca^{2+}-dependent cell–cell interactions and has been shown to play an important role in embryonic development and morphogenesis. In later stages, E-cadherin is specifically expressed in epithelial tissues. The functional importance of E-cadherin in preserving epithelial tissue integrity was demonstrated by the use of antibodies against E-cadherin, leading to dissociation of epithelial cell layers in cell culture and, more significantly, to an increased invasive potential of cells. Increased invasive behavior can also be induced by introducing E-cadherin antisense DNA into cells. Conversely, introduction of E-cadherin cDNA, by means of transfection, into invasive cells

resulted in differentiation of carcinomas. These studies provide evidence that E-cadherin can act as an invasion suppressor. Invasiveness may be acquired by down-regulation of E-cadherin at the DNA, RNA or protein level. In recent years various laboratories have studied the expression of E-cadherin in a great number of different human and animal cell lines and carcinomas and found a reduced expression of E-cadherin correlating with poor differentiation of human tumors, suggesting an important role for E-cadherin in the maintenance of the differentiated phenotype of carcinomas (for a review, see reference 21).

We first studied the expression of E-cadherin in a rat prostatic cancer model system[22] and we found that down-regulation of E-cadherin mRNA expression was associated with the invasive capacity of the sublines studied. We then assessed E-cadherin expression in human prostatic cancer specimens by immunohistochemical analysis. In these human cancer specimens a correlation with Gleason grade was found[23,24]. Moreover, within the Gleason scores of 6, 7 and 8, E-cadherin differentiated two types, i.e. normal staining vs. aberrant staining (heterogeneous or negative). A correlation with survival was strongly suggested from the limited follow-up of the patients[24].

Not all types of adhesion deficiencies in invasive carcinomas are caused by decreased E-cadherin expression. Loss of E-cadherin function may also be due to loss of, or reduced contact with the cytoskeleton. Interactions between the cytoskeleton and adhesion molecules have been shown to be essential for a variety of cellular functions, including cell–cell and cell–matrix interactions and cell motility. Normally, the highly conserved cytoplasmic domain of E-cadherin associates with three independent proteins, called α-, β- and γ-catenin. Significant changes in the cadherin–catenin complex have been shown to disturb the junctional complex, thereby affecting the greater motility of invasive cells[21]. Preliminary studies, using immunohistochemical analysis on human prostate cancer specimens, showed that α-catenin expression is often down-regulated in high-grade prostate cancer (R. Umbas and colleagues, personal communication). Furthermore, these studies indicate that α-catenin may provide additional prognostic information for prostate cancer. However, large prospective studies will have to reveal the clinical value of both E-cadherin and α-catenin as prognostic factors. It is interesting that the α-catenin gene maps to chromosome 5q, a chromosomal region that is also frequently lost in prostatic tumors (25%).

Candidate progression markers for prostate cancer

The detection of circulating tumor cells is also based on advanced methodologies based on the polymerase chain reaction (PCR) and despite equivocal reports to date this may be an important addition in the accurate assessment of the stage of the disease. New candidate tissue markers are cathepsin D, plasminogen activators (uPA, tPA, PAI-1, uPA-R), *bcl*-2 and frequency of allelic loss.

Molecular diagnostics: perspectives

It is clear that through elucidation of the molecular cascade that leads to prostate cancer the use of this information can lead to a better assessment of the biological potential of prostate tumors.

The exact place of all these new markers in the diagnostic armamentarium can be determined only in well-controlled, prospective clinical evaluations, in which methods are standardized. The multifocality and heterogeneity that are so characteristic of prostate cancer will undoubtedly complicate interpretation, particularly for biopsy material. The intrinsic sampling artifact will often result in biopsies that are poorly representative of the entire malignant process, as mapped in the radical prostatectomy specimens. Ironically, therefore, the value of pre-surgical molecular diagnostic procedures will be critically dependent on the development of clinical imaging tools that allow the urologist adequately to biopsy the most malignant area in the prostate.

References

1. Brothman, A. R., Peehl, D. M., Patel, A. M. and McNeal, J. E. (1990). Frequency and pattern of karyotypic abnormalities in human prostate cancer. *Cancer Res.*, **50**, 3795–803
2. Baker, S. J., Fearon, E. R., Nigro, J. M., Hamilton, S. R., Preisinger, A. C., Yessup, J. M., Van Tuinen, P., Ledbetter, D. H., Barker, D. F., Nakamura, Y. and Vogelstein, B. (1989). Chromosome 17 deletions and p53 mutations in colorectal carcinomas. *Science*, **244**, 217–21
3. Carter, B. S., Ewing, C. M., Ward, W. S., Treiger, B. F., Aalders, T. W., Schalken, J. A., Epstein, J. I. and Isaacs, W. B. (1990). Allelic loss of chromosomes 16q and 10q in human prostate cancer. *Proc. Natl. Acad. Sci. USA*, **87**, 8751–5
4. Kunimi, K., Bergerheim, U. S. R., Larsson, I.-L., Ekman, P. and Collins, V. P. (1991). Allelic loss of human prostatic adenocarcinoma. *Genomics*, **11**, 530–6
5. Bergerheim, U. S. R., Kunimi, K., Collins, V. P. and Ekman, P. (1991). Deletion mapping of chromosomes 8, 10 and 16 in human prostatic carcinoma. *Genes Chromosomes Cancer*, **3**, 215–20

6. Bova, G. S., Carter, B. S., Bussemakers, M. J. G., Emi, M., Fujiwara, Y., Kyprianou, N., Jacobs, S. C., Robinson, J. C., Epstein, J. I., Walsch, P. C. and Isaacs, W. B. (1993). Homozygous deletion and frequent allelic loss of chromosome 8p22 loci in human prostate cancer. *Cancer Res.*, **53**, 3869–73
7. MacGrogan, D., Levy, A., Bostwick, D., Wagner, M., Wells, D. and Bookstein, R. (1994). Loss of chromosomal arm 8p loci in prostate cancer: mapping by quantitative allelic loss. *Genes Chromosomes Cancer*, **10**, 151–9
8. Trapman, J., Sleddens, H. F., Van der Weiden, M. M., Dinjens, W. N., Konig, J. J., Schroder, F. H., Faber, P. W. and Bosman, F. T. (1994). Loss of heterozygosity of chromosome 8 microsatellite loci implicates a candidate tumor suppressor gene between the loci D8S87 and D8S133 in human prostate cancer. *Cancer Res,*. **54**, 6061–4
9. Schalken, J. A., Ebeling, S. B., Isaacs, J. T., Treiger, B., Bussemakers, M. J. G., De Jong, M. E. M. and Van de Ven, W. J. M. (1988). Down

modulation of fibronectin mRNA in metastasizing rat prostatic cancer cells revealed by differential hybridization analysis. *Cancer Res.*, **48**, 2042–8

10. Bussemakers, M. J. G., Van de Ven, W. J. M., Debruyne, F. M. J. and Schalken, J. A. (1991). Identification of high mobility group protein I(Y) as a potential marker for prostate cancer by differential hybridization analysis. *Cancer Res.*, **51**, 606–11

11. Bussemakers, M. J. G., Verhaegh, G. W. C. T., Van Bokhoven, A., Debruyne, F. M. J. and Schalken, J. A. (1992). Differential expression of vimentin in rat prostatic tumors. *Biochem. Biophys. Res. Commun.*, **182**, 1254–9

12. Tamimi, Y., Van der Poel, H. G., Denyn, M. M., Umbas, R., Karthaus, H. F., Debryne, F. M. J. and Schalken, J. A. (1993). Increased expression of high mobility group protein I(Y) in high grade prostatic cancer determined by *in situ* hybridization. *Cancer Res.*, **53**, 5512–16

13. Liang, P. and Pardee, A. B. (1992). Differential display of eucaryotic messenger RNA by means of the polymerase chain reaction. *Science*, **257**, 967–71

14. Lee, W. H., Morton, R. A., Epstein, J. I., Brooks, J. D., Campbell, P. A., Bova, G. S., Hsieh, W. S., Isaacs, W. B. and Nelson, W. G. (1994). Cytidine methylation of regulatory sequences near the pi-class glutathione S-transferase gene accompanies human prostatic carcinogenesis. *Proc. Natl. Acad. Sci. USA*, **91**, 11733–7

15. Bookstein,, R., MacGrogan, D., Milsenbeck, S. G., Sharkey, F. and Allred, D. C. (1993). p53 is mutated in a subset of advanced-stage prostate cancer. *Cancer Res.*, **53**, 3369–73

16. Dinjens, W. N., Van der Weiden, M. M., Schroeder, F. H., Bosman, F. T. and Trapman, J. (1994). Frequency and characterization of p53 mutations in primary and metastatic human prostate cancer. *Int. J. Cancer*, **56**, 630–3

17. Gumerlock, P. H., Poonamallee, U. R., Meyers, F. J. and Devere White, R. W. (1991). Activated *ras* alleles in human carcinoma of the prostate are rare. *Cancer Res.*, **51**, 1632–7

18. Konishi, N., Enomoto, T., Buzard, G., Ohshima, M., Ward, J. M. and Rice, J. M. (1992). K-*ras* activation and *ras* p21 expression in latent prostatic carcinoma in Japanese men. *Cancer*, **69**, 2293–9

19. Anwar, K., Nakakuki, K., Shiraishi, T., Naiki, H., Yatani, R. and Inuzuka, M. (1992). Presence of *ras* oncogene mutations and human papilloma virus DNA in human prostate carcinoma. *Cancer Res.*, **52**, 5991–6

20. Carter, B. S., Bova, G. S., Beaty, T. H., Steinberg, G. D., Childs, B., Isaacs, W. B. and Walsh, P. C. (1993). Hereditary prostate cancer: epidemiology and clinical features. *J. Urol.*, **150**, 797–802

21. Birchmeier, W. and Behrens, J. (1994). Cadherin expression in carcinomas: role in formation of cell junctions and the prevention of invasiveness. *Biochem. Biophys. Acta*, **1198**, 11–26

22. Bussemakers, M. J. G., Van Moorselaar, R. J. A., Giroldi, L. A., Ichikawa, T., Isaacs, J. T., Takeichi, M., Debruyne, F. M. J. and Schalken, J. A. (1992). Decreased expression of E-cadherin in the progression of rat prostatic cancer. *Cancer Res.*, **52**, 2916–22

23. Umbas, R., Schalken, J. A., Aalders, T. W., Carter, B. S., Debruyne, F. M. J. and Isaacs, W. B. (1992). Decreased expression of E-cadherin in high grade prostate cancer. *Cancer Res.*, **52**, 5104–9

24. Umbas, R., Isaacs, W. B., Bringuier, P. P., Schaafsma, H. E., Karthaus, H. F., Oosterhof, G. O., Debruyne, F. M. J. and Schalken, J. A. (1994). Decreased E-cadherin expression is associated with poor prognosis in patients with prostate cancer. *Cancer Res.*, **54**, 3929–33

Can we safely exclude patients with confined prostate cancer from treatment?

29

G. J. Miller and S. J. Pfister

Introduction

Prostate cancer incidence and prevalence continue to rise throughout North America[1]. An important and characteristic feature of this disease is its heterogeneity both in morphology and clinical behavior. In addition, the disease displays an unusually slow progression in some patients. There is, for example, about a 15-fold greater chance of having a prostatic carcinoma found at autopsy than there is of dying from the disease[2]. On the other hand, it is well recognized that once it is metastatic, prostatic cancer carries a poor prognosis with devastating clinical consequences[3]. Unfortunately, many patients who undergo surgical removal of the prostate in an attempt to effect a cure are still found to have locally invasive or metastatic disease[4]. Concern over our lack of ability to treat prostate cancer once it has spread beyond the confines of the gland have led to an intensified interest in detecting the disease at earlier stages. However, as stated above, it is recognized that there is a large reservoir of relatively quiescent tumors that will not harm the average patient during his lifetime. Once these are found, we are left with a dilemma regarding how to distinguish those tumors that are biologically aggressive and require radical therapy from those that should be left alone. Ultimately, the answer to this dilemma depends on a full understanding of the natural history of prostatic carcinoma and elucidation of the specific changes in prostatic carcinoma cells that allow them to invade and/or metastasize.

Lessons learned from prostatectomies

In the last 10 years, there has been an unprecedented opportunity to study the natural history of prostatic carcinoma afforded by the clinical popularity of radical prostatectomy. The study of radical prostatectomy specimens has provided us with considerable new information about the interrelationships of tumor volume, grade and pathological stage[5,6].

We have recently described our findings on a series of radical prostatectomy specimens that were studied by the whole-mount technique[7]. These specimens have provided us with a tool to define the precise points at which carcinomas of the prostate begin to display the features of invasion that would identify them as being a clinical threat. Using computer reconstruction of 151 cases, we identified 293 spatially independent foci of carcinoma. There were an average of 1.9 carcinomas per case with a range of 1–6 separate lesions per prostate. Only 66 of 151 prostates contained what was interpreted as a unifocal carcinoma. In addition, since these 66 tumors were of relatively high volume (mean 6.52 cm^3) it is possible that at least some of these actually represented collisions between smaller multifocal lesions. Prostatic cancer is, therefore, a highly multifocal disease.

Previous workers[5,6] have emphasized a relationship between prostatic cancer volume and histological grade; a measure of malignant potential. However, in our series, we have found only a modest correlation ($r_s = 0.4868$) between these two variables. Moreover, tumors with Gleason sums of 2–10 were found with volumes of < 1 cm^3. These findings are consistent with the conclusion that prostatic cancer grade is a relatively stable feature of its natural history. Specifically, it appears that tumors can originate with 'high-grade' morphologies and this is not a feature that needs to be acquired during tumor progression.

Of the low-grade (Gleason sum = 2) tumors, 92% were confined within the prostatic capsule. In contrast, high-grade carcinomas (Gleason sums of ≥ 7) frequently (86%) invaded through the prostatic capsule. It would appear, therefore, that the extremes of Gleason sum have predictive value regarding local invasion. However, 198/293 (67.6%) carcinomas had Gleason sums of 3–6. Of these, 66% were confined within the prostatic capsule, making intermediate Gleason scores inadequate for prediction of local invasion. The amount of capsule perforation in a given case was related to the volume of carcinoma present. However, capsule perforation did not occur exclusively in high-volume tumors. Among 185 carcinomas with volume of < 1 cm^3, 30 (16%) had measurable capsule penetration (up to 1.3 cm^2). Although a higher percentage (89.3%) of tumors with Gleason sums of 2–4 were confined within the prostate compared to those with Gleason sums of 8–10 (40%), 43% of all tumors that had penetrated through the capsule were of low grade. This indicates that it is not necessary for tumors to attain either high volume or high grade before they can demonstrate a cardinal feature of malignancy: invasion.

It would seem, therefore, that the most widely accepted prognostic variables that are currently available are only partially predictive of the malignant potential of prostatic carcinomas. Consistent with the basic definitions of malignancy, carcinomas of the prostate, regardless of their grade, can display an invasive phenotype. Prediction of any given patient's clinical course is further complicated by the fact that prostatic cancer is a multifocal disease.

Time and metastasis

The growth rates and doubling times of prostatic carcinomas are recognized to be quite prolonged. Even patients with advanced-stage disease can progress with calculated doubling times of up to 4 years[8]. Using such reported doubling times, we have recently calculated[9] that approximately 16 years could elapse between the time that the first metastatic cells arrive at a lymph node and the time at which a lymph node metastasis reaches a volume of 1 cm^3. This would imply that a primary tumor should be able to begin its process of metastatic dissemination relatively early in its course, possibly at a volume of less than 0.5 cm^3.

Since it is recognized that vascular and/or lymphatic invasion is required for dissemination of prostatic carcinoma cells, we have recently attempted to determine the size of tumors directly, where this process begins[10]. Fifty-three prostatectomy specimens were selected in which the total tumor volume for a given case was less than 5 cm^3. Sixty-three independent carcinomas were present in these cases. Fifteen per cent of organ-confined carcinomas were found to have focal areas of vascular invasion. Of most importance, tumors as small as 0.29 cm^3 contained areas in which malignant cells invaded into veins and/or lymphatic channels, well within the prostatic parenchyma. However, tumors with volumes of less than 0.2 cm^3 failed to demonstrate invasion into vascular spaces. Although vascular invasion was more common (44%) in higher-grade tumors (Gleason sums 7 and 8), it did occur (14%) in tumors with Gleason sums of 2–4. Again, these findings are consistent with the concept that prostatic carcinomas do not have to attain large volumes or high histological grades before they display the attributes of malignancy.

Summary and conclusions

Prostatic carcinoma is clearly a multifocal disease. Whether all of the lesions in a given patient's prostate share common molecular changes is not fully known, but it is most likely that these represent relatively unique events, each with their own biological and malignant potentials. The earliest evidence of invasiveness occurs in relatively small-volume lesions of $< 1\ cm^3$. The extremes of histological grade are informative regarding the likelihood of a tumor being confined within the prostate. Unfortunately, intermediate-grade tumors comprise a spectrum of lesions with great variability in their malignant potentials. For these lesions, grade, by itself, does not provide a reliable indicator of the presence or absence of capsular perforation.

Finally, in view of the long doubling times reported for advanced-stage prostatic carcinomas, it is likely that the process of metastasis begins when primary tumors are relatively young and of small volume. Study of intraprostatic vascular invasion reveals that malignant cells can be found invading into potential routes of metastasis in tumors with volumes as low as $0.29\ cm^3$. All of these findings are consistent with a model in which the malignant phenotype of carcinomas is expressed very early, perhaps at the genesis of these lesions. This being the case, as soon as prostatic carcinoma cells have reached a route of egress from the prostate, they can be shed into the vascular or lymphatic systems. The likelihood that a given patient will eventually die of metastatic disease is then dependent on two separate components, each of which is related to time.

The first component is the probability that metastatic colonization has occurred. This is a function of access to a metastatic route, the rate of cell shedding, the ability of cells to colonize and the length of time that the patient is exposed to his risk. The second component is the length of time that a patient continues to live after metastatic deposits have become established. Given adequate time, even small metastases would attain sufficient size to be of clinical consequence.

The answer to the question of whether or not localized prostate carcinomas need to be treated is, therefore, as much a factor of the host's permissiveness to the development of the disease as it is of the inherent properties of the malignant cells themselves. By definition, all carcinomas of the prostate are 'malignant'. Consistent with this paradigm, we have found that the malignant phenotype of invasion is expressed in relatively small-volume tumors, even those of low histological grade. We can conclude that the definition of any given tumor as 'clinically significant' or 'clinically insignificant' must include a meaningful analysis of the host context in which that tumor exists. The precise means of integrating such information into clinical planning remains to be established. Until the criteria are better defined, it is difficult to be certain that any patient who is able to tolerate definitive therapy should be denied appropriate treatment.

References

1. Parker, S. L., Tong, T., Bolden, S. and Wingo, P. A. (1996). Cancer statistics, 1996. *CA Cancer J. Clin.*, **46**, 5–27
2. Scardino, P. T, Weaver, R. and Huscon, M. A. (1992). Early detection of prostate cancer. *Hum. Pathol.*, **23**, 211–22
3. Prostate Cancer Trialists' Collaborative Group (1995). Maximum androgen blockade in advanced prostate cancer: an overview of 22 randomized trials with 3283 deaths in 5710 patients. *Lancet*, **346**, 265–9
4. Voges, G. E., McNeal, J. E., Redwine, E. A., Freiha, F. A. and Stamey, T. S. (1992). Morphologic analysis of surgical margins with positive findings in prostatectomy for adenocarcinoma of the prostate. *Cancer*, **69**, 520–6
5. McNeal, J. E., Bostwick, D. G., Kindrachuk, R. A., Redwine, E. A., Freiha, F. S. and Stamey, T. A. (1986). Patterns of progression in prostate cancer. *Lancet*, **1**, 60–3
6. Stamey, T. A., McNeal, J. E., Freiha, F. S. and Redwine, E. (1988). Morphometric and clinical

studies on 68 consecutive radical prostatectomies. *J. Urol.*, **139**, 1235–41

7. Miller, G. J. and Cygan, J. M. (1994). Morphology of prostate cancer: the effects of multifocality on histological grade, tumor volume and capsule penetration. *J. Urol.*, **152**, 1709–13

8. Schmid, H. P., McNeal, J. E. and Stamey, T. A. (1993). Observations on the doubling time of prostate cancer. The use of serial prostate-specific antigen in patients with untreated disease as a measure of increasing cancer volume. *Cancer*, **71**, 2031–40

9. Miller, G. J. (1995). Pathology in prostate cancer: limitations with current techniques. *Cancer Control*, **2**, 27–32

10. Pfister, S. J. and Miller, G. J. (1996). Intraprostatic invasion by prostatic carcinoma. *Am. J. Pathol.*, in press

Interactive Voting System

1   At what volume do prostate carcinomas become 'aggressive'?

Response	*Option*
30%	0.05 cm^3.
24%	0.10 cm^3.
15%	0.20 cm^3.
27%	0.50 cm^3.
4%	1.00 cm^3.

Number of votes: 97

2   At what volume do prostate carcinomas become clinically 'significant'?

5%	0.05 cm^3.
8%	0.10 cm^3.
17%	0.20 cm^3.
55%	0.50 cm^3.
15%	1.00 cm^3.

Number of votes: 100

Watchful waiting as a treatment option in the management of clinically localized prostate cancer

30

G. W. Chodak

Introduction

In recent years, the management of clinically localized prostate cancer has come under increasing scrutiny. In part because of the widespread use of prostate specific antigen (PSA) for screening, the detection of localized disease has increased substantially. Since a survival benefit from local therapy has yet to be demonstrated in a randomized controlled trial, the question of whether to treat or observe has become more important. Although two randomized studies are currently under way, definitive results will not be available for at least 10 years. In the interim, watchful waiting as a treatment modality needs to be addressed in terms of its known risks and benefits, so that patients can make comparisons with the other treatment options available.

Management by watchful waiting

By definition, watchful waiting means not administering local therapy (radiation or surgery). Patients are treated expectantly, i.e. they are treated if and when they develop clinical symptoms or signs of progression. Before the development of PSA testing, patients managed by watchful waiting would undergo some combination of a digital rectal examination, bone scan or bone X-rays and serum acid phosphatase measurement at varying intervals. Local therapy such as transurethral resection of the prostate (TURP) was provided for local symptoms such as urinary retention or voiding dysfunction, and hormone therapy was used for ureteral obstruc-

tion or symptomatic metastatic disease. With the development of PSA testing, however, watchful waiting is now more likely to involve performing only a digital examination and PSA measurement at regular intervals until high PSA levels occur. Some patients who initially choose watchful waiting may do so until the PSA level reaches a 'critical' value, at which point local therapy may then be desired. Since there is no evidence for the impact of delayed local therapy or for the critical PSA level at which local therapy is both necessary and beneficial, patients choosing watchful waiting should really understand that this option means neither radiation therapy to the prostate nor radical prostatectomy are ever given. Although the natural history of this disease is quite variable, patients nevertheless need to know that prostate cancer will invariably grow and the PSA level will rise at a variable rate. Until more information is available and since considerable patient and physician anxiety is likely to coincide with the rise in PSA level, perhaps the best solution for now may be to perform this test less often.

Benefits and risks of watchful waiting

In presenting patients with information about watchful waiting, one could begin with the potential benefits. These may include maintaining one's immediate quality of life, especially if no symptoms of the disease are present, and avoiding the potential complications that can occur following radiation or surgery. On the basis of the long-term results from this approach, some men may avoid therapy entirely, depending on the progression rate of their tumor and their remaining life expectancy. In addition, since no clear scientific proof exists that surgery and radiation significantly reduce the morbidity and mortality of the disease, purists could argue that patients benefit by not undergoing a treatment of unproven benefit.

The risks of watchful waiting are quite obvious. First, patients may miss a chance to be cured of their disease. The cancer may then progress and eventually metastasize, causing considerable pain and suffering, and ultimately cause death, resulting in a loss of normal life expectancy. Although hormone therapy most often produces a clinical remission once metastases develop, men need to understand that most patients who develop metastases ultimately will die of their disease with at least the last 6–12 months almost invariably associated with a poor quality of life. Essentially, the decision about watchful waiting is a decision about trade-offs; the adverse consequences of treatment are immediate and may last many years, whereas the benefits may be quite delayed and potentially of limited duration, because patients may die of some other disease. This trade-off between risks and benefits requires individualization of the decision regarding this therapy, since no physician can really understand the goals, fears and motivation of each patient. Although physicians are clearly expected to make a recommendation for treatment, it is still the physician's responsibility to present an objective assessment of the outcomes of watchful waiting, so that patients are sufficiently well informed to help decide on a course of action.

Outcomes following watchful waiting

To date, only one randomized study comparing watchful waiting to local therapy has ever been performed[1], and the results are unreliable, due to many methodological flaws. Therefore, the relative outcomes from this therapy compared to other treatments can be defined only from uncontrolled studies. Over the past 10 years, several reports have appeared; however, three fundamental problems are associated with these reports which include patient selection bias, a larger proportion of men with low-grade disease than is seen in men undergoing radical prostatectomy and an older age at diagnosis. Rather than focusing on any single paper with its inherent biases, the treatment guidelines panel of the American Urological Association attempted to compare treatments by performing a meta-analysis of the published literature[2]. This analysis revealed that the 95% confidence intervals for the 10-year cancer-specific survival rate could not be distinguished from the rates for radical prostatectomy or radiation therapy. These results led the panel to conclude that watchful waiting needed to be included in the presentation of choices when patients with localized disease were counselled. Unfortunately, this meta-analysis did not stratify the outcomes of each treatment according to significant prognostic factors such as tumor grade, because such a task was not really possible based on the data included in each report.

In an attempt to address some of the potential problems inherent in the single-institution reports, another attempt was made to compile the data from different watchful waiting studies into a 'pooled analysis', using original case data rather than published results. A comparison of the results from a conventional meta-analysis and a pooled analysis has demonstrated that more reliable outcomes are obtained with a pooled analysis[3]. One major advantage of the pooled analysis is that it permits an assessment of the outcomes stratified for significant risk factors and the impact of specific biases on the outcomes.

With the use of this approach and the Kaplan–Meier method for determining survival curves, 828 patients from six studies originating from four countries were included in the analysis[4]. The study found that tumor grade was the most important prognostic factor. When the results were stratified by grade, the cancer-specific survival 10 years after diagnosis was 87%, 87% and 34%, and the metastases-free survival was 81%, 58% and 26% for grade 1 (Gleason 2–4), grade 2 (Gleason 5–7) and grade 3 tumors (Gleason 8–10), respectively. Age-adjusted overall survival was comparable to the normal survival for the respective populations, suggesting that no significant loss of life expectancy occurred following watchful waiting. The importance of age and clinical stage at diagnosis, and the impact of delayed local therapy (radiation or surgery) were assessed and found not to influence the outcomes significantly. This report refined the outcomes that might be expected with watchful waiting, providing the most reliable estimates to date.

Nevertheless, since they were not based on a randomized study, the data must be interpreted cautiously. Perhaps the most significant deficiency in this study was the absence of a centralized review of the pathology. To compensate for this, a Cox regression analysis was performed to compare the outcomes from the six different centers to each other, before the data were combined together, in order to minimize the possibility that the results would be unduly influenced by differences in pathology. Importantly, the results from only one of the reports differed from the other five and the overall results with and without these men included did not differ significantly.

These findings were partially substantiated by a subsequent report by Albertson[5], in which he reviewed the results for men aged 65–75 at diagnosis who were treated by watchful waiting in the state of Connecticut and followed long term. In contrast to the pooled analysis study, the report by Albertson for the first time contained 15-year outcomes following watchful waiting. Strengthening these results is the fact that all the pathological samples were re-analyzed by a single pathologist. At 10 and 15 years, respectively, the cancer-specific survival rates were 91% and 91%, 76% and 72%, and 58% and 48% for Gleason 2–4, 5–7 and 8–10 cancers. These results were slightly better for well- and poorly differentiated cancer and slightly worse for moderately differentiated cancer, compared to the pooled analysis study. Once again they confirmed that while significant percentages of men may die of their disease, prostate cancer does not invariably lead to premature death.

Another important feature of this study was an estimate of the average loss of life expectancy that might be expected with watchful waiting, which is 0 years for men with well-differentiated cancer, 4–5 years for men with moderately differentiated cancer and 6–8 years for men with poorly differentiated cancer. One must keep in mind that this patient population included only men aged between 65 and 75 years at diagnosis. Thus, for younger men who usually have a longer average life expectancy, the average number of years that might be lost following watchful waiting is probably higher. Also, neither the pooled analysis nor the Connecticut study included men with stage T_{1C} cancer who were diagnosed by PSA testing. Because of lead time bias, all of the above survival rates are likely to be higher in patients with these cancers.

With the best estimates of the outcomes from watchful waiting defined, the question is how these results compare to radical prostatectomy or radiation therapy. The criticisms suggested for the individual watchful waiting studies apply equally to the studies involving surgery or radiation. Until one of the ongoing randomized trials has been completed, the only valid method for comparing therapies is to perform a similar pooled analysis of the other treatments. A preliminary report of this methodology for radical prostatectomy was reported at the American Urological Association in 1995[6] and further analysis is now under way to make a comparison of similar groups of patients. One preliminary finding is that the non-cancer survival of the men treated by surgery (and radiation) is higher than that for men treated by watchful waiting. A second finding is that surgery appears to offer a survival advantage for men with poorly differentiated cancers, an observation not previously substantiated in the literature.

Adverse consequences of watchful waiting

In addition to a potential reduction in life expectancy, another disadvantage of watchful waiting is progression of the cancer, resulting in the need for additional therapy. This may take the form of urinary obstruction, requiring transurethral resection; ureteral obstruction, causing renal impairment, which requires percutaneous nephrostomy; and bone metastases, requiring hormone therapy, focal radiation therapy and/or high-dose analgesia. The likelihood of receiving additional therapy in the pre-PSA era was approximately 25–30% for men managed by watchful waiting. In contrast, for men undergoing radical prostatectomy, the frequency of receiving additional cancer therapy ranged from 15% for well-differentiated cancer to 42% for poorly differentiated disease[7]. Once again, the longer a patient survives, the greater the likelihood of requiring therapy for symptomatic progression.

Making decisions about watchful waiting

On the basis of currently available information, how can physicians help patients come to a decision about whether to select watchful waiting or local therapy? First, patients need to be made aware of the relative risk of the cancer, which primarily depends on tumor grade and life expectancy. For those with a life expectancy of 10 years or less, few men are likely to live longer as a result of local treatment, unless they have a poorly differentiated cancer. Therefore, these men are clearly the best candidates for watchful waiting. For those diagnosed by PSA alone or those with a well- or moderately differentiated cancer, a life expectancy of 13–15 years may be needed to derive a survival benefit from treatment, because of the lead time of diagnosis. However, by 10 years, patients should recognize that watchful waiting may result in a slightly greater chance of having metastatic disease.

The real dilemma about managing localized prostate cancer is the inability to identify which patients truly need local therapy and will also benefit from it. Consequently, for men hoping to maximize their survival and minimize their risks from prostate cancer, they must receive local therapy even though this will invariably result in some men being treated unnecessarily. On the other hand, watchful waiting is best for men who are more concerned about their immediate quality of life, with the recognition that they might be deprived of several years of life expectancy and a poorer quality of life. Since the quality of most men's lives is worse at the end of their life span than at the time of diagnosis, many men may feel that the potential gain in survival is not worth the price, and therefore watchful waiting should be selected. In the final analysis, this decision will be affected by the fears and goals of each patient and their family members, by cultural factors specific for each country and by the biases of counselling physicians. Hopefully, the ongoing clinical trials will provide even better information about the relative risks and benefits of surgery compared to watchful waiting. Until that time, patient education should lead to the best opportunity for patients to make informed decisions.

References

1. Madsen, P. O., Graversen, P. H., Gasser, T. C. and Corle, D. K. (1988). Treatment of localized prostatic cancer: radical prostatectomy versus placebo: a 15-year follow-up. *Scand. J. Urol. Nephrol.*, (Suppl 1) **10**, 95–100
2. Middleton, R. G., Thompson, I. M., Austenfeld, M. S., Cooner, W. H., Correa, R. J., Gibbons, P. *et al.* (1995). Prostate clinical guidelines panel summary report on the management of clinically localized prostate cancer. *J. Urol.*, **154**, 2144–8
3. Chodak, G. W. and Thisted, R. A. for the Prostate Cancer Pooled Analysis Group. (1996). Comparison of cancer specific survival (CSS) following radical prostatectomy (RP) or Watchful Waiting (WW) based on two multi-institutional pooled analysis. *J. Urol.*, **155**(5), 559A

4. Chodak, G. W., Thisted, R. A., Gerber, G. S., *et al.* (1994). Results of conservative management of clinically localized prostate cancer. *N. Engl. J. Med., 330,* 242–8

5. Albertsen, P. C., Fryback, D. G., Stomer, B. G., Kolon, T. F. and Fine, J. (1995). Long-term survival among men with conservatively treated localized prostate cancer. *J. Am. Med. Assoc.,* **274,** 626–31

6. Gerber, G. S., Thisted, R. A., Chodak, G. W., *et al.* (1995). Results of radical prostatectomy in men with clinically localized prostate cancer: multi-institutional analysis. *J. Urol.,* **153,** 252A

7. Lu-Yao, G. L., Potosky, A. L. and Albertsen, P. C. (1995). Secondary cancer treatments after radical prostatectomy among patients with prostate cancer. *J. Urol.,* **153,** 253A

Interactive Voting System

1   For every 100 men aged 68 with a well-differentiated stage T_2 prostate cancer, how many will live longer if treated by radical prostatectomy compared to watchful waiting?

Response	Options
Response	*Options*
20%	None.
33%	10.
14%	20.
20%	30.
13%	More than 50.

Number of votes: 110

2   To avoid the possibility of a 10% chance of bothersome incontinence and a 25% chance of impotence, what percentage reduction in cancer mortality would you require to select radical prostatectomy over watchful waiting?

2%	0–5%.
28%	5–10%.
27%	10–20%.
25%	20–30%.
18%	More than 30%.

Number of votes: 108

The PSA response following radical radiation therapy for localized prostate cancer

31

A. L. Zietman, C. T. Smith and W. U. Shipley

Introduction

The two most commonly employed therapeutic alternatives for clinically localized T_{1-2} N_x M_0 prostate carcinoma are radical prostatectomy and radical radiation therapy. Each modality has its proponents and a vigorous debate about the relative efficacy of each is currently being conducted. Careful stratification by Gleason grade and pre-treatment level of prostate specific antigen (PSA), coupled with the use of sensitive indicators of disease control such as post-therapy PSA and rebiopsy, have recently made it clear that neither therapy is quite as effective as was previously assumed[1]. Both treatments are associated with relatively high rates of failure, and both are, for some categories of patients, clearly insufficient. This paper aims to define those patients within the rather heterogeneous T_1–T_2 group who are most likely to be cured by radical radiation as a monotherapy. Those who cannot be cured by this method may be better served by either surgery or new radiation techniques (such as high-dose conformal therapy or brachytherapy), or by some form of combined modality employing radiation with surgery or with neo-adjuvant androgen suppression.

Defining failure following radical radiation therapy

Clinical endpoints

The only truly valid and unequivocal endpoints in prostate cancer are overall survival, cancer-specific survival and freedom from symptomatic failure. These reflect the influence of prostate cancer on both length and quality of life[2].

It has proved difficult to ascertain any overall survival advantage for men treated with radical therapy compared with those managed by observation. This is because most men are currently being diagnosed in their sixties or seventies with a disease that may be protracted over decades. There is a significant competing mortality within this age group and men succumb to cardiac and other ailments at a rate of 3% per year. Thus, overall survival amongst prostate cancer patients may only be marginally improved, even by a therapy that was 100% effective[3].

Cancer-specific survival assesses the likelihood of death from cancer if a man does not die from another cause. This is a better measure of the efficacy of a treatment than overall survival, because it is not confounded by other causes of death. As a result, it is used in most prospective studies. Unfortunately, 10 or more years of follow-up are required to obtain evaluable results.

Despite the competing causes of death, freedom from clinical failure is a relevant endpoint that can be meaningfully assessed with less than a decade of follow-up. Failure may not be life threatening yet still be symptomatic and greatly affect the patient's quality of life. In addition, it will usually be followed by androgen suppression with its attendant psychological and physical discomforts.

Early (surrogate) endpoints of failure

Early endpoints of failure are currently being sought, more rapidly to assess the efficacy of the many therapies available. Two techniques for early evaluation now in common use are the post-radiation prostate rebiopsy and serum PSA measurement. These surrogates are good measures of the ability of radiation to eradicate tumor, whether it has an impact on the subsequent well-being of the patient or not.

Prostatic rebiopsy Many studies have demonstrated that, in the absence of a palpable local failure, prostate glands may harbor occult disease on rebiopsy several years after radiation therapy. A positive rebiopsy after 2 or more years is associated with higher subsequent rates of local failure and of distant metastasis[4-7]. In one study reported by Kuban and colleagues[7], those with positive rebiopsies experienced clinical failure over 70% of the time as compared to only 20% in those whose biopsies were negative. The significance of a positive rebiopsy is determined by the time at which it was performed after the radiation therapy. Prostate cancer cells take many months and sometimes years to die following radiation and, therefore, men who have a positive rebiopsy after 1 year will not necessarily still have a positive rebiopsy at 2 or 3 years[8]. The incidence of positive rebiopsy in the literature ranges between 10 and 91%[9]. This disparity can be entirely accounted for by a careful examination of the reasons men were selected for rebiopsy. Positive rebiopsies are far more likely in T_3 disease than in T_1 or T_2 disease, and more likely when there is a rising serum PSA pattern and no evidence of distant metastatic disease. The only careful prospective study in the literature was recently reported by Crook and colleagues[10]. Men were rebiopsied annually following radiation, and at 3 years, approximately 20% of T_1 patients were positive, as were 30% of the T_2 patients. These figures correspond very closely with the anticipated 10-year rates of clinical local failure.

The fact that a positive rebiopsy in conjunction with a palpably normal gland is associated with a high metastatic rate raises the possibility that the metastases arose from locally persistent disease. This suggests a need for improved radiation techniques to increase pathological as well as clinical local control.

Rising PSA Following radical prostatectomy, when all tumor and healthy prostatic tissues have been removed, the serum PSA level should decline to zero within a month. Any detectable PSA unambiguously reflects persistent cancer. Following radiation therapy, the situation is far less clear. Firstly, the PSA level takes a highly variable time to normalize[11]. Prostatic tumors regress slowly and may still produce PSA until regression is complete. The median time to reach the lowest (nadir) PSA level following radiation therapy at our institution is 17 months, although some patients continue to decline for up to 3 years. Secondly, it is uncertain just how far the PSA level should fall for a patient to be declared biochemically disease-free. There is little doubt that the prostate gland, like other protein- and peptide-secreting glands, such as the pituitary or thyroid, is functionally affected by radiation therapy. In a series of bladder and rectal cancer patients without prostate cancer, who received incidental prostatic irradiation as part of their therapy, the median PSA level was found to be 0.6 ng/ml with 78% having a PSA level below 1.0 ng/ml[12]. This compares with a median value amongst age-matched men that was significantly higher at 1.1 ng/ml (Figure 1). It is, therefore, too much to demand that the PSA level following radiation for prostate cancer come down to undetectable levels, as the normal prostatic tissue is still able to produce some PSA, though at a reduced rate. Hanks and co-workers[13] have argued for an upper limit of normal for the PSA level to be set at 1.5 ng/ml, 2 or more years after radiation. We have erred on the side of caution, only declaring our patients disease-free when their PSA level was below 1.0 ng/ml[14]. Neither definition of biochemical failure is in fact the whole truth, as there are undoubtedly patients with PSA values higher than this, whose values never rise and who are truly disease-free[12]. There are also those

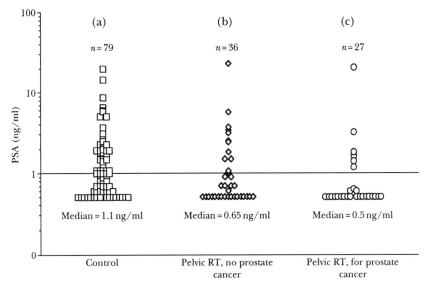

Figure 1 Serum PSA values in three groups of men: (a) age-matched control men without prostate cancer or prostatic irradiation; (b) those who had radiation therapy (RT) for bladder or rectal cancer and whose treatment included the prostate; (c) those who had RT for prostate cancer 10 or more years previously and who are clinically free from disease

with PSA values below these arbitrary levels, whose profile is rising and who are destined to fail.

Some groups have been using even earlier endpoints, such as serum PSA level at 6–12 months, or the rate of PSA decline. These endpoints are probably measured too early to be of reliable prognostic significance and encourage the publication of very immature series.

The only biochemical endpoint that is now generally agreed upon as having reliability and relevance is a rising PSA profile. But how many measurements are necessary to establish a rise? We have found that once a nadir has been reached, two rises are followed by a third rise only 54% of the time. However, when there have been three consecutive rises, a fourth rise occurs 84% of the time. Three consecutive rises, therefore, seems to be a relatively secure endpoint of failure. Sometimes it is possible to call failure with fewer rises than this, if a single rise exceeds 50% of the previous PSA value or if a single rise exceeds 1 ng/ml. The only problem with the successive rises criterion is that it is simply not possible to analyze the results of a radiation treated series with less than 3 years of follow-up.

It takes 1 to 2 years for the PSA level to normalize, and then, if the patient is being seen in 6-monthly follow-up, another few years to document failure. We have tested the ability of the PSA nadir to predict a subsequently rising PSA profile. Those who achieved a nadir of less than 0.5 ng/ml have a 94% chance of remaining free from a rising PSA level at 4 years. Those who achieve a nadir in excess of 1.0 ng/ml have only a 30% chance of remaining free from a rising PSA level in 4 years.

It has been argued that a rising PSA level, although representing failure of primary therapy, is not relevant to the patient, unless it inevitably predicts clinical relapse within his lifetime. This would be a valid argument, except that, in the USA, when the PSA level starts to rise, androgen suppression is very likely to follow, even in the absence of symptoms. Whether the impetus for this comes from the patient, who cannot stand to watch a rising PSA and remain untreated, or from urologists, who propose early intervention, is uncertain. For this reason PSA failure has real clinical relevance for patients, as it is probably a prelude to medical or surgical castration (Figure 2).

243

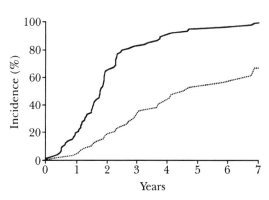

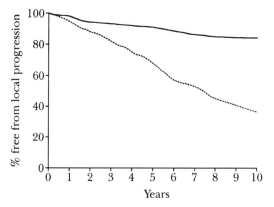

Figure 2 Analysis of patients biochemically failing radiation treatment. Cumulative plot demonstrates the probability of androgen suppression following biochemical failure. Solid line, rising prostate specific antigen levels; dotted line, androgen deprivation

Figure 3 The probability of men with clinically localized prostate cancer remaining free from local progression by initial mode of management. Data for radiation treatment (solid line) are from the Patterns of Care Studies[16]; data for observation (dashed line) are from reference 15

Results of conventional external-beam radiation therapy

Most patients selected by virtue of their early stage and low-grade disease for a policy of watchful waiting will, in time, progress locally. Whitmore and co-workers[15] documented local progression in 90% of patients managed expectantly over 15 years of observation. The likelihood of clinical (palpable) local failure in radiation-treated T_1 and T_2 patients has been thoroughly evaluated, and in most 10–15 year series stands at 25% or less (Figure 3)[16]. Even if there were no survival advantage to radiation-treated patients, there is little doubt that the majority would benefit in terms of freedom from local progression.

Whether true cancer control has been achieved or not is best determined by examining the biochemical failure rates following radical radiation therapy. At the Massachusetts General Hospital we have recently evaluated the outcome for 346 men treated between 1986 and 1993 with a median follow-up of 4 years. The results clearly demonstrate the heterogeneity of the T_1–T_2 N_x group (Figure 4). Patients with well-differentiated disease fared substantially better than those with poorly differentiated disease in terms of 6-year disease-free survival

(58% and 27%, respectively). A pre-treatment prognostic indicator of equal importance is the initial serum PSA level. Those who begin with serum PSA values of 4 ng/ml or less have an 89% chance of remaining biochemically disease free at 6 years. This declines to 59% for those with 4–10 ng/ml, 38% for those with 10–20 ng/ml and 18% for those with a serum PSA level over 20 ng/ml.

Figure 5 shows that those with T_1T_{2A} disease and a serum PSA value of less than 10 ng/ml have a high likelihood of cure with conventional radiation therapy. These are the patients who are now being identified in large numbers by screening programs across the USA. Other T_{1-2} patients, however, fare substantially less well. Though they have a high chance of clinical local control and clinical freedom from metastasis over the same period of time, they are much more likely to have a rising PSA level, with all that it portends for the future.

When conventional external-beam radiation series are compared with radical prostatectomy series, the selection biases that are inherent within these groups must be taken into account. Those with larger tumors (T_{2B-C}) or higher PSA values are more likely to receive radiation[1]. Surgical series also screen out those patients

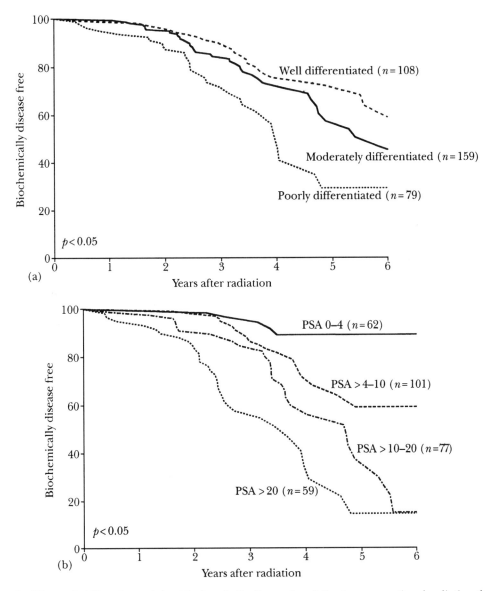

Figure 4   The probability of remaining biochemically disease free following conventional radiation therapy. Men treated at the Massachusetts General Hospital 1986–93. Influence of Gleason grade (a) and pre-treatment prostate specific antigen (PSA) level (ng/ml) (b)

who are node-positive, although this represents a shrinking proportion of men in the era of early detection. Table 1 shows the results of conventional radiation therapy that was performed at the MD Anderson Hospital and the Massachusetts General Hospital when stratified by initial PSA level[17]. There is agreement about the high probability of biochemical disease control in men with initial PSA levels of less than 10 ng/ml, and these figures compare well with the Johns Hopkins and the UCLA surgical series[18,19]. Both modalities are, however, relatively ineffective as monotherapies for men with PSA values above this level. There is considerable disagreement among radiation oncologists about the initial PSA level above

Table 1 Likelihood of biochemical disease-free survival in men treated either by external beam radiation or radical prostatectomy.

| | MGH radiation | | M. D. Anderson radiation | | Johns Hopkins prostatectomy | |
Pretreatment PSA (ng/ml)	No. of patients	5-year FFRBP (CI)	No. of patients	5-year FFRBP (CI)	No. of patients	5-year FFRBP (CI)
≤ 4	62	89 (80–98)	117	91 (78–97)	284	92 (86–95)
4.1–10.0	101	59 (42–76)	169	69 (55–80)	237	83 (76–89)
10.1–20.0	77	38 (20–56)	118	62 (47–75)	105	56 (42–69)
> 20	59	15 (0–32)	57	38 (25–53)	40	45 (26–63)

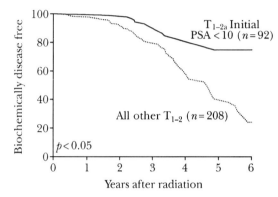

Figure 5 The probability of remaining biochemically disease free following conventional radiation therapy. Men treated at the Massachusetts General Hospital 1986–93. those with T_{1-2A} and serum prostate specific antigen (PSA) values of less than 10 ng/ml represent a favorable subset

Table 2 PSA doubling times following the failure of radical therapies

	Median	(range)
Prostatectomy (UCLA 1994)	10.2	(1–99)
Radiation (MGH 1995)	11.1	(1–100)

which cure is unlikely and an alternative strategy necessary.

Stamey and co-workers have leveled a number of serious charges against the use of radiation therapy for prostate cancer, arguing that only 20% are cured and the remaining 80% demonstrate rapidly rising PSA rates on failure, implying disease acceleration[20]. The implication is that these patients would have been better off being managed by watchful waiting. That 80% failed in the small series examined by Stamey and colleagues is true. This is to be expected, as almost half of the group had T_{3-4} or nodal disease and were being treated with palliative intent and without a view to cure. A reanalysis by the Stanford radiation oncologists of all patients treated around the era described in the report by Stamey and colleagues demonstrated 62% failure[21]. When, however, one ex-

amines patients with true early-stage disease, these high failure rates are simply not seen (Figure 5). The second, perhaps more serious, charge deserves close examination. Men who fail after radiation are usually those with prognostically unfavorable T_{1-2} N_x disease and are many years more advanced in their disease at the time of failure. Therefore, to compare their PSA doubling times with those selected (often by virtue of a low PSA doubling time) for watchful waiting is inappropriate. In addition, when one examines doubling times following radical prostatectomy failure, their median value and range compare closely with those seen after radiation (Table 2).

The implication of Dr Stamey's argument is that radiation accelerates cancer, and therefore an excess of metastatic disease and cancer-specific death will be seen with sufficient follow-up. A comparison between the rates of these events in our radiation-treated series and those seen in the observation series reported in a meta-analysis by Chodak and co-workers shows no excess of cancer death or of metastasis at 12 years[22,23]. The predicted wave of failure late in the first decade did not occur (Figure 6).

Bagshaw and associates[24] have reported a very mature series of men treated by radical

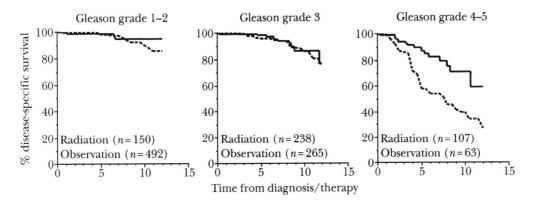

Figure 6 A comparison of disease-specific survival between men treated with radiation therapy at the Massachusetts General Hospital (solid lines; data from reference 22) or managed expectantly, as reported in a meta-analysis by Chodak and colleagues (dashed lines, data from reference 23)

radiation therapy. When survival rates are compared with those expected in an age-matched population, there is no difference for those with T_1 or T_{2A} disease. There is a small decrease in survival seen in the second decade for those with T_{2B} and T_{2C} disease. These figures differ little from those few long-term radical prostatectomy series that have been reported.

A small case-controlled study performed by Freiha at Stanford University compared radiation and surgically treated patients and found no significant difference in overall or cancer-specific survival at 10 years[25]. Although there is no proven survival advantage for men treated by radical prostatectomy over radiation therapy, the former is more commonly offered to younger men, on the supposition that such an advantage may ultimately emerge. It is also possible that men who have developed a prostate cancer relatively early in life have an epithelial field change that will predispose them to further prostatic cancer in the future, even if the first is eradicated by radiation.

Modern management of aggressive $T_{1–2}$ disease

As can be seen from the preceding section, it is evident that there are men who, although their condition has been effectively palliated at the primary site by conventional radiation therapy, are infrequently cured. These are men with high

Gleason grades, bulky T_2 tumors and serum PSA values in excess of 10–20 ng/ml. Although the treatment in many of these men fails because of occult metastatic disease, a substantial proportion will have local failure. Dugan and co-workers[26] showed that those with a rising serum PSA level after radiation and no evidence of metastatic disease on bone scan had positive rebiopsies in 68% of cases.

Efforts to improve local control have taken two forms (Figure 7). The first is to increase the radiation dose delivered. This necessarily carries risks to the surrounding normal tissues and can only be achieved by using modern conformal three-dimensional planning techniques or by the use of brachytherapy. The alternative is to cytoreduce the tumor prior to radiation, using neo-adjuvant androgen suppression. This does not carry the same risks as dose escalation and is far more applicable to the radiotherapeutic community at large.

Dose escalation

The relationship between delivered radiation dose and tumor control probability is central to the practice of modern radiotherapy. The Patterns of Care Studies have shown an apparent dose response forLee prostate tumors over the range 60–70 Gy with clinical local control as the endpoint[16]. Dose escalation above 70 Gy would probably increase this further, but can only be

247

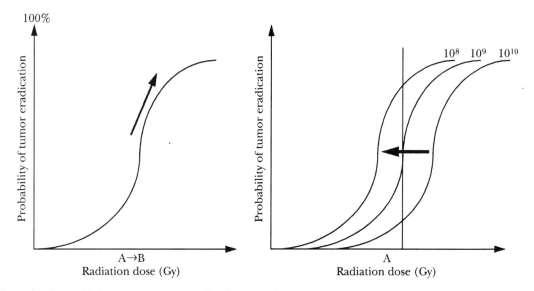

Figure 7 Sigmoid dose–response curves for theoretical tumors treated by radiation. Dose escalation (left) seeks to increase tumor control probability by increasing the radiation dose delivered. Cytoreduction (right) seeks to reduce the volume of tumor (number of tumor clonogens) prior to radiation. This has the effect of shifting the curve to the left and increasing the tumor control probability for the same radiation dose

safely achieved by using conformal techniques with or without three-dimensional planning.

Leibel and associates[27] presented interesting early results from a phase I dose-escalation study. Three hundred and twenty-four patients received doses ranging from 65 to 81 Gy with 237 being treated to at least 70 Gy. The 3-year actuarial probability of surviving with a normal PSA level was 97% for stages T_{1C-2A}, 86% for T_{2B}, 60% for T_{2C} and 43% for T_3. Encouraging as these results are for early disease, those obtained for T_{2B-3} patients leave much to be desired. They are likely to decline even further with time.

The only randomized study to address dose escalation comprehensively was reported by Shipley and associates[28]. Two hundred and two T_{3-4} N_x M_0 patients were given 50.4 Gy by conventional four-field external-beam photons and were then randomized to receive either a photon boost to 67.2 Gy or a conformal boost with a perineal proton field to 75.6 cobalt gray equivalent (CGE). The results with a median of 5 years' follow-up are shown in Table 3. No significant differences were seen between the treatment arms in terms of local control, disease-free survival, or overall survival. There was a trend

towards an improvement in local control for those receiving a high dose. Subset analysis showed that this resulted from a significant improvement in local control amongst those with poorly differentiated tumors. The rate of positive rebiopsy in patients whose digital rectal examination had normalized following treatment and who underwent prostate rebiopsy was lower for the high-dose than the low-dose arm (28% vs. 45%) but this also did not reach a level of significance.

The fact that this trial was largely negative should not deter us from a further exploration of dose escalation. It is possible that the dose tested was not high enough. It is also probable that a large number of men with occult metastatic disease and nothing to gain from dose escalation were included in the trial. Future studies will exclude those who are known to be node-positive and those with exceedingly high serum PSA values. The latter was not available at the initiation of this study to discriminate the highest risk subgroups.

Leibel, Soffen and Lichter and their colleagues appeared to demonstrate that dose escalation can be achieved with minimal rectal toxicity when conformal techniques are employed[27,29,30]. A note of warning, however, has been sounded by the Massachusetts General Hospital randomized trial. This study, with considerably longer follow-up than any other reported, showed a 27% level of grade 1–2 late rectal bleeding when 75.6 Gy was given in a randomized trial as compared with only 9% when the dose was 67.2 Gy[31]. The vast majority of the bleeding was only grade 1 or 2 and was temporary. This may not be too high a price to pay for a higher likelihood of cure, if it were actually proven to exist.

Recent work by Corn and colleagues[32] with only short follow-up seems to show an advantage, in terms of early biochemical control, with conformal radiation over conventional techniques without any increase in total given dose. This raises the possibility that more cure may be achieved simply by improved targeting.

Neo-adjuvant cytoreduction

When seeking to improve local control the alternative to giving a higher radiation dose to the same tumor is to give the same radiation dose to a tumor made smaller by pre-radiation therapy. The relationship between decreasing tumor volume and increasing tumor control is well established in both the clinic and the laboratory[33]. Androgen suppression reliably reduces the volume of over 90% of prostate carcinomas and looks theoretically attractive in this regard. A recent study using serial transrectal ultrasound showed an average volume reduction of 37% over 3 months[34]. Several studies have also shown a considerable reduction in the incidence of positive margins when 3–4 months of androgen suppression precede radical surgery for T_{2B-3} disease[35,36]. Whether this represents true downstaging or merely a diffuse reduction in the number of tumor cells ('downsizing') is of importance to the surgeon but is not relevant to the radiation oncologist. Either could result in improved local control with radiation. Cytoreduction is more attractive than dose escalation to many radiation oncologists, because it raises

the hope of improved local control without the risks of increased normal tissue damage.

The most compelling data currently available on the use of radiation in combination with neo-adjuvant suppression (NAS) come from RTOG protocol 8610[37]. This study evaluated the efficacy and the safety of the combination of goserelin acetate (3.6 mg subcutaneously 4-weekly) and flutamide (250 mg orally, three times a day), administered prior to and during radiation in patients with bulky, locally advanced (T_{2C}, T_3, and T_4) prostate cancer. Androgen suppression began 8 weeks prior to irradiation and continued through it for a total of 16 weeks.

A total of 471 patients were enrolled and randomized with a median follow-up of 4.5 years. The results demonstrated some remarkable differences between the two treatment arms. The estimated cumulative incidence of local failure at 5 years was 71% of control patients but only 54% of experimental patients ($p = < 0.001$). Interestingly, the two cumulative incidence curves appear to be diverging, suggesting that this advantage to the experimental arm may increase with the passage of further time. This study is the first convincing demonstration that eradication of prostatic tumor is enhanced by prior cytoreduction. It also answers the theoretical criticism that androgen suppression might put tumor cells into a more resistant phase of the cell cycle and thus render them more resistant to radiation.

It is of note that the local failure rates are higher in the control arm than in many other series reporting results with radiation alone for similar stages of tumor. This most probably reflects the use of more rigorous failure criteria, in particular the rebiopsy of many, but not all, patients with clinically negative glands. It is also based on the presumption that those with biochemical failure and no clinical evidence of distant metastases have local failure which may well overestimate the incidence of the latter.

There was also a strong trend towards a reduction in the cumulative incidence of distant metastases at 5 years between the treatment and control groups (34% and 41%, $p = 0.09$). It is not yet clear whether this results from the improved local control or whether it is the result of the systemic action of the androgen suppression on occult micrometastases.

The biochemical disease-free survival data are the most informative. The estimated incidence of disease-free survival at 5 years was only 15% in the control group but 36% for the experimental group ($p < 0.001$). It is likely that the clinical disease-free survival figures with approximately 6–10 years of follow-up will reflect these numbers. The 21% gain in biochemical disease-free survival mirrors the gain in local control (25%), suggesting that it is here that, to date, most of the advantage of the addition of androgen suppression has been felt. Subgroup analysis is not yet available to determine whether one particular TN-stage or tumor grade benefits more than another.

An interim analysis of a randomized trial from Quebec has recently been reported[38]. Patients were randomized to receive either radiation alone, 3 months of NAS then radiation, or 3 months of NAS followed by radiation and a further 6 months of androgen suppression. One hundred and twenty patients have so far reached 2 years on the trial and undergone prostate rebiopsies. The rates of positive rebiopsy were 64%, 28% and 8%, respectively. A long-term gain from the addition of as little as 3 months of androgen suppression is once again demonstrated.

A recent study of 'intermediate-risk' men with prostate cancer reported by Duchesne and co-workers[39] noted that those patients who had neo-adjuvant androgen suppression (cyproterone acetate from diagnosis for a varia-ble time until the end of radiation) were significantly more likely to be free from an elevated PSA level (> 10 ng/ml) at 4 years than those who had not (83% vs. 25%). Although this study was not randomized, the neo-adjuvant group had a higher average initial PSA level (22 vs. 10 ng/ml), suggesting that any bias was not in its favor.

The duration of neo-adjuvant therapy has yet to be established. Gleave and colleagues[40] have used an ultrasensitive PSA assay to show that, although the bulk of the PSA decline takes place over the first 3 months, a slower decline may be detected for up to 6 months more. They have shown that this has a clinical correlate in that the positive margin rate after radical surgery for T_{1-3} disease was reduced from 10–32% to 4% when neo-adjuvant therapy was extended from 3 to 8 months. A new Canadian randomized study is testing 3 and 8 months of neo-adjuvant therapy prior to radiation for T_{2B-4} disease.

Conclusions

Men with T_{1-2A} N_x prostate cancer and serum PSA values of less than 10 ng/ml have a high probability of cure with conventional radiation therapy. Those with T_{2B} disease or larger and those with initial PSA values in excess of 10 ng/ml may benefit from conventional radiation therapy in terms of local control, but are unlikely to be cured. These patients should be managed by more modern approaches, such as conformal therapy with dose-escalation or in protocols employing neo-adjuvant androgen suppression.

References

1. Zietman, A. L., Shipley, W. U. and Coen, J. J. (1994). Radical prostatectomy and radical radiation therapy for clinical T1–2 adenocarcinoma of the prostate: new insights into outcome from rebiopsy and PSA follow-up. *J. Urol.*, **152**, 1806–12

2. Zietman, A. L. and Shipley, W. U. (1993). Randomized trials in loco-regionally confined prostate cancer: past, present, and future. *Semin. Radiat. Oncol.*, **3**, 210–20

3. Barry, M. J., Fleming, C., Coley, C. M., Wasson, J. H., Fahs, M. C. and Oesterling, J. E. (1995).

Should Medicare provide reimbursement for prostate specific antigen testing for early detection of prostate cancer? Part I: framing the debate. *Urology*, **46**, 2–13

4. Scardino, P. T. and Wheeler, T. M. (1988). Local control of prostate cancer with radiotherapy: frequency and prognostic significance of positive results of post-irradiation prostate biopsy. *NCI Monogr.*, **7**, 95–103

5. Schellhammer, P. F., El-Mahdi, A. M., Higgins, E. M., Schultheiss, T. E., Ladage, L. E. and Babb, T. J. (1987). Prostate biopsy after definitive treatment by interstitial ^{125}Iodine implant or external beam radiation therapy. *J. Urol.*, **137**, 897–901

6. Kabalin, J. N., Hodge, K. K., McNeal, J. E., Freima, F. S. and Stamey, T. A. (1989). Identification of residual cancer in the prostate following radiation therapy: role of transrectal ultrasound guided biopsy and prostate specific antigen. *J. Urol.*, **142**, 326–31

7. Kuban, D. A., El-Madhi, A. M. and Schellhammer, P. (1991). The significance of post-irradiation prostate biopsy with long-term follow-up (Abstr.). *Int. J. Radiat. Oncol. Biol. Phys.*, **21** (Suppl. 1), 191

8. Cox, J. D. and Kline, R. W. (1983). The lack of prognostic significance of biopsies after radiotherapy for prostatic cancer. *Semin. Urol.*, **1**, 237–42

9. Zietman, A. L., Shipley, W. U. and Willett, C. G. (1993). Residual disease following radical surgery or radiation therapy for prostate cancer: clinical significance and therapeutic implications. *Cancer*, **71**, 959–69

10. Crook, J., Robertson, S., Collin, G., Zaleski, V. and Esche, B. Clinical relevance of transrectal ultrasound, biopsy, and serum PSA following external beam radiotherapy for carcinoma of the prostate. *Int. J. Radiat. Oncol. Biol. Phys.*, **27**, 31–7

11. Zagars, G. K. (1993). Serum PSA as a tumor marker for patients undergoing definitive radiation therapy. *Urol. Clin. North Am.*, **20**, 737–47

12. Willett, C. G., Zietman, A. L., Shipley, W. U. and Coen, J. J. (1993). The effect of pelvic radiation therapy on serum levels of prostatic specific antigen. *J. Urol.*, **151**, 1579–81

13. Hanks, G. E., Lee, W. R. and Schultheiss, T. E. (1995). Clinical and biochemical evidence of control of prostate cancer at five years after external beam radiation. *J. Urol.*, **154**, 456–9

14. Zietman, A. L., Coen, J. J., Shipley, W. U., Willett, C. G., and Efird, J. T. (1994). Radical radiation therapy in the management of prostatic adenocarcinoma: the initial prostate specific antigen value as a predictor of treatment outcome. *J. Urol.*, **151**, 640–5

15. Whitmore, W. F., Warner, J. A. and Thompson, I. M. (1991). Expectant management of localized prostatic cancer. *Cancer*, **67**, 1091–6

16. Hanks, G. E., Diamond, J. J. and Krall, J. M. (1987). A ten year follow-up of 682 patients treated for prostate cancer with radiation therapy in the United States. *Int. J. Radiat. Oncol. Biol. Phys.*, **13**, 499–505

17. Zagars, G. K. and Pollack, A. (1995). Radiation therapy for T1 and T2 prostate cancer: prostate specific antigen and disease outcome. *Urology*, **45**, 476–83

18. Partin, A. W., Pound, C. R., Clemens, J. Q., Epstein, J. L. and Walsh, P. C. (1993). Serum PSA after anatomic radical prostatectomy: the Johns Hopkins experience after 10 years. *Urol. Clin. North Am.*, **20**, 713–25

19. Trapasso, J. G., DeKernion, J. B., Smith, R. B. and Dorey, F. (1994). The incidence and significance of detectable levels of prostate specific antigen after radical prostatectomy. *J. Urol.*, **152**, 1821–5

20. Stamey, T. A., Ferrari, M. K. and Schmid, H.-P. The value of serial PSA determinations 5 years after radiotherapy: steeply increasing values characterize 80% of patients. *J. Urol.*, **150**, 1856–9

21. Hancock, S. L., Cox, R. S. and Bagshaw, M. A. (1995). Prostate specific antigen after radiotherapy for prostate cancer: re-evaluation of long-term biochemical control and kinetics of recurrence in patients treated at Stanford University. *J. Urol.*, **154**, 1412–17

22. Zietman, A. L., Coen, J. J., Dallow, K. A. and Shipley, W. U. (1995). The treatment of prostate cancer by conventional radiation therapy: an analysis of long term outcome. *Int. J. Radiat. Oncol. Biol. Phys.*, **32**, 287–92

23. Chodak, G. W., Thirsted, R. A., Gerber, G. S., Johansson, J.-E., Adolfsson, J., Jones, G. W., Chisholm, G. D., Moskovitz, B., Livne, P. M. and Warner, J. (1994). Results of conservative management of clinically localized prostate cancer. *N. Engl. J. Med.*, **330**, 242–8

24. Bagshaw, M. J., Cox, R. S. and Hancock, S. L. (1994). Control of prostate cancer with radiotherapy: long-term results. *J. Urol.*, **152**, 1781–5

25. Freiha, F. S. (1995). A comparative study of external beam radiation therapy and radical retropubic prostatectomy in men with clinically localized prostate cancer and pathologically negative lymph nodes. Ten year follow-up. In Murphy, G., Khouy, S., Chaterlain, C. and Denis, L. (eds.) *Proceedings of the Fourth International*

Symposium on Recent Advances in Urologic Cancer, Diagnosis and Treatment, vol. 4, pp. 1–8. (Jersey, UK: Scientific Communication International)

26. Dugan, T. C., Verhey, L. J. and Shipley, W. U. (1990). Post-irradiation biopsy of the prostate in stage T3 prostatic cancer: correlation with original histologic grade and with current PSA values. *Int. J. Radiat. Oncol. Biol. Phys.*, **19**, 198–9

27. Leibel, S. A., Zelefsky, M. J., Kutcher, G. J., Burman, C. M., Kelson, S. and Fuks, Z. (1994). Three-dimensional conformal radiation therapy in localized carcinoma of the prostate: interim report of a phase I dose–escalation study. *J. Urol.*, **152**, 1792–8

28. Shipley, W. U., Verhey, L. J., Munzenrider, J. E., Suit, H. D., Urie, M. M., McManus, P. L., Young, R. H., Shipley, J. W., Zietman, A. L., Biggs, P. J., Heney, N. M. and Goitein, M. (1995). Advanced prostate cancer: the results of a randomized comparative trial of high dose irradiation boosting with conformal protons compared with conventional dose irradiation using photons alone. *Int. J. Radiat. Oncol. Biol. Phys.*, **32**, 3–12

29. Soffen, E. M., Hanks, G. E., Hunt, M. A. and Epstein, B. E. (1992). Conformal static field radiation therapy treatment of early prostate cancer versus non-conformal techniques: a reduction in acute morbidity. *Int. J. Radiat. Oncol. Biol. Phys.*, **24**, 485–91

30. Lichter, A. S., Sandler, H. M., Robertson, J. M., Lawrence, T. S., Ten Haken, R. K., McShan, D. L. and Frass, B. A. (1992). Clinical experience with three-dimensional planning. *Sem. Rad. Oncol.*, **2**, 257–63

31. Benk, V. A., Adams, J. A., Shipley, W. U., Urie, M. M., McManus, P. L., Efird, J. T. and Willett, C. G. (1993). Late rectal bleeding following combined x-ray and proton high dose irradiation for patients with stages T3-4 prostatic carcinoma. *Int. J. Radiat. Oncol. Biol. Phys.*, **26**, 551–7

32. Corn, B. W., Hanks, G. E., Schultheiss, T. E., Hunt, M. A., Lee, T. R. and Coia, L. R. (1995). Conformal treatment of prostate cancer with improved targeting: superior prostate-specific antigen response compared to standard treatment. *Int. J. Radiat. Oncol. Biol. Phys.*, **32**, 325–30

33. Suit, H. D., Shalek, R. J. and Wette, R. (1965). Radiation response to C3H mouse mammary carcinoma evaluated in terms of cellular radiosensitivity. In Shalek, R. J. *et al.* (eds.) *Cellular Radiation Biology*, pp. 5114–530. (Baltimore: Williams and Wilkins)

34. Sneller, Z., Hop, Carpentier, P., Hop, W. C. J. and Schröder, F. H. (1992). Prognosis and prostate volume changes during endocrine management of prostate carcinoma: a longitudinal study. *J. Urol.*, **147**, 962

35. Labrie, F., Dupont, A., Cusan, L., Gomez, J. L., Diamond, P., Koutsilieris, M., Suburu, R., Fradet, Y., Lemay, M. and Tetu, B. (1993). Downstaging of localized prostate cancer by neoadjuvant therapy with flutamide and lupron: the first controlled and randomized trial. *Clin. Invest. Med.*, **16**, 499

36. Fair, W. R., Aprikian, A., Sogani, P., Reuter, V. and Whitmore, W. F. (1993). The role of neoadjuvant hormonal manipulation in localized prostate cancer. *Cancer*, **71**, 1031

37. Pilepich, M. V., Krall, J. M., Al-Sarraf, M., Scotte-Doggett, R. L., Sause, W. T., Lawton, C. A., Abrams, R. A., Rotman, M., Rubin, P., Shipley, W. U., Grignon, D., Caplan, R. and Cox, J. D. (1995). Androgen deprivation with radiation therapy alone for locally advanced prostatic carcinoma: a randomized comparative trial of the Radiation Therapy Oncology Group. *Urology*, **45**, 616–23

38. Laverdiere, J., Gomez, J. L., Cusan, L., Suburu, E. R., Diamond, P., Lemay, M., Candas, B. and Labrie, F. (1995). Beneficial effect of combination therapy administered prior and following external beam radiation in localized prostate cancer (Abstr.). *Int. J. Radiat. Oncol. Biol. Phys.*, **32** (Suppl. 1), 189

39. Duchesne, G. M., Bloomfield, D. and Wall, P. (1996). Identification of intermediate-risk prostate cancer patients treated with radical radiotherapy suitable for neoadjuvant hormone studies. *Radiother. Oncol.*, **38**, 7–12

40. Gleave, M. E., Goldenberg, S. L., Jones, E. C., Bruchovsky, N. and Sullivan, L. (1996). Biochemical and pathological effects of 8 months of neoadjuvant androgen withdrawal therapy before radical prostatectomy in patients with clinically confined prostate cancer. *J. Urol.*, **155**, 213–19

Early vs. delayed endocrine treatment of prostate cancer

32

K. H. Kurth

Screening, early detection and treatment are the central tenets of cancer control, but as yet they are unproven in prostate cancer. Central to the debate concerning the need for immediate treatment is the biological behavior of the tumor itself. Concepts regarding the natural history of prostate cancer have undergone some revision over the past years. The disease has been judged to be unpredictable with regard to its behavior and to have multiple alternatives of natural expression. Such concepts evolved in part because of the striking variance between the clinical expression and pathological prevalence of the disease[1].

When prostate cancer is clinically manifested, parameters such as prostate specific antigen (PSA), stage and tumor grade have significant predictive value with regard to the incidence of lymph node metastases[2], yet with regard to apparent clinical course a sense of variance and unpredictability has been perceived.

Undoubtedly tumor grade and tumor volume are of predictive value in estimating the potential for metastatic disease. Unfortunately, tumor volume cannot be calculated precisely by applying methods for imaging the prostatic gland, but only in radical prostatectomy specimens[3,4].

Observational studies referred to as deferred/delayed treatment or 'watchful waiting' have been, and certainly will remain for some time to come, the subject of debate. A patient who finds himself diagnosed with prostate cancer in 1996 is likely to discover that experts disagree on the best course in his particular case, especially when the tumor was detected at an early stage. Since PSA measurement

became widely available in 1986, a constant increase in the number of men diagnosed with prostate cancer has been observed. Although more cases are detected at an early stage, prostate cancers diagnosed by PSA-driven screening had an average volume of 7.12 ml[5].

Authors considering non-invasive treatment for localized disease generally excluded distant metastases (by bone scan, chest X-ray and computerized tomography (CT) scan), but the status of regional lymph nodes in the pelvis remained unknown[6-8]. Initial surveillance was followed by endocrine treatment when the tumors metastasized. Johansson and co-workers[7] followed 223 patients (mean age 72 years at diagnosis) who had localized prostate cancer T_1/T_2. At the end of 10 years, 124 patients had died, but only in 19 of them (8.5%) was death due to prostate cancer. Bone metastases developed in 12%. In this study prostatic carcinoma was poorly differentiated in only 4%. In a second Swedish study reported by Adolfsson and colleagues[8], again only T_{1-2} tumors (diagnosed by cytological aspirate – all well and moderately differentiated) were included. Of 122 patients (median age 68 years), 109 had T_2 (89%) and the tumors were well differentiated in 77 (63%).

After a median follow-up of 7.5 years, 47 patients had died, nine (7%) due to prostatic cancer, and 17 patients (14%) developed distant metastases. For patients with clinically localized tumors the disease-specific survival at 10 years was found to be 84%[8] and 85%[7]. Because of the lack of large randomized studies comparing invasive treatment (radical prostatectomy) with surveillance, decision models and meta-analyses have been performed to compare the outcomes that result from each treatment. Such a decision model was used in a study reported by Fleming and colleagues for the Prostate Patient Outcomes Research Team (PORT). Data on treatment outcomes in the existing medical literature were used to try to calculate risks and benefits of treatment for men who were older than 60 years[9]. The PORT group members concluded that for patients with well differentiated localized prostate cancer, treatment offered little benefit over 'watchful waiting', whereas for patients with moderately or poorly differentiated tumors, treatment might increase by less than 1 year the quality-adjusted life expectancy.

Chodak and co-workers[10] analyzed published data from six trials (828 patients), in which men with localized cancer (T_{1-2}) received no immediate therapy. The disease-specific survival at 10 years was 87% for patients with well or moderately differentiated tumors and 34% for patients with poorly differentiated tumors. The metastasis-free survival at 10 years was 81%, 58% and 26% for patients with well, moderately or poorly differentiated tumors, respectively.

Miles and Kattan[11] repeated the PORT analysis using the model the PORT team provided but substituting the metastatic rates for each grade with those from the series of conservatively managed patients reported by Chodak and associates[10]. The metastatic rates in the report by Chodak and co-workers were 3.3–7.8 times higher than those of the PORT analysis and, at these metastatic rates, treatment added 2.68 quality-adjusted life years for a 65-year-old man with grade 3 cancer. Furthermore, all grades would benefit from treatment and not just grades 2 and 3, as in the PORT report, regardless of quality of life adjustments (disutilities) or complications of therapy[11]. Differences between the outcomes in the PORT study and those in the report by Chodak and co-workers, who used the same model, were explained by the inclusion of a large group of pT_A patients (345 of 617 patients; 55.9%) in the PORT study. Patients with incidental prostatic carcinoma stage pT_A (less than 5% of the tissue removed

on transurethral resection of the prostate or open prostatectomy was cancer) are not representative of the patients treated for localized disease. For modelling purposes, metastatic rates of untreated patients should include only those patients who would be considered for curative therapy, i.e. those with T_{1B}, T_{1C} and T_2[11].

All studies referred to are far from definitive. The Swedish surveillance studies may be criticized because not all patients were selected randomly but chosen specifically because they had well differentiated tumors. Furthermore, a large number of patients were elderly and/or had other chronic disorders. Therefore, the conclusion drawn cannot be applied to men who have moderately or poorly differentiated cancer, who are young or who are healthy except for the presence of prostate cancer. Similarly, the study by Chodak and co-workers[10], containing mainly elderly patients, limits its applicability to younger individuals.

Recently the Medical Research Council (MRC) of the UK has launched a study to compare radical prostatectomy with radiotherapy and 'watchful waiting' in patients with localized prostatic carcinoma. The European Organization for Research and Treatment of Cancer Genitourinary Group (EORTC GU group) has adopted this study for their members. Participants, who are more in favor of either radiotherapy or radical prostatectomy, can recruit patients for a second or third option, where 'watchful waiting' is compared with only one of the aforementioned treatment forms. Many urologists – including myself – are looking forward to seeing this trial recruiting well. However, I am sceptical about whether patients of 65 years or younger are ready to accept not being cured but being treated palliatively whenever progression is documented. On the other hand, patients of 70 years or older may refuse to undergo surgery when informed that the risk of dying due to prostatic carcinoma will probably differ only marginally after either radical prostatectomy or deferred endocrine therapy. Therefore, one can only hope that the MRC trial will be conducted in a satisfactory manner and will recruit enough patients in an acceptable timeframe.

Early or delayed treatment in patients with prostatic carcinoma metastasized to the lymph nodes

Whereas 'watchful waiting' or invasive treatment are very controversially discussed treatment forms for localized prostatic carcinoma, this may be less the case for those patients with nodal disease found during staging lymphadenectomy, mostly prior to a planned radical prostatectomy. In 1986, the EORTC GU group launched a prospective trial in which patients with positive lymph nodes are randomized to either early endocrine treatment (goserelin acetate monthly and cyproterone acetate 50 mg daily during the first 4 weeks of treatment) or delayed endocrine treatment when objective progression (usually the appearance of distant metastases) is observed. For an interim period, patients refusing to be randomized could be treated according to their personal preference. Patient recruitment in the past 10 years was slow, but at a constant rate. Three centers (Rotterdam, Oslo and Amsterdam) contributed 72% of the 250 patients recruited as of September 1995. This study is still ongoing and will be closed when 320 evaluable patients are entered.

Patients in this study are followed at 3-monthly intervals during the first 2 years and every 6 months during further follow-up. Follow-up consists of physical examination, including digital rectal examination, ultrasonography of the prostate, determination of serum alkaline phosphatase, prostatic acid phosphatase (PAP) or PSA levels (the latter since 1988). Computerized tomography and bone scanning are carried out only on indication of increasing serum markers or specific complaints of the patients.

Progression is defined as the occurrence of metastases proved by bone scans and imaging. An elevation of serum markers alone is not considered as progression. While the policy of the EORTC does not allow for publication of results on a study still open for recruitment, subgroups of the patients recruited were subjects of several side-studies published recently[12-14].

The impact of ploidy on time to progression was investigated by Van den Ouden and co-workers[12]. In 87 patients (mean age 63.9 years, mean follow-up 33.4 months), in whom the ploidy of the lymph nodes and/or the primary was evaluable, the tumors were classified as diploid in 45 (52%), tetraploid in 13 (15%) and aneuploid in 29 (33%). From the 63 patients in whom the ploidy of the primary tumors was evaluable, aneuploid tumors were found in only 12 (19%), whereas the lymph nodes of 71 patients showed aneuploidy in 25 (29%). In 46 patients the ploidy of both the primary and the lymph node metastases could be obtained. Aneuploidy again was present in a higher percentage in the lymph nodes (30.4%) than in the primary (19.5%). The likelihood of aneuploidy in the lymph nodes was highest for patients with aneuploidy in the primary (89%). Aneuploid tumors were equally distributed between moderately differentiated and undifferentiated lesions.

A Cox multivariate regression analysis for the different prognostic factors for interval to progression (grade, stage, ploidy of the primary and lymph node, $</>$ 4% S phase, $</>$ 6% $G_2 + S$ phase, early or delayed treatment) revealed that therapy is the most important factor. This was the case for progression of the primary ($p = 0.0004$) and for progression to distant disease ($p = 0.005$). However, irrespective of the treatment, the ploidy of the primary tumor was significantly correlated with progression ($p = 0.01$), whereas the grade was not.

Therefore, in conclusion, stage (1982 TNM classification) and grade in the presence of lymph node metastases were not significantly correlated with interval to progression, whereas DNA ploidy (as percentage of cells in the S phase or $S + G_2$ phases of the cell cycle) and treatment indicated a significant difference for interval to progression.

In a second study, the impact of T and pN categories, grade, tumor volume and PSA level on interval to progression was studied in 61 patients with node-positive prostate cancer, and prospectively followed without adjuvant treatment. The mean patient age was 65 years, and mean follow-up 41 months (range 12–82). Again, as mentioned above, hormonal treatment was initiated only when objective progression was documented (increase of tumor volume greater than 25%, appearance of distant metastases on bone scan or soft tissue masses on CT scan). Of the 61 patients, 30 (49%) had objective progression during the study period (local or metastatic disease) and nine patients had local subjective progression (outflow obstruction, perineal pain). The median interval to progression was 18 months (range 3–45); 21 patients (54%) had metastatic progression.

A higher T stage at entry into the study was associated with an increased risk of progression ($p = 0.04$). Grade at presentation was a strong predictor of progression. When both T stage and grade were subjected to multivariate analysis, only grade remained significantly related to progression.

In 40 patients, baseline PSA levels were measured at entry into the study. The median level at entry was 37 ng/ml, range 4–360 ng/ml. The baseline level was not significantly different between patients with and without progression. At some time during the study, 53 patients had two or more PSA measurements recorded, thus allowing PSA doubling times to be calculated. The median doubling time for the entire group was 20 months, in 58% (31 patients) less than 24 months and in 26% (14 patients) longer than 60 months. Although not significantly related, doubling time was influenced by grade, with 27 months for grades 1 plus 2 and 14 months for grade 3. The 21 patients not showing progression during the observation period had a significantly greater PSA doubling time ($p < 0.0001$) than the 32 with progression (median 52 and 13 months, respectively) (Table 1).

In patients with available baseline PSA measurements, the relationship between PSA increase and progression could be calculated. When the PSA level increased 20% or more over baseline the risk of progression was 4.9 times

Table 1 PSA doubling times (medians) in patients with nodal disease left without treatment until progression. Baseline PSA level 37 ng/ml (range 4–360 ng/ml). Based on reference 13

	Doubling time (months)	Patients	
		n	%
All patients	20	53	100
	< 24	31	58
	> 60	14	26
Grades 1 plus 2	27		
Grade 3	14		
Without progression	52	21	39.7
With progression	13	32	60.3

higher than in those with no increase or < 20% increase. Interestingly, increases in PSA level of > 50%, 75% and 100% did not significantly increase the rate of progression over that of a 20% PSA increase.

From this study and other published reports[16–18], one can conclude:

(1) When left untreated, patients with nodal disease develop distant metastases after a median interval of 12 to 22 months;

(2) The expected rate of distant metastases is 65% after 3 years and 76% after 5 years;

(3) Some patients (11/61 in the study of Davidson and co-workers[13]) remain without evidence of progression for a long period (> 36 months);

(4) The likelihood of progression increases in patients with high grade and stage;

(5) The likelihood of progression is small as long as the PSA level remains stable or increases by less than 20%;

(6) Surprisingly, and in contrast to other authors, the degree of nodal involvement does not correlate with risk of progression[19–23]; and

(7) The question of whether early or delayed endocrine therapy in patients with nodal disease is associated with an advantage in survival cannot yet be answered.

Quality of life

Clinicians typically focus on outcome indicators when treating prostatic carcinoma, although relatively little systematic attention is paid to how treatment affects the quality of life.

We examined the impact of immediate or delayed treatment in patients with prostatic carcinoma stage T_{1-3}, N_{1-3}, M_0 on quality of life parameters[15]. Most patients were recruited from the aforementioned EORTC study. An extended questionnaire was constructed, containing 59 items, consisting of the EORTC Core Quality of Life Questionnaire (EORTC-QOL-C30), a global measurement of quality of life (Selby Uniscale), the IPSS, the sexual behavior questionnaire[24] and questions about the side effects of hormonal treatment. Furthermore, we examined the correlation between PSA level and quality of life parameters by comparing the results of the questionnaire of patients with different cut-off levels of PSA. A total of 47 patients participated in this study and they all completed the self-administered questionnaire twice (1994 and 1995). The comparison between the affective and the cognitive component of quality of life in prostate cancer patients with or without treatment did not show

significant differences except for psychological distress, hot flushes, erectile dysfunction and lessening of sexual activity, interest and enjoyment, all of which were more experienced by treated patients. The premise that active treatment would improve the psychological quality of life was not sustained (Table 2). The no-therapy group has better psychic and sexual functioning. Analysis of the questionnaire results of the hormonally treated patients with the use of a PSA cut-off value of 20 ng/ml showed significant differences in physical, role, emotional, cognitive and social functioning as well as the overall quality of life, fatigue, energy and sexual pleasure. The patients with a PSA level of > 20 ng/ml always showed less favorable results than patients with a PSA level of < 20 ng/ml. Analysis in the rest of the groups with respect to the various PSA cut-off values did not show significant differences in any of the items. Therefore, the main question of whether patients with nodal disease are better with treatment that is immediate or delayed to increase survival remains unanswered. However, measurement of quality of life functions reveals that untreated patients judge their condition similarly to or better than treated patients[14].

Table 2 Quality of life in patients receiving no therapy vs. hormone therapy – questionnaire 1994. From reference 15

Quality of life scale	No therapy (n = 20)	Hormone therapy (n = 27)	Student's t-test	p-Value
Physical function	93.0	86.7	1.36	NS
Role function	89.5	92.6	< 1.0	NS
Emotional function	95.6	87.9	3.25	0.002
Cognitive function	94.1	93.2	< 1.0	NS
Social function	96.7	91.4	1.28	NS
Overall quality of life	81.3	79.0	< 1.0	NS
Fatigue	11.7	16.9	< 1.0	NS
Pain	5.8	9.9	< 1.0	NS
Energy	85.2	71.0	< 1.0	NS
Erections	1.3	1.9	6.29	0.000
Sexual interest	0.8	2.0	4.25	0.000
Sexual activity	0.9	2.7	6.43	0.000
Sexual enjoyment	0.8	2.2	4.03	0.000
IPPS	8.1	7.0	< 1.0	NS
Hot flushes	2.8	39.6	6.29	0.001

NS, not significant; IPPS, International Prostate Symptom Score

References

1. Stamey, T. A. (1983). Cancer of the prostate. *Monogr. Urol.*, **4**, 68–92
2. Kleer, E., Larson-Keller, J. J., Zincke, H. and Oesterling, J. E. (1993). Ability of preoperative serum prostate specific antigen value to predict pathologic stage and DNA ploidy. *Urology*, **41**, 207–16
3. Stamey, T. A., McNeal, J. E., Freiha, F. S. *et al.* (1988). Morphometric and clinical studies on 68 consecutive radical prostatectomies. *J. Urol.*, **139**, 1235–41
4. McNeal, J. E., Kindrachuck, R. A., Freiha, F. S. *et al.* (1986). Patterns of progression in prostate cancer. *Lancet*, **1**, 60–3
5. Scardino, P. T., Weaver, R. and Hudson, M. A. (1992). Early detection of prostate cancer. *Hum. Pathol.*, **23**, 211–22
6. George, N. J. R. (1988). Natural history of localised prostatic cancer managed by conservative therapy alone. *Lancet*, **1**, 494–7
7. Johansson, J. E., Adami, H. O., Andersson, S. O. *et al.* (1992). High 10-year survival in patients with early untreated prostatic cancer. *J. Am. Med. Assoc.*, **267**, 2191–6
8. Adolfsson, J., Carstensen, J. and Löwhagen, T. (1992). Deferred treatment in clinically localized prostatic carcinoma. *Br. J. Urol.*, **69**, 183–7
9. Fleming, C., Wasson, J. H., Albertsen, P. C., Barry, M. J. and Wennberg, J. E. (1993). A decision analysis of alternative treatment strategies for clinical localized prostate cancer. Prostate Patient Outcomes Research Team. *J. Am. Med. Assoc.*, **269**, 2650–8
10. Chodak, G., Thiested, R., Gerber, G. *et al.* (1994). Outcome following conservative management of patients with clinically localized prostate cancer. *N. Engl. J. Med.*, **330**, 242–8
11. Miles, B. J. and Kattan, M. W. (1995). Computer modeling of prostate cancer: a paradigm for oncologic management? *Surg. Oncol. Clin. North Am.*, **4**, 361–72
12. Van den Ouden, D., Tribukait, B., Blom, J. H. M., Fossa, S. D., Kurth, K. H., Ten Kate, F. J. W., Heiden, T., Wang, H., Schröder, F. H. and Members of the EORTC GU group (1993). Deoxyribonucleic acid ploidy of core biopsies and metastatic lymph nodes of prostate cancer patients: impact on time to progression. *J. Urol.*, **150**, 400–6
13. Davidson, P. J. T., Hop, W., Kurth, K. H., Fossa, S. D., Waehre, H., Schröder, F. H. and the members of the EORTC GU group (1995). Progression in untreated carcinoma of the prostate metastatic to regional lymph nodes (stage T0 to 4, N1 to 3, M0, D1). *J. Urol.*, **154**, 2118–22
14. Kurth, K. H., De Reijke, T. M. and De Haes, H. (1995). Quality of life assessment in patients with prostatic carcinoma category T1-3N1-3M0, who received or did not receive hormonal treatment. *J. Urol.*, **153** (Suppl.), 238A
15. Kurth, K. H., Van Andel, G., De Reijke, T. M. and De Haes, H. (1995). Quality of life assessment in patients with prostatic carcinoma category T1-3N1-3M0, receiving or not receiving hormonal treatment. 'AMC meets Mayo' proceedings. *Excerpta Med.*, 39–40
16. De Vere White, R. (1983). Radiation and chemotherapy for stage D1 prostate cancer. *Semin. Urol.*, **1**, 261
17. Paulson, D. F., Cline, W. A., Jr, Koefoot, R. B., Jr, Hinshaw, W., Stephani, S. and Uro-Oncologic Research Group (1982). Extended field radiation therapy versus delayed hormonal therapy in node positive prostatic adenocarcinoma. *J. Urol.*, **127**, 935
18. Kramer, S. A., Cline, W. A., Jr, Farnham, R., Carson, C. C., Cox, E. B., Hinshaw, W. and Paulson, D. F. (1981). Prognosis of patients with stage D1 prostatic adenocarcinoma. *J. Urol.*, **125**, 817
19. DeKernion, J. B., Neuwirth, H., Stein, A., Dorey, F., Stenzl, A., Hannah, J. and Blyth, B. (1990). Prognosis of patients with stage D1 prostate carcinoma following radical prostatectomy with and without early endocrine therapy. *J. Urol.*, **144**, 700
20. Golimbu, M., Provet, J., Al-Askari, S. and Morales, P. (1987). Radical prostatectomy for stage D1 prostate cancer. Prognostic variables and results of treatment. *Urology*, **30**, 427
21. Steinberg, G. D., Epstein, J. I., Piantadosi, S. and Walsh, P. C. (1990). Management of stage D1 adenocarcinoma of the prostate: the Johns Hopkins experience 1974 to 1987. *J. Urol.*, **144**, 1425
22. Prout, G. R., Jr, Heaney, J. A., Griffin, P. P., Daly, J. J. and Shipley, W. U. (1980). Nodal involvement as a prognostic indicator in patients with prostatic carcinoma. *J. Urol.*, **124**, 226
23. Anscher, M. S. and Prosnitz, L. R. (1992). Prognostic significance of extent of nodal involvement in stage D1 prostate cancer treated with radiotherapy. *Urology*, **39**, 39
24. Derogatis, L. R. (1977). *The SCL-90 Manual.* (Baltimore: Johns Hopkins University Press)

Interactive Voting System

1   When you find nodal disease in your 60-year-old patient planned for radical prostatectomy, would you go on with:

Response	Option
8%	Radical prostatectomy.
22%	Orchidectomy.
9%	Both of the above.
61%	Termination of surgery and ask your patient to participate in an early vs. immediate randomized trial.

Number of votes: 95

2   Assuming your patient with nodal disease refused to be randomized and asked you for advice, what would be your preference?

54%	Immediate hormonal treatment.
46%	Delayed treatment when progression is documented.

Number of votes: 101

How to handle the patient with a rising PSA level (all stages)

33

P. J. Van Cangh

Introduction

The management of the patient with a rising level of serum prostate specific antigen (PSA) is controversial. Suggestions vary widely and common recommendations include benign negligence, watchful waiting ('wawa': initial surveillance and initiation of therapy upon appearance of symptoms)[1,2], or immediate administration of adjuvant therapy, such as endocrine or radiation treatment. Unequivocal evidence of the superiority of any one option in a given situation is bitterly lacking, and divergence of opinion is therefore common. It is not unusual for the inquisitive patient to be offered the whole spectrum of options upon presenting his unique personal data to various physicians.

Significant data are, however, available to help the puzzled patient to make an informed decision. The question eventually amounts to how to handle asymptomatic progressive cancer: what is the best timing to start treatment (earlier, at the time of diagnosis, or later, when symptoms appear), and what is the best therapeutic modality?

This review presumes that the rise of the PSA level is real and progressive, has been verified and is secondary to prostate cancer. PSA progression is considered in the following situations: (1) untreated vs. recurrent disease; and (2) localized vs. advanced cancer.

Untreated, localized prostatic cancer

Few uro-oncological subjects have been so hotly debated as the management of early prostate cancer[3]. Supporters of a delayed conservative attitude stress the benign evolution of many cases, the risk of overdiagnosis and overtreatment, and the significant incidence and severity of complications of a therapy that is of unproven value. On the other hand, equally enthusiastic defendents of early aggressive treatment advance the following arguments: (1) only localized prostate cancer can be cured; disseminated disease is incurable; (2) active treatment improves cancer-specific survival, as illustrated after radical prostatectomy (93%) vs. watchful waiting (75%); (3) early treatment decreases local and systemic progression rates; (4) the only chance of cure for high-grade cancer (g3) is radical prostatectomy when the tumor is still confined to the prostate.

Faced with this controversy, recent data on the natural history of the disease and on serum PSA kinetics are useful when treatment strategy is discussed in an individual patient with a rising PSA level. PSA is the best non-invasive marker of the extent of prostate cancer; the serum PSA level is directly related to tumor volume: 1 cm³ of cancer elevates the serum PSA level by 3.6 ng/ml, about 10 times as much as 1 cm³ of benign hypertrophy[4,5]. The patterns of chronological changes in PSA levels have been evaluated in the Baltimore Longitudinal Study of Aging, and were found to be sensitive and specific markers for the development of prostate cancer[6,7]. Although only a small number ($n = 18$) of prostate cancer patients have been followed, on a population level, they exhibited an early slow linear phase followed by a rapid exponential increase proportional to the extent of disease. PSA levels began to increase years before diagnosis, on average 7.3 years in local/regional disease and 9.2 years in advanced/metastatic disease. It took an average of ± 2 years to change from local to advanced disease. In contrast, no exponential increase was seen in men with benign prostatic hyperplasia, (BPH) who showed a gradual acceleration in the range of change in PSA level, nor in men with normal prostates who exhibited a slow linear increase. For an individual patient, however, serial PSA data were *not* predictive of tumor behavior and clinical outcome, because of the multiplicity of uncontrollable extraneous factors such as associated benign hypertrophy, inflammation, androgen levels and growth factors. Although the PSA level at diagnosis was significantly higher in the poor outcome group, a low serum PSA level or a slow doubling time did not exclude an aggressive tumor.

Therapeutic considerations

Stage T_{1A} or A_1 Scandinavian studies have shown a low (14%) progression rate of low-grade T_1 tumors in older men and a 6% cancer-specific mortality rate after 8–10 years[2]. In our series 10% of pT_{1A} patients progressed after a median of 65 months' follow-up (range 19–97)[8]. PSA data have greatly simplified the counselling of those patients and reduced the need for repeated transurethral resection of the prostate (TURP) and rebiopsy[9]. Watchful waiting is an option when the PSA level is ≤ 1 ng/ml, the digital rectal examination (DRE) si normal and the tumor is well differentiated, as the risk of progression is low[10]. Conversely, if the PSA level increases, a more aggressive therapy should be considered, especially in younger men, whose longer life expectancy increases the risk of recurrence. In addition, the presence of residual cancer and/or multifocal cancer in the peripheral zone in up to 20% of T_{1A} cases is disturbing and invites vigilance and possibly more aggressive intervention[11].

Stage T_{1B} or A_2 These patients have a high progression rate if left untreated, and should be managed positively in a similar way to the treatment for stage T_2. In our own series as many as 25% of untreated pT_{1B} patients had already progressed after a median follow-up of only 3.5 years[8].

Stage ≥ T_2 In a highly selected group of 75/4000 patients with T_2 prostate cancer managed expectantly, the overall median intervals for local progression, development of metastases and death were 78, 186 and 156 months, respectively. There was a mean interval of 108 months or 9 years to initiation of any treatment[12]. In selected older patients, watchful waiting is therefore acceptable. In the majority of patients, however, it is potentially harmful, as progression is certain, as illustrated by a short PSA doubling time[13] and a 30–50% metastatic rate at 10 years[1].

Stage T_{1C} The natural history of 'PSA-detected' prostate cancer is not well defined. As many as 50% of these are significant tumors that are locally confined when discovered, and therefore potentially curable; approximately 15% are insignificant, and 35% are advanced. By using a combination of criteria including PSA, volume and pathological findings of the needle biopsy, 73% of the insignificant tumors could be accurately predicted and become potential candidates to (very) careful 'watchful waiting'[11]. The amount of modification in the 'watched' parameters triggering a change in attitude is undetermined.

Stage $pN+ M_0$ The majority of men with untreated pN+ M0 prostate cancer progress rapidly. A small number will have stable asymptomatic disease for a prolonged period of time: i.e. those with initial low-grade low-stage cancer as well as < 20% PSA increase. In a recent series, grades 1 and 2 tumors required a median of 40 months to progress, compared to only 12 months for grade 3 tumors. Once the PSA level had increased by > 20% over baseline, the rate of progression was ± 5 times that of patients whose PSA level remained stable or increased by less than 20%[14]. It is of importance that disease progression can occur in as much as one-third of pN+ M$_0$ patients without significant PSA increase; additional diagnostic tools should be used if early detection of progression is deemed desirable[15].

After treatment for localized disease

After radical prostatectomy

After a successful cancer-eradicating radical prostatectomy, serum PSA should be *undetectable* after 3 weeks. In practice, PSA becomes undetectable in only 90% of patients with organ-confined disease, 80% with positive surgical margins and 30% with invasion of seminal vesicles and/or lymph nodes[16,17]. *Detectable* PSA after radical prostatectomy is a sensitive (but not absolute – see below) marker of persistent carcinoma and precedes clinical progression by years[17–19]. Very low levels of PSA are difficult to measure accurately, and no consensus exists on a simple definition of 'undetectable' PSA. Various threshold values have been recommended, especially since the development of new hypersensitive assays: 0.008, 0.1, 0.2, 0.3, 0.4 and 0.6 ng/ml have all been considered[20]. At the time of this writing, the significance of a very low PSA level (< 0.1 ng/ml) is unclear[21]. New technologies such as reverse transcriptase polymerase chain reaction (RT-PCR) are becoming available to help in defining the true significance of a detectable postoperative PSA level, but their value remains highly debated[22]. Extraprostatic sources of PSA are well documented, but these are unlikely to influence the serum PSA level significantly. If PSA is found to be detectable postoperatively, a safe recommendation would be to repeat the dosage and to document a progressive rise, thereby eliminating laboratory errors and technical problems such as retained benign elements.

A *rising* PSA level after radical prostatectomy is a frequent problem; in the most recent series, up to 50% of such patients will exhibit this finding in their lifetime[23,24–26]. It is an interesting albeit sobering observation that the published PSA failure rate is increasing with the length of follow-up. A documented rise in serum PSA level is a sign of failure of the radical operation, with few exceptions; in men with undetectable postoperative PSA, a persistent elevation of PSA level above 0.1 ng/ml will always continue to rise[17]. Conversely, men with persistently undetectable postoperative PSA have a good prognosis: if PSA remains undetectable at 3 years, the risk of subsequent failure is only 8%[27]. Post-prostatectomy PSA doubling time can help to predict the pattern or site of clinical failure, thereby helping in selecting therapy[25]. PSA doubling time was found to be significantly shorter in patients who experienced metastatic disease (median 4.3 months) than in those with local recurrence, or PSA elevation only (median 11.7 months)[26]. A combination of the range of change in PSA level, pathological stage and histological grade help to distinguish local vs. distant failure[25,28,29].

The time interval between elevation of PSA (> 0.1 ng/ml) and clinical progression is variable: many patients remain asymptomatic and without clinical evidence of disease for many years; the decision to treat is therefore controversial, because of the side effects of therapy and the absence of evidence that treatment prolongs survival. The median PSA (> 0.1 ng/ml) lead time is approximately 4–5 years, but varies with grade: the worse the differentiation, the shorter the PSA lead time. The mean interval between elevation of the PSA level after 1 ng/ml and clinical progression is approximately 1 year[30]. Rarely, cancer recurrence has been observed in hormonally intact patients after radical prostatectomy who have an undetectable or stable PSA level[17,31–33]. Their tumors are characterized by marked histological dedifferentiation. Such patients need diagnostic tests such as DRE and imaging studies in addition to PSA determination to achieve early diagnosis, as clinical progression precedes biochemical evidence.

Therapeutic considerations. 1. Adjuvant radiation therapy

When the PSA level rises after radical prostatectomy and local recurrence appears likely, the option of adjuvant radiation therapy must be discussed. *Advocates* insist on immediate delivery of adjuvant radiation therapy, because

46–75% of T_3 will relapse within 5 years after radical prostatectomy. Adjuvant radiation therapy has been shown to decrease and/or delay local recurrences, which in turn might be beneficial, as local control decreases the risk of secondary metastatic dissemination[18,34]. Morbidity is present, but usually mild and transient in the hands of experts, provided that treatment is delayed for 3–4 months until complete healing without stricture has occurred and continence has been regained[32].

On the other hand, *opponents* insist that not all T_3 will fail (up to 50% do not need adjuvant radiation therapy) and that small recurrences can be eradicated by irradiation, even when palpable, thereby allowing radiation therapy to be postponed until DRE becomes positive[35]. In addition, they insist on the potentially serious complications, such as impotence, incontinence, as well as bladder neck and urethral strictures. Finally, they stress the fact that so far no advantage in survival has been demonstrated, despite a decrease in the rate of local recurrences. Adjuvant radiation therapy reduces PSA sometimes to normal levels, but the response is durable in only 10–40% of patients, and only in those whose PSA level becomes undetectable. In a recent series, the failure rate at more than 2 years was 30% when PSA became undetectable after radical prostatectomy, as opposed to 80% in less than 1 year when PSA remained detectable[36].

This controversy cannot be solved at the present time and firm guidelines are not available; practical recommendations based on actual inconclusive experience are summarized hereafter. Adjuvant radiotherapy is probably *not indicated* in the following circumstances: (1) in case of high probability of systemic failure such as: (a) when the PSA level does not return to normal postoperatively, or when the PSA level rises rapidly and doubling time is short, (b) in N+ disease and (c) in seminal vesicle invasion (pT$_3$c), as these cases are usually already disseminated; (2) in case of low probability of local failure where no treatment is needed, such as: microscopic capsular penetration of Gleason score ≤ 6[35,36].

Adjuvant radiotherapy is a *valid option* when PSA becomes undetectable postoperatively and there is a high risk of persistent disease (positive margins, capsular penetration and high grade (> 6) Gleason score as radiation therapy is most effective against low-volume disease[16]. When local biopsy of the vesicourethral anastomosis is positive, most authors recommend adjuvant radiation therapy, even when systemic failure is likely[32]. In addition, if the PSA doubling time is long, adjuvant radiation therapy may be indicated even if a biopsy is negative, as a negative biopsy does not rule out the possibility of local residual disease, and the response in this selected group appears to be durable[32]. Under those circumstances, adjuvant radiation therapy led to a decrease of PSA in 90% of patients, thereby suggesting a locoregional source for the detectable PSA[37]. In the future, if radioimmunodetection holds its promise, selection may become facilitated[38].

The somewhat pessimistic and defeatist concept that regular follow-up after radical prostatectomy is superfluous, as no effective salvage therapy exists for local as well as distant recurrences, may well have to be revised. In contemporary series a larger proportion of patients are treated at an earlier stage as soon as the PSA level increases, and it is reasonable to expect definitive local control of minimal disease to be achieved with early treatment. Although no statistically significant survival advantage has been demonstrated so far, it is possible that some subgroups may benefit, possibly those with extracapsular disease and undetectable PSA postoperatively.

Ongoing randomized studies such as EORTC 22911 and INT-0086 should be encouraged.

Therapeutic considerations. 2. Adjuvant hormonal therapy Antiandrogens will delay clinical recurrence, but there is so far no evidence of survival advantage. On the other hand, pure antiandrogens have minimal side effects on the quality of life. Possible indications include failure of adjuvant radiation therapy, positive nodes (N+), and PSA progression after radical prostatectomy. Adjuvant hormonal therapy will remain controversial until a clear superiority of early vs. delayed treatment is demonstrated. The recently initiated EORTC 30943 trial will address and hopefully help to solve this dilemma.

Alternatively, new forms of hormonal therapy using 5α-reductase inhibitors are being actively pursued; preliminary results have shown a delay in PSA progression, and a possible anti-tumor effect has been postulated[39,40].

After radiation therapy

After radiation therapy, the serum PSA level reflects the presence of the irradiated prostate, consisting of normal, tumoral and adenomatous tissue in undetermined proportion. A unique definition of biochemical recurrence, or 'PSA failure', after radiation therapy is lacking; commonly reported cut-off values include (1) > 1 ng/ml; (2) above the upper limit of normal (4 ng/ml); and (3) secondary rise after a nadir has been reached[41].

The prevalence of a rising PSA level after radical radiation therapy varies from 25 to 50%, depending on patient selection and length of follow-up. When the PSA level starts rising after radiation therapy, it is progressive and a clear hallmark of recurrence in more than 90% of cases[42]. Under these circumstances, a positive prostate biopsy has been found in 70–100% of cases, and progression to metastatic disease in 50–100%, depending upon the length of follow-up. The lead time between biochemical and clinical failure is usually measured in months (mean 10–14 months) rather than in years; it is shorter for distant failure (± 10 months) than for local recurrence (± 21 months)[41,43]. Despite some controversial evidence[44], PSA doubling times appear to be equivalent after radical prostatectomy and radiation therapy; significant and equivalent differences were noted between local and distant failure, with a shorter delay in the latter[43].

The pre-treatment PSA level is an important factor predicting PSA changes after radiation therapy; 15 ng/ml is a useful cut-off value, segregating good- and poor-risk patients[45]. However,

the rate of fall does not appear to have prognostic significance. The mean time to reach the lowest PSA value (nadir-PSA) is approximately 12 months. The level of nadir-PSA also has a useful predictive value: recurrence rates amount to < 35%, 63% and 91% for undetectable nadir-PSA, PSA between 0.4 and 4 ng/ml and PSA > 4 ng/ml, respectively[42,46].

Therapeutic considerations Most patients with local progression will require one or more transurethral resections for relief of obstructive symptoms. Hormonal therapy is widely used, but is only of temporary benefit. Additional radiation therapy, by the external route or by brachytherapy, has not gained widespread popularity, due to its limited efficacy and significant morbidity. Preliminary studies on cryotherapy have demonstrated a palliative benefit, associated at times with significant morbidity.

Salvage radical prostatectomy is an option when the disease appears to be still localized. Prognostic factors and thus selection criteria have been identified: favorable characteristics include a pre-radiation stage of ≤ T₂, a Gleason score of < 7 and a PSA level of < 20 ng/ml. In a recent report, more than half of the patients with clinically localized disease (≤ T₂) and three-quarters of those with PSA failure only and no palpable evidence of local progression had pathologically confined disease, and are considered potentially cured[47]. As a whole, however, few patients benefit and the late morbidity of the procedure is not insignificant. In the Stanford experience, 99 of the 139 patients with a positive post-irradiation biopsy received a secondary treatment, and experienced a decreased survival compared to the 40 patients who were observed without further intervention[48].

Advanced disease (hormonal therapy)

First line (primary) hormonal therapy

Pre-treatment PSA level correlates with the extent of disease, not always with prognosis; although for several authors the initial PSA level is a valid prognostic index[5,10,49], and for many others it was not helpful in predicting the response to hormonal treatment, improved survival, or even prolonged disease-free survival[50]. In a recent study that included a sizeable number of patients with localized disease, treated initially with androgen ablation ($n = 245$) rather than surgery or radiotherapy, a direct correlation was found between initial PSA level and the time to PSA failure, but only in patients with localized cancer, and not in those with metastatic disease[51]. *PSA doubling time* can provide significant guidance for further therapy: it was found to be significantly shorter in patients who developed new metastases (mean 2.5 months) than those who did not (mean 7.5 months)[13,51].

PSA response to treatment is an excellent prognostic factor, with significant predictive value. The following criteria were found to be good predictors of favorable response: a return to normal, a fast rate of fall and an early achievement of nadir value (2–6 weeks). Normalization of PSA level at 3 months was the strongest prognosticator of response. In a recent study mean time to progression was 45.9, 16.7 and 12.5 months for PSA minima of < 1, between 1 and 10, and > 10 ng/ml, respectively[52]. In another similar series, in which PSA evolution was studied after androgen deprivation, a *PSA nadir* of < 1 ng/ml was of favorable prognosis in patients with localized as well as in those with metastatic disease, although fewer patients in the latter category reached such a favorably low level[51]. A low serum PSA level in patients receiving hormonal therapy must be interpreted with caution: androgen deprivation may have a direct influence on serum PSA expression, independent of an antitumor effect. A low serum PSA value cannot be taken as synonymous with absence of disease: some patients may have a serum PSA level in the normal range, despite active metastatic disease[53].

A new therapeutic perspective has emerged from the recognition of the antiandrogen withdrawal syndrome. From 15 to 40% of patients progressing on combination therapy will experience a biological as well as a clinical remission when the antiandrogen is withdrawn[54,55].

Although the exact mechanism of this phenomenon remains controversial, its therapeutic implications are obvious, suggesting the need for antiandrogen discontinuation under these circumstances, as well as for documentation of progression off antiandrogen before initiation of an alternative treatment.

Refractory (hormone-resistant) disease

A rising PSA level while receiving hormonal therapy is a sign of progression, usually preceding clinical progression by 6–12 months; this delay may represent an ideal opportunity for intervention, because of the hopefully limited volume of disease present at that time. The PSA doubling time was found to be useful for assessing progression after relapse: patients with a PSA doubling time higher than 80 days had a significantly better prognosis than those with a shorter doubling time[13].

In hormone-resistant prostate cancer, however, PSA is a less reliable marker after hormonal relapse, as normal PSA levels have been observed in 15–20% of progressing patients. A low PSA level in hormone-resistant disease may be a token of biological aggressiveness (a large amount of undifferentiated cells incapable of producing PSA). In second-line hormonal therapy and chemotherapy, PSA changes correlate with clinical outcome, but only major (> 80–90%) variations can be considered to be significant[56,57].

Arguments in favor of early hormonal therapy

Few authors systematically recommend immediate endocrine therapy in early-stage disease. In contrast, in locally advanced or disseminated cancer, strong arguments have been presented in favor of early administration of hormonal treatment. These are as follows. (1) It is preferable to treat the tumor when it is small, thereby preventing complications from uncontrolled tumor growth. (2) Current drugs have few side effects; pure antiandrogens do not reduce potency. Arguments against early treatment originating in VACURG studies (1967) are no longer valid. (3) In advanced T_3 cases, one can hope to delay progression from locally advanced to metastatic disease, even if no survival advantage can be demonstrated. (4) It is not certain that endocrine therapy does not have a beneficial impact on survival. Some studies indeed show that complete androgen suppression provides some advantage over simple castration (NCI-036 and EORTC 30853), thereby suggesting that effective hormonal treatment has a beneficial impact on survival. (5) There is no proof in clinical practice that selection of hormone-resistant clones occur. (6) If hormone-resistant cells develop from hormone-sensitive cells, then early treatment might prevent this change. (7) Patients do not understand watchful waiting; they worry about their PSA, and do not care about cost.

Arguments in favor of delayed hormonal therapy
Conversely, many authors recommend delaying treatment until the appearance of symptoms. The commonly invoked clinical arguments are: (1) many cancers do not lead to death or symptoms, and therefore need no therapy; (2) no universally accepted study definitely demonstrates a survival benefit from early vs. delayed hormonal treatment; (3) endocrine treatment provides good palliation, and palliation should only be given when there is something to palliate; (4) side effects from endocrine treatment are not insignificant, and deferred hormonal treatment offers the best quality of life. Deleterious effects of endocrine therapy are not confined to libido and sexuality, but are also manifest as hot flushes, decreased mental alertness, aggressiveness and appetite for life; (5) increased cost.

In addition, several theoretical considerations support delayed initiation of therapy. In the *adaptation model*, cells will adapt to surviving in a hormone-free milieu; hormonal treatment should therefore be withheld until symptoms demand intervention. In the *clonal selection model*, both hormone-dependent and hormone-independent cells coexist in a tumor; only the majority of hormone-dependent cells are influenced, whereas hormone-independent cells continue to grow. Early treatment selects hormone-resistant clones, and hormonal treatment becomes ineffective when needed at the time of objective or symptomatic progression. If effective chemotherapy existed for hormone-independent cells, early treatment would be advisable; as this is not so, delayed treatment is preferable. In the theory of *clonal stability and equilibrium*, prostate cancer cells grow faster in castrated than in non-castrated nude mice; secondary to hormonal therapy, competitive inhibition is lost and hormone-independent cells grow faster, as competition has disappeared; early hormonal treatment may therefore be deleterious to the patient.

Conclusion

The final answer to the original question must remain individually tailored with a major emphasis on quality of life, as no conclusive evidence of prolongation of life from early therapy exists. Thirty years later, Whitmore's aphorisms remain of actuality there is a subset of patients who progress slowly and they are going to die of other causes before their cancer progresses; another subset of patients already has metastatic disease and they will die of cancer despite all our efforts. The striving to avoid overdiagnosis as well as overtreatment must continue.

Fortunately, prognostic factors of significant disease are becoming more accurate, hopefully allowing identification of individuals at risk. The presence of neuroendocrine cells in the tumor and active angiogenesis has been correlated with prognosis. Molecular biology is thriving to isolate genes influencing growth rate and metastatic potential, as well as growth factors and/or mutations involved in the transformation of indolent into aggressive cancers. Earlier identification of micrometastases, before clinical or simple biological evidence, may be under way; radiolabelled monoclonal antibodies as well as RT-PCR appear capable of detecting circulating prostatic cells, although their real significance remains unknown[22]. Finally, prevention of prostate cancer by dietary regimen, or innovative hormonal manipulations, is being actively investigated[39,58].

Recently, 5α-reductase inhibitors have been observed to delay the rise of PSA level after radical prostatectomy and to reduce local and distant recurrences; a direct antitumor effect has been postulated. In addition, intermittent androgen ablation has theoretical as well as clinical appeal, with a probable improvement in the quality of life and a possible prolongation of prostate cancer survival[59].

Although PSA progression signifies eventual albeit sometimes remote failure, the absence of PSA progression does not rule out cancer evolution; in as many as 30% of pN+ M_0 patients and heavily hormonally treated patients, tumor continues to grow despite a stable low PSA.

Until a clear advantage has been ascertained for a specific therapy and timing of administration, answers to the title's fundamental question – outside controlled randomized studies – must be individually selected between patient and physician, based on imperfect but existing information.

References

1. Chodak, G. W., Thisted, R. A., Gerber, G. S., Johansson, J. E., Adolfsson, J., Jones, G. W., Chisholm, G. D., Moskovitz, B., Livne, P. M. and Warner, J. (1994). Results of conservative management of clinically localized prostate cancer. *N. Engl. J. Med.*, **330**, 242–8

2. Johansson, J. E., Adami, H. O., Andersson, S. O., Bergstrom, R., Holmberg, L. and Krusemo, U. B. (1992). High 10-year survival rate in patients with early, untreated prostatic cancer. *J. Am. Med. Assoc.*, **267**, 2191–6

3. Woolf, S. H. (1995). Screening for prostate cancer with prostate-specific antigen. *N. Engl. J. Med.*, **333**, 1401–5

4. Oesterling, J. E. (1991). Prostate-specific antigen: a critical assessment of the most useful tumor marker for adenocarcinoma of the prostate. *J. Urol.*, **145**, 907

5. Kabalin, J. N., McNeal, J. E., Johnstone, I. M. and Stamey, T. A. (1995). Serum prostate-specific antigen and the biologic progression of prostate cancer. *Urology*, **46**, 65–70

6. Pearson, J. D. and Carter, H. B. (1994). Natural history of changes in prostate-specific antigen in early stage prostate cancer. *J. Urol.*, **152**, 1743–8

7. Carter, H. B., Pearson, J. D., Metter, J., Brant, L. J., Chan, D. W., Andres, R., Fozard, J. L. and Walsh, P. C. (1992). Longitudinal evaluation of prostate-specific antigen levels in men with and without prostate disease. *J. Am. Med. Assoc.*, **267**, 2215–20

8. Tombal, B., Van Cangh, P. J., De Visscher, L., Lorge, F., Wese, F. X. and Opsomer, R. J. (1996). Stage A (pT1) prostate cancer: 10 years followup. *J. Urol.*, **155**, 603A

9. Carter, H. B., Partin, A. W., Epstein, J. I., Chan, D. W. and Walsh, P. C. (1990). The relationship of prostate-specific antigen levels and residual tumor volume in stage A prostate cancer. *J. Urol.*, **144**, 1167–71

10. Cooper, E. H., Armitage, T. G., Robinson, M. R. G. *et al.* (1990). Prostatic specific antigen and the prediction of prognosis in metastatic prostatic cancer. *Cancer*, **66**, 1025–8

11. Epstein, J. I., Walsh, P. C. and Brendler, C. B. (1994). Radical prostatectomy for impalpable prostate cancer: the Johns Hopkins experience with tumors found on transurethral resection (Stages T1a and T1b) and on needle biopsy (Stage T1c). *J. Urol.*, **152**, 1721–9

12. Warner, J. and Whitmore, W. F. (1994). Expectant management of clinically localized prostatic cancer. *J. Urol.*, **152**, 1761–5

13. Akimoto, S., Masai, M., Akakura, K. and Shimazaki, J. (1995). Tumor marker doubling time in patients with prostate cancer: determination of prostate specific antigen and prostatic acid phosphatase doubling time. *Eur. Urol.*, **27**, 207–12

14. Davidson, P. J., Hop, W., Kurth, K. H., Fossa, S. D., Waehre, H., Schröder, F. H. and the EORTC genitourinary group (1995). Progression in untreated carcinoma of the prostate metastatic to regional lymph nodes (Stage T0 to 4, N1 to 3, M0, D1). *J. Urol.*, **154**, 2118–22

15. Josefsen, D., Waehre, H., Paus, E. and Fossa, S. D. (1995). Increase of serum prostatic specific antigen and clinical progression in pN+ M0 prostate cancer. *Br. J. Urol.*, **75**, 502–6

16. McCarthy, J. F., Catalona, W. J. and Hudson, M. A. (1994). Effect of radiation therapy on detectable serum prostate-specific antigen levels following radical prostatectomy: early versus delayed treatment. *J. Urol.*, **151**, 1575–8

17. Lange, P. H., Ercole, C. J., Lightner, D. J., Fraley, E. E. and Vessella, R. (1989). The value of serum prostate-specific antigen determinations before and after radical prostatectomy. *J. Urol.*, **141**, 873–9

18. Frazier, H. A., Robertson, J. E., Humphrey, P. A. and Paulson, D. F. (1993). Is prostate-specific antigen of clinical importance in evaluating outcome after radical prostatectomy? *J. Urol.*, **149**, 516–18

19. Ferguson, J. K. and Oesterling, J. E. (1994). Patient evaluation if prostate-specific antigen becomes elevated following radical prostatectomy or radiation therapy. *Urol. Clin. North Am.*, **21**, 677–85

20. Prestigiacomo, A. F. and Stamey, T. A. (1995). A comparison of 4 ultrasensitive prostate-specific antigen assays for early detection of residual cancer after radical prostatectomy. *J. Urol.*, **152**, 1515–19

21. Stamey, T. A., Graves, H. C., Wehner, N., Ferrari, M. and Freiha, F. S. (1993). Early detection of residual prostate cancer after radical prostatectomy by an ultrasensitive assay for prostate-specific antigen. *J. Urol.*, **149**, 787

22. Cama, C., Olsson, C. A., Raffo, A. J., Perlman, H., Buttyan, R., O'Toole, K., McMahon, D., Benson, M. C. and Katz, A. E. (1995). Molecular staging of prostate cancer. II. A comparison of the application of an enhanced reverse transcriptase polymerase chain reaction assay for prostate specific antigen versus prostate specific membrane antigen. *J. Urol.*, **153**, 1373–8

23. Hale, B. D., Kaplan, C. R., Keane, T. E., Petros, J. A. and Graham, S. D. (1994). Value of prostate-specific antigen levels in detecting recurrences after radical prostatectomy (Abstr. 118). *J. Urol.*, **151**, 257A

24. D'Amico, A. V., Whittington, R., Malkowicz, S. B., Schultz, D., Schnall, M., Tomaszewski, J. E. and Wein, A. (1995). A multivariate analysis of clinical and pathological factors that predict for prostate-specific antigen failure after radical prostatectomy for prostate cancer. *J. Urol.*, **154**, 131–8

25. Partin, A. W., Pearson, J. D., Landis, P. K., Carter, H. B., Pound, C. R., Clemens, J. Q., Epstein, J. I. and Walsh, P. C. (1994). Evaluation of serum prostate-specific antigen velocity after radical prostatectomy to distinguish local recurrence from distant metastases. *Urology*, **43**, 649–59

26. Trapasso, J. G., Dekernion, J. B., Smith, R. B. and Dorey, F. (1994). The incidence and significance of detectable levels of serum prostate-specific antigen after radical prostatectomy. *J. Urol.*, **152**, 1821–5

27. Stein, A., deKernion, J. B., Smith, R. B., Dorey, F. and Patel, H. (1992). Prostate-specific antigen levels after radical prostatectomy in patients with organ confined and locally extensive prostate cancer. *J. Urol.*, **147**, 942

28. Bangma, C. H., Blijenberg, B. G. and Schröder, F. H. (1995). Single and serial PSA determinations in the detection and follow up of prostatic cancer. *Eur. Urol. Update Ser.*, **4**, 2–7

29. Weldon, V. E., Travel, F. R., Neurwirth, H. and Cohen, R. (1995). Patterns of positive specimen margins and detectable prostate-specific antigen after radical perineal prostatectomy. *J. Urol.*, **153**, 1565–9

30. Bentvelsen, F. M., Van den Ouden, D. and Schröder, F. H. (1993). Prostate-specific antigen in screening for recurrence following radical prostatectomy for localized prostatic cancer. *Br. J. Urol.*, **72**, 88–91

31. Goldrath, D. E. and Messsing, E. M. (1989). Prostate-specific antigen: not detectable despite tumor progression after radical prostatectomy. *J. Urol.*, **142**, 1082–4

32. Takayama, T. K. and Lange, P. H. (1994). Radiation therapy for local recurrence of prostate cancer after radical prostatectomy. *Urol. Clin. North Am.*, **21**, 687–700

33. Oefelein, M. G., Smith, N., Carter, M., Dalton, D. and Schaeffer, A. (1995). The incidence of prostate cancer progression with undetectable serum prostate-specific antigen in a series of 394 radical prostatectomies. *J. Urol.*, **154**, 2128–31

34. Haab, F., Meulemans, A., Boccon-Gibod, L., Dauge, M. C., Delmas, V., Hennequin, C., Benbunan, D. and Boccan-Gibod, L. (1995). Effect of radiation therapy after radical prostatectomy on serum prostate-specific antigen measured by an ultrasensitive assay. *Urology*, **45**, 1022–7

35. Gibbons, R. P. and Jonsson, E. (1995). Adjuvant radiation therapy following radical prostatectomy for pathologic stage C prostate cancer. *Eur. Urol.*, **27** (Suppl. 2), 24–5

36. Coetzee, L. J., Hars, V. and Paulson, D. F. (1995). Postoperative prostate-specific antigen as a prognostic indicator in patients with margin-positive prostate cancer, undergoing adjuvant radiotherapy after radical prostatectomy. *Urology*, **47**, 232–5

37. Lange, P. H., Lightner, D. J., Medini, E. and Reddy, P. K. (1990). The effect of radiation therapy after radical prostatectomy in patients with elevated prostate-specific antigen levels. *J. Urol.*, **144**, 917–20

38. Kahn, D., Miller, S., Gerstbrein, J., Maguire, R. and Williams, R. D. (1995). Accuracy of In-111 capromab pendetide Mab scan for detecting

prostate fossa tumor recurrence following radical prostatectomy. *J. Urol.*, **153**, 519A

39. Andriole, G., Lieber, M., Smith, J., Soloway, M., Schroeder, F., Kadmon, D., De Kernion, J., Rajfer, J., Boake, R., Crawford, D., Ramsey, E., Perreault, J., Trachtenberg, J., Fradet, Y., Block, N., Middleton, R., Ng, J., Ferguson, D. and Gormley, G. (1995). Treatment with finasteride following radical prostatectomy for prostate cancer. *Urology*, **45**, 491–7

40. Bologna, M., Muzi, P., Biordi, L., Festuccia, C. and Vicentini, C. (1995). Finasteride dose-dependently reduces the proliferation rate of the LnCap human prostatic cancer cell line *in vitro*. *Urology*, **45**, 282–90

41. Van Cangh, P. J. and Richard, F. (1994). Prostate-specific antigen after definitive radiation therapy. *Curr. Opin. Urol.*, **4**, 256–60

42. Zagars, G. K. and Von Eschenbach, A. C. (1993). Prostate-specific antigen: an important marker for prostate cancer treated by external beam radiation therapy. *Cancer*, **72**, 538–48

43. Fowler, J. E., Pandey, P., Braswell, N. T. and Seaver, L. E. (1994). Prostate-specific antigen progression rates after radical prostatectomy or radiation therapy for localized prostate cancer. *Surgery*, **116**, 302

44. Stamey, T. A., Ferrari, M. K. and Schmid, H. P. (1993). The value of serial prostate-specific antigen determinations 5 years after radiotherapy: steeply increasing values characterize 80% of patients. *J. Urol.*, **150**, 1856–9

45. Teshima, T., Hanlon, A. M. and Hanks, G. E. (1995). Pretreatment prostate-specific antigen values in patients with prostate cancer: 1989 patterns of care study process survey. *Int. J. Rad. Oncol. Biol.*, **33**, 809–14

46. Zagars, G. K. (1994). Prostate-specific antigen as an outcome variable for T1 and T2 prostate cancer treated by radiation therapy. *J. Urol.*, **152**, 1786–91

47. Lerner, S. E., Blute, M. L. and Zincke, H. (1995). Critical evaluation of salvage surgery for rdio recurrent resistant prostate cancer. *J. Urol.*, **154**, 1103–9

48. Bagshaw, M. A., Cox, R. S. and Hancock, S. L. (1994). Control of prostate cancer with radiotherapy: long term results. *J. Urol.*, **152**, 1781–5

49. Matzkin, H., Eber, P., Todd, B., van der Zwaag, R. and Soloway, M. (1992). Prognostic significance of changes in prostate-specific markers after endocrine treatment of stage D2 prostatic cancer. *Cancer*, **70**, 2302–9

50. Petros, J. A. and Andriole, G. L. (1993). Serum PSA after antiandrogen therapy. *Urol. Clin. North Am.*, **20**, 749–55

51. Fowler, J. E., Pandey, P., Seaver, L. E., Feliz, T. P. and Braswell, N. T. (1995). Prostate-specific antigen regression and progression after androgen deprivation for localized and metastatic prostate cancer. *J. Urol.*, **153**, 1860–5

52. Riedl, C. D., Huebner, W. A., Mossig, H., Ogris, E. and Pflueger, H. (1995). Prognostic value of prostate-specific antigen minimum after orchidectomy in patients with stage C and D prostatic carcinoma. *Br. J. Urol.*, **76**, 34–40

53. Leo, M. E., Bilhartz, D. L., Bergstralh, E. J. and Oesterling, J. E. (1991). Prostate-specific antigen in hormonally treated stage D2 prostate cancer: is it always an accurate indicator of disease status? *J. Urol.*, **145**, 802–6

54. Scher, H. I. and Kelly, W. K. (1993). Flutamide withdrawal syndrome: its impact on clinical trials in hormone-refractory prostate cancer. *J. Clin. Oncol.*, **11**, 1566–72

55. Small, E. J. and Srinivas, S. (1995). The antiandrogen withdrawal syndrome: experience in a large cohort of unselected patients with advanced prostate cancer. *Cancer*, **76**, 1428–34

56. Fossa, S. D., Waehre, H. and Paus, E. (1992). The prognostic significance of prostate-specific antigen in metastatic hormone-resistant prostate cancer. *Br. J. Cancer*, **66**, 181–4

57. Matzkin, H. and Soloway, M. S. (1992). Response to second-line hormonal manipulation monitored by serum PSA in stage D2 prostate cancer. *Urology*, **40**, 78–80

58. Thompson, I., Coltman, C. A., Brawley, O. W. and Ryan, A. (1995). Chemoprevention of prostate cancer. *Semin. Urol.*, **13**, 122–9

59. Goldenberg, S. L., Bruchovsky, M., Gleave, M. E., Sullivan, L. D. and Akakura, K (1995). Intermittent androgen suppression in the treatment of prostate cancer: a preliminary report. *Urol.*, **45**, 839–44

Interactive Voting System

1   I know my serum PSA level.

Response	*Option*
24%	Yes.
76%	No.

Number of votes: 99

2   I wish I knew my serum PSA level.

29%	Yes.
71%	No.

Number of votes: 84

Radical prostatectomy in the treatment of locally confined prostate cancer: issues defined

34

R. P. Myers

Is cure necessary?

Willet F. Whitmore Jr, 1988[1]

New data for 1996 reveal in the United States an estimated 317 100 new prostate cancer diagnoses and 41 400 expected deaths[2]. Every year in the recent past, both of these values have risen. In 1980, the values were 66 000 new cases and 22 000 deaths[3]. The age-adjusted death rate per 100 000 population has risen from 14.5 in 1974–75 to 17.5 in 1990–93. The more than doubling in new cases is directly attributable to several factors: (1) increased public awareness about the prevalence of prostate cancer; (2) the use of serum prostate specific antigen (PSA) in screening, despite no consensus to do so; and (3) greater impetus among physicians to diagnose prostate cancer, because a case has been established that there may be benefit from early diagnosis. The plethora of articles about localized prostate cancer and what to do about it reflect (1) its widespread prevalence; (2) its virtually unpredictable threat in many individuals; (3) controversy as to the best therapy, for example, radical prostatectomy, radiation, or watchful waiting; (4) the quality of life if treated; and (5) the lifetime cost of diagnosis and treatment, i.e. its economic impact.

When Whitmore[1] emphasized the virtually identical 15-year survivals for stage B (T_{2A}) nodule cancer, whether treated aggressively or conservatively, and furthermore noted that treatment has not diminished the mortality from prostate cancer, as evidenced above in a rising age-adjusted death rate, he brilliantly asked his two now famous questions:

(1) Is cure necessary in those in whom it is possible?

(2) Is cure possible in those in whom it is necessary?

Background

Historically, the majority of prostate cancer patients presented with advanced disease, a phenomenon still true in countries that do not conduct the same level of diagnostic vigilance practiced currently in the United States. The breakdown of the original Veteran's Administration Cooperative Urological Research Group (VACURG) patient population of 2316, as reported in 1967 for stages I, II, III and IV was 5.2%, 7.7%, 47.9% and 39.2%, respectively, comprising 74% of all previously untreated patients with prostate cancer[4]. (Not included were 26% because of health that was too poor for study, secondary malignancy, or lack of co-operation in a randomized protocol.) In that era of the mid-1960s and before, relatively few patients were identified as candidates for potentially curative therapy such as radical prostatectomy; it took a positive biopsy after suspicious digital rectal examination, and then severely limiting criteria for operation, that is low grade 1 or 2 cancer with nodules no larger than 1–1.5 cm[5,6].

The VACURG study heightened public awareness about prostate cancer, because a shift occurred to finding a far greater percentage with apparently localized cancer. Evidence for this comes in 1970–73 data, revealing the stage at diagnosis as local (61%), regional (13%) or distant (21%)[3]. Little change is evident roughly 15 years later in 1986–91 data[2]: local (57%), regional (17%) and distant (14%). (Sites do not add up to 100%, because of insufficient information.) Both of these distributions stand in vivid contrast to the VACURG patients, in whom only 13% had apparently organ-confined disease at diagnosis. With many more patients found with 'local' disease, the 1970s and 1980s saw a jump in candidates for radical prostatectomy as well as radiotherapy, and interest in radical prostatectomy took a particular significant boost from the introduction by Walsh and colleagues[7] of the cavernous nerve-preserving radical retropubic prostatectomy, which emphasized an extraordinary anatomic dissection. In the United States, the rate of radical prostatectomy increased 5.75 times from 1984 to 1990[8]. From the mid-1960s onward, the criteria for operation became progressively liberalized, from strict guidelines as to nodule size, to no more than half a gland[9], to a state that has included virtually any stage of cancer in mobile ('operable') prostate glands[10]. Neither early clinical stage C[11,12] nor stage D_1 (T_1–T_3 N_1 M_0)[13] have been a deterrent, despite significant controversy.

The trend (maintained) towards early diagnosis afforded by both the VACURG studies and Walsh's operation was given another significant lift from the rapidly increasing use of PSA and publicity with respect to PSA screening, beginning at the end of the 1980s. The proportion of patients with non-palpable stage T_{1C} coming to radical prostatectomy has steadily increased to almost 30% (M. L. Blute, unpublished data). Furthermore, these are being identified in a much younger and healthier patient population with longer life expectancy, which is now ripe for testing the hypothesis that early intervention with curative intent, for example radical prostatectomy, can reduce progression to metastatic disease and mortality from prostate cancer. In two studies, PSA testing has resulted in significant lead times of 5.5 and 6.7 years, respectively, with regard to much earlier diagnosis[14,15]. The eventual outcome of these T_{1C} patients treated with curative intent[16,17], the majority of whom have been diagnosed and treated in the 1990s, is not accounted for in current statistical projections. Of additional note is the observation that the incidence of unsuspected lymph node metastases has dropped dramatically in patients who elect to undergo radical prostatectomy, presumably on the basis of more aggressive diagnosis[18].

Controversy

The increase in diagnosis and use of radical prostatectomy as opposed to conservative therapy has been met with significant counter-argument in numerous Markov model decision analyses, quality of life 'disutility' outcomes and epidemiological studies[19–23]. Despite an excellent study showing exactly the opposite conclusion (more than 90% of prostate cancers identified by PSA 'appeared to be serious cancers in terms of tumor volume and/or grade'[24], there is the counter-concept that PSA screening might overdiagnose too many cancers that would otherwise be insignificant during the lifetime of many patients[25]. This concept of overdiagnosis of non-threatening cancers provides impetus for the conservative, economically advantageous program of 'watchful waiting': (1) because radical prostatectomy and radiotherapy have not been proven by prospective, randomized study to be superior; and (2) because quality of life is 'better', owing to the absence of specific risks of therapy, such as urinary incontinence and impotence, or even such frightening prospects as perioperative mortality. In a consideration of quality of life, radical prostatectomy was shown to be of marginal benefit when the Patient Prostate Outcomes Research Team (PORT) study[20] showed 'quality-adjusted life years' for well-, moderately and poorly differentiated disease as −0.34, +0.33 and +1.00 years, respectively. That is, there was very little gain from operating, and a negative result for well-differentiated cancer. Parenthetically, it is just such well-differentiated nodule cases that formed Culp's basic criteria for operation[5] and for which Whitmore found no impact in terms of 15-year survival, whether the patient underwent operation or not[1]. From the PORT data, the gleam of slightly increased quality-of-life years is present, but limited to those with moderate or poorly differentiated cancer, which, as importantly noted below, make up the preponderant proportion of cases of localized cancer.

The PORT study was subsequently criticized for the following reasons: (1) progression and metastatic rates were unreasonably 'low-end'; (2) treatment 'disutilities' were improperly weighted, e.g. incontinence was given greater weight than metastatic disease; and (3) perhaps most significantly the patient groups studied were not contemporary[26,27]. Radical prostatectomy was shown to improve considerably with respect to additional quality-of-life years when more realistic metastatic rates from Chodak and colleagues[28] and progression rates from Baylor[26] were substituted into the PORT scheme (Table 1). Importantly, there are 'PORT II' studies currently in progress to introduce contemporary series of patients into the PORT model (M. L. Blute, unpublished data).

It is pertinent that quality-of-life models need to include health-related quality of life, including the psychosocial consequences of having cancer[23,28]. Patient insecurity can be a significant disutility of watchful waiting. As Hall[29] stated 'The knowledge of harboring untreated cancer is an intolerable burden for some men'. While it is easy for a panel of 'experts' to give a high 'disutility' to the side effects of radical

Table 1 Quality-adjusted life years for radical prostatectomy, seen to improve for well-(WD), moderately (MD) and poorly (PD) differentiated cancer over PORT results[20] after more realistic data are substituted from Chodak and colleagues[28] or Baylor[26]. Data obtained from Beck and co-workers[26]

Grade	Port	Chodak et al	Baylor
WD	−0.34	+1.01	+1.81
MD	+0.33	+2.41	+2.94
PD	+1.00	+2.68	+2.34

prostatectomy, patients do not always feel the same way. In a published testimonial, Howe[30] exclaimed, 'I am satisfied with my decision to undergo radical surgery and am more than willing to live with the side effects in return for an apparent cure'. In a United States Medicare opinion survey[31] ($n = 731$), 86% were delighted, please, or mostly satisfied with surgery, and, in 217 of 757 (28.7%) wearing pads or clamps for urinary incontinence, 68% were positive about results with 86% saying they would choose surgery again. In the office setting, most patients with prostate cancer present as desperate human beings. They look for cure of their affliction, and *curative effort is appreciated even if the effort, in the end, is not curative*. They want something done and are intensely skeptical about 'watching it'. For patients confronted with a decision about their localized disease, the possibility of complete cure by radical prostatectomy is very powerful and compelling when weighed against the insecurity of living with cancer posed by watchful waiting. What surgery offers that no other treatment confers is the immensely satisfying concept, both to the surgeon and to the patient, of possible complete excision. Watchful waiting entails unnerving symbiosis, and radiotherapy with 80% at risk for biochemical failure within 5 years involves a similar live-with-cancer, hope-radiotherapy-works anxiety, with only 20% achieving long-term control[32]. Hanks and colleagues[33] were slightly more 'encouraging' with 61% and 50% biochemical failure at 5 years for conventional and conformal radiotherapy, respectively. In fairness, biochemical failure does not necessarily translate into clinical failure, and androgen deprivation is available as follow-up treatment to retard disease progression. Whether radiotherapy provides clonagenic advantage to radioresistant subpopulations with an accelerated growth rate remains unsettled[32,33].

Comorbidity

There is no question that comorbidity or potentially life-threatening disease other than prostate cancer increases with age and affects the choice of treatment. In a recent population-based study from the Connecticut Tumor Registry (CTR) with mean follow-up of 15.5 years, comorbidity was a powerful independent predictor of survival[32–34]. Furthermore, the age-adjusted survival for patients aged 65–75 treated conservatively was no different for the general population if they had Gleason score 2–4 tumors. This information and Swedish data[35], heavily skewed to indolent cancer in older patients, have become grist for condemning radical prostatectomy. It is of special note that the CTR lost-life expectancy was 4–5 years for Gleason score 5–7, and 6–8 years for Gleason score 8–10. The CTR study would be particularly meaningful from the standpoint of cost and quality of life, and argues for conservative therapy if a significant number of patients aged 65–75 had had low-stage, low-grade organ-confined cancer, but only 44 of 451 or 9.7% fit this profile, leaving 290 of 451 (64.3%) with potentially life-limiting disease, had they no competing comorbidity. In patients with estimated 10-year survival and without significant comorbidity, this study argues for aggressive therapy with curative intent and against watchful waiting for patients with Gleason scores 5–10 in the age range 65–75. The preponderance of cases in the moderately to poorly differentiated category (64.2%) in the CTR study is of significant contrast to Johannson's Örebro study[35] of 223 patients with 148 or 66.4% grade 1, 29.6% grade 2 and 4% grade 3, i.e. a gross aberration from typical United States clinical practice.

Significant vs. insignificant cancer

In the United States, patients with low Gleason score undergoing surgery at responsible institutions represent a very thin percentage of the total patients population. A recent Mayo Clinic study[36] of 337 radical prostatectomy patients carefully assessed by whole-mount step section demonstrated Gleason scores of 4 in 3%, 5–6 in 33.5% and 7–9 in 63.6%. Therefore, 97% fit the CTR study criteria[34] for life-limiting Gleason score disease. Furthermore, based on: (1) 1990 Life Table analysis; (2) a range of assumed dou-

bling times at 2, 3, 4 and 6 years; and (3) Gleason score, all men under age 60 ($n = 69$) had potentially significant cancer. Assuming a doubling time of 4 years or less, 91.5% of men aged 60–69 ($n = 175$) and 89.3% of those aged 70–79 ($n = 93$) had potentially significant cancer and were considered to be treated appropriately by surgery. Parenthetically, it is important to state in general that these Mayo patients were healthy and selected over a wide age range without, in general, significant competing comorbidity, and their apparent life expectancy exceeded normal expectation.

Surgeons are clearly motivated to operate upon what they consider to be significant cancer. Stamey and colleagues[37] have defined significant cancer in terms of volume greater than 0.5 cm^3 without using life-table analysis or Gleason score. Taking into consideration age, allowable Gleason score as a function of decade of life and a range of assumed doubling times, one can construct a table of insignificant cancer volumes (Table 2). Tumor volumes of less than 0.5 cm^3 may be significant, depending upon age at diagnosis, Gleason score and assumed doubling time. The clinician's dilemma is the inability accurately to predict tumor volume before surgery in any individual patient. Digital rectal examination, percentage of cores and number of cores containing cancer, preoperative PSA level, PSA density and ultrasound volume of cancer have all been used to defined insignificant cancer[16,37–40]. Even

Table 2 Volumes of cancer (cm^3) that define insignificant cancer at three different doubling times, taking into account age at four different decades. Any cancer of volume greater than tabulated value would be considered significant cancer for that doubling time. As years of life expectancy decrease, allowable Gleason score (GS) increases as a function of decade. Data adapted from Dugan and colleagues[36]

Age	Years	GS	Doubling time		
			2 year	4 year	6 year
50	26	< 5	0	0	1
60	18	< 6	0	1	2
70	12	< 7	0	2	5
80	7	< 8	2	6	9

magnetic resonance images with endorectal coil providing sharp detail (Figure 1) and a means for volume determination for unifocal, well-defined lesions, fail to provide certainty with respect to volume or extracapsular extension of cancer. Furthermore, multifocality and/or high-grade, infiltrative cancers make any

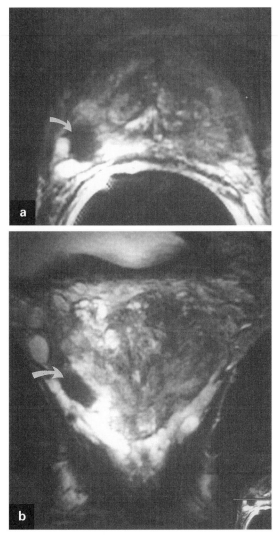

Figure 1 Endorectal coil magnetic resonance image (MRI) of prostate with well circumscribed cancer (arrow). (a) axial plane – lesion peripheral right; (b) coronal plane with axial inset. This lesion on examination of the radical prostatectomy specimen was intracapsular, even though it appears not to be, in the MRI. Two other focal cancers in this prostate were not apparent on MRI

sensible estimate of tumor volume virtually impossible. Because insignificant volume cannot be identified preoperatively, patients cannot be excluded from surgery on the basis of any currently reliable means to assess volume.

One of the limitations of the Mayo study[36] was the assumption of linear growth in each doubling time category. Insignificant cancer was defined as a lesion not expected to reach 20 cm^3 during the expected life of the patient based on 1990 life tables; 20 cm^3 was chosen as the level on average associated with metastasis. The assumption of linear growth may have been too conservative by failing to allow for malignant degeneration; the actual numbers of significant cancers may have been even greater. Malignant degeneration both in histology and change in ploidy has been established[41] and led Whitmore[42] in 1990 to remark, 'Since progression of grade and ploidy occurs with increasing tumor volume, it is logical to treat the tumor at earliest recognition'.

Radical prostatectomy in 1996

It is widely recognized and sad that there are no valid contemporary, prospective, randomized trials with published long-term results comparing the efficacy of surgery (radical prostatectomy) to either radiation or watchful waiting. Retrospective comparisons are statistically invalid. The survey[43] in which the Mayo Clinic 15-year disease-specific survival after radical prostatectomy[44] is compared with Stanford radiotherapy[45] for the same endpoint is primarily of interest. That the differences are truly real cannot be established from data obtained retrospectively. With respect to radical prostatectomy, disease-specific 15-year survivals at 93%, 82% and 71% for Gleason score groups 2–3, 4–6 and 7–10, respectively, make surgery inviting as a treatment choice for operable localized disease in selected patients. The 'comparable' 15-year Stanford radiotherapy survivals stand at 85%, 60% and 40% for the same three Gleason score groupings.

If patients with apparently organ-confined disease are in otherwise good health with expected survival of at least 10 years, and the operation is performed with skill, urinary incontinence should be negligible, potency can be managed if not saved and mortality should be virtually non-existent. In the absence of comorbidity, no other treatment to date has been shown to provide higher probability for cure or freedom from metastases than radical prostatectomy. Hospitalization has been reduced to a matter of a few days[46]. Lifetime hospitalization for patients treated initially by radical prostatectomy has not been reported. The burden posed by conservative therapy is substantial[47], and the need for hospital care (average of 5 weeks) due to prostate cancer for patients treated expectantly with non-curative intent is of serious concern[48]. It would be pertinent to show, as might be possible, that the life-time cost associated with definitive therapy is significantly less than that of expectant management.

Candidates for surgery also include patients in whom external beam radiotherapy has failed, and those who have biopsy-proven cancer, progressively rising PSA levels and established satisfactory continence zones; these patients comprise a subset undergoing 'salvage' radical prostatectomy; urinary incontinence presents significant morbidity[49].

Limitations of radical prostatectomy

Radical prostatectomy is eminently successful for small organ-confined cancer that has no metastatic potential at the time the prostate is removed. Risk factors for failure have been analyzed[50,51]. Failure increases with increasing tumor volume, which is reflected in both clinical and pathological stage, local lymph node metastasis and preoperative serum PSA level. The greater the volume the more likely there will be seminal vesicle involvement, which has been associated with poor prognosis. However, in multivariate analysis using the Cox proportional hazards model, four risk factors, which clearly independently and adversely affect prognosis, include preoperative serum PSA level, histology (Gleason score), a non-diploid number of chromosomes and microvessel density

(angiogenesis)[52]. The reason that these four variables are so powerful is that they appear to be most closely associated with metastasis. Large volume of cancer, advanced local stage, seminal vesicle involvement and positive surgical margins are not necessarily associated with poor prognosis, because they are not always associated with metastatic disease. In multivariate analysis, they do not generally achieve a level of statistical significance when the above four independent risk factors are considered.

Attempts have been made to improve the outlook for patients undergoing elective radical prostatectomy by a program of preoperative androgen deprivation (neo-adjuvant therapy)[53–55], but long-term follow-up is lacking with regard to lowering the incidence of biochemical relapse, i.e. rising PSA level. Maximal apoptotic regression may take 8 months of androgen deprivation prior to surgery[56]. Skeptics may say that the only effect is to make a fat octopus into a skinny one; the legs are still there in unrecognizable, dormant pyknotic nuclei just waiting for androgen stimulation.

Whether the prostate is taken out retropubically or perineally, the process is an exacting anatomic challenge. Because the prostate is closely invested by the levator ani laterally, the dorsal vein complex anteriorly, the rectum posteriorly, the bladder superiorly and the membranous urethra with its striated sphincter distally, there is really very little leeway for so-called 'wide' resection. Margins are a matter of millimeters from critical abutting tissue that is best spared as much as possible. There is a fine line between preserving function, urinary continence and potency, the latter when indicated, on the one hand, and negative margins of resection on the other. Tissues must be manipulated with exceptional care. Hemostasis is essential for satisfactory visualization and dissection. Surgeons must be very carefully trained, skilled with the use of their instruments and fully knowledgeable about individual anatomic variation and how to cope with it. On the wall of the Anatomy Museum in Basel, Switzerland, there is a plaque that quotes Tiedemann, 'Ärzte ohne Anatomie gleichen Maulwürfen: sie arbeiten im

Dunklen, und ihrer Hände Tagewerk sind-Erd-hügel', i.e. 'Surgeons without (knowledge of) anatomy are like moles; they work in the dark and create piles of dirt'. Time and experience are great allies in the quest for good results. The morbidity of contemporary radical prostatectomy has decreased dramatically as the operation becomes increasingly refined[57]. Lack of operative skill and experience can be the most serious obstacle to successful radical prostatectomy.

Conclusion

In summary, if we ignore the psychologically detrimental thought of living with cancer posed by conservative therapy, current studies tell us that the value of radical prostatectomy is inversely proportional to age and increasing co-morbidity, for example, cardiovascular disease. The risk of dying of prostate cancer is substantial for localized disease[58–60], but depends directly on the characteristics of the patient population. Patients are diagnosed over a wide age range and with variable comorbidity and aspirations about quality of life. As Whitmore so succinctly put it, 'There is no single best method of treatment for all patients'[1]. Currently, the emphasis is directed towards identifying cancer in young men at a time when cure may be possible, in the previously unobtainable 'window of opportunity', beyond which delayed diagnosis results in reduced life expectancy from prostate cancer death. It is widely recognized that efforts must be directed towards finding significant organ-confined disease of such a nature that prostate removal can be accomplished without loss of either urinary control or potency, or any other diminution in quality of life. This does not mean that the same care and concern should not be extended to older patients; it is just that with increasing age considerations change, other competing diseases creep into the equation and the treatment choices must be tailored after frank discussion with the patient concerning the pluses and minuses of the different treatment strategies.

As a final sobering note, questions of therapy including surgery for localized disease could become moot in the face of discovery of practical chemoprevention[61] or genetic modulation of tumor growth as demonstrated recently *in vitro* for breast and ovarian tumor cell lines by retroviral transfer of the wild-type *BRCA1* gene[62]. Active research of tumor or metastasis suppressor genes on chromosomes 11, 12 and 17, with a 17q site distal to *BRCA1* in prostate cancer recently identified[63], holds promise for future novel therapies for prostate cancer, a disease so very complex from the standpoint of genetic and epigenetic factors.

It is fitting that this overview end with a quotation from that most wonderful and engaging teacher to us all, Willet Francis Whitmore Jr (see below), so gifted in capturing in words and speech the essence of the issues related to prostate cancer, whose life was consumed by the very

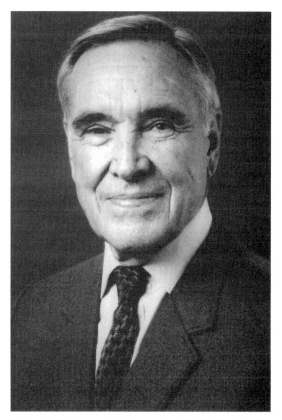

Willet F. Whitmore, Jr. December 13, 1917 – May 8, 1995

disease of which we speak, and to whom this manuscript is dedicated. In 1956, or 40 years ago, he wrote poignantly, 'The general aim of treatment is to prolong life with comfort when possible, and at the least to provide comfort if life cannot be prolonged'[64].

References

1. Whitmore, W. F. Jr (1988). Clinical management of prostate cancer. *Am. J. Clin. Oncol.*, **11** (Suppl. 2), S88–S97

2. Parker, S. L., Tong, T., Bolden, S. and Wingo, P. A. (1996). Cancer statistics, 1996. *CA Cancer J. Clin.*, **65**, 5–27

3. Silverberg, E. (1980). Cancer statistics, 1980. *CA Cancer J. Clin.*, **30**, 23–38

4. Veteran Administration Cooperative Urological Research Group (1967). Carcinoma of the prostate: treatment options. *J. Urol.*, **98**, 516–22

5. Culp, O. S. (1968). Radical perineal prostatectomy: its past, present, and possible future. *J. Urol.*, **98**, 618–26

6. Jewett, H. J., Bridge, R. W., Gray, G. F. Jr and Shelley, W. M. (1968). The palpable nodule of prostatic cancer. *J. Am. Med. Assoc.*, **203**, 115–18

7. Walsh, P. C., Lepor, H. and Eggleston, J. C. (1983). Radical prostatectomy with preservation of sexual function: anatomical and pathological considerations. *Prostate*, **4**, 473–85

8. Lu-Yao, G. L., McLerran, D., Wasson, J. and Wennberg, J. E. (1993). An assessment of radical prostatectomy: time trends, geographic variations and outcomes. *J. Am. Med. Assoc.*, **269**, 2633–6

9. Jewett, H. J. (1975). The present status of radical prostatectomy for Stages A and B prostatic cancer. *Urol. Clin. North Am.*, **2**, 105–24

10. Hudson, H. C. and Howland, R. L. Jr (1972). Radical retropubic prostatectomy for cancer of the prostate. *J. Urol.*, **108**, 944–7

11. Tomlinson, R. L., Currie, D. P. and Boyce, W. H. (1977). Radical prostatectomy: palliation for Stage C carcinoma of the prostate. *J. Urol.*, **117**, 85–7

12. Cheng, W. S., Frydenberg, M., Bergstralh, E. J., Larson-Keller, J. J. and Zincke, H. (1993). Radical prostatectomy for pathologic stage C prostate cancer: influence of pathologic variables and adjuvant treatment in disease outcome. *Urology*, **42**, 283–91

13. Zincke, H., Bergstralh, E. J., Larson-Keller, J. J., Farrow, G. M., Myers, R. P., Lieber, M. M., Barrett, D. M., Rife, C. C. and Gonchoroff, N. J. (1992). Stage D1 prostate cancer treated by radi-

cal prostatectomy and adjuvant hormonal treatment. *Cancer*, **70** (Suppl.), 311–23

14. Gann, P. H., Hennekens, C. H. and Stampfer, M. J. (1995). A prospective evaluation of plasma prostate-specific antigen for detection of prostatic cancer. *J. Am. Med. Assoc.*, **273**, 289–94

15. Tibblin, G., Welin, L., Bergström, R., Ronquist, G., Norlén, B. J. and Adami, H. O. (1995). The value of prostate specific antigen in early diagnosis of prostate cancer: the study of men born in 1913. *J. Urol.*, **154**, 1386–9

16. Epstein, J. I., Walsh, P. C., Carmichael, M. and Brendler, C. B. (1994). Pathologic and clinical findings to predict tumor extent of nonpalpable (Stage T1c) prostate cancer. *J. Am. Med. Assoc.*, **271**, 368–74

17. Lerner, S. E., Seay, T. M., Blute, M. L., Bergstralh, E. J., Barrett, D. and Zincke, H. (1996). Prostate specific antigen detected prostate cancer (clinical Stage T1c): an interim analysis. *J. Urol.*, **155**, 821–6

18. Petros, J. A. and Catalona, W. J. (1992). Lower incidence of unsuspected lymph node metastases in 521 consecutive patients with clinically localized prostate cancer. *J. Urol.*, **147**, 1574–5

19. Mold, J. W., Holtgrave, D. R., Bisanni, R. S., Marley, D. S., Wright, R. A. and Spann, S. J. (1992). The evaluation and treatment of men with asymptomatic prostate nodules in primary care: a decision analysis. *J. Fam. Pract.*, **34**, 561–8

20. Fleming, C., Wasson, J. H., Albertson, P. C., Barry, M. J. and Wennberg, J. E. (1993). A decision analysis of alternative treatment strategies for clinically localized prostate cancer. *J. Am. Med. Assoc.*, **269**, 2650–8

21. Krahn, M. D., Mahoney, J. E., Eckman, M. H., Trachtenberg, J., Pauker, S. G. and Detsky, A. S. (1994). Screening for prostate cancer. A decision analytic view. *J. Am. Med. Assoc.*, **272**, 773–80

22. Harwood, R. H. (1995). Management of localized prostate cancer: an epidemiological perspective. *Clin. Oncol.*, **7**, 151–9

23. Litwin, M. S., Hays, R. D., Fink, A., Ganz, P. A., Leake, B., Leach, G. E. and Brook, R. H. (1995). Quality-of-life outcomes in men treated for

localized prostate cancer. *J. Am. Med. Assoc.*, **273**, 129–35

24. Catalona, W. J., Smith, D. S., Ratliff, T. L. and Baster, J. W. (1993). Detection of organ-confined prostate cancer is increased through prostate-specific antigen-based screening. *J. Am. Med. Assoc.*, **270**, 948–54

25. Brawer, M. K. (1994). Screening for prostate cancer. *Mongr. Urol.*, **15**, 1–24

26. Beck, R. J., Kattan, M. W. and Miles, B. J. (1994). A critique of the decision analysis for clinically localized prostate cancer. *J. Urol.*, **152**, 1894–9

27. Gerber, G. (1994). Conservative approach to the management of prostate cancer. *Eur. Urol.*, **26**, 271–5

28. Chodak, G. W., Thisted, R. A., Gerber, G. S., Johansson, J. E., Adolfsson, J., Jones, G. W., Chisholm, G. D., Moskovitz, B., Livne, P. M. and Warner, J. (1994). Results of conservative management of clinically localized prostate cancer. *N. Engl. J. Med.*, **330**, 242–8

29. Hall, R. R. (1994). Radical prostatectomy and prostate cancer screening: the need for national audit and research. *Am. R. Coll. Surg. Engl.*, **76**, 367–72

30. Howe, R. J. (1994). Prostate cancer: a patient's perspective. *J. Urol.*, **152**, 1700–3

31. Fowler, F. J., Barry, M. J., Lu-Yao, G., Wasson, J., Roman, A. and Wennberg, J. (1995). Effect of radical prostatectomy for prostate cancer on patient quality of life: results from a Medicare survey. *Urology*, **45**, 1007–15

32. Stamey, T. A., Ferrari, M. K. and Schmid, H. P. (1993). The value of serial prostate specific antigen determinations 5 years after radiotherapy: steeply increasing values characterize 80% of patients. *J. Urol.*, **150**, 1856–9

33. Hanks, G. E., Lee, W. R. and Schultheiss, T. E. (1995). Clinical and biochemical evidence of prostate cancer at 5 years after external beam radiation. *J. Urol.*, **154**, 456–9

34. Albertson, P. C., Fryback, D. G., Storer, B. E., Kolon, T. F. and Fine, J. (1995). Long-term survival among men with conservatively treated localized prostate cancer. *J. Am. Med. Assoc.*, **274**, 626–31

35. Johansson, J. E. (1994). Expectant management of early stage prostatic cancer: Swedish experience. *J. Urol.*, **152**, 1753–6

36. Dugan, J. A., Bostwick, D. G., Myers, R. P., Qian, J., Bergstralh, E. J. and Oesterling, J. E. (1996). The definition and preoperative predication of clinically insignificant prostate cancer. *J. Am. Med. Assoc.*, **275**, 288–94

37. Stamey, T. A., Freiha, F. S., McNeal, J. E., Red-wine, E. A., Whittemore, A. S. and Schmid, H. (1993). Localized prostate cancer: relationship of tumor volume to clinical significance for the treatment of prostate cancer. *Cancer*, **71** (Suppl.), 933–8

38. Palken, M., Cobb, O. E., Warren, B. H. and Hoak, D. C. (1990). Prostate cancer: correlation of digital rectal exam, transrectal ultrasound, and prostate specific antigen levels with tumor volumes in radical retropubic prostatectomy specimens. *J. Urol.*, **143**, 1155–62

39. Cupp, M. R., Bostwick, D. G., Myers, R. P. and Oesterling, J. E. (1995). The volume of prostate cancer in the biopsy specimen cannot reliably predict the quantity of cancer in radical prostatectomy on an individual basis. *J. Urol.*, **153**, 1543–8

40. Terris, M. K., Haney, D. J., Johnstone, I. M., McNeal, J. E. and Stamey, T. A. (1995). Prediction of prostate cancer volume using prostate-specific antigen levels, transrectal ultrasound, and systematic sextant biopsies. *Urology*, **45**, 75–80

41. Adolfsson, J. and Tribukait, B. (1990). Evaluation of tumor progression by repeated fine needle biopsies in prostate adenocarcinoma: modal deoxyribonucleic acid value and cytological differentiation. *J. Urol.*, **144**, 1408–10

42. Whitmore, W. F. Jr (1990). *Prostate Cancer Overview. Current Advances in the Management of Prostatic Disease*, Snowbird, Utah, July 26–29

43. Menon, M., Parulkar, B. G. and Baker, S. (1995). Should we treat localized prostate cancer? An opinion. *Urology*, **46**, 607–16

44. Zincke, H., Oesterling, J. E., Blute, M. L., Bergstralh, E. J., Myers, R. P. and Barrett, D. M. (1994). Long term (15 years) results after radical prostatectomy for clinically localized (Stage T2 or lower) prostate cancer. *J. Urol.*, **152**, 1850–7

45. Bagshaw, M. A., Cox, R. S. and Hancock, S. L. (1994). Control of prostate cancer with radiotherapy: long term results. *J. Urol.*, **152**, 1781–5

46. Palmer, J. S., Worwag, E. M., Conrad, W. G., Blitz, B. F. and Chodak, G. W. (1996). Same day surgery for radical prostatectomy: is it an attainable goal? *Urology*, **47**, 23–8

47. Otnes, B., Harvei, S. and Fosså, S. D. (1995). The burden of prostate cancer from diagnosis until death. *Br. J. Urol.*, **76**, 587–94

48. Aus, G., Hugosson, J. and Norlén, L. (1995). Need for hospital care and palliative treatment for prostate cancer treated with non-curative intent. *J. Urol.* **154**, 466–9

49. Lerner, S. E., Blute, M. L. and Zincke, H. (1995). Critical evaluation of salvage surgery for radio-recurrent/resistant prostate cancer. *J. Urol.*, **154**, 1103–9

50. Ackerman, D. A., Barry, J. M., Wicklund, R. A., Olson, N. and Lowe, B. A. (1993). Analysis of risk

factors associated with prostate cancer extension to the surgical margin and pelvic node metastasis at radical prostatectomy. *J. Urol.*, **150**, 1845–50

51. Lerner, S. E., Blute, M. L. and Zincke, H. (1996). Risk factors for progression in patients with prostate cancer treated with radical prostatectomy. *J. Urol.*, in press

52. Brawer, M. K., Deering, R. E., Brown, M., Preston, S. D. and Bigler, S. A. (1994). Predictors of pathologic stage in prostatic carcinoma: the role of neovascularity. *Cancer*, **73**, 678–87

53. Labrie, F., Cusan, L., Gomez, J. L., Diamond, P. and Candas, B. (1995). Combination of screening and preoperative endocrine therapy: the potential for an important decrease in prostate cancer mortality. *J. Clin. Endocrinol. Metab.*, **80**, 2002–13

54. Soloway, M. S., Sharifi, R., Wajsman, Z., McLeod, D., Wood, D. P. Jr and Puras-Baez, A. (1995). Randomized prospective study comparing radical prostatectomy alone versus radical prostatectomy preceded by androgen blockade in clinical stage B2 (T2bNxMo) prostate cancer. *J. Urol.*, **154**, 424–8

55. Van Poppel, H., De Ridder, D., Elgamal, A. A., Van de Voorde, W., Werbrouck, P., Ackaert, K., Oyen, R., Pittomvils, G., Baert, L. *et al.* (1995). Neoadjuvant hormonal therapy before radical prostatectomy decreases the number of positive surgical margins in Stage T2 prostate cancer: interim results of a prospective randomized trial. *J. Urol.*, **154**, 429–34

56. Gleave, M. E., Goldenberg, S. L., Jones, E. C., Bruchovsky, N. and Sullivan, L. D. (1996). Biochemical and pathologic effects of 8 months of neoadjuvant androgen withdrawal therapy before radical prostatectomy in patients with clinically combined prostate cancer. *J. Urol.*, **155**, 213–19

57. Lerner, S. E., Blute, M. L., Lieber, M. M. and Zincke, H. (1995). Morbidity of radical retropubic prostatectomy for localized prostate cancer. *Oncology*, **9**, 379–89

58. Hanash, K. A., Utz, D. C., Cook, E. N., Taylor, W. F. and Titus, J. I. (1972). Carcinoma of the prostate: a 15-year followup. *J. Urol.*, **107**, 450–3

59. Lerner, S. P., Seale-Hawkins, C., Carlton, C. E. Jr and Scardino, P. T. (1991). The risk of dying of prostate cancer in patients with clinically localized disease. *J. Urol.*, **146**, 1040–5

60. Aus, G., Hugosson, J. and Norlén, L. (1995). Long-term survival and mortality in prostate cancer treated with noncurative intent. *J. Urol.*, **154**, 460–5

61. Bostwick, D. G. (1994). Target populations and strategies for chemoprevention trials of prostate cancer. *J. Cell. Biochem.* (Suppl.), **19**, 191–6

62. Holt, J. T., Thompson, M. E., Szabo, C., Robinson-Benion, C., Arteaga, C. L., King, M. C. and Jensen, R. A. (1996). Growth retardation and tumor inhibition by BCRA1. *Nature Gen.*, **12**, 298–302

63. Williams, B. J., Jones, E., Zhu, X. L., Steele, M. R., Stephenson, R. A., Rohr, L. R. and Brothman, A. R. (1996). Evidence for a tumor suppressor gene distal to BRCA1 in prostate cancer. *J. Urol.*, **155**, 720–5

64. Whitmore, W. F. Jr. (1956). Hormone therapy in prostatic cancer. *Am. J. Med.*, **21**, 697–713

Index

LIBRARY & HERITAGE SERVICE

Online Services
www.kingston.gov.uk

Renew a book (5 times)   Request a book
Change of address   Email a branch
Library news and updates   Get your PIN
Search the catalogue   Access reference sites

New Malden Library
48 Kingston Road
New Malden
KT3 3LY

Five interesting things about Rachel Gibson:

1. Growing up, I didn't like to read. I liked to play tetherball and wanted to be a tetherball champion.
2. I have a deadly fear of grasshoppers.
3. I am a shoe-aholic. I think ugly shoes are an abomination of biblical proportion.
4. I love to read the tabloids. Especially the ones featuring stories such as Bat Boy and women having Big Foot's baby.
5. I write romance novels, but I hate overly sentimental movies and sappy love songs.

TANGLED UP IN YOU

Maddie Jones doesn't like bars — she doesn't like the noise, the smoke or the trouble you find there. But she's got questions about her past, questions to which she's determined to find answers, and Hennessy's bar of Truly, Idaho, is where she'll find them. Of course, the bar also holds owner Mick Hennessy, and he's the kind of head-turning, heart-stopping, bad — but oh-so-good — kind of distraction that Maddie could do without. Mick, on the other hand, plans to get very distracted by Ms Jones. But then he doesn't know why she's really in town . . .

RACHEL GIBSON

TANGLED
UP IN YOU

Complete and Unabridged

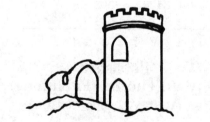

ULVERSCROFT
Leicester

First published in Great Britain in 2007 by
Little Black Dress
an imprint of Headline Publishing Group, London

First Large Print Edition
published 2009
by arrangement with
Headline Publishing Group
An Hachette Livre UK Company, London

The moral right of the author has been asserted

British Library CIP Data

Gibson, Rachel
    Tangled up in you.—Large print ed.—
    Ulverscroft large print series: romance
    1. Idaho—Social life and customs—Fiction
    2. Love stories 3. Large type books
    I. Title
    813.6 [F]

    ISBN 978–1–84782–590–2

Published by
F. A. Thorpe (Publishing)
Anstey, Leicestershire

Set by Words & Graphics Ltd.
Anstey, Leicestershire
Printed and bound in Great Britain by
T. J. International Ltd., Padstow, Cornwall

This book is printed on acid-free paper

1

The glowing white neon above Mort's Bar pulsed and vibrated and attracted the thirsty masses of Truly, Idaho, like a bug light. But Mort's was more than a beer magnet. More than just a place to drink cold Coors and get into a fight on Friday nights. Mort's had historical significance — kind of like the Alamo. While other establishments came and went in the small town, Mort's had always stayed the same.

Until about a year ago when the new owner had spruced the place up with gallons of Lysol and paint and had instituted a strict no-panty-tossing policy. Before that, women throwing their undies like a ring toss up onto the row of antlers above the bar had been encouraged as a sort of indoor sporting event. Now, if a woman felt the urge to toss, she got tossed out on her bare ass.

Ah, the good old days.

Maddie Jones stood on the sidewalk in front of Mort's and stared up at the sign, completely immune to the subliminal lure that the light sent out through the impending darkness. An indistinguishable hum of voices

1

and music leached through the cracks in the old building sandwiched between Ace Hardware and the Panda Restaurant.

A couple in jeans and tank tops brushed past Maddie. The door opened and the sound of voices and the unmistakable twang of country music spilled out onto Main Street. The door closed and Maddie remained standing outside. She adjusted the purse strap on her shoulder, then pulled up the zipper on her bulky blue sweater. She hadn't lived in Truly for twenty-nine years, and she'd forgotten how cool it got at night. Even in July.

Her hand lifted toward the old door, then dropped to her side. A surprising rush of apprehension raised the hair on the back of her neck and tilted her stomach. She'd done this dozens of times. So why the apprehension? Why now? she asked herself, even though she knew the answer. Because it was personal this time, and once she opened that door, once she took the first step, there was no going back.

If her friends could see her, standing there as if her feet were set in the concrete, they'd be shocked. She'd interviewed serial killers and cold-blooded murderers, but chatting up nut jobs with antisocial personality disorders was a piece of cake compared to what waited for her inside Mort's. Beyond the NO ONE

2

UNDER 21 sign, her past waited for her, and as she'd learned recently, digging into other people's pasts was a hell of a lot easier than digging into her own.

'For God's sake,' she muttered and reached for the door. She was a little disgusted with herself for being such a wimp and a weenie, and she squelched her apprehension under the heavy fist of her strong will. Nothing was going to happen that she did not want to happen. She was in control. As always.

The heavy thump of the jukebox and the smell of hops and tobacco assaulted her as she stepped inside. The door shut behind her and she paused to let her eyes adjust to the dim light. Mort's was just a bar. Like a thousand others she'd been in across the country. Nothing special, not even the array of antlers hanging above the long mahogany bar was anything out of the ordinary.

Maddie didn't like bars. Especially cowboy bars. The smoke, the music, the steady stream of beer. She didn't particularly care for cowboys either. As far as she was concerned, a pair of snug Wranglers on a tight cowboy butt couldn't quite make up for the boots, the buckles, the wads of chew. She liked her men in suits and Italian leather shoes. Not that she'd had a man, or even a date, in about four years.

She studied the crowd as she wove her way to the middle of the long oak bar and the only empty stool. Her gaze took in cowboy hats and trucker caps, a few crew cuts, and a mullet or two. She noticed ponytails, shoulder-length bobs, and some of the worst perms and flipped bangs to ever come out of the eighties. What she didn't see was the one person she'd come searching for, although she didn't really expect to see him sitting at one of the tables.

She wedged herself onto the stool between a man in a blue T-shirt and a woman with overprocessed hair. Behind the cash register and bottles of alcohol, a mirror ran the length of the bar while two bartenders pulled beers and blended drinks. Neither was the owner of this fine establishment.

'That little gal was into AC/DC, if you know what I mean,' said the man on her left, and Maddie figured he wasn't talking about *Back in Black* or *Highway to Hell*. The guy in question was about sixty, sported a battered trucker's hat and a beer belly the size of a pony keg. Through the mirror Maddie watched several men down the row nod, paying rapt attention to beer-belly guy.

One of the bartenders set a napkin in front of her and asked what she'd like to drink. He looked to be about nineteen, although she

4

supposed he had to be at least twenty-one. Old enough to pour liquor within the layers of tobacco smoke and knee-deep bullshit.

'Sapphire martini. Extra dry, three olives,' she said, calculating the carbs in the olives. She pulled her purse into her lap and watched the bartender turn and reach for the good gin and vermouth.

'I told that little gal she could keep her girlfriend, so long as she brought her over once in a while,' the guy on her left added.

'Damn right!'

'That's what I'm talking about!'

Then again, this was small-town Idaho, where things like liquor laws were sometimes overlooked and some people considered a good bullshit story a form of literature.

Maddie rolled her eyes and bit her lip to keep her comments to herself. She had a habit of saying what she thought. She didn't necessarily consider it a *bad* habit, but not everyone appreciated it.

Through the mirror, her gaze moved up, then down the bar, searching for the owner, not that she thought she'd see him plopped down on a stool any more than sitting at a table. When she'd called the other bar he owned in town, she'd been told that he would be here tonight, and she figured he was probably in his office examining his books or, if he was like his father, the inner thigh of a barmaid.

'I pay for everything,' the woman on Maddie's opposite side wailed to her friend. 'I even bought my own birthday card and had J.W. sign it, thinking he'd feel bad and get the hint.'

'Oh, geez,' Maddie couldn't help but mutter and looked at the woman through the mirror. Between bottles of Absolut and Skyy vodka, she could make out big blond hair falling to chubby shoulders and breasts spilling out of a red tank top with rhinestones on it.

'He didn't feel bad at all! Just complained that he didn't like mushy cards like the one I bought.' She took a drink of something with an umbrella in it. 'He wants me to come over when his mother goes out of town next weekend and make him dinner.' She brushed moisture from beneath her eyes and sniffed. 'I'm thinking of telling him no.'

Maddie's brows drew together and a stunned, 'Are you shitting me?' escaped her mouth before she knew she'd uttered a word.

'Excuse me?' the bartender asked as he set the drink in front of her.

She shook her head. 'Nothing.' She reached into her purse and paid for her drink as a song about a Honky Tonk Badonkadonk, whatever the hell that meant, thumped from the glowing neon jukebox and coalesced with the steady hum of conversation.

She pulled back the sleeve of her sweater and reached for her martini. She read the glowing hands of her watch as she raised the glass to her lips. Nine o'clock. The owner was bound to show his face sooner or later. If not tonight, there was always tomorrow. She took a sip and the gin and vermouth warmed a path all the way to her stomach.

She really hoped he'd show up sooner rather than later. Before she had too many martinis and forgot why she was sitting on a barstool eavesdropping on needy passive-aggressive women and delusional men. Not that listening in on people with lives more pathetic than hers couldn't be highly entertaining at times.

She set the glass back on the bar. Eavesdropping wasn't her first choice. She much preferred the straightforward approach: digging into people's lives and plumbing their dirty little secrets without distraction. Some people gave up their secrets without protest, eager to tell all. Others forced her to reach deep, rattle them loose or rip them out by the roots. Her work was sometimes messy, always gritty, but she loved writing about serial killers, mass murderers, and your everyday run-of-the-mill psychopaths.

Really, a girl had to excel at something, and Maddie, writing as Madeline Dupree, was one of the best true crime writers in the genre. She wrote blood and gore. About the sick and disturbed, and there were those who thought, her friends among them, that what she wrote warped her personality. She liked to think it added to her charm.

The truth was somewhere in the middle. The things she'd seen and written about did affect her. No matter the barrier she placed between her sanity and the people she interviewed and researched, their sickness sometimes seeped through the cracks, leaving behind a black tacky film that was hard as hell to scrub clean.

Her job made her see the world a little differently than those who'd never sat across from a serial killer while he got off on the retelling of his 'work'. But those same things also made her a strong woman who didn't take crap from anyone. Very little intimidated her, and she didn't have any illusions about mankind. In her head, she knew that most people were decent. That given the choice, they would do the right thing, but she also knew about the others. The fifteen percent who were only interested in their own selfish and warped pleasure. Out of that fifteen percent, only about two percent were actual serial killers. The other social deviants were just your everyday rapists, murderers, thugs, and corporate executives secretly plundering their employees' 401(k) accounts.

And if there was one thing she knew as certainly as she knew the sun would rise in the east and set in the west, it was that everyone had secrets. She had a few of her own. She just held hers closer to the vest than most people.

She raised the glass to her lips and her gaze was drawn to the end of the bar. A door in the back opened and a man stepped from the lit alley and into the dark hall.

Maddie knew him. Knew him before he walked from the shadows. Before the shadows slid up the wide chest and shoulders of his black T-shirt. Knew him before the light slipped across his chin and nose and shone in his hair as black as the night from which he'd come.

He moved behind the bar, wrapping a red bar apron around his hips and tying the strings above his fly. She'd never met him. Never been in the same room, but she knew he was thirty-five, a year older than herself. She knew he was six-two, one hundred and ninety pounds. For twelve years he'd served in the army, flying helicopters and raining

Hellfire missiles. He'd been named after his father, Lochlyn Michael Hennessy, but he went by Mick. Like his father, he was an obscenely good-looking man. The kind of good-looking that turned heads, stopped hearts, and gave women bad thoughts. Thoughts of hot mouths and hands and tangled clothes. The whisper of warm breath against the arch of a woman's throat and the touch of flesh in the backseat of a car.

Not that Maddie was susceptible to those thoughts.

He had an older sister Meg, and he owned two bars in town, Mort's and Hennessy's. The latter had been in his family longer than he'd been alive. Hennessy's, the bar where Maddie's mother had worked. Where she'd met Loch Hennessy and where she'd died.

As if he felt her gaze, he glanced up from the strings of the apron. He stopped a few feet from Maddie and his eyes met hers. She choked on the gin that refused to go down her throat. From his driver's license, she knew his eyes were blue, but they were more a deep turquoise. Like the Caribbean Sea, and seeing them looking back at her was a shock. She lowered her glass and raised a hand to her mouth.

The last strains of the honky-tonk song died out as he finished tying the strings, and he stepped closer until only a few feet of mahogany separated his gaze from hers. 'You going to live?' His deep voice cut through the noise around them.

She swallowed and coughed one last time. 'I believe so.'

'Hey, Mick,' the blonde on the next stool called out.

'Hey, Darla. How're things?'

'Could be better.'

'Isn't that always the case?' he said as he gazed at the woman. 'Are you planning on behaving yourself?'

'You know me.' Darla laughed. 'I always plan on it. Course, I can always be persuaded to misbehave.'

'You're going to keep your underwear on tonight, though. Right?' he asked with a lift of one dark brow.

'You never can tell about me.' She leaned forward. 'You never know what I might do. Sometimes I'm crazy.'

Just sometimes? Buying her own birthday card for her boyfriend to sign suggested a passive/aggressive disorder that bordered on crazy as hell.

'Just keep your panties on so I don't have to toss you out on your bare butt again.'

Again? Meaning it had happened before? Maddie took a drink and slid her gaze to

11

Darla's considerable behind squeezed into a pair of Wranglers.

'I just bet you all would love to see that!' Darla said with a toss of her hair.

For the second time that night, Maddie choked on her drink.

Mick's deep chuckle drew Maddie's attention to the amusement shining through his startling blue eyes. 'Honey, do you need some water?' he asked.

She shook her head and cleared her throat.

'That drink too strong for you?'

'No. It's fine.' She coughed one last time and set her glass on the bar. 'I just got a horrifying visual.'

The corners of his lips turned up into a knowing smile that made two dents in his tan cheeks. 'I haven't seen you in here before. You just passing through?'

She forced the image of Darla's big bare butt from her head and her mind back on the reason she was in Mort's. She'd expected to dislike Mick Hennessy on sight. She didn't. 'No. I bought a house out on Red Squirrel Road.'

'Nice area. Are you on the lake?'

'Yes.' She wondered if Mick had inherited his father's charm along with his looks. From what Maddie had been able to gather, Loch Hennessy had charmed women into the sack with little more than a look in their direction. He'd certainly charmed her mother.

'Are you here for the summer, then?'

'Yes.'

He tilted his head to one side and studied her face. His gaze slid from her eyes to her mouth and lingered for several heartbeats before he looked back up. 'What's your name, brown eyes?'

'Maddie,' she answered, holding a breath as she waited for him to connect her with the past. His past.

'Just Maddie?'

'Dupree,' she answered, using her pen name.

Someone down the bar called his name and he glanced away for a moment before returning his attention to her. He gave her an easy smile. One that brought out those dimples of his and softened his masculine face. He didn't recognize her. 'I'm Mick Hennessy.' The music started once more and he said, 'Welcome to Truly. Maybe I'll see you around.'

She watched him walk away without telling him the reason she was in town and why she was sitting in Mort's. Now wasn't the best time or place, but there was no 'maybe' about it. He didn't know it yet, but Mick Hennessy would be seeing a lot of her. Next time he might not be so welcoming.

The sounds and smells of the bar pressed in on her and she hung her purse over her shoulder. She slid from the stool and wove her way through the dimly lit crowd. At the door, she looked over her shoulder toward the bar and Mick. Beneath the lights above him, he tilted his head back a little and smiled. She paused and her grasp on the handle tightened as he turned and poured a beer from a row of spigots.

While she stood there, the juke playing something about whiskey for men and beer for horses, her gaze took in his dark hair at the back of his neck and his wide shoulders in his black T-shirt. He turned and placed a glass on the bar. As she watched him, he laughed at something, and until that moment Maddie hadn't known what she'd expected of Mick Hennessy, but whatever it had been, this living, breathing man who laughed and smiled hadn't been it.

Through the dark bar and cigarette haze, his gaze landed on her. She could almost feel it reach across the room and touch her, which she knew was pure illusion. She stood in the darkened entrance and it would be near impossible for him to distinguish her from the crowd. She opened the door and stepped outside into the cool evening air. While she'd been in Mort's, night had descended on Truly like a heavy black curtain. The only relief a few lit business signs and the occasional streetlamp.

Her black Mercedes was parked across the street in front of Tina's Mountain Skivvies and the Rock Hound Art Gallery. She waited for a yellow Hummer to pass before she stepped from the curb and walked from beneath the glow of Mort's neon sign.

A keyless transponder in her purse unlocked the driver's-side door as she approached, and she opened it and slid inside the cool leather interior. Normally, she wasn't materialistic. She didn't care about clothes or shoes. Since no one ever saw her underwear these days, she didn't care if her bra matched her panties and she didn't own expensive jewelry. Before purchasing the Mercedes two months ago, Maddie had put over two hundred thousand miles on her Nissan Sentra. She'd needed a new vehicle and had been looking at a Volvo SUV when she'd turned around and locked eyes on the black S600 sedan. The showroom lights had been shining down on the car like a signal from God, and she could have sworn she heard angels singing hallelujahs like the Mormon Tabernacle Choir. Who was she to ignore a message from the Lord? A few hours after

15

walking into the dealership, she'd driven the car out of the showroom and into the garage of her home down in Boise.

She pressed the start button on the shifter and hit the lights. The CD in her stereo system filled the Mercedes with Warren Zevon's *Excitable Boy*. She pulled away from the curb and flipped a U in the middle of Main Street. There was something brilliant and disturbing about Warren Zevon's lyrics. A little like looking into the mind of someone who stood at the line between crazy and sane and occasionally pushed one toe over. Toying with the line, testing it, then pulling back just before getting sucked into looneyville. In Maddie's line of work, there weren't many who pulled back in time.

The Mercedes' headlights cut through the inky night as she turned left at the only traffic signal in town. The very first car she'd ever owned had been a Volkswagen Rabbit, so battered the seats had been held together with duct tape. She'd come a long way since then. A long way from the Roundup Trailer Court where she'd lived with her mother, and the cramped little house in Boise where she'd been raised by her great-aunt Martha.

Until the day of her retirement, Martha had worked the front counter at Rexall Drug, and they'd lived off her small paycheck and

16

Maddie's Social Security checks. Money had always been tight, but Martha kept half a dozen cats at any given time. The house had always smelled like Friskies and litter boxes. To this day, Maddie hated cats. Well, maybe not her good friend Lucy's cat, Mr Snookums. Snookie was cool. For a cat.

She drove for a mile around the east side of the lake before turning into her driveway lined with thick towering pines and pulling to stop in front of the two-story home she'd bought a few months ago. She didn't know how long she'd keep the house. One year. Three. Five. She'd bought rather than leased for the investment. Property around Truly was hot, and when or if she sold the place, she stood to make a nice profit.

Maddie cut the Mercedes' headlights and the darkness pressed in on her. She ignored the apprehension in her chest as she got out of the car and walked up the steps and onto the wraparound porch lit up with numerous sixty-watt bulbs. She wasn't afraid of anything. Certainly not the dark, but she knew bad things did happen to women who weren't as aware and as cautious as Maddie. Women who didn't have a small arsenal of safety devices in their shoulder bags. Things like a Taser and Mace, a personal alarm, and brass knuckles, just to name a few. A girl could never be too careful, especially at night in a town where it was difficult to see your hand in front of your face. In a town set smack-dab in the middle of dense forest where wildlife rustled from trees and underbrush. Where rodents with beady little eyes waited for a girl to go to bed before ransacking the pantry. Maddie had never had to use any of her personal safety devices, but lately she'd been wondering if she was a good enough shot to zap a marauding mouse with her Taser.

Lights burned from within the house as Maddie unlocked the forest-green door, stepped inside, and flipped the deadbolt behind her. Nothing scurried from the corners as she tossed her purse on a red velvet chair by the door. A large fireplace dominated the middle of the big living room and divided it into what was meant to be the dining room but what Maddie used as her office.

On a coffee table in front of the velvet sofa sat Maddie's research files and an old five-by-seven photograph in a silver frame. She reached for the picture and looked into the face of her mother, at her blond hair, blue eyes, and big smile. It had been taken a few months before Alice Jones had died. A photo of a happy twenty-four-year-old, so vibrant and alive, and like the yellowed photograph in the expensive frame, most of Maddie's memories had faded too. She recalled bits of this and snatches of that. She had a faint memory of watching her mother put on makeup and brush her hair before leaving for work. She recalled her old blue Samsonite suitcase and moving from place to place. Through the watery prism of twenty-nine years, she had a very faint memory of the last time her mother had packed up their Chevy Maverick and the two-hour drive north to Truly. Moving into their trailer house and orange shag carpet.

The clearest memory Maddie had of her mother was the scent of her skin. She'd smelled like almond lotion. But mostly she recalled the morning her great-aunt had arrived at the Roundup Trailer Court to tell her that her mother was dead.

Maddie set the photo back on the table and moved across the hardwood floor into the kitchen. She grabbed a Diet Coke out of the refrigerator and unscrewed the cap. Martha had always said that Alice was flighty. Flitting like a butterfly from place to place, from man to man, searching for somewhere to belong and looking for love. Finding both for a time before moving on to the next place or newest man.

Maddie drank from the bottle, then replaced the cap. She was nothing like her mother. She knew her place in the world. She was comfortable with who she was, and she certainly didn't need a man to love her. In fact, she'd never been in love. Not the romantic kind that her good friend Clare wrote about for a living. And not the foolish, mad-for-the-man kind that had ruled and ultimately taken her mother's life.

No, Maddie had no interest in a man's *love*. His body was a different matter, and she did want an occasional boyfriend. A man to come over several times a week to have sex. He didn't have to be a great conversationalist. Hell, he didn't even have to take her to dinner. Her ideal man would just take her to bed, then leave. But there were two problems with finding her ideal man. First, any man who just wanted sex from a woman was most likely a jerk. Second, it was difficult to find a willing man who was good in bed rather than who just thought he was good. The chore of sorting through men to find what she wanted had become such a hassle, she'd given up four years ago.

She hooked the top of the Coke bottle between two fingers and moved from the kitchen. Her flip-flops slapped the bottoms of her feet as she walked through the living room and passed the fireplace to her office. Her laptop sat on an L-shaped desk shoved up against the wall and she flipped on the lamp clamped to the hutch of her desk. Two sixty-watt bulbs lit up a stack of diaries, her laptop, and her 'Taking Names and Kicking Ass' sticky notes. Altogether there were ten diaries in various shapes and colors. Red. Blue. Pink. Two of the diaries had locks, while one of the others was nothing more than a yellow spiral notebook with the word 'Diary' written in black marker. All of them had belonged to her mother.

Maddie tapped the Diet Coke bottle against her thigh as she gazed at the top white book. She hadn't known they'd even existed until her great-aunt Martha's death a few months ago. She didn't believe Martha had purposely kept the diaries from her. More than likely she'd intended to give them to Maddie someday but had completely forgotten. Alice hadn't been the only flighty female on the Jones family tree.

As Martha's only living relative, it had been up to Maddie to settle her affairs, see to her funeral, and clean out her house. She'd managed to find homes for her aunt's cats and had planned to donate most everything else to Goodwill. In one of the last cartons she'd sorted through, she'd come across old shoes, outdated purses, and a battered boot box. She'd almost tossed the battered box without lifting the top. A part of her almost wished that she had. Wished she'd spared herself the pain of staring down into the box and feeling her heart shoved into her throat. As a child she'd longed for a connection with her mother. Some little something that she could have and hold. She'd dreamed of having something she could take out from time to time that tied her to the woman who'd given her life. She'd spent her childhood longing for something . . . something that had been a few feet away in the top of a closet the whole time. Waiting for her in a Tony Lama box.

The box had contained the diaries, her mother's obituary, and newspaper articles about her death. It had also held a satin bag filled with jewelry. Cheap stuff, mostly. A Foxy Lady necklace, several turquoise rings, a pair of silver hoop earrings, and a tiny pink band from St. Luke's Hospital with the words 'Baby Jones' printed on it.

Standing in her old bedroom that day, unable to breathe as her chest imploded, she'd felt like a kid again. Scared and alone. Afraid to reach out and make the connection, but at the same time excited to finally have something tangible that had belonged to a mother she hardly remembered.

Maddie set her Coke on the top of her desk and spun her office chair around. That day, she'd taken the boot box home and placed the silk bag in her jewelry box. Then she'd sat down and read the diaries. She'd read every word, devouring them in one day. The diaries had started on her mother's twelfth birthday. Some of them had been bigger and taken her mother longer to fill. Through them she'd gotten to know Alice Jones.

She'd gotten to know her as a child of twelve who'd longed to grow up and be an actress like Anne Francis. A teen who longed to find true love on *The Dating Game*, and a woman who looked for love in all the wrong places.

Maddie had found something to connect her to her mother, but the more she'd read, the more she'd felt at loose ends. She'd gotten her childhood wish and she'd never felt so alone.

2

Mick Hennessy slipped a rubber band about a stack of cash and set it next to a pile of credit card and debit receipts. The sound of the electric coin sorter sitting on his desk filled the small office in the back of Mort's. Everyone but Mick had gone home for the evening and he was just balancing the tills before he headed that way himself.

Owning and running bars was in Mick's blood. Mick's great-grandfather had made and sold cheap grain alcohol during Prohibition and opened Hennessy's two months after the Eighteenth Amendment was repealed and the spigots once again flowed in the United States. The bar had been in his family ever since.

Mick didn't particularly care for belligerent drunks, but he did like the flexible hours that came with being his own boss. He didn't have to take orders or answer to anyone, and when he walked into one of his bars, he had a feeling of possession that he'd never felt with anything else in his life. His bars were loud and raucous and chaotic, but it was a chaos he controlled.

More than the hours and feeling of possession, Mick liked making money. During the summer months, he made tons of money from tourists and from the people who lived in Boise but owned cabins on the lake in Truly.

The coin sorter stopped and Mick slid stacks of coins into paper sleeves. An image of a dark-haired, red-lipped woman entered his head. He wasn't surprised that he'd noticed Maddie Dupree within seconds of stepping behind the bar. It only would have surprised him if he hadn't noticed her. With her beautiful smooth skin and seductive brown eyes, she was just the sort of woman who drew his attention. That small mole at the corner of her full lips had reminded him just how long it had been since he'd kissed a mouth like hers and worked his way south. Down her chin and the arch of her throat to all the soft places and sweet parts.

Since his move back to Truly two years ago, his sex life had suffered more than he liked. Which sucked. Truly was a small town where people went to church on Sundays and married young. They tended to stay married and if not, looked to remarry real quick. Mick never messed with married women or women with marriage on their minds. Never even thought twice about it.

Not that there weren't plenty of unmarried

women in Truly. Owning two bars in town, he came in contact with a lot of available women. A good share of them let him know they were interested in more than his cocktail list. Some of them he'd known all of his life. They knew the stories and gossip and thought they knew him too. They didn't, or they would know he preferred to spend time with women who didn't know him or the past. Who didn't know the sordid details of his parents' lives.

Mick shoved the money and receipts into deposit bags and zipped them closed. The clock on the wall above his desk read 2:05. Travis's latest school photograph sat on a polished oak desk; a sprinkling of brown freckles scattered across the boy's cheeks and nose. Mick's nephew was seven going on fourteen and had too much Hennessy in him for his own good. The innocent smile didn't fool Mick one bit. Travis had his ancestors' dark hair and blue eyes and wild ways. If left unchecked, he'd inherit their fondness for fighting, booze, and women. Any one of those traits by themselves wasn't necessarily bad in moderation, but generations of Hennessys had never cared squat about moderation, and the combination had sometimes proved lethal.

He moved across the office and set the

money on the top shelf of the safe, next to the printout of that night's transactions. He swung the heavy door shut, pushed down the steel handle, and spun the combination lock. The tick-tick of the lock filled the silence of the small office in the back of Mort's.

Travis was giving Meg hell, that was for sure, and Mick's sister had little understanding of boys. She just didn't get why boys threw rocks, made weapons out of everything they touched, and punched each other for no apparent reason. It was up to Mick to be the buffer in Travis's life and to help Meg raise him. To give the boy someone to talk to and to teach him how to be a good man. Not that Mick was an expert or a shining example of what made a good man. But he did have first-hand knowledge and some experience in what made an asshole.

He grabbed a set of keys off the desktop and headed out of the office. The heels of his boots thudded against the hardwood floor, sounding inordinately loud in the empty bar.

When he was a kid, no one had been around for him to talk to or teach him how to be a man. He'd been raised by his grandmother and sister, and he'd had to learn for himself. Most often than not, he learned the hard way. He didn't want the same for Travis.

Mick flipped the light switches off and headed out the back door. The cold morning air brushed his face and neck as he stuck a key in the deadbolt and locked it behind him. Right out of high school he'd left Truly to attended Boise State down in the capital city. But after three years of aimless pursuits and a rotten attitude, he'd enlisted in the army. At the time, seeing the world from the inside of a tank had sounded like a real smart plan.

A red Dodge Ram was parked next to the Dumpster and he climbed inside. He'd certainly seen the world. Sometimes more of it than he cared to remember, but not from the inside of a tank. Instead he'd viewed it from thousands of feet in the air within the cockpits of Apache helicopters. He'd flown birds for the U.S government before getting out and moving back to Truly. The army had given him more than a kick-ass career and a chance to live a good life. It had taught him how to be a man in a way that living in a house of women had not. When to stand up and when to shut the hell up. When to fight and when to walk away. What mattered and what wasn't worth his time.

Mick started the truck and waited a few moments for the vehicle to warm up. He owned two bars, and he figured it was a very good thing that he'd learned to deal with belligerent drunks and assorted dipshits in a way that didn't require throwing fists and cracking heads. Otherwise, he'd get little else done. He'd be in one fight after another, walking around with a black eye and busted lip like he had growing up. Back then he hadn't known how to handle the dipshits of the world. Back then he'd been forced to live with the scandal his parents had created. He'd had to live with the whispers when he walked into a room. The sideways glances at church or the Valley Grocery Store. The taunts from other children at school or, worse, the birthday parties he and Meg had not been invited to. Back then, he'd handled every slight with his fists. Meg had retreated within herself.

Mick flipped on the headlights and shoved the truck into reverse. The Ram's taillights lit up the alley as he looked over his shoulder and backed out of the parking space. In a larger town, the salacious lives of Loch and Rose Hennessy would have been forgotten within a few weeks. Front-page news for a day or two, then eclipsed by something more shocking. Something bigger to talk about over morning coffee. But in a town the size of Truly, where the juiciest scandal usually involved such nefarious deeds as a stolen bicycle or Sid Grimes poaching out of season, the sordidness of Loch and Rose Hennessy had kept the town talking for years. Speculating and rehashing every tragic detail had become a favorite pastime. Right up there with holiday parades, the ice-sculpting contest, and raising money for the town's various causes. But unlike decorating floats and instituting after-school just-say-no-to-drugs programs, what everyone seemed to forget, or perhaps didn't care about, was that within the wreckage that Rose and Loch had created, there had been two innocent children just trying to live it all down.

He shoved the truck into drive and rolled out of the alley and onto a dimly lit street. A lot of his childhood memories were old and faded and thankfully forgotten. Others were so crystal clear he could recall every detail. Like the night he and Meg had been woken up by a county sheriff, told to grab a few things, and taken to their grandmother Loraine's house. He remembered sitting in the back of the squad car in his T-shirt, underwear, and sneakers, holding his Tonka truck, while Meg sat next to him, crying as if their world had just ended. And it had. He remembered all the squawk and adrenaline-laced voices on the police radio, and he remembered something about someone checking up on the other little girl.

Leaving the few city lights behind, Mick drove through the pitch-darkness for two miles before turning onto his dirt street. He drove past the house where he and Meg had been raised after the death of their parents. His grandmother Loraine Hennessy had been affectionate and loving in her own way. She'd made sure he and Meg had things like winter boots and gloves and were always filled with comfort food. But she'd completely neglected what they'd really needed. The most normal life possible.

She'd refused to sell the old farmhouse where he and Meg had lived with their parents. For years it sat abandoned on the outskirts of town, becoming a haven for mice and a constant reminder of the family that had once lived there. A person couldn't enter town without seeing it. Without seeing the overgrown weeds, the peeling white paint, and the sagging clothesline.

And Monday through Friday, for nine months out of every year, Mick and Meg had been forced to pass it on their way to school. While the other children on the bus chatted about the latest episode of *The Dukes Of Hazzard* or checked out the contents of their lunch boxes, he and Meg turned their heads away from the window. Their stomachs got heavy and they held their breath, praying to

God no one noticed their old house. God hadn't always answered and the bus would fill with the latest gossip the kids had overheard about their parents.

The bus trip to school had been a daily hell. A routine torture — until a cold October night in 1986 when the farmhouse erupted in a huge orange fireball and burned completely to the ground. Arson had been determined as the cause of the fire, and there'd been a big investigation. Almost everyone in town had been questioned, but the person responsible for dousing the place with kerosene had never been caught. Everyone in town thought they knew who'd done it, but no one had known for sure.

After Loraine's death three years ago, Mick sold the property to the Allegrezza boys and he'd thought about selling the family bar too, but in the end he decided to move back and run the place. Meg needed him. Travis needed him, and to his surprise, when he'd returned to Truly, no one really talked about the scandal anymore. Whispers no longer followed him, or if they did, he no longer heard them.

He slowed the truck and made another left, turning into his long driveway and heading up a hill seated at the base of Shaw Mountain. He'd bought the two-story house shortly after he'd moved back to Truly. It had a great view of the town and the rugged mountains surrounding the lake. He parked in the garage next to his twenty-one-foot ski boat and entered the house through the laundry room. The light in his office was on and he turned it off as he passed. He moved through the dark living room and took the stairs two at a time.

For the most part, Mick didn't really think of the past that had been such a focus in his childhood. Truly didn't talk about it anymore, which was ironic as hell, because he just didn't give a shit what people said and thought about him these days. He walked into his bedroom at the far end of the hall and moved through the moonlight pouring through the open slats of his wooden blinds. Shadow and muted strips of light touched his face and chest as he reached for his back pocket. He tossed his wallet on his dresser, then grabbed two fistfuls of his T-shirt and pulled it over his head. But just because he didn't give a shit about the past, didn't mean that Meg was over it. She had her good days and bad days. Since the death of their grandmother, her bad days were getting worse, and that was just no way for Travis to live.

Moonlight and shadow spilled across the

green quilt and solid oak posts of Mick's bed. He dropped the shirt by his feet, then walked across the room. Sometimes he felt that moving back to Truly had been a mistake. It felt as if he were standing in one place, unable to move forward, and he didn't know why he felt that way. He'd bought a new bar and was thinking of starting a helicopter service with his friend Steve. He had money and success and he belonged in Truly with his family. The only family he had. The only family he was ever likely to have, but sometimes . . . sometimes he couldn't shake the feeling that he was standing in one place. As if maybe he was waiting for something.

The mattress dipped as he sat on the edge and pulled off his boots and socks. Meg thought all he needed was to meet a nice woman to make him a good wife, but he just couldn't see himself married. Not now. He'd had a few good relationships in his life. Good right up until the moment that they weren't. None had lasted more than a year or two. Partly because he'd been gone so much. Mostly because he didn't want to buy a ring and walk down the aisle.

He stood and stripped to his underwear. Meg thought he was afraid of marriage because their parents' had been so bad, but that wasn't true. The truth was that he didn't remember his parents all that much. Just a few watery memories of family picnics at the lake and his parents cuddling on the sofa. His mother crying at the kitchen table and an old heavy telephone thrown through the television screen.

No, the problem wasn't the memories of his parents' fucked-up relationship. He'd just never loved one woman enough to want to spend the rest of his life with her. Which he didn't consider a problem at all.

He pulled back the quilt and lay between the cool sheets. For the second time that night, he thought about Maddie Dupree, and he laughed into the darkness. She'd been a smart-ass, but he'd never held that against a woman. If fact, he liked a woman who could stand up to a man. Who gave as good as she got and didn't need a man to take care of her. Who wasn't needy or weepy or crazy as hell. Whose moods didn't swing like a pendulum.

Mick turned on his side and glanced at the clock on his nightstand. He'd set his alarm for ten A.M. and was ready for a full seven hours of uninterrupted shut-eye. Unfortunately, he didn't get it.

The next morning, the ringing of the telephone brought him out of a deep sleep. He opened his eyes and squinted against the morning sun pouring across his bed. He glanced at the caller ID and reached for the cordless receiver.

'You better be spurting blood,' he said and pushed the covers down his naked chest. 'I told you not to call before ten unless it's an emergency.'

'Mom's at work and I need some fireworks,' his nephew informed him.

'At eight-thirty in the morning?' He sat up and ran his fingers through one side of his hair. 'Is your sitter there with you?'

'Yeah. Tomorrow's the Fourth of July and I don't got no fireworks.'

'You just realized this?' There was more to the story. With Travis, there was always more to the story. 'Why didn't your mom get you your fireworks?' There was a long pause and Mick added, 'You might as well tell me the truth because I'm going to ask Meg.'

'She said I have a potty mouth.'

Mick stood and his feet sank into thick beige carpeting as he walked across the room toward a dresser. He was almost afraid to ask. 'Why?'

'Well . . . she made meatloaf again. She knows I hate meatloaf.'

He didn't blame the kid there. The Hennessy women were notorious for their shitty meatloaf. He opened the second dresser drawer and prompted, 'And?'

'I said it tasted like shit. I said you thought so too.'

Mick paused in the act of pulling out a white T-shirt and glanced into his reflection above the dresser. 'Did you use the real s-word?'

'Uh-huh, and she said I can't have fireworks, but you say the s-word all the dang time.'

That was true. He hung the shirt over one shoulder and leaned forward to look into his bloodshot eyes. 'We talked about words I can say and words you can say.'

'I know, but it just slipped out.'

'You need to watch what slips out of your mouth.'

Travis sighed. 'I know. I said I was sorry, even though I'm not really. Just like you said I should say to girls. Even the stupid ones. Even when I'm right and they're wrong.'

That wasn't quite what he'd said. 'You didn't tell Meg I said that, though.' He pulled a pair of Levi's out of the dresser and added, 'Right?'

'Right.'

He couldn't countermand his sister, but at the same time, a boy shouldn't be punished for speaking the truth. 'I can't buy you fireworks if your mom says no, but we'll see if we can't work something out.'

An hour later, Mick shoved a bag of fireworks behind the driver's seat of his truck. He'd bought a small variety pack as well as a few sparklers and snakes from the Safe and Sane stand in the parking lot of Handy Man Hardware. He hadn't bought them for Travis. He'd bought them to take to Louie Allegrezza's Fourth of July barbeque. If anyone asked, that was the story, but he doubted anyone would believe him. Like all other residents of the pyrotechnically obsessed town, he had a big box of illegals just waiting to be shot over the lake. Adults didn't buy Safe and Sanes unless they had kids. Legal fireworks were kind of like training wheels.

Travis and Louie's son Pete Allegrezza were buddies, and days ago, Meg had agreed that Travis could go to the barbeque with Mick if he stayed out of trouble. The barbeque was tomorrow, and Mick figured Travis should be able to control his behavior for one more day. Mick shut the door to his truck, and he and Travis headed across the parking lot toward the hardware store. 'If you behave yourself, maybe you can hold a sparkler.'

'Man,' Travis whined. 'Sparklers are for little kids.'

'With your track record, you'll be lucky if you're not in bed before dark.' Sunlight shone in his nephew's short black hair and across the shoulders of his red Spider-Man T-shirt. 'You're having a hard time controlling yourself lately.' He opened the door and waved to the owner standing behind the counter. 'Meg's still pretty mad at us both, but I have a plan.' For several months, Meg had complained about a leaky pipe beneath her kitchen sink. If he and Travis fixed her S trap so that she didn't have to keep emptying a pan of water, maybe she'd be in a more forgiving mood. But with Meg, a person never knew. She wasn't always the most forgiving person.

The soles of Travis's sneakers scuffed alongside Mick's boots as they walked to the plumbing section. The store was quiet except for a couple looking at garden hoses and Mrs Vaughn, his first-grade teacher, rooting through a bin of assorted drawer handles. He was always amazed to see Laverne Vaughn still alive and walking around. She had to be older than dirt.

While Mick grabbed a PVC pipe and plastic washers, his nephew picked up a caulking gun and aimed it at a bird feeder at the end of the aisle as if it were a .45 Magnum.

'We don't need that,' Mick told him as he reached for some plumber's tape.

Travis popped off a few rounds, then tossed the gun back onto the shelf. 'I'm gonna go look at the deer,' he said and disappeared around the corner of the aisle. Handy Man's had a big selection of plastic animals that people could display in their yards. Although why you would want to do that when the real thing was likely to roam through was beyond Mick.

He stuck the pipe beneath one arm and went in search of his nephew, who didn't usually go looking for trouble, but like most seven-year-old boys seemed to find it anyway. He moved through the store, glanced down each crammed row, and paused next to a display of mops.

A smile of pure male appreciation curved the corners of his mouth. Maddie Dupree stood in the middle of aisle six, a neon-yellow box in her hands. Her brown hair was in one of those claws and looked like someone had stuck a dark feather duster on the back of her head. His gaze moved down her smooth profile, past her throat and shoulder, and stopped dead on her black T-shirt. Last night, he hadn't been able to get a good look at her. Today, the fluorescent lighting of Handy Man Hardware lit her up like a walking, talking, breathing centerfold. Like an old-school playmate before eating disorders and silicone. Desire stirred in the pit of his stomach. He didn't even know her well enough to be feeling a thing. Didn't know if she was married or single, had a man in her life and ten kids waiting at home. Apparently it didn't matter, because she drew him down the aisle like a magnet.

'Looks like you got problems with some mice,' he said.

'What?' Her head snapped up and her gaze flew to his like he'd caught her doing something she shouldn't. 'Christ almighty.' Her lips parted and she sucked in a breath, drawing his attention to the mole at the corner of her mouth. 'You startled me.'

'Sorry,' he said, but he really wasn't. She looked good all wide-eyed and breathy and a little off balance. He glanced up and pointed with the PVC to the box in her hand. 'Mice troubles?'

'One actually ran across my foot this morning while I was making coffee.' She crinkled her nose. 'It slid under the pantry door and disappeared. It's probably in there right now feasting on my granola bars.'

'Don't worry.' Mick laughed. 'He probably won't eat much.'

'I don't want him to eat anything at all.

Except maybe some poison.' She turned her attention back to the box in her hand. Fine dark hair clung to the side of her neck and Mick thought he smelled strawberries.

At the far end of the aisle, Travis turned the corner and stopped in his tracks. His mouth got a little slack as he stared at Maddie. Mick knew the feeling.

'It says here that odor problems can occur if rodents expire in inaccessible areas. I really don't want to have to search for stinking mice.' She looked up at him out of the corners of her eyes. 'I wonder if there isn't something better I could use.'

'I wouldn't recommend the tape.' He pointed to a box of glue boards. 'Mice get stuck on it and squeak a lot.' There it was again. Strawberries, and he wondered if Handy's had some scented feeders for hummingbirds. 'You could use traps,' he suggested.

'Really? Aren't traps kind of . . . violent?'

'They can snap a mouse in half,' Travis said as he came to stand beside Mick. He rocked back on his heels and grinned. 'Sometimes their head pops off when they go for the cheese.'

'Good Lord, kid.' Maddie's brows drew together as she lowered her gaze to Travis. 'That's gruesome.'

'Uh-huh.'

Mick stuck the pipe under his arm and placed his free hand on top of Travis's head. 'This gruesome guy is my nephew, Travis Hennessy. Travis, say hello to Maddie Dupree.'

Maddie stuck out her palm and shook Travis's hand. 'It's a pleasure to meet you, Travis.'

'Yeah. You too.'

'And thanks for telling me about the traps,' she continued and released him. 'I'll keep them in mind if I decide on decapitation.'

Travis's smile grew to show off his missing front tooth. 'Last year I killed tons of mice,' he boasted, employing his special brand of seven-year-old charm. 'Call me.'

Mick glanced down at his nephew and wasn't sure, but he thought Travis was puffing up his skinny chest. 'The best way to get rid of mice,' he said, saving Travis from embarrassing himself further, 'is to get a cat.'

Maddie shook her head and her brown eyes looked into his, all warm and soft and liquid. 'Cats and I don't get along.' His gaze slid to her mouth and he again wondered how long it had been since he'd kissed a mouth that good. 'I'd rather have severed heads in my kitchen or hidden carcasses stinking up the place.'

She was talking about severed heads and stinking carcasses and he was getting turned on. Right there in Handy Man Hardware, like he was sixteen again and couldn't control himself. He'd been with a lot of beautiful women and wasn't a kid. He'd saved Travis from embarrassing himself, but who was going to save him?

'We've got some plumbing to do.' He held up the sealant and took a step back. 'Good luck with those mice.'

'See you boys around.'

'Yeah,' Travis said and followed him to the check-out counter. 'She was nice,' he whispered. 'I like the color of her hair.'

Mick chuckled and set the PVC next to the register. The kid was only seven, but he was a Hennessy.

3

September 5, 1976

Dan said he was going to leave his wife for me!! He said he'd been sleeping on the couch since May. I just found out she got pregnant in June. I've been cheated and lied to!! When is it my turn for happiness? The only person who loves me is my baby girl. She's three now and tells me every day that she loves me. She deserves a better life.

Why can't Jesus drop-kick us somewhere nice?

Maddie closed her eyes and leaned her head back in her office chair. In reading the diaries, not only had Maddie discovered her mother's passion for exclamation marks, but her fondness for other women's husbands as well. Counting Loch Hennessy, she'd had three of them in her twenty-four years. Not counting Loch, each had vowed to leave his wife for her, but in the end, they'd all *cheated and lied!!*

Maddie tossed the diary on her desk and

45

stretched her arms above her head. Besides the husbands, Alice had dated single men also. In the end, they'd all cheated and lied and left her for someone else. All except Loch. Although, if the affair hadn't been cut short, Maddie was sure Loch would have cheated and lied like all the others. Single or married, her mother had chosen men who left her heartbroken.

Through the open windows, the noise from her neighbors' barbeque carried on a slight breeze. It was the Fourth of July, and Truly was in full celebration mode. In town, buildings were decked out in red, white, and blue bunting, and that morning there'd been a parade down Main Street. Maddie had read in the local paper about the big celebration planned in Shaw Park and the town's 'impressive fireworks show' to begin 'at full dark.'

Maddie stood and walked into the bathroom. Although really, how 'impressive' could the show be in such a small town? Boise, the capital city, hadn't had a decent show in years.

She plugged the drain in the deep jetted tub and turned on the water. As she undressed, her neighbors' laughter carried though the small window above the toilet. Earlier in the day, Louie and Lisa Allegrezza had come over to invite her to their barbeque, but even at her best, she wasn't very good at making polite conversation with people she didn't know. And lately, Maddie had not been at her best. Finding the diaries had been a real mixed blessing. The diaries had answered some important questions for her. Questions that most people knew from birth. She'd learned that her father was from Madrid and that her mother had become pregnant with Maddie the summer after graduating from high school. Her father had been in the States visiting family, and they'd both fallen madly in 'luv'. At the end of the summer, Alejandro had returned to Spain. Alice had written him several letters to tell him about her pregnancy, but she'd never heard from him. Apparently, their 'luv' had been one-sided.

Maddie swept her hair up and clamped it on top of her head with a big claw. She'd come to terms with the fact long ago that she would never know her father. That she would never know his face or the sound of his voice. That he'd never teach her to ride a bike or drive a car, but like everything else, reading the diaries had brought it all to the surface again and she wondered if Alejandro was dead or alive and what he might think of her. Not that she would ever know.

Maddie poured German chocolate cake

47

bubble bath into the running water and set a tube of chocolate-cake-scented body scrub on the side of the tub. She might not care about matching underwear or the brand name on her shoes, but she loved bath products. Scented potions and lotions were her passion. Give her a creamy scrub and body butter over designer clothes any day.

Naked, she stepped into the tub and lowered herself into the warm scented water. 'Ahh,' she sighed as she slid beneath the suds. She leaned back against the cool porcelain and closed her eyes. She owned every scent imaginable. Everything from roses to apples, espresso to cake, and years ago she'd made peace and learned how to live with her inner hedonist.

There'd been a time in her life when she'd binged on almost anything that gave her pleasure. Men, dessert, and expensive lotions had featured high on her list. As a result of all that bingeing she'd developed a narrow view of men and a large behind. A very soft and smooth behind, but a big butt nonetheless. As a child, she'd been overweight and the horrors of once again hauling a wide load had forced her to change her life. The realization had happened on the morning of her thirtieth birthday when she'd woken up with a cheesecake hangover and a guy named

Derrick. The cheesecake had been mediocre and Derrick a real disappointment.

These days she was still a hedonist at heart, but she was a *nonpracticing* hedonist. She still over-indulged on lotions and bath products, but she needed those to relax and destress and to stave off dry, flaky skin.

She sank farther beneath the water and attempted to find a little peace for herself. Her body succumbed to the bubbles and warm water, but her mind wasn't so easily quieted and continued to roam over the past few weeks. She was making real progress on her time-line and notes. She had a list of people mentioned in her mother's last diary, the few friends she'd made in Truly and people with whom she'd worked. The county coroner from 1978 had died, but the sheriff still lived in Truly. He was retired, but Maddie was sure he could provide valuable information. She had newspaper accounts, police reports, the coroner's findings, and as much information on the Hennessy family as she could possibly dig up. Now all she had to do was talk to anyone connected to her mother's life and death.

She'd discovered that two women her mother had worked with still lived in town and she planned to start with them tomorrow morning. It was past time she talked to

49

people in town and started unearthing information.

The warm water and scented bubbles slid over her stomach and the bottom swell of her breasts. Reading those diaries, she could almost hear her mother's voice for the first time in twenty-nine years. Alice wrote about her fear at finding herself alone and pregnant and her excitement over Maddie's birth. Reading about her hopes and dreams for herself and her baby had been heartbreaking and so bittersweet. But with the heartbreaking and bittersweet discoveries, she'd learned that her mother wasn't the blond-haired, blue-eyed angel she'd created in her child's head and heart. Alice had been the sort of woman who had to have a man in her life or she'd felt worthless. She'd been needy and naive and eternally optimistic. Maddie had never been needy, nor could she recall a time when she'd been naive or overly optimistic about anything. Not even as a child. Discovering that she had absolutely nothing in common with the woman who'd given her birth, nothing that tied her to her mother, left her empty inside.

Early in life, Maddie had developed a hard shell around her soul. Her tough exterior had always been an asset while doing her job, but she didn't feel so tough today. She felt raw and vulnerable. Vulnerable to what, she didn't know, but she hated the feeling. It would be so much easier if she tossed the diaries and wrote about a psychopath by the name of Roddy Durban. She'd been writing about the nasty little bastard who'd killed more than twenty-three prostitutes right before she'd found the diaries. Writing about Roddy would be a hell of a lot easier than writing about her mother, but the night that Maddie had taken the diaries home and read them, she knew there was no turning back. Her career, while not always carefully calculated, had not been random. She was a true crime writer for a reason, and as she'd pored over her mother's overly feminine handwriting, she knew the time had come to sit down and write about the crime that had left her mother dead.

She turned off the water with her foot and reached for the body scrub on the side of the tub. She squirted the thick sugar scrub into her palm and the scent of chocolate cake filled her nose. With it came the unbidden memory of standing on a chair next to her mother and stirring chocolate pudding on the stove. She didn't know how old she'd been or where they'd lived. The memory was as tangible as a wisp of smoke, but it managed to deliver a punch to the lonely place next to her heart.

Bubbles clung to her breasts as she sat up and lifted her feet over the side of the tub. Obviously, she'd failed to find the calm and comfort she usually found in her bath, and she quickly exfoliated her arms and legs. When she was through, she got out of the tub and dried off, then she rubbed chocolate-scented lotion into her skin.

She tossed her clothes in the hamper and walked into her bedroom. Her three closest friends lived in Boise, and she missed meeting them for lunch or dinner or impromptu bitch sessions. Her friends Lucy, Clare, and Adele were the closest thing she had to a family, and the only people for whom she would consider giving a kidney or loaning money. She was fairly certain they would return the favor.

Last year when her friend Clare had discovered her fiancé with another man, the other three friends had rushed to her house to talk her off the ledge. Out of the four women, Clare was the most kind-hearted and easily hurt. She was also a romance writer who'd always believed in true love. For a time after her fiancé's betrayal, she'd lost her faith in the happy-ever-after until a reporter by the name of Sebastian Vaughan came into her life and restored her faith. He was her very own romance hero, and the two were getting married in September. Maddie had to drive to Boise in a few days to be fitted for her bridesmaid dress.

Once again she was allowing one of her friends to deck her out in a ridiculous dress and make her stand up at the front of a church. The year before she'd been a bridesmaid at Lucy's wedding. Lucy was a mystery writer and had met her husband Quinn when he'd mistaken her for a serial killer. Long story short, he hadn't let a little thing like homicide stand in the way of his pursuit of Lucy.

Out of the four friends, that left herself and Adele still single. Maddie pulled on a pair of black cotton panties and tossed the towel on the bed. Adele wrote fantasy novels for a living, and although she had her own man troubles, Maddie figured it was a lot more likely that Adele would marry before she would herself.

Maddie fit the large cups of her bra over her breasts and fastened it in back. In fact, she just didn't see herself getting married. She wanted a kid about as much as she wanted a cat. The only time a man came in handy was when she needed someone to do some heavy lifting or when she desired a warm naked body next to hers. But she owned a sturdy hand truck and big Carlos, and when she had need of heavy lifting or sexual release she reached for one of them. Admittedly, neither was as good as the real thing, but the hand truck went back in the garage when she was through, and big Carlos got shoved back into her bedside table. Both of them stayed put and didn't give her crap, play games with her heart, or cheat on her. Pretty much a win-win.

She stepped into a pair of jeans and then shoved her arms through the sleeves of her most comfortable hooded sweatshirt. She just didn't have the same burning desires, or instincts, or clocks that drove other women into matrimony and childbirth. Which wasn't to say that she didn't get lonely sometimes. She absolutely did.

Shoving her feet into a pair of flip-flops, she moved from the bedroom, though the living room, to the kitchen. The noise from the neighbors' party grew louder and she reached into the refrigerator. Voices floated in through her open windows as she pulled out a bottle of carb-reduced merlot. She was alone and lonely and apparently feeling quite sorry for herself too. Which really wasn't like her. She never felt sorry for herself. There were too many people in the world with real problems.

The shrill screech of at least a half dozen Piccolo Petes sliced through the air, and

Maddie almost dropped the corkscrew. 'Damn it,' she cursed and placed her free hand over her heart. Beyond the French doors leading out to her deck, she could see the pale shadows of dusk and the darkening surface of the usually emerald-green lake. She poured red wine into a glass and carried it outside to the deck and set it on the chest-high railing. A dozen or so people stood on the neighbors' deck and the beach below. Along the water's edge three mortar tubes stuck out of the sand and pointed toward the sky. Several children held sparklers while men supervised, lit more Piccolo Petes and something that flashed like little strobe lights. Smoke from bombs of every color clouded the beach, and the children ran through the paisley haze like genies from a bottle.

Against the smoke and chaos, Mick Hennessy stood in profile with a punk between his teeth like a long thin cigarette. She recognized his wide shoulders and black hair and the boy who stood gazing up at him. He handed his nephew a lit sparkler and Travis spun on one foot and waved it about. Mick took the punk from between his teeth, said something, and Travis immediately stopped and held the firework in front of him like a statue.

Maddie took a sip of her wine. Yesterday,

seeing him at the hardware store had been a real shock. She'd been so intent on her box of poison that she hadn't noticed him until he'd stood right next to her. Looking up into those blue eyes so close and so much like his father's had forced a stunned 'Christ almighty' out of her.

She lowered the glass and set it on the railing as she watched Mick with his nephew. She really didn't know what to think about him. Not that she knew enough to form an opinion or that it even mattered. The book she planned to write had nothing to do with him and everything to do with the love triangle between Loch, Rose, and Alice. Like Maddie, Mick had been just another innocent victim.

Louie Allegrezza and two other men knelt close to the water and stuck bottle rockets into several soda bottles. They lit one fuse right after the other, and Maddie watched the rockets fly up high over the water and explode with soft pop-pop-pops.

'Be careful with those around the kids,' Lisa called down to her husband.

'These never hurt anyone,' he called back as he once again loaded up the bottles. Four of the rockets flew straight up, while the fifth flew straight at Maddie. She ducked as it whizzed past her head.

56

'Shit!'

The rocket landed behind her and exploded on her deck. With her heart pounding in her ears, she straightened to peer over the railing.

'Sorry about that,' Louie called out.

Through the light wash of gray night, Mick Hennessy looked up and stared at her for several seconds. His dark brows lifted as if surprised to see her standing there. Then he rocked back on his heels and laughed like the whole thing was horribly funny. The dimples denting his cheeks and the amusement in his shining blue eyes gave the illusion that he was as trustworthy and harmless as a Boy Scout. But harmless Boy Scouts wore their beige shirts buttoned and tucked into their pants. A Boy Scout didn't leave his shirt hanging open, showing off washboard abs and a lickable happy trail running down his sternum, circling his navel, and disappearing behind the waistband of his Levi's. Not that she was in any danger of licking any part of him. But just because he was who he was and she was who she was didn't mean she was blind.

'Louie, warn us before you set those things off,' Lisa said above the noise. 'Maddie, come over here. You'll be safer.'

Maddie tore her gaze from Mick's chest

and looked across the ten feet of yard at her neighbor. When it came to safety, trading her deck for theirs didn't make a bit of sense, but since staring at Mick's chest was the biggest thrill she'd had in weeks, she was obviously bored and sick of her own company.

She grabbed her glass and walked the short distance. She was quickly introduced to Louie's daughter Sofie and her friends who lived in Boise and attended BSU but were in Truly for the weekend. She met several neighbors from farther down the beach, Tanya King, a petite blonde who looked like she hung from her heels and did crunchies all day, and Suzanne Porter, whose husband Glenn and teenage son Donald were on the beach setting off fireworks. After that, she lost track of names and couldn't remember who was whom, where they lived, or how long they'd lived in town. They all blurred together except for Louie's mother and aunt Narcisa, who sat at a table wearing equally disarming scowls of disapproval and speaking to each other in rapid Basque. No way could she forget those women.

'Would you like more wine?' Lisa asked. 'I've got Basque Red and Chablis. Or you can have beer or a Coke.'

'No, thanks.' She held up her half-full glass and looked at it. 'I'm a cheap date tonight.'

She needed to get up early and get to work, and wine tended to give her a headache.

'Before I married Louie and had Pete, these Fourth of July barbeques were out of control. Lots of drunks and dangerous fireworks.'

As far as Maddie could see, not a lot had changed.

The last person she was introduced to was Lisa's sister-in-law, Delaney, who looked about twelve months pregnant.

'I'm not due until September,' Delaney said as if she'd read Maddie's mind.

'You're joking.'

'No.' Delaney laughed and her blond ponytail brushed her shoulder as she shook her head. 'I'm having twin girls.' She pointed toward the beach. 'That's my husband, Nick, down there with Louie. He's going to be a great dad.'

As if on cue, the great dad-to-be turned and his gaze sought his wife. He was tall and unbelievably handsome, and the only other guy around who gave Mick Hennessy any competition whatsoever in the looks department. Then his intense gaze found his wife and the competition was over. There was just nothing sexier than a man who only had eyes for one woman. Especially when that woman looked like Buddha.

'Are you okay?' Nick Allegrezza called out.

'For goodness' sake,' Delaney grumbled, then yelled, 'Yes.'

'Maybe you should sit down,' Nick suggested.

She spread her arms. 'I'm fine.'

Maddie's gaze slid to Mick, who knelt on one knee as he helped Travis light a flashing strobe. She wondered if he had ever looked that way at any one woman, or if he was more like his father and had eyes for a lot of women.

'Fire in the hole,' Louie yelled, and Maddie's gaze flew to the bottle rockets whizzing upward. This time none of the rockets buzzed Maddie's head and instead exploded above the lake. Relief calmed her beating heart. A few years ago, she'd volunteered to be Tasered in one of her self-defense classes. She wasn't a chicken, but those flying missiles worried her.

'Last week I started to have a few contractions, and the doctor said the babies are probably going to come early,' Delaney said, drawing Maddie's attention. 'Nick's totally freaking out about it, but I'm not worried. We've been through hell to have these girls. The hard part is over and everything else will be fine.'

Maddie had spent her adult life trying *not*

to get pregnant and wondered what Delaney had been through, but she didn't know her well enough to ask.

'You two did go through hell.' Lisa rubbed her sister-in-law's belly, then dropped her hands to her sides. 'But I have a feeling that having two thirteen-year-old girls in the same house at the same time is going to give new meaning to the word hell.'

'Not a problem. Nick's not going to let the girls out of his sight until they're twenty-one for fear they'll run into boys like him.'

Suzanne raised a glass of white wine and laughed. 'I never thought Nick would settle down and get married. Growing up, he was as wild as Louie was crazy.'

'Louie wasn't crazy,' Lisa defended her husband, and her brows lowered over her blue eyes.

'Everyone called him Crazy Louie for a reason,' Delaney reminded her sister-in-law. 'He stole his first car when he was, what? Ten?'

'Yeah, well, Nick was right there in the passenger seat with Louie.' Lisa sniffed. 'And he really didn't steal cars. He just borrowed them for a few hours.'

Delaney's brows lowered. 'Are you listening to yourself?'

Lisa shrugged. 'It's true. Besides, Nick

came up with lots of bad ideas all on his own. Remember those horrid snowball fights?'

'Of course, but Nick doesn't have to throw things at me to get my attention these days.' Delaney smiled and rested her hands on top of her big belly. 'He's still a little wild sometimes, but nothing like he was in school.'

'Every class had at least one bad boy. Class of 1990 it was Mick Hennessy,' Suzanne said. 'He was always in trouble. In the eighth grade, he punched Mr Shockey in the face.'

Maddie casually took a sip of her wine as if her ears hadn't perked up.

'I'm sure Mr Shockey deserved it,' Lisa defended Mick. 'He used to make us run track even when we had period cramps. Sadistic bastard.'

'Lisa, you were always having cramps,' Delaney reminded her sister-in-law. 'Even in the first grade. And I swear you'd defend the devil.'

Lisa shrugged. 'All I'm saying is that considering what Mick had to deal with growing up, he turned out pretty good.'

Maddie didn't know what Mick had dealt with as a child, but she could guess.

'I didn't know Mick growing up, but I've heard the stories.' Tanya raised her glass and took a drink. 'And he turned out *real* good.' Behind the glass, one corner of Tanya's lips lifted, leaving little doubt that she knew just how 'real good' Mick was.

'Be careful, Tanya, Mick is like his daddy,' Suzanne warned. 'He isn't the kind of guy to stay with one woman. Last year Cinda Larson thought she had him all to herself, but he was seeing a few other women at the same time.'

The difference being, Maddie thought, Mick wasn't married like his daddy had been.

'I just got divorced last year.' Tanya wore a strapless sundress on her tiny body, and she shrugged one bare shoulder. 'I'm not looking for an exclusive relationship,'

Maddie took a drink of her wine and made a mental note. Not that Mick's relationships with women were of interest to her, personally or professionally. His and Meg's personal relationships would not end up in the book any more than hers, but she was curious. Curious if their childhood had been any better than hers. From the little she'd just heard, she'd say no.

Suzanne moved to the rail and yelled down, 'Donald, make sure you point the big ones over the lake.' Then she turned back and her green eyes settled on Maddie. 'Do you have children?' she asked.

'No.' If she hadn't been standing next to a pregnant lady, she might have added that she didn't think she'd ever want children either.

'What do you do for a living?'

If Maddie answered truthfully, she'd open herself up to questions she wasn't so sure she wanted to answer at a Fourth of July barbeque. Not yet, and especially not with Mick and Travis walking up the beach toward her. The ends of Mick's shirt slightly billowing about his chest and hips as he moved, drawing her and every other female's attention to his Levi's hanging low on his bare waist.

There was no doubt about it. Mick Hennessy was so blatantly all man that it hit a woman like a brick to the forehead. He was headed straight for her, and she'd be lying to herself if she pretended that he wasn't hot as hell. While she had no problem lying to other people, she could never lie to herself.

4

'Fire in the hole!' Louie shouted and set off several screeching rockets, saving Maddie the effort of thinking up a half-truth or full-out lie. Four rockets flew up instead of at her head and her pulse steadied.

These rockets were a little bigger than the last and exploded in small bursts of color. Louie had broken out heavier artillery, yet still no one seemed in the least worried. No one except Maddie.

'I want to stay down there,' Travis grumbled as he, Mick, and Pete moved up the steps of the deck.

'The big show's about to start,' Mick said, 'and you know kids have to move where it's safe.'

Big show? She raised her wine and drained the glass. She wondered if Mick was going to put Tanya out of her misery and button his shirt. Sure, it had been hot earlier, but it was getting fairly nippy now.

'Donald is a kid,' Pete complained.

'Donald is fourteen,' Lisa said. 'If you're going to argue, you can go sit by your grandmother and Tia Narcisa.'

Pete quickly plopped his behind down on the steps. 'I'll sit here.' Travis sat next to him, but neither appeared happy about being confined to the deck.

'Hey, Mick,' Tanya called out to him.

He glanced up from Travis, but his gaze met Maddie's. His blue eyes looked into hers for several heartbeats before he turned his attention to the petite woman on Maddie's left. 'Hey, there, Tanya. How's it going?'

'Good. I still have some Bushmills Malt 21. What are you doing after the show?'

'I've got to take Travis home, then head to work,' he said. 'Maybe some other time.' He moved past them to a cooler and bent at the waist. He lifted the white lid and his shirt fell open. Naturally. 'Yo, Travis and Pete,' he called out. 'Do you boys want a root beer?'

As one, the two boys turned at the waist. 'Yeah.'

'Sure.'

Ice and water sloshed in the cooler as he grabbed two cans of Hires and lobbed them into the boys' waiting hands. He pulled out a Red Bull, then closed the cooler's lid.

'Maddie, have you met Mick Hennessy?' Lisa asked.

Out of habit, she held out her hand, 'Yes, we've met.'

He wiped his hand on his pants, then took

her fingers in his cool wet palm. 'Kill any mice today?'

'No.' His thumb brushed her bare ring finger and he smiled. Intentional or not, she didn't know, but the light touch spread hot itchy little tingles to her wrist. It was the closest she'd come to real sex in years. 'No dead mice yet, but I'm hoping they're experiencing death rattles even as we speak.' She pulled her hand back before she forgot who he was and why she was in town. Once he found out, she doubted there would be any more handshakes and tingles. Not that she particularly wanted either.

'Call an exterminator,' Tanya said.

Maddie had called an exterminator and he couldn't get to her house for a month.

'Be careful who you call,' Lisa warned. 'Carpenters and exterminators work on Miller time around here and they have a habit of just up and leaving at three o'clock.'

'I take it three o'clock is Miller time.'

'Pretty much.' Lisa's mother-in-law called her name and she grimaced. 'Excuse me.'

'Better her than me,' Delaney uttered as Lisa walked away.

'I could give you the number of someone who might actually arrive when he says he will.' Mick popped the top to his Red Bull. 'And stay until the job is finished.'

'Have your husband or boyfriend take care of your mice problem,' Tanya suggested.

She looked at Tanya and suddenly didn't get a nice neighborly vibe. The energy had changed since Mick had walked onto the deck. She wasn't sure, but she guessed that Tanya wasn't going to be her new bff. 'Don't have a boyfriend and I've never been married.'

'Never?' Tanya raised a brow as if Maddie were a freak, and Maddie would have laughed if it wasn't so ridiculous.

'Hard to believe, isn't it?' she said. Tanya need not worry. The very last man on the planet she would ever get involved with was Mick Hennessy. Despite his nice abs and killer happy trail. 'I'm such a great catch.'

Mick chuckled and took a drink of his Red Bull. Through the darkening shadows of nightfall, she could just see the laugh lines creasing the corners of his blue eyes as he looked at her over the bottom of the silver can.

She smiled back and decided it was past time to change the subject. 'Did you have to toss Darla out of Mora's on her bare behind?'

He lowered the can and sucked moisture from his bottom lip. 'Nah. She behaved.'

'Are women still tossing their panties?' Delaney asked.

'Not as much. Thank God.' Mick shook his

head and grinned, a flash of white against the dark. 'Believe me, tossing drunk, half-naked women from my bar isn't as fun as it sounds.'

Maddie laughed. Never in a million years would she have thought she'd find Mick Hennessy so utterly likable. 'Does that happen very often?' Then again, he was his father's son.

'Mort's used to be a really wild place before I took over, and some people are having a hard time adjusting.'

'They've never adjusted to Jackson's Texaco taking over for Grover's Gas and Go, and that was about six years ago.' Delaney drew in a breath and let it out slowly. 'My feet are killing me.'

'Fire in the hole!' Louie yelled seconds before sending up another barrage. Maddie spun around and her gaze flew to the rockets soaring straight up.

Behind her, Mick's deep laughter was almost drowned out by the rockets' pop-pop-pops. When she turned back, he'd moved to help Delaney find a chair. Tanya trailed after them and Maddie wasn't sorry to see her go. The woman had gone from perfectly pleasant to bitchy over a man, something Maddie had never understood. There were so many available men on the planet, why get all uptight over one? Especially if that one had a reputation for never getting involved. For loving and leaving. Not that Maddie ever held that against anyone. She didn't understand women who got so attached so easily. After a few dates or good sex, they were in love. How did that happen? How was that even possible?

Sofie Allegrezza and her friends moved to the railing beside Maddie for a better view of her father's fireworks show. Maddie set her glass on the railing and watched Louie load up the three big mortar tubes. She'd never needed a man in order to feel good about herself or to make her life complete. Not like her mother.

'Fire in the hole.' This time there was an audible whoosh seconds before the three rounds shot from tubes and exploded with three loud booms. Startled, Maddie jumped back and collided with something solid. A pair of big hands grabbed her arms as green, gold, and red bursts of fire rained down toward the lake. 'Sorry.' She turned her head and looked up into the shadows resting on Mick's face.

'Not a problem.' Instead of pushing her away, he held her right where she'd landed. 'Tell me something.'

'What?'

He lowered his face and spoke just above her ear. 'If you're a great catch, why haven't you been caught?'

His warm breath touched the side of her head and slipped down her neck. 'Probably for the same reason you haven't.'

'Which is?'

'You don't want to be caught.'

'Honey, all women want to be caught.' His hands slid to her elbows, then up again, bunching her sweatshirt. 'All women want a white wedding, picket fence, and a baby maker.'

'Have you met all women?'

She thought she felt him smile. 'I've met my share.'

'So I hear.'

'You shouldn't believe everything you hear.'

'And you shouldn't believe all women want you for their own personal baby maker.'

'You don't want me for your own personal baby maker?'

'Shocking, isn't it?'

He laughed. A low rumble against the side of her head. 'You smell good.' Against her back, she felt him draw in a deep breath.

'German chocolate cake.'

'What?'

'I smell like German chocolate cake body scrub.'

'I haven't had chocolate cake in a long time.' She'd been mistaken about his hand-shake being like the best sex she'd had in years. This, his soft breath in her hair and his hands on her arms, was practically orgasmic. Which she figured made her particularly pathetic. 'You're making me hungry,' he said next to her ear.

'For cake?'

His hands slid to her shoulders, then back down to her elbows. 'For starters.'

'Uncle Mick,' Travis called out as he stood. 'When are the town fireworks going to start?'

Mick looked up. His hands tightened a fraction, then dropped to his sides. 'Any minute,' he answered and took a step back. As if on cue, several enormous booms shook the ground and the night sky lit up with huge bursts of color. Sofie Allegrezza pushed play on her small sound system and Jimi Hendrix's sonic guitar wailed 'The Star Spangled Banner' into the night. Forest critters scrambled for cover as around the lake fireworks exploded from the beaches, competing with the town's pyrotechnic eruptions.

Welcome to Truly. The original shock and awe.

★　★　★

'Did you have fun, Travis?'

A huge yawn came from the other side of the dark truck. 'Yeah. Maybe next year I can blow off bigger fireworks.'

'Maybe, if you stay out of trouble.'

'Mom said if I stay out of trouble, I can get a puppy.'

Mick turned the Ram into Meg's driveway and pulled to a stop next to her Ford Taurus. A dog was a good idea. A boy needed a dog. 'What kind of puppy?'

'I like black ones with white spots.'

Lights burned from within the house and a single bulb lit the porch. Together they climbed out of the truck and walked up the front steps. It was close to eleven-thirty and Travis's feet were dragging. 'How long do you have to be good?'

'For one month.'

The kid couldn't stay out of trouble with his mother for one week. 'Well, just watch your mouth and you might make it.' He shoved his keys into his pants pocket and opened the door for his nephew.

Meg sat on the couch in her white nightgown and pink fuzzy robe. Tears shone in her green eyes as she looked up from something she held in her hand. A forced smile curved her lips and dread settled on Mick's shoulders. It was going to be one of those nights.

'Did you see the fireworks, Mom?' If Travis noticed, he didn't seem bothered.

'No, honey, I didn't go outside. But I heard

73

them.' She stood and Travis wrapped his arms around her waist. 'They were huge!'

'Did you behave yourself?' She placed her hand on her son's head and looked over at Mick.

'Yes,' Travis answered, and Mick confirmed it with a nod.

'That's my good boy.'

Travis looked up. 'Pete said maybe I could spend the night and his mom said, 'Some other time.''

'We'll see.' Like their mother, Meg was a beautiful woman, with smooth white skin and long black hair. And as with their mother, her moods were unpredictable as hell. 'Go get your pajamas on and get in bed. I'll be in to kiss you good night in a minute.'

'Okay,' Travis said through a yawn. 'Good night, Uncle Mick.'

'Night, buddy.' An almost overwhelming urge to turn away pulled at Mick and he actually took a step back. Away from what he knew was to come and toward the cool night air.

Meg watched her son leave the room, then she held out her hand and opened her palm. 'I found Mom's wedding ring.'

'Meg.'

'She took it off and left it on her nightstand before she went to the bar that night. She never took it off.'

'I thought you weren't going to go through her things anymore.'

'I wasn't.' She closed her hand around the ring and bit her thumbnail. 'It was packed away with Grandmother Loraine's jewelry, and I found it when I was looking for her four leaf clover necklace. The one she used to wear all the time because it brought her luck. I wanted to wear it to work tomorrow.'

God, he hated when his sister got like this. He was five years younger than Meg, but he'd always felt like the older brother.

Her big green eyes looked across at him and her hand fell to her side. 'Was Daddy really going to leave us?'

Hell, Mick didn't know. No one knew but Loch, and he was long dead. Dead and gone and in the past. Why couldn't Meg leave it alone?

Maybe because she'd just turned ten a few months before the night their mother had loaded a snubnosed .38 and emptied five chambers into Mick's father and a young waitress by the name of Alice Jones. Meg remembered a hell of a lot more about that night twenty-nine years ago when their mother had killed more than Loch and his latest lover. More about the night their mother had put the short barrel into her own mouth, pulled the trigger, and killed more than herself too. She'd blown apart the lives of her two children, and Meg had never really recovered.

'I don't know, Meggie. Grandmother didn't think so.' But that wasn't saying anything. Loraine had always turned a blind eye and deaf ear to her own husband's and son's many affairs and offenses and later to everything Mick had done. She lived her whole life in denial. It had been easier for her to pretend everything was wonderful. Especially when it wasn't.

'But Grandmother didn't live with us then. She didn't know what it was like. You didn't either. You were too little. You don't remember.'

'I remember enough.' He raised his hands and scrubbed his face. They'd had this conversation before and it never resolved anything. 'What does it matter now?'

'Did he stop loving us, Mick?'

He dropped his hands to his sides and felt the back of his skull get tight. *Please stop.*

Tears streamed down her cheeks. 'If he still loved us, why did she shoot him? He'd had affairs before. According to everyone in town, he'd had lots of affairs.'

He walked to his sister and put his hands on the shoulders of her fuzzy pink robe. 'Let it go.'

'I've tried. I've tried to be like you, and sometimes I can, but . . . why wasn't she buried with her wedding ring?'

The bigger question was, why had she loaded the .38? Had she really meant to kill anyone or just scare the piss out of Loch and his young lover? Who knew, but thinking about it didn't serve any purpose but to drive a person crazy. 'It doesn't matter now. Our life isn't in the past, Meg.'

She took a deep breath. 'You're right. I'll put the ring away and forget about it.' She shook her head. 'It's just that sometimes I can't turn it off.'

He pulled her to his chest and held her tight. 'I know.'

'I get so afraid.'

He got afraid too. Afraid that she'd fall into the downward spiral that had claimed their mother and that she'd never climb out. Mick had always wondered if his mother had given a second of thought to him and Meg. If she'd thought about the devastation and loss she was about to leave behind on a barroom floor. As she'd loaded the gun that night, had it crossed her mind that she was about to leave her children orphans or that her actions would force them to live within the horrible fallout of her action? As she'd driven to Hennessy's, had she thought about them and not cared? 'Have you been taking your medicine?'

'It makes me tired.'

'You have to take it.' He pulled back and looked down into her face. 'Travis depends on you. And I depend on you too.'

She sighed. 'You do not, and Travis would probably be better off without me.'

'Meg.' He looked deep into her eyes. 'You of all people know that isn't true.'

'I know.' She pushed her hair out of her face. 'I just meant that raising a boy is so hard.'

He hoped like hell that's what she meant. 'That's why you have me.' He smiled, even though he felt ten years older than he had before walking into the house. 'I'm not going anywhere. Even though you do make the world's shittiest meatloaf.'

She smiled, and just like that, her mood changed. Like someone reached into her head and flipped a switch. 'I like my meatloaf.'

'I know.' He dropped his hands and reached into his pocket for his keys. 'But you like old-lady food.' Meg cooked like their grandmother had. Like she was baking a casserole for a potluck at the senior center.

'You're evil and a bad influence on Travis.' She laughed and folded her arms across her chest. 'But you always make me feel better.'

'Good night,' he said and headed for the door. Cool night air brushed across his face and neck as he walked to his truck, and he took a deep breath and let it out. He'd always made Meg feel better. Always. And afterward, he always felt like shit. She'd have a breakdown, and when it was over, she'd be fine. Never seeming to notice the broken bits and pieces she'd left in the wake of her unpredictable moods.

Having been gone for twelve years, he'd almost forgotten what those moods were like. Sometimes he wished he'd just stayed gone.

5

Maddie reached for a bottle of Diet Coke sitting on her desk and unscrewed the cap. She took a long drink, then returned the cap. The instant she'd opened her eyes that morning, she'd known where the book had to open. In the past, she'd always opened each book with chilling facts.

This time she sat down and wrote:

'I promise it's going to be different this time, baby.' Alice Jones glanced at her young daughter, then returned her gaze to the road. 'You're going to love Truly. It's a little like heaven, and it's about damn time Jesus dropkicked us into a better life.'

Baby didn't say anything. She'd heard it before. The excitement in her mother's voice and the promises of a better life. The only thing that ever changed was their address.

Like always, baby wanted to believe her mother. Really she did, but she'd just turned five. Old enough to realize that nothing ever got better. Nothing ever changed.

'We're going to live in a nice trailer house.' She unfolded her arms from across her chest as she looked out the windshield at the pine trees whizzing by. A trailer house? She'd never lived in a house.

'And a swing set in the front yard.'

A swing set? She'd never had a swing set. She turned her gaze to her mother and the sunlight shining in her blond hair. Her mother looked like an angel on a Christmas card. Like she should be standing on top of a Christmas tree, and baby let herself believe. She let herself believe in the dream of finding heaven. She let herself believe in a better life, and for five months it had been better — right up until the night an enraged wife pumped a set of .38 hollow points into Alice Jones's young body and turned the dream into a nightmare.

Maddie pushed her chair back from her desk and stood. The sleeves of her cotton pajamas slid to her elbows as she raised her arms over her head and stretched. It was a little after noon and she hadn't showered. Her good friend Clare showered and put on makeup every day before she sat down to write. Not Maddie. Of course, that meant that occasionally she got caught by FedEx looking like complete crap. Something she really didn't worry about.

She jumped in the shower and thought about the rest of her day. She had a list of names and addresses with respective relationships to the case. First on the list was a visit to Value Rite Drug, where Carleen Dawson worked. Carleen had been a waitress at Hennessy's at the same time as Maddie's mother. She wanted to set up a time to interview the woman and asking in person had advantages over asking on the telephone.

After her shower, she rubbed almond-scented lotion into her skin and put on a black dress that wrapped around and tied at the side of her waist. She pulled her hair back from her face, applied a little mascara and a deep red lipstick. She wore red sandals and slid a notebook into her slim leather briefcase. Not that she planned to use anything in the briefcase, but it gave the right impression.

Value Rite Drug was located a few blocks off Main Street next to Helen's Hair Hut. Potted geraniums and yellow awnings gave the outside of the store splashes of color. The inside was stuffed with everything from Band-Aids and aspirin to wooden statues of elk, moose, and bear carved by locals. She asked at the front register where she might find Carleen and was pointed to the snack food aisle.

'Are you Carleen Dawson?' she asked a short woman wearing a white blouse and blue and red apron, and who was bent over a cart of marshmallows and Pop Smart.

She straightened and looked at Maddie through a pair of bifocal lenses. 'Yes.'

'Hello, my name is Madeline Dupree and I am a writer.' She handed Carleen a business card. 'I am hoping that you'll give me a few moments of your time.'

'I'm not on break.'

'I know.' Carleen's hair was processed within an inch of its life, and Maddie wondered briefly what was up with some of the locals and bad hair. 'I thought we could set up a time when you're off work.'

Carleen looked down at the black and silver card, then back up. 'True crime? You write true crime? Like Ann Rule?'

That hack. 'Yes. Exactly.'

'I don't know how I can help you. We don't have serial killers in Truly. There was one in Boise a few years ago, a female one, of all things. If you can believe that.'

Actually Maddie could believe it, since her friend Lucy had been a suspect, and since Maddie planned to write about the murderous rampage in the future.

'Nothing ever happens around here,' Carleen added and stuffed a bag of marshmallows on the shelf.

'I'm not writing about a serial killer.'

'What, then?'

Maddie's grasp on her briefcase tightened and she placed her other hand in the pocket of her dress. 'Twenty-nine years ago you worked in Hennessy's Bar when Rose Hennessy shot and killed her husband, a cocktail waitress named Alice Jones, then turned the handgun on herself.'

Carleen stilled. 'I wasn't there.'

'I know. You'd already gone home for the night.'

'That was a long time ago. Why do you want to write about that?'

Because it's my life. 'Because not all interesting true crime stories are about serial killers. Sometimes the best stories are about real people. Normal people who snap and commit horrible crimes.'

'I guess.'

'Did you know Alice Jones?'

'Yeah, I knew her. I knew Rose too, but I don't think I should talk about that. It was a real sad situation and people have moved on.' She shoved the business card back at Maddie. 'Sorry, I can't help you.'

Maddie knew when to press and when to take a step back. For now. 'Well, think about it.' She smiled and kept one hand in her pocket and the other wrapped around the handle of her briefcase. 'And if you change your mind, give me a call.'

Carleen slid the card into the front pocket of her blue apron. 'I won't change my mind. Some things are better left buried in the past.'

Perhaps, but what Carleen didn't know but would find out was that Maddie rarely took no for an answer.

★   ★   ★

'No. I can't help you.'

Maddie stood on the pockmarked porch of Jewel Finley, a second cocktail waitress, who had worked at Hennessy's at the time of Alice's death. 'It'll just take a few moments.'

'I'm busy.' Jewel's hair was in pink rollers and Maddie thought she detected the aroma of Dippity-do. Lord, did they still sell Dippity-do? 'Rose was my good friend and I'm not goin' to talk against her,' Jewel said. 'What happened to her was a tragedy. I'm not goin' to exploit her misfortune.'

Her misfortune? 'My purpose is not to exploit anyone, but to tell everyone's side of the story.'

'Your purpose is to make money.'

'Believe me, there are easier ways to make money.' Maddie felt her temper rise, but she wisely held back. 'Is there a better time for me to come back?'

'No.'

'Perhaps when you're not quite so busy.'

'I'm not goin' to talk to you about Rose, and I doubt anyone else will talk to you neither.' She stepped back into her house. 'Good-bye,' she said and shut the door.

Maddie stuck a business card in the porch screen and walked toward her Mercedes parked at the curb. Not only did Maddie not take no for an answer, she was like the damn Terminator and she'd be back.

★ ★ ★

'Do you know when he'll be back?'

'That depends on if the fish are biting. Tomorrow, if it's bad. Who knows, if it's good.' Levana Potter looked at Maddie's business card and turned it over. 'But I can tell you that he remembers everything about that night.' The wife of the retired sheriff looked up. 'It still haunts him.' She'd found Levana digging in the flower bed in the front of her ranch-style home, and the good news was that the sheriff would more than likely be willing to talk to Maddie. The bad news was her interview would have to wait on the capricious lake trout. 'Did you know the parties involved?'

'Sure.' Levana stuck the business card in

the pocket of her shirt, then shoved her hand back inside her gardening glove. 'The Hennessys have lived in this valley for generations. I didn't know Alice much. Just chatted the few times she came into the little ice-cream and gift store I used to own off Third. Pretty thing and seemed kind of sweet. Looked like an angel. She had a little girl, I know that. After Alice died, her aunt came and took her. I don't know whatever happened to her.'

Maddie smiled a little. 'Do you remember her name?'

Levana shook her head and her white permed hair wafted a bit in the breeze. 'Heavens, no. That was twenty-nine years ago and I only saw her a few times. Heck, I have a hard time remembering my own name sometimes.'

'Alice lived at the Roundup Trailer Court.'

'Heck, that was torn down years ago.'

'Yes, I know. But I can't find any records of people who might have lived there at the same time as Alice and her daughter.' In her diaries, Alice had mentioned a few women by their first names. 'Do you recall a woman named Trina who may have lived next door to Alice?'

'Hmm.' Levana shook her head. 'That doesn't ring any bells. Bill will know,' she said referring to her husband. 'He remembers everyone who ever lived in this town. I'll give him your card when he gets back from his fishing trip.'

'Thank you. I'm not going to be here in town tomorrow, but I'll be back the day after.'

'I'll tell him, but it might be next week.'

Fabulous. 'Thank you for your time.'

On the way home from the Potters', Maddie stopped off at the grocery store and bought a roasted deli chicken and some Excedrin. Carleen had been guarded and uncooperative and Jewel had been openly hostile. Her head pounded, she was frustrated by her lack of progress, and she had an urge to put someone in a headlock.

With a blue basket hanging off one arm, she took her place in line at checkout number three. The next time she spoke to Carleen and Jewel, she'd try a less businesslike tactic. She'd try the nice-as-pie, friendly approach. If that didn't work, she'd go all Jerry Springer on their hillbilly asses.

'I saw you at Value Rite earlier,' a woman in the next line over said.

Maddie looked up from putting her basket on the conveyor belt. 'Are you talking to me?'

'Yeah.' The other woman had short dark hair and wore a T-shirt with a picture of her grandkids on the front. 'Carleen said you were askin' about Rose and Loch Hennessy.'

Wow, word really did travel fast in small towns. 'That's right.'

'I grew up with Rose and she had a few problems, but she was a good person.'

A few problems. Is that what they all called pumping lead into two people? Maddie would call it a psychotic breakdown. 'I'm sure she was.'

'That little waitress got what she deserved for messing with a married man.'

Tired, frustrated, and now pissed off, Maddie said, 'So you think that every woman who gets involved with a married man deserves to die on a barroom floor?'

The woman tossed a bag of potatoes on the conveyor belt in front of her. 'Well, I just mean that if you mess around with another woman's man, you might get hurt. That's all.'

No, that wasn't all, but Maddie wisely held her tongue.

★ ★ ★

Maddie tossed her briefcase on the sofa and glanced at the photo of the mother sitting on the coffee table. 'Well, that was a waste of makeup.' She kicked off her shoes and put the photograph face down. She couldn't look at her mother's cheery smile when her day had been a bust.

Barefoot, she walked into the kitchen and reached into the refrigerator for the bottle of merlot she'd opened the day before. She thought better of it and grabbed the Skyy vodka, diet tonic, and a lime. Sometimes a girl needed a drink, even if she was alone. While she poured vodka into a highball glass and added the tonic, the George Thorogood song 'I Drink Alone' ran through her head. She'd never liked that song. Perhaps it was the writer in her, but the chorus was redundant. Of course when you drink alone you drink with nobody else.

Just as she slid ice and a slice of lime into the glass, the doorbell rang. She grabbed her drink and raised it to her lips as she moved through the living room. She certainly wasn't expecting anyone, and the person on the other side of the door was the last person she expected.

She looked through her peephole at Mick Hennessy, and she unlocked the deadbolt and opened the door. The late afternoon sun cut across Mick's cheek and one corner of his mouth. He wore a wife beater beneath a blue plaid shirt that he'd hacked the sleeves off just above the bulge of his biceps. The pale blue in the plaids matched his eyes and set off his tan skin and black hair like he belonged on the cover of a magazine, selling sex and breaking hearts.

'Hello, Maddie,' he said, his voice a low rumble. He held a business card between the fingers of one raised hand.

Shit! The last thing she needed today was a confrontation with Mick. She took another fortifying drink and waited for him to start yelling. Instead he flashed her a killer grin.

'I told you I'd give you the name of a good exterminator.' He held the business card toward her. It was white, not black, and had a rat on it.

She hadn't realized she'd felt a little anxious until relief curved the corners of her lips into a smile. She took the card from him. 'You didn't have to come all the way out here to give this to me.'

'I know.' He handed her an orange and yellow box. 'I thought you could use this until Ernie's Pest Control can get out here. It's easier than hunting for a smelly carcass.'

'Thanks. No man has ever given me . . . ' she paused and looked at the box. 'A Mouse Motel 500.'

He chuckled. 'They had a Mouse Motel 200, but I thought you deserved the best.'

She opened the door wide. 'Would you like to come in?' She should tell him why she was in Truly, but not right now. She just wasn't in the mood for another confrontation.

'I can't stay long.' He stepped past her, bringing with him the scent of the outdoors and woodsy soap. 'My sister is expecting me for dinner.'

'I always wanted a sister.' Somewhere to go for holidays besides a friend's house.

'If you knew Meg, you might consider yourself lucky.'

She shut the door and moved into the living room beside him. She had to admit, it was strange having him in her house. Not just because he was Mick Hennessy, but because it had been a long time since she'd let a man in her home. The energy seemed to change, the air to sexually charge. 'Why?'

'Meg can be . . . ' He smiled and glanced about the room. 'A horrible cook,' he said, but Maddie got the feeling that wasn't what he'd been about to say. 'The kind of cook who thinks she's a lot better than she actually is, which means she'll never get better. If she's thrown peas in a casserole and calls it dinner, I'm out of there.' His gaze returned to hers and he pointed to her drink. 'Hard day?'

'Yeah.'

'More mice feasting on your granola bars?'

She shook her head. He'd remembered that?

'What happened?'

She was fairly certain he'd hear about it soon enough. 'Nothing important. Do you have time for a drink?'

'Do you have a beer?'

'Just ultra.'

He made a face. 'Don't tell me you count carbs.'

'Oh, yeah.' She moved into the kitchen and he followed close behind. 'If I don't, I get a huge behind.' She looked over her shoulder and watched his gaze slide down her back to her butt.

'You look pretty good to me.'

'Exactly.' As if he had all day, his gaze slid back up to her face. 'I have vodka, gin, and Crown Royal.'

His lids lowered a fraction over his blue eyes, making his dark lashes look very long. 'Crown.'

She opened a cupboard and raised onto the balls of her feet. Maddie recognized the look in his eyes. She hadn't had sex in four years, but she remembered that look.

'I'll get that,' he said as he moved close behind her and reached to the top shelf.

She dropped to her heels and turned. He was so close that if she leaned forward just a little, she could bury her nose in his neck. The sides of his open shirt brushed her breasts and she held her breath.

He looked into her eyes as he handed her the old-fashioned glass. 'Here you go.' He took a step back.

'Thank you.' She moved around him and opened the freezer. The cold air felt good against her heated cheeks. This absolutely could not be happening. Not with him, and if he'd been any other man, she could not be held responsible for how badly she might use and abuse his body.

'Are you from Idaho?' he asked as he leaned a hip into the counter and folded his arms across his chest. 'Or are you a transplant?'

'I was born and raised in Boise.' Except for the five months she'd lived in Truly and the six years she'd lived in Southern California attending UCLA. She tossed a few ice cubes into the glass.

'Your folks live in Boise?'

'I never knew my father.' She shut the freezer and set the glass on the counter. 'I was raised by my aunt and she passed away a few months ago.'

'Where's your mother?'

The same place as his. Buried about five miles away. 'She died when I was young.' Maddie bent at the waist and pulled the bottle of whiskey from her booze cabinet.

'I'm sorry to hear that.'

'I hardly remember her.' She waited for him to say something about losing his parents when he'd been a boy. He didn't and she straightened and handed him the Crown Royal. 'Sorry. It isn't as good as Bushmills 21.'

He took the bottle from her and unscrewed the cap. 'Company is better, though.' He poured three fingers of whiskey over the ice.

'You don't know me.'

He put the bottle on the counter and raised the glass to his lips. 'That's one of the things I like about you.' He took a drink, then added, 'I didn't sit next to you in second grade. Your sister isn't friends with my sister and your mama wasn't best friends with my mama.'

No, but she'd been pretty good friends with your daddy. 'Tanya wasn't raised around here.'

'True, but she's too uptight. She can't just relax and have a good time.' He lowered his glass and looked out into the living room. 'This is one of the older houses on the lake.'

'The realtor said it was built in the forties.'

He leaned forward a little and looked down the hall toward the bathroom and bedrooms. 'It looks different from the last time I was here.'

'I was told that the kitchen and the

bathrooms were remodeled last year.' Maddie took a drink. 'When were you here last?'

'Oh, I don't know.' He straightened and looked down into her face. 'I was probably about fifteen. So about twenty years ago.'

'Did you have a friend who lived here?'

'You could say that. Although I don't know if I'd call Brandy Green a *friend*.' A smile tugged at one corner of his mouth as he added, 'Her parents were at the Pendleton Rodeo in Oregon.'

'And you had your own private rodeo?'

The little smile turned into a wicked grin. 'You could say that.'

She frowned. 'Which room was Brandy's?' He'd probably carved his initials into the ceiling beam.

'Can't say.' He rattled the ice in his glass, then raised the glass to his lips. 'Spent most of our time in her parents' room. Their bed was bigger.'

'Oh, my God! You've had sex in my bedroom.' She put her hand on her chest. 'I haven't even had sex in that bedroom.' The second she blurted that out, she wished the floor would open up and she would fall through. She didn't embarrass herself often, but she hated when it happened. Especially when he tipped his head back and laughed. 'It's not funny.'

'Yes, it is.' After a few more moments of hilarity on his part, he said, 'Honey, we could take care of that right now.'

If his offer had felt the least bit threatening or smarmy, she would have kicked him out of her house. Instead it was simple and straightforward and made her smile even when she didn't want to. 'No, thanks.'

'You sure?' He took another drink, then set his glass on the counter.

'I'm sure.'

'I'm a lot better at it than the last time I was here.' The smile he gave her was filled with an irresistible mix of charm, confidence, and pure sin. 'I've had lots of practice since then.'

She hadn't had any practice lately. A fact brought home to her by the tightening in her breasts and the warm tug in her stomach. Mick was the last man on earth for whom she should fall off the sexual wagon. Her head knew that, but her body didn't seem to care.

He reached for her hand and brushed his thumb across the backs of her knuckles. 'Do you know what I like best about you?'

'My Crown?'

He shook his head.

'That I don't want a white wedding, picket fence, and a baby maker?'

97

'Besides that.' He pulled her toward him. 'You smell good.'

She set her glass on the counter and thought back to the lotion she'd put on earlier.

He lifted her hand and smelled the inside of her wrist. 'Like cherries, maybe.'

'Almonds.'

'Yesterday it was chocolate. Today it's almonds. It makes me wonder what you'll smell like tomorrow.' He put her hand on his shoulder.

'Peaches.' Probably.

He pushed one side of her hair back and lowered his face to the side of her neck. 'I like peaches about as much as I like chocolate and almonds. You make me hungry.'

She knew the feeling. 'Maybe you should hurry over to your sister's for some pea casserole.' She felt his soft laughter against her skin a moment before he placed hot openmouthed kisses on the side of her throat. A shiver ran down her spine and her head fell to one side. She'd have to stop him, but not now. In a minute.

'Maybe I should just eat you.'

Her eyes closed and she knew she was in trouble. This couldn't be happening. Mick Hennessy could not be in her house, telling her he wanted to eat her and giving her bad suggestions about where he should start. Making her want to run her hand up his chest and her fingers through his hair.

'Do you know what I'd do to you if I had more time?' His hands grasped her waist and he drew her against him. She felt the swell beneath his button fly, and she had a pretty good idea.

She swallowed hard as he lightly bit her earlobe. 'Try to get another look at the master bedroom?'

He raised his head and his sexy blue eyes had gone all sleepy with desire. 'Who needs a bedroom?'

That was true. Her hand slid across his shoulder and up the side of his neck. Perhaps it had been a mistake to go without sex for so long. The press of his body felt so incredible she didn't want him to stop. But he had to, of course. In a minute.

'You're a beautiful woman, Maddie.' He brushed his lips lightly across hers. 'If I had more time, I'd untie your dress for you.'

'I can untie my own dress.'

One side of his mouth lifted at the corner. 'It's more fun if I do it.' Then he kissed her, a soft and tantalizing press of his mouth. He teased her, drawing out the kiss until her fingers combed through his short hair to the back of his head and her lips parted. His tongue entered her mouth, wet and so good; he tasted like whiskey and lust. Liquid heat pooled between her thighs, and she slid her free hand up his flat stomach, feeling the hard contours of his chest. It had been so long. So long since she'd touched a man like this. Kissed him. Wanted to glue herself to him. Since her skin felt itchy and tight and made her want to tear at his clothes and feel the press of naked skin. It had been a long time. Partly because she'd given up on this, and partly because no man had tempted her like Mick.

His hands slipped up the sides of her waist. His grasp tightened and his thumbs pressed into her stomach just below her breasts. He tilted his head to one side and lightly sucked her tongue into his mouth, where he was warm and slick. Her fingers curled in his hair and she pressed herself against his hard body. Her nipples tightened against his hard chest and he groaned deep in his throat. This was quickly spinning out of control. A whirling cyclone of need and greed and long-denied pleasure, building deep inside and working its way out. Growing and threatening to overpower her.

She pulled back. 'Stop.'

He looked as dazed as she felt. 'Why?'

'Because . . . ' She took a deep breath and

let it out slowly. *Because you don't know who I am and when you find out you'll hate me.* 'Because you have to go have dinner with your sister.'

He opened his mouth to argue, but then his brows lowered as if he'd forgotten. 'Damn.' His grasp on her tightened a fraction before he took a step back and dropped his hands to his sides. 'I didn't mean to start something I can't finish.'

'I didn't mean to start anything at all.' Maddie licked her lips and debated whether to come clean. Right there. Right now. Before he heard it from someone in town. 'This is definitely not a good idea.'

'You're wrong about that.' He reached for her hand and pulled her along with him toward the front door. 'The only thing wrong is my timing.'

'But you don't know me,' she protested as she moved beside him to the entry.

'What's the rush?' He opened the door, but stopped in the threshold. He looked down into her face and let out a heavy breath. 'Okay, what do I need to know?'

And she chickened out. Or rather, decided that telling him while her body still craved his wasn't the best timing. Instead she chose another approach. 'I'm kind of sexually abstinent.'

'Kind of?' He looked down into her face. 'How can you be 'kind of sexually abstinent'?'

Yeah. How? 'I just haven't had sex with a man in a very long time.'

His brows drew together. 'Are you a lesbian?'

'No.'

'I didn't think so. You don't kiss like a lesbian.'

'How do you know?'

One second she was looking up into his blue eyes, and in the next she was up against his body. His mouth closed over hers and he fed her kisses so hot she felt it in the pit of her stomach. He pulled the oxygen from her lungs and made her dizzy. Lord, she couldn't breathe or think. She was going to pass out from pleasure.

He let go of her and she fell back against the doorframe. 'That's how I know,' he said.

'My God, you're like a tornado,' she gasped. She placed her fingers on her bottom lip. Her mouth felt numb. 'Sucking up everything around you.'

'Not everything.' He stepped out onto the porch and into the sunlight. 'And not yet.'

6

Maddie stood with her hands sticking straight out from her shoulders as Nan, the seam-stress, pinned peach satin beneath her armpits. The other two bridesmaids stood on either side of her in various degrees of undress while being pinned and poked.

'You owe me,' she said to her friend Clare, the blushing bride-to-be. She'd driven down from Truly that morning and planned to go out with her friends before driving back the next day.

'Look at it this way,' Clare said from her position on the couch inside of Nan's Bridal. 'At least the dresses aren't all froufrou like the dresses Lucy made us wear for her wedding.'

'Hey. Those were beautiful,' Lucy protested, defending her choice of froufrou while a second seamstress pinned her hem.

'We looked like prom escapees,' Adele argued. Adele held up her thick curly hair as a woman pinned the back of her dress. 'But I've seen worse. My cousin Jolene made her bridesmaids wear purple and white toile de Jouy.'

Clare, the arbiter of exquisite taste, gasped.

'Toile like the postural prints you see on chairs and wallpaper?' Maddie asked.

'Yep. They looked like sofas. Especially Jolene's friend who was a little roomier than the other girls.'

'That's sad.' Lucy turned so the seamstress could work on the back of the hem.

'Criminal,' Adele added. 'Some things should just be against the law. Or if not, there should be some reparation for putting a person through emotional stress.'

'What did Dwayne do now?' Clare asked, referring to Adele's old boyfriend.

For two years Adele had dated Dwayne Larkin and had thought she just might end up as Mrs Larkin. She'd overlooked his more undesirable habits, like smelling the armpits of his shirts before he put them on because he'd been buff and very hot. She'd put up with his beer-swilling, *Star Wars*-obsessed ways, because not everyone was perfect. But the moment when he'd told her she was getting a 'fat ass' like her mother, she'd kicked him out of her life. No one used the *f*-word in relation to her behind or insulted her mama. But Dwayne wouldn't go completely. Every few weeks, Adele would find on her porch one or two of the presents she'd given to him or things she'd left at his house.

The stuff would just be lying there. No note. No Dwayne. Just random-as-hell items.

'For his birthday, I gave him a limited-edition Darth Vader.' Adele dropped her hands and her thick blond hair fell down her back. 'I found it on my porch with the head cut off.'

Maddie was kind of with Dwayne on this issue but for different reasons. If she opened a birthday present and found a Darth Vader, limited edition or not, she'd get fairly pissed off. But still, any sort of violence should never be taken lightly. 'You need to get an alarm system. Do you still have the stun gun I got you?'

Adele held still as the seamstress measured the circumference of her arm. 'Somewhere.'

'You need to find it and zap him with it.' Nan moved to Maddie's bodice and she dropped her arms to her sides. 'Or better yet, let me get you a Cobra like I have, and you can Taser his ass with fifty thousand volts.'

Without moving her body, Adele turned her head and looked at Maddie like she was the crazy one. 'Won't that kill him?'

Maddie thought a moment. 'Does he have a heart condition?'

'I don't think so.'

'Then no,' Maddie answered. Nan took a step back to eye her progress. 'He'll convulse like you're killing him, though.'

Adele's and Clare's mouths fell open in shock, as if she'd lost what little mind she had left, but Lucy nodded. She'd fought for her life against a serial killer and knew firsthand the importance of personal safety devices. 'And when you have him on the ground, douse him with pepper spray.'

'Dwayne is an idiot, but he's not violent,' Adele said. 'Although seeing the Darth Vader did remind me of something horrible.'

'What?' If Dwayne had ever hit Adele, Maddie would hunt him down and zap him herself.

'He has my Princess Leia slave costume.'

Clare scooted to the edge of the couch. 'You have a slave costume?'

Maddie only had one question. 'Are you shitting me?'

Lucy had two. 'What's that?' And, 'Do you mean a metal bikini?'

As if a metal slave bikini were a normal part of a woman's wardrobe, Adele nodded. 'Yeah. And I'd really like to have it back in one piece.' She thought a moment, then added, 'Well, the two pieces . . . and the armbands and collar.' She must have noticed her friends' expressions, ranging from appalled to worried, because she added, 'Hey, I spent a lot of money on that costume and I want it back.' The seamstress stepped away to write down a measurement and Adele folded her arms under her breasts. 'Don't tell me you girls have never role-played.'

Lucy shook her head. 'No, but I used to pretend that an old boyfriend was Jude Law. He didn't know it, though, so I don't think that counts.'

Clare, who always tried to make everyone feel better, said, 'Well, I told Sebastian once that I had costumes and handcuffs.' She sat back on the sofa. 'But I lied. Sorry.'

Maddie glanced at the three seamstresses to see their reactions. They looked as poker-faced as Sunday school teachers. They'd probably heard worse. She turned her gaze to Adele, who'd tilted her head to one side as if she were waiting for something.

'What?' Maddie asked.

'I know you've done kinky stuff.'

Mostly Maddie was just talk. 'I've never dressed up.' She thought a moment and in an effort to sooth Adele she confessed, 'But if it makes you feel better, I've been tied up.'

'Me too.'

'Of course.'

'Big deal.' Adele didn't look placated. 'Everyone's been tied up.'

'That's true,' Nan the seamstress added. She plucked a pin from the cushion on her wrist and glanced over at Adele. 'And if it makes you feel better, every now and again I dress up as Little Red Riding Hood.'

'Thank you, Nan.'

'You're welcome.' She made a spinning motion with her finger. 'Turn, please.'

After the bridesmaids were done with their fittings, the four friends drove to their favorite place to meet for lunch. Café Olé didn't have the best Mexican food in town, but it did have the best pitchers of margaritas. They were shown to one of their favorite booths, and over piped-in mariachi Muzak, they caught up. They talked about Clare's wedding and Lucy's plans to start a family with her hunk of a husband Quinn. And they wanted to hear all about Maddie's life, one hundred miles north in Truly.

'It's actually not as bad as I'd thought,' she said as she raised her drink to her lips. 'It's very beautiful and quiet — well, except on the Fourth. Half the women in town have really bad hair, and the other half look great. I'm trying to figure out if it's a native vs. snowbird thing, but so far I can't tell.' She shrugged. 'I thought spending so much time cooped up in my house would drive me insane, but it hasn't.'

'You know I love you,' Lucy said, which was always followed by a but. 'But you are already totally insane.'

Probably that was true.

'How's the book?' Clare asked as a waitress brought their food.

'Slow.' She'd ordered a chicken tostada salad and picked up her fork as soon as the waitress left. She'd only told her friends about her plans to write about her mother's death a few weeks ago, long after she'd found the diaries and bought her house in Truly. She didn't know why she'd waited. She usually wasn't shy about sharing the details of her personal life with her friends, sometimes to their shock and horror, but reading her mother's diaries had left her so raw, she'd needed time to adjust and take it all in before she talked about it with anyone.

'Have you met the Hennessys?' Adele asked as she dug into an enchilada oozing with cheese and topped with sour cream. Adele worked out every day, and as a result could eat whatever she wanted. Maddie, on the other hand, hated exercise.

'I've met Mick and his nephew Travis.'

'What was Mick's reaction to your writing the book?'

'Well, he doesn't know.' She took a bite of her salad, then added, 'The time just hasn't been right to talk to him about it.'

'So.' Lucy's brows drew together. 'What

have you talked to him about?'

That neither of them could see themselves married and that he liked her butt and the way she smelled. 'Mice, mostly.' Which was kind of the truth.

'Wait.' Adele held up one hand. 'He knows who you are, who your mother was, and he just wants to chat about mice?'

'I haven't told him who I am.' All three friends paused in the act of eating to stare at her. 'While he's working in his bar, or when everyone's standing around a barbeque, isn't the place to walk up to him and say, 'My name is Maddie Jones and your mother killed mine.'' Her friends nodded in agreement and went back to their meals. 'And yesterday was just bad timing all around. I'd had a crappy day. He was nice and brought me the Mouse Motel and then he kissed me.' She speared a piece of chicken and avocado. 'After that, I just forget.'

All three friends paused once again.

'To borrow your favorite phrase,' Lucy said, 'are you shitting me?'

Maddie shook her head. Maybe she should have kept that one to herself. Too late now.

Now it was Clare's turn to hold up one hand. 'Wait. Clear something up for me.'

'Yes.' Maddie answered what she thought was the next logical question. The one she would have asked. 'He's really hot and he's good. My thighs about went up in flames.'

'That wasn't the question.' Clare glanced around, as she always tended to do when she thought Maddie was being inappropriate in a public place. 'You made out with Mick Hennessy and he has no idea who you are? What do you think is going to happen when he finds out?'

'I imagine he's going to be really pissed off.'

Clare leaned forward. 'You imagine?'

'I don't know him well enough to predict how he'll feel.' But she did. She knew he was going to be angry, and she knew she sort of deserved it. Although, to be fair to herself, there really hadn't been a good time to tell him. And she hadn't come to his house and kissed him breathless. He'd done that to her.

'When you do tell him, make sure you have your Cobra,' Lucy advised.

'He's not a violent guy. I won't need to Taser him.'

'You don't know him.' Adele pointed her fork at Maddie and pointed out the obvious. 'His mother killed yours.'

'And as you are always pointing out to us, it's the sane-looking ones you have to watch out for,' Clare reminded Maddie.

'And that without personal safety devices,

we're all sitting ducks.' Lucy laughed and lifted her drink. "And the next thing you know, some guy is wearing your head for a hat."

'Remind me again why I'm friends with you three?' Maybe because they were the only people alive who cared about her. 'I'll tell him. I'm just picking my moment.'

Clare sat back against the seat. 'Oh, my God.'

'What?'

'You're afraid.'

Maddie picked up her margarita and took a long drink until the backs of her eyeballs froze. 'I call it being a little apprehensive.' She placed a warm palm on her brow. 'I'm not *afraid* of anything.'

★ ★ ★

The black metal frame on a pair of Revo high-resolution sunglasses sat on the bridge of Mick's nose while the blue mirrored lenses shaded his eyes from the scorching six o'clock sun. As he walked across the school parking lot, his gaze was intent on player number twelve in the blue Hennessy's T-shirt and the red batter's helmet. He'd been busy going over the books and ordering beer from the distributor and he'd missed the first inning.

112

'Come on, Travis,' he called out and sat on the bottom row of bleacher seats. He leaned forward to place his forearms on the tops of his thighs.

Travis rested the bat on one shoulder as he approached the black rubber T. He took several practice swings like his coach had shown him as the opposing team, Brooks Insurance, stood in the field, mitts at the ready. Travis got into the perfect batter's stance, swung, and completely missed.

'That's okay, buddy,' Mick called out to him.

'You'll get it this time, Travis,' Meg yelled down from where she sat in the top row next to her good friends and fellow T-ball moms.

Mick glanced up at his sister before returning his gaze to the plate. Last night's dinner at her house had been perfectly fine. She'd made steak and baked potatoes and had been the fun-loving Meg most people knew. And the whole time, he hadn't wanted to be there. He'd wanted to be across town. In a house on the lake with a woman he knew nothing about. Talking about mice and burying his nose in the side of her neck.

There was something about Maddie Dupree. Something besides the beautiful face, the hot body, and the smell of her skin. Something that made him think about her when he should be thinking about other things. Distracted while he looked over his accounting system for errors.

Travis once again got into stance and took a swing. This time he connected and sent the ball hurling between second and third base. He dropped the bat and took off for first and his helmet slid back and forth on his head as he ran. The ball bounced and rolled past the outfielder, who took off after it. The first base coach urged Travis to keep going and he made it all the way to third before the outfielder picked up the ball and threw it a few feet. Travis took off again and did a beauty of a slider into home while the outfielder and second baseman fought over the ball.

Mick hollered and gave Travis the thumbs-up. Extremely proud as if he were the boy's daddy instead of his uncle. For the time being, he was the male in Travis's life. Travis hadn't seen his father in four years, and Meg didn't know where he was. Or, more likely, she didn't want to know where the deadbeat was. Mick had met Gavin Black one time, at Meg's wedding. He'd summed him up in one glance as a loser, and he'd been right.

Travis brushed off his pants and handed his coach the helmet. He high-fived his teammates, then took a seat on the team bench. He looked over at Mick and grinned, his one missing tooth a black shadow in his small mouth. If Gavin Black had been standing in front of Mick, he would have kicked his ass all over the schoolyard. How could any man run out on his son? Especially after raising him for two years. And how could his sister have married such a loser?

Mick placed his hands on his knees as the next batter struck out and Travis's team took the field. The best thing for Travis and Meg would be for her to find a nice dependable man. Someone who would be good to her and Travis. Someone stable.

He loved Travis and would always look out for him. Just as he'd looked out for Meg when they'd been kids. But he was tired now. It seemed to him that the more time he gave her, the more she took. In some ways, she'd become their grandmother, and he'd stayed away for twelve years to get away from Loraine. If he let Meg, he was afraid she'd become too dependent on him. He didn't want that. After a life of turmoil, whether as a child or living in war zones, he wanted some peace and calm. Well, as peaceful and calming as could be expected owning two bars.

Meg was the sort of woman who needed a man in her life, someone to balance her out, but it couldn't be him. He thought of Maddie and her assertion that she wasn't looking for a husband. He'd heard that claim before, but with her, he believed it. He didn't know what she did for a living, if anything, but she obviously didn't need a man to support her.

Mick rose and moved to the batter's cage to get a better look at Travis standing out in center field with his mitt held up in the air as if he expected a ball from heaven to land inside.

He hadn't planned to kiss Maddie yesterday. He'd brought her Ernie's card and the Mouse Motel, and he'd planned to leave. But the second she'd opened the door, his plans got shot all to hell. The black dress had clung to her sexy curves and all he'd been able to think about was untying it. Pulling the strings and unwrapping her like a birthday gift. Touching and tasting her all over.

He raised his hands and grasped the chain link in front of his face. Yesterday his timing had been bad, but there wasn't a doubt in his mind. He was going to kiss Maddie again.

'Hi, Mick.'

He looked across his shoulder as Jewel Finley walked toward him. Jewel had been one of his mother's friends. She had two obnoxious twin boys, Scoot and Wes, and a whiny crybaby girl named Belinda whom everyone called Boo. Growing up, Mick had hit Boo with a Nerf ball and she'd acted like she'd been mortally injured. According to Meg, Belinda wasn't quite the crybaby these days, but the twins were obnoxious as ever.

'Hello, Mrs Finley. Do you have a grandkid playing tonight?'

Jewel pointed toward the opposing bench. 'My daughter's son, Frankie, is playin' outfield for Brooks Insurance.'

Ah. The boy who threw like a girl. Figured.

'What are Scoot and Wes up to these days?' he asked to be polite. Not that he gave a shit.

'Well, after their fish farm failed, they both got their commercial driver's licenses and now they drive big rigs for a movin' company.'

He turned his attention to the field and Travis, who was now tossing his mitt in the air and catching it. 'Which company?' If he had to move, he wanted to know who *not* to call.

'York Transfer and Storage. But they're gettin' tired of the long haul. So as soon as they save up enough money, they're thinkin' about starting one of those house-flippin' businesses. Like on TV'

Mick figured it would take the twins less than a year of working for themselves before they filed for bankruptcy. To say the boys weren't the sharpest knives in the drawer was an understatement.

117

'There's good money in flippin' houses.'

'Uh-huh.' He was going to have to talk to Travis about paying attention to the game.

'As much as fifty grand a month. That's what Scooter says.'

'Uh-huh.' Geez-us. Now the kid was turned completely around and watching cars drive by in the street.

'Have you talked to that writer yet?'

He probably shouldn't yell at Travis to watch the game, but he wanted to. 'What writer?'

'The one who's writin' a book about your parents and that waitress, Alice Jones.'

7

Maddie tossed her overnight bag on her bed and unzipped it. She had a slight headache, and she wasn't sure if it was due to her lack of sleep, drinking too much with Adele, or listening to her friend's stories about her fractured love life.

After she'd had lunch at Café Olé, she and Adele had gone back to her house in Boise to catch up. Adele always had really funny stories about her love life — although she sometimes didn't mean for them to be quite so entertaining — and like a good friend, Maddie had listened and poured the wine. It had been a long time since Maddie had been able to reciprocate with funny and entertaining stories of her own, so mostly she'd just listened and offered occasional advice.

Before leaving Boise, she'd invited Adele to spend the following weekend with her. Adele agreed to come and, knowing her friend, Maddie was sure she'd have several more dating horror stories to share.

Maddie took her dirty clothes from the bag and tossed them into her hamper. It was just after noon and she was starving. She ate a chicken breast and some celery with cream cheese while she checked and answered her e-mails. She checked her answering machine, but there was only one message, and that was from a carpet cleaner. No word from Sheriff Potter.

Later, she planned to find Mick and tell him who she was and why she was in town. It was the right thing to do, and she wanted him to hear if from her first. She figured she could find him at one of his two bars, and she hoped he was working at Mort's tonight. She really wasn't looking forward to walking into Hennessy's, although she would have to at some point. She'd never been inside the bar where her mother had died. To her, Hennessy's wasn't just another old crime scene. One she had to visit for her book. She would have to go to note the changes and observe the place. And while she certainly *wasn't* afraid, she was apprehensive.

As she rinsed her plate in the sink and put it in the dishwasher, she wondered exactly how angry Mick was likely to get. Until her friends had mentioned it, she hadn't thought of packing her Taser when she told him. While he seemed perfectly nonviolent, he had shot Hellfire missiles from helicopters. And of course his mother had been a nut job, and while Maddie liked to think she had a special psycho radar, honed after years of meeting with them while they'd been chained to a table, it never hurt to error on the side of caution and a really good pepper spray.

The doorbell rang, and this time she wasn't surprised to see Mick standing on her porch. Just like last time, he held a business card between two fingers, but there was no mistaking that the card was hers.

He stared at her from behind the blue lenses of his sunglasses, and his lips were set in a flat line. He wasn't wearing a happy face, but he didn't look too angry. She probably wouldn't have to hose him with the pepper spray. Not that she even had it on her.

Maddie lowered her gaze to the card. 'Where did you get that?'

'Jewel Finley.'

Crap. She really hadn't meant for him to find out that way, but she wasn't surprised. 'When?'

'Last night at Travis's T-ball game.'

'I'm sorry you heard about it like that.' Maddie didn't invite him inside, but he didn't wait for an invitation.

'Why didn't *you* tell me?' he asked as he brushed past her, six feet two, one hundred and ninety pounds, of determined man. Trying to stop him would have been as futile as trying to stop a tank.

Maddie closed the door and followed. 'You didn't want to know anything about me. Remember?'

'That's a bunch of bullshit.' Light from outside flowed in through the large windows, over the back of the sofa and coffee table and across the hardwood floor. Mick stopped within the spill of light and took off his sunglasses. Maddie had been wrong about his anger. It burned like blue fire in his eyes. 'I didn't want to know about your old boyfriends, your favorite chocolate chip cookie recipe, or who you sat next to in the second grade.' He held up the card. 'This is different, and don't pretend that it's not.'

She pushed her hair behind her ears. He had a right to be angry. 'That first night at Mort's, I went there to introduce myself and to tell you who I was and why I was in town. But the bar was busy and it wasn't a good time. When I saw you at the hardware store and on the Fourth, Travis was with you and I didn't think it an appropriate time then either.'

'And when I was here alone?' He frowned and stuck his glasses on top of his head.

'I tried to tell you that day.'

'Is that so?' He slid the card in the pocket of his black Mort's Bar polo shirt. 'Before or after you stuck your tongue down my throat?'

Maddie gasped. Yeah, he had a right to be angry, but not to rewrite history. 'You kissed me!'

'An *appropriate time*,' he said as if she hadn't protested, 'might have been before you glued yourself to my chest.'

'Glued? You pulled me in to your chest.' Her gaze narrowed, but she wouldn't allow herself to get angry. 'I told you that you didn't know me.'

'And instead of you telling me the important shit like you're in town to write a book about my parents, you thought I would be more interested in knowing that you're 'kind of sexually abstinent'.' He rested his weight on one foot and tilted his head to one side as he looked down at her. 'You weren't planning to tell me.'

'Don't be absurd.' She folded her arms beneath her breasts. 'This is a small town and I knew you'd find out.'

'And until I did, were you planning to fuck me for information?'

Don't get mad, she told herself. *If you get mad, you might get out the Taser.* 'There are two problems with your theory.' She held up a hand and raised one finger. 'That I need you to give me information. I don't.' She raised a second finger. 'And that I was planning to fuck you. I wasn't.'

He took a step toward her and smiled. Not one of his nice, charming smiles either. 'If I'd had more time, you would have been flat on your back.'

'You're dreaming.'

'And you're lying. To me and to yourself.'

'I never lie to myself.' She looked into his eyes, not in the least intimidated by his size or anger. 'And I never lied to you.'

His gaze narrowed. 'You purposely hid the truth, which is the same damn thing.'

'Oh, that's rich. A morality lesson by you. Tell me, Mick, do all the women you sleep with know about each other?'

'I don't lie to women.'

'No, you just bring mousetraps thinking that will get you into their pants.'

'That isn't the reason I brought you the trap.'

'Now who's lying?' She pointed toward the door. 'It's time for you to leave.'

He didn't budge. 'You can't do this, Maddie. You can't write about my family.'

'Yes, I can, and I'm going to.' She didn't wait for him but walked to the door and opened it.

'Why? I've read all about you,' he said as he moved toward her, his boot heels an angry thud across the hardwood. 'You write about serial killers. My mother wasn't a serial killer.

She was a housewife who'd had enough of a cheating husband. She flipped out and killed him and herself. There's no big villain here. No sick bastards like Ted Bundy or Jeffrey Dahmer. What happened to my mother and father is hardly the sensational sort of stuff that people want to read about.'

'I think I'm a little more qualified to determine that than you.'

He stopped on the threshold and turned to face her. 'My mother was just a sad woman who snapped one night and left her children orphaned, victims of her mental illness.'

'All this talk of you and your family, you seem to forget there was another innocent victim.'

'That little waitress was hardly innocent.'

Actually, she'd been talking about herself. 'So you're like everyone else in this town and think Alice Jones got what she deserved.'

'No one got what they deserved, but she was screwing around with a married man.'

Now. Now she was truly good and angry. 'So your mother was perfectly justified in shooting her in the face.'

His head jerked back as if she'd slapped him. Obviously he hadn't seen the photos or read the report.

'And your father may have been a cheater, but did he deserve to be shot three times and bleed to death on a barroom floor while your mother watched?'

His voice rose for the first time. 'You're full of shit. She wouldn't have watched my father die.'

If he hadn't told her she was full of shit, she would have spared him, no matter her own anger. 'Her bloody footprints were all over the bar. And she didn't get up and walk around after she shot herself.'

His mouth clamped shut.

'Alice Jones had a child too. Did she deserve to lose her mother? Did she deserve to be made an orphan?' Maddie placed her hand in the center of his chest and pushed. 'So don't tell me that your mother was just some sad housewife who'd been pushed too far. She had other options. Lots of other options that didn't involve murder.' He took a step back out onto her porch. 'And don't come here and think you can tell me what to do. I really don't give a damn if you like it or not. I'm going to write the book.' She tried to shut the door, but his arm shot out and kept it open.

'You do that.' With his free hand, he took his sunglasses from the top of his head and slid them in place, covering the anger in his blue eyes. 'But you stay away from me,' he said and dropped his hand from the door.

'And you stay the hell away from my family.'

Maddie slammed the door and pushed her hair from her face. Damn. That hadn't gone well. He'd been angry. She'd gotten angry. Heck, she was still angry.

She heard him start his truck, and out of habit, she locked her front door. She didn't need him or his family in order to write the book, but realistically, it'd be nice if she had their cooperation. Especially since she needed to get into the lives of Loch and Rose.

'Well, that sucked,' she said and walked into the living room. She would have to write the book without their input. Her mother's photograph sat on the coffee table. She'd been so young and filled with so many dreams. Maddie picked up the photo and touched the glass above her mother's lips. It had been sitting there the whole time while Mick had been there, and he hadn't noticed.

She'd planned to tell him that she was more than just an author interested in writing a book. That his mother had left her an orphan too. Now he wanted nothing to do with her, and who she really was just didn't seem to matter anymore.

★　★　★

Mick pulled his truck to a stop in front of the Shore View Diner where Meg worked five days a week waiting tables and pulling in tips. He was still so angry he felt like hitting something or someone. Like picking Maddie Dupree up by her shoulders and shaking her until she agreed to pack up and go away. Like forgetting she'd ever heard of the Hennessys and their messed-up lives. But she'd made it really clear she wasn't going anywhere, and now he had to tell Meg before she heard it from someone else.

He turned off the truck and leaned his head back. His mother had watched his father die? He hadn't known that. Wished he didn't know it now. How could he possibly reconcile the woman who'd killed two people with the mother who'd made him peanut butter and strawberry jelly sandwiches, cut the crusts off, and sliced the bread at an angle just as he'd liked it? The loving mother who bathed him and washed his hair and tucked him in at night, with the woman who'd left footprints in her husband's blood all over his bar? How could that even be the same woman?

He rubbed his face with his hands and slid his fingers beneath his sunglasses to rub his eyes. He was so damn tired. After Jewel had given him Maddie's business card, he'd gone to his office in Hennessy's and locked himself in. He'd searched the Internet for information about Maddie, and there'd been a lot. She'd published five books, and he'd discovered head shots of her and photos of her at book signings. There was no mistaking that the Maddie Dupree whom he'd been planning to get to know better was the woman who wrote about psychotic killers. The Madeline Dupree who was in town to write about the night his mother had killed his father. He opened the door to his truck and stepped outside. And there wasn't a damn thing he could do to stop her.

From as far back as he could remember, the Shore View Diner had smelled the same. Like grease and eggs and tobacco. The diner was one of the last places in America where a person could have a cup of coffee and a Camel or Lucky Strike, depending on his or her poison. As a result, it was always filled with smokers. Mick had tried to talk Meg into working someplace where she wasn't likely to get lung cancer from secondhand smoke, but she insisted that the tips were too good to work anyplace else.

It was around two in the afternoon and the diner was half empty when Mick entered. Meg stood behind the front counter, filling Lloyd Brunner's cup of coffee and laughing at something he'd said. her black hair was pulled back into a ponytail, and she wore a bright pink blouse beneath a white apron. She looked up and waved at him.

'Hey, there. Are you hungry?' she asked.

'No.' He took a seat at the counter and pushed his Revos to the top of his head. 'I was hoping you could get off early.'

'Why?' Her smile fell and she set the coffee carafe on the counter. 'Has something happened? Is it Travis?'

'Travis is fine. I just wanted to talk to you about something.'

She looked into his eyes as if she could read his mind. 'I'll be right back,' she said and walked into the kitchen. When she returned, she had her purse.

Mick rose and followed her outside. As soon as the door to the diner swung shut behind them, she asked, 'What is it?'

'There's a woman in town. She's a true crime writer.'

Meg squinted against the bright sun as they walked across the gravel lot to his truck. 'What's her name?'

'Madeline Dupree.'

Her jaw dropped. 'Madeline Dupree? She wrote *In Her Place*, the story of Patrick Wayne Dobbs. The serial killer who killed women and then wore their clothes under his business suit. That book scared me so much I couldn't sleep for a week.' Meg shook her head. 'What is she doing in Truly?'

He slid his sunglasses down to cover his eyes. 'Apparently, she's going to write about what happened with Mom and Dad.'

Meg stopped. 'What?'

'You heard me.'

'Why?'

'God, I don't know.' He raised a hand, then dropped it to his side. 'If she writes about serial killers, I don't know what she finds so damn interesting about mom and dad.'

Meg folded her arms across the front of her apron and they continued to walk. 'What does she know about what happened?'

'I don't know, Meg.' They stopped by his truck and he leaned a hip into the front fender. 'She knows Mom shot that waitress in the head.' His sister didn't bat an eye. 'Did you know that?'

Meg shrugged and bit her thumbnail. 'Yeah. I heard the sheriff tell Grandma Loraine.'

He looked into his sister's eyes and wondered what else she knew that he didn't. He wondered if she knew that their mother hadn't killed herself right away. He supposed it didn't matter. She was taking the news better than he'd expected. 'Are you going to be okay?'

She nodded. 'Is there anything we can do to stop her?'

'I doubt it.'

She leaned back into the driver's-side door and sighed. 'Maybe you can go talk to her.'

'I did. She's going to write it, and she doesn't care what we have to say about it.'

'Shit.'

'Yeah.'

'Everyone is going to start talking about it again.'

'Yep.'

'She'll say bad stuff about Mom.'

'Probably about all three of them. But what can she say? The only people who know what really happened that night are dead.'

Meg glanced away.

'Do you know something that happened that night?'

She dropped her hand. 'Just that Mom had been pushed too far and she killed Dad and that waitress.'

He wasn't so sure he believed her, but what difference did it make twenty-nine years later? Meg hadn't been there. She'd been home with him when the sheriff had arrived at their house that night.

He looked up at the clear blue sky. 'I'd forgotten that the waitress had a little girl.'

'Yeah, I can't remember her name, though.'

Meg returned her gaze to Mick. 'Not that I care. Her mother was a whore.'

'That wasn't the girl's fault, Meg. She was left without a mother.'

'She was probably better off. Alice Jones was cheating with our father and didn't care who knew. She flaunted their relationship in front of the whole town, so don't expect me to feel sorry for some nameless, faceless orphan girl.'

Mick didn't know if there'd been any flaunting, and if there had been, he figured their dad had to take the majority of the blame, since he'd been the married one.

'Are you going to be okay with this?'

'No, but what can I do about it?' She adjusted her purse on her shoulder. 'I'll survive, just like I did before.'

'I told her to stay away from you and Travis, so I don't think she'll be bothering you with questions.'

Meg raised a brow. 'Is she going to be bothering you with questions?'

There was more than one way a woman could bother a man. *And don't come here and think you can tell me what to do. I really don't give a damn if you like it or not. I'm going to write the book.* She'd been mad and obstinate and sexy as hell. Her big brown eyes had gotten kind of squinted at the corners just before she'd slammed the door in his face. 'No,' he answered. 'She won't be bothering me with questions.'

★ ★ ★

Meg waited until Mick's truck pulled out of the parking lot before she let out a breath and raised her hands to the sides of her face. She pressed her fingers into her temples and closed her eyes against the pressure building in her head. Madeline Dupree was in town to write a book about her parents. There had to be something someone could do to stop her. A person shouldn't be allowed to just ... just ruin lives. There should be a law against snooping around and ... digging into someone's past.

Meg opened her eyes and stared down at her white Reeboks. It wouldn't be long before everyone in town knew about it. Before they started talking and gossiping and looking at her as if she were liable to go off at any time. Even her brother sometimes looked at her as if she were crazy. Mick thought he was so good at forgetting the past, but there were some things even he'd never been able to forget. Tears clouded her vision and dropped on the gravel by the instep of her shoe. Mick also mistook emotion for mental illness. Not that she really blamed him. Growing up with their parents had been an emotional tug-of-war ending in their death.

A second truck pulled into the parking lot and Meg raised her gaze as Steve Castle opened the door of his Tacoma and got out. Steve was Mick's buddy and manager of Hennessy's. Meg didn't know much about him, other than he'd flown helicopters in the army with Mick, and there'd been some sort of accident in which Steve had lost his right leg beneath the knee.

'Hey, there, Meg,' he called out, his deep voice booming across the lot as he moved toward her.

'Hey.' Meg hurriedly wiped beneath her eyes, then dropped her hands to her sides. Steve was a big guy and shaved his head completely bald. He was tall and broad-chested and so . . . so manly that Meg felt a little intimidated by his size.

'Having a rough day?'

She could feel her cheeks get hot as she looked up into his deep blue eyes. 'Sorry. I know men don't like to see women cry.'

'Tears don't bother me. I've seen tough Marines cry like little girls.' He folded his arms across the dogs playing poker on the front of his T-shirt. 'Now, what's got you so upset, sweetheart?'

135

Meg usually didn't share her feelings with people she didn't know, but there was something about Steve. While his size intimidated her, he also made her feel safe at the same time. Or perhaps it was just because he'd called her 'sweetheart', but she opened her mouth and confided, 'Mick was just here, and he told me that there's a writer in town and she's going to write about the night our mother killed our father.'

'Yeah. I heard about that.'

'Already? How did you find out?'

'The Finley boys were in Hennessy's last night talking about it.'

She raised a hand and chewed on her thumbnail. 'Then I think it's safe to assume the whole town knows, and everybody is going to be talking about it and speculating.'

'What are you going to do about it?'

She dropped her hand to her side and shook her head. 'What can I do?'

'Maybe you can talk to her.'

'Mick tried that. She's going to write the book no matter what we think about it.' She looked down at her shoes. 'Mick told her to stay away from me and Travis.'

'Why avoid her? Why don't you tell her your side of things?'

She looked up into his eyes and the sunlight bouncing off his shiny head. 'I don't know if she'd care about my side.'

'Maybe, but you won't know that unless you talk to the woman.' He unfolded his arms and rested one big hand on her shoulder. 'If there is one thing I know, it's that you have to confront something head-on. You can get through anything if you know what you're facing.'

Which she was sure was true and very good advice, but she couldn't think past the weight of his hand on her shoulder. The solid feel and the warmth of his touch spread to her stomach. She hadn't felt warmth from a man since her ex-husband. The men in town talked to her and flirted with her, but they never seemed to want more than a coffee refill.

Steve slid his palm down her arm and grasped her hand. 'I've wondered something since I moved to town.'

'What's that?'

He tilted his head to one side and studied her. 'Why you don't have a boyfriend.'

'I think the men in this town are half afraid of me.'

His brows lowered over his eyes and then he burst out laughing. A deep booming laugh lit his face.

'It's not funny,' she said, but at that moment, surrounded by Steve Castle's laughter, it was kind of funny. And standing so close, with her hand in his, was kind of . . . nice.

8

The fishing at upper Payette Lake had been so good, Sheriff Potter hadn't returned until the following Tuesday, but once he'd been given Maddie's card he'd called her immediately and set up a meeting for the next day at his house. If there was one thing in Maddie's line of work that she could always count on, it was cops. Whether an LAPD detective or a small-town sheriff, cops loved to talk about old cases.

'I'll never forget that night,' the retired sheriff said as he looked at the old crime scene photos through a pair of reading glasses. Unlike the stereotypical retired sheriff who'd gone to fat, Bill Potter was still quite thin and had a full head of white hair. 'That scene was a mess.'

Maddie scooted the small tape recorder closer to the baby-blue La-Z-Boy recliner where Sheriff Potter sat. The inside of the Potters' home was a fusion of floral prints and wildlife art that clashed on so many different levels that Maddie feared her eyes would cross before the day was through.

'I'd known Loch and Rose since they were

kids,' Bill Potter continued. 'I'm a few years older, but in a town this size, especially back in the seventies, everyone knows everyone. Rose was one of the most beautiful women I'd ever seen, and it was a shock to see what she'd done to those two people and then to herself.'

'How many homicide cases had you investigated before the Hennessy case?' she asked.

'One, but it was nothing like the Hennessy case. Old Man Jenner got shot in a dispute over a dog. Mostly we get accidental shootings, and those are usually around hunting season.'

'The first officer on the scene was a . . .' Maddie paused to look at the report. 'Officer Grey Tipton.'

'Yep. He left the department a few months after that and moved away,' the sheriff said. 'And I hear he died a few years ago.'

Which was just one of the many hurdles she was always coming up against in this town. Either people weren't willing to talk about what happened or they were dead. At least she had Officer Tipton's report and notes. 'Yes, he died in an ATV accident in 1981. Did the shooting have anything to do with him leaving the department?'

Sheriff Potter shuffled the photos. 'It had

139

everything to do with it. Grey had been really good friends with Loch, and seeing him shot like that haunted him so bad he couldn't sleep.' He held up the photo of Rose lying beside her dead husband. 'It was the first time any of us had seen anything like that. I'd responded to plenty of automobile accidents that were bloody as hell, but they weren't personal.'

Since there would be no trial to write about, Maddie had to get as much personal information as possible. And since the Hennessys weren't talking, she had to rely on other sources.

'Grey had such a hard time with it. He had to quit. Just goes to show you that you don't know how you'll deal with a situation until you're knee-deep in blood.'

For the next hour, they talked about the crime scene. The photos and reports answered the who, what, where, and when, but the why was still fuzzy. Maddie changed the tape in the little recorder, then asked, 'You knew both Loch and Rose. What do you think happened that night?' In every case like this, there was always a catalyst. A stressor was introduced that pushed the perpetrator over the edge. 'From what I've heard and read, Alice Jones wasn't Loch's one and only affair.'

'No. She wasn't. That marriage had been like a roller coaster for years.' The sheriff shook his head and removed his glasses. 'Before they moved into that farmhouse right outside of town, they used to live down by the lake on Pine Nut. Every few months I'd get a call from one of their neighbors and I'd have to drive over there.'

'What did you find once you arrived?'

'Screaming and yelling, mostly. A few times Loch'd have his clothes torn or a red mark on his face.' Bill chuckled. 'One time I got there and the front window was busted out and a skillet was lying in the yard.'

'Was anyone ever arrested?'

'Nah. Then the next time you'd see the two of them, they'd be all lovey-dovey and happy as pie.'

And when they weren't lovey-dovey, they pulled other people into their messed-up marriage. 'But once they moved into the farmhouse, the calls to your office stopped?'

'Yeah. No more neighbors around, you know.'

'Where is the farmhouse now?'

'Burned down . . . ' He paused in thought and deep grooves wrinkled his forehead. 'Must have been about twenty years ago. One night, someone went over there, doused it with kerosene, and lit it up good.'

'Was anyone hurt?'

'No one lived there at the time.' He frowned and shook his head. 'Never did find out who started it. Always had my suspicions, though.'

'Who?'

'Only a couple of people wanted that house gone bad enough to do such a good job. Kids just playin' around with matches don't torch a place like that.'

'Mick?'

'And his sister, although I could never prove it. Didn't actually want to prove it, if truth be told. Growing up, Mick was always in trouble. A constant pain in the ass, but I always felt bad for him. He had a real hard life.'

'Lots of children lose their parents and don't turn to arson.'

The sheriff leaned forward. 'Lots of kids don't live the life Rose Hennessy left behind for her kids.'

That was true, but Maddie knew a bit about that life. She flipped a page in her notebook and said, 'Alice Jones lived in the Roundup Trailer Court. Do you know a woman by the name of Trina who may have lived in the same trailer court in 1978?'

'Hmm, that doesn't sound familiar.' He thought a moment, then leaned forward. 'You might talk to Harriet Landers. She lived in that trailer court for years. When the land was sold to a developer, she had to be practically hog tied and carried away.'

'Where does Harriet live now?'

'Levana,' he called to his wife. When she appeared from the back of the house he asked, 'Where is Harriet Landers living these days?'

'I believe she lives at the Samaritan Villa.' Levana looked at Maddie and added, 'That's a retirement center off of Whitetail and Fifth. She's a little hard of hearing these days.'

★ ★ ★

'What?' Harriet Landers yelled from her wheelchair. 'Speak up, for pity's sake.'

Maddie sat in an old iron chair in the small garden at the Samaritan Villa. Looking at the old woman, it was hard to gauge her age. Maddie would guess somewhere between one foot in the grave and fossilized. 'My name is Maddie Dupree! I wonder if I might be — '

'You're that writer,' Harriet interrupted. 'I heard you're here to write a book about them Hennessys.'

Wow, news traveled fast even on the nursing home circuit. 'Yes. I was told that you once lived at the Roundup Trailer Court.'

'For about fifty years.' She'd lost almost all of her white hair and most of her teeth and she wore a pink housecoat with white lace and snaps. But there didn't seem to be anything wrong with her mind. 'I don't know what I could talk to you about.'

'How about living at the Roundup?'

'Humpf.' She raised a knobby and gnarled hand and swiped at a bee in front of her face. 'Not a lot to say about that, that anyone wants to hear. Folks think that people who live in trailer houses are poor trailer trash, but I always liked my trailer. Always liked having the option of packing up the house and moving the whole damn thing if I wanted.' She shrugged a bony shoulder. 'Guess I never did, though.'

'People can be very cruel and dismissive,' Maddie said. 'When I was little, we lived in a trailer, and I thought it was the best.' Which was true, mostly because the trailer had been such an improvement over the other places she and her mother had lived. 'We certainly weren't trash.'

Harriet's sunken blue eyes gave Maddie the once-over. 'You lived in a trailer?'

'Yes, ma'am.' Maddie held up the tape recorder. 'Do you mind if I record our conversation?'

'What for?'

'So that I don't misquote you.'

Harriet put her skinny elbows on the arms of her wheelchair and leaned forward. 'Go ahead.' She pointed at the recorder. 'What do you want to know?'

'Do you recall the summer that Alice Jones lived at the Roundup?'

'Sure, although I lived down the road from her and not next door. But I'd see her sometimes as I was driving past. She was a real pretty thing and had a little girl. That little girl used to swing all day and half the night on the swing set in her front yard.'

Yes, that part Maddie knew. She remembered swinging so high, she thought her toes touched the sky. 'Did you ever talk to Alice Jones? Have friendly conversations?'

A frown pulled at the wrinkles in her forehead. 'Not that I can recall. That was a long time ago and my memory isn't so good these days.'

'I understand. My memory isn't always in the best of shape either.' She looked down at her notes as if to remind herself of what to ask next. 'Do you recall a woman by the name of Trina who may have lived at the Roundup at that time?'

'That would probably be Trina Olsen. Betty Olsen's middle girl. She had flaming red hair and freckles.'

145

Maddie wrote down the last name and circled it. 'Do you know if Trina still lives in Truly?'

'No. Betty's dead, though. Died of liver cancer.'

'I'm sorry.'

'Why, did you know her?'

'Ah . . . no.' She put the cap back on her pen. 'Is there anything else you can remember from around the time Alice Jones lived at the Roundup?'

'I remember lots of things.' She shifted a little in her chair, then said, 'I remember Galvin Hennessy, that's for sure.'

'Loch's father?' Maddie asked, just to clarify. What could Galvin have to do with Maddie's mother?

'Yep. He was a handsome devil, just like all the Hennessy men.' She shook her head and sighed. 'But a girl would have to be an idiot to marry a Hennessy.'

Maddie skimmed her notes looking for Galvin's name. She thumbed past a Founders Day flyer she'd been handed at the front desk, but as far as she could recall, he'd never been mentioned in any of the police reports.

'I dated that man off and on until the day he dropped dead in the backseat of my Ford Rambler.'

Maddie's head came up. 'Pardon me?'

Harriet laughed, a crackling, rattling sound that left her in a fit of coughing. Maddie became so concerned, she set her notes on the grass and rose to thump Harriet on the back. When Harriet got herself under control, Maddie asked, 'Are you okay?' Gee, Harriet was old, but Maddie didn't want to be the reason she keeled over.

'I wish you could have seen your face. I didn't think it was possible to shock anyone in this town anymore. Not at my age.' Harriet chuckled.

'So?' Maddie sat back down. 'Did Galvin have anything to do with what happened at Hennessy's Bar?'

'No. He was dead before all that happened. Loraine never forgave me for Galvin dying in the back of my car, but shoot, you can't throw a rock in this town without hitting some woman who hasn't had an affair with a Hennessy.'

'Why?' Maddie asked. Lots of men had looks and charm. 'What makes the Hennessy men so irresistible to the women of Truly?'

'They're beautiful to look at, but mostly on account of what they got in their pants.'

'You mean they've got . . . ' Maddie paused and held up a hand as if she couldn't think of the word. She could, of course. Her favorite word, heft, came to mind, but for some reason she just couldn't say it in front of an old woman.

'They're blessed,' Harriot provided. Then, over the next hour, she proceeded to give Maddie the details of her long and illustrious affair with Galvin Hennessy. Apparently, Harriet was one of *those* girls. No matter that she was well into her nineties and no more than a raisin with eyes, Harriet Landers was one of *those* girls who loved to talk about their sex lives with a perfect stranger.

And Maddie, lucky girl, got it all on tape.

★ ★ ★

Wednesday night at Hennessy's was Hump Night. In an effort to help the citizens get past the hump in the week, Hennessy's offered half-price well drinks and dollar drafts until seven. After seven, a few people left, but most stayed and paid full price for their booze. Galvin Hennessy had been the brains behind Hennessy's Hump Night, and the custom had been carried through the following generations.

There were those who'd feared the demise of Hump Night when Mick had taken over the place. After all, he'd done away with panty-tossing at Mort's, but after two years of cheap well drinks and dollar beers, Truly could breathe easier knowing that some traditions were still sacred.

Mick stood at the far end of the bar, weight resting on one booted foot and pool cue in hand as Steve Castle bent over the table and took a shot. Steve was slightly taller than Mick and wore a baby-blue ATTENTION LADIES: I LOVED THE NOTE-BOOK T-shirt stretched across his barrel chest. Mick had known Steve since flight training. Back then, Steve had had a full head of blond hair. These days he was as bald as the billiard he sent down on the table.

When Mick had gotten out of the army, Steve had stayed in until his Black Hawk had been shot down over Fallujah by an SA-7 shoulder-fired missile. In the crash that had killed five soldiers and wounded seven, Steve had lost his leg. After months of rehabilitation and a new prosthesis, he'd gone home to Northern California to find his marriage in ruins. He'd gone through a real rough time and a bad divorce, and when Mick had asked him to move to Truly and manage Hennessy's, he'd climbed into his truck and arrived in days. Mick had never expected him to last in the small town, but that was a year and a half ago, and Steve had just bought a house near the lake.

Steve was the closest thing Mick had to a

brother. The two shared the same experiences and visceral memories. They'd shared a life that civilians did not understand, and their time in the military was something they never talked about in public.

The six ball landed in the corner pocket and Steve lined up the two ball. 'Meg was in here yesterday looking for you,' he said. 'I guess the whole town is buzzing like a wasp nest because that writer talked to Sheriff Potter and Harriet Landers.'

'Meg called me about it last night.' Steve was the only person Mick had ever spoken to about Meg's unpredictable emotional outbursts and mood swings. 'She isn't as upset about this whole book business as I thought she'd be.' At least she hadn't freaked out, which was what Mick had expected from the woman who'd been known to lose it over the sight of a wedding ring.

'Maybe she's stronger than you give her credit for.'

Maybe, but Mick doubted it.

Steve shot, but the two hit the corner of the pocket and bounced back. 'I meant to do that.'

'Uh-huh.' Mick chalked his cue and hit the remaining ten ball into a side pocket.

'I better get back behind the bar,' Steve said as he placed his cue in the rack. 'Are you going to be here until close?'

'No.' Mick put his cue next to Steve's and looked out over the bar. On weeknights, both Hennessy's and Mort's closed at midnight. 'I want to see how the new bartender is doing at Mort's.'

'How's he working out so far?'

'A hell of a lot better than the last one. I should have known better than to hire Ronnie Van Damme in the first place. Most of the Van Dammes are worthless.' Mick had had to fire Ronnie two weeks ago for always coming in late and standing around jerking his gherkin when he had been there. 'The new guy used to manage a bar in Boise, so I'm hoping he works out.' Eventually Mick's goal was to find a manager for Mort's so he could work less and make more money. He didn't trust government pensions or Social Security to provide for him for the rest of his life and he'd made his own investments.

'Let me know if you need help,' Steve said as he walked away, his limp barely noticeable. Mick hadn't been in Iraq when Steve's bird had been shot down, but he'd had a few close calls and been forced to make an emergency landing in Afghanistan when a rocket-propelled grenade hit his Apache. The landing hadn't been pretty, but he'd survived.

He'd loved flying and it was one of the

things he missed most about his former life. But he didn't miss the sand and dust and the politics of army life. He'd take getting fired at over the tedium of sitting around waiting for orders, only to gear up and have the mission scrubbed at the last moment.

These days he lived in a small town where nothing much happened, but he was never bored. Especially lately.

Mick looked out at the empty dance floor at the other end of the bar. On the weekends, he usually hired a band and the floor was packed. Tonight a few people stood around talking, others sat at tables and at the bar. By nine on Hump Nights the bar usually cleared out except for a few stragglers. As he was growing up, his dad had brought him and Meg to the bar occasionally and let them pour root beer into mugs. He taught them how to pour the perfect head. Looking back, that hadn't been the best thing to teach your kids, but he and Meg had loved it.

Your father may have been a cheater, Maddie had said, *but did he deserve to be shot three times and bleed to death on a barroom floor while your mother watched?*

He'd thought more about his father in the past two days than he had in the past five years. If Maddie was right, his mother watched his father die, and he just couldn't get that image out of his head.

He sat on the edge of the pool table and crossed one booted foot over the other as he watched Steve grab a Heineken from the refrigerator and twist off the top. Mick knew that the waitress, Alice Jones, had been killed behind the bar, while his mother and father had both died in front of the bar. He'd never seen photos or read the reports, but throughout the years he'd certainly heard enough talk about the night his mother had killed his father and Alice Jones that he thought he'd heard it all. Now he guessed he hadn't.

Over the past thirty-five years, he'd been in this bar thousands of times. Meg had a photograph of him at the age of three sitting on a barstool with his father. Generations of Hennessys had worked their asses off in the bar, and after his parents' deaths, the place had been completely renovated and any trace of what had happened that night had long since been removed. When he walked through the back door, he never thought about what his mother had done to his father and Alice Jones.

Until now.

So your mother was perfectly justified in shooting her in the face, Maddie had said. For some reason, he couldn't get Maddie

Dupree and her damn crime book out of his mind. The last thing in the world he wanted to occupy his thoughts was the deaths of his parents. His past was best left buried, and the last person he wanted stuck in his head was the woman responsible for digging it all up again. She was a one-woman backhoe, uncovering things that were best left covered. But short of tying her up and shoving her in a closet, there wasn't anything he could do to stop her. Although tying her up did have a certain appeal that had nothing to do with stopping her from writing.

My God, you're like a tornado. Sucking up everything around you, she'd said, and it didn't seem to matter that she was the last person in the world that he should want. The memory of her lips beneath his, and the sight of her looking thoroughly kissed and gasping for breath, were trapped in the center of his brain.

Mick rose from the table and moved past the dance floor toward the bar. Reuben Sawyer sat on his regular stool, looking old and pickled. Reuben had lost his wife thirty years ago, and for the last three decades, he'd sat on the same stool almost every night drowning his sorrows. Mick didn't believe in soul mates and didn't understand that kind of sorrow. As far as he was concerned, if you're that lonely for a woman, do something about it that doesn't involve a bottle of Jack Daniel's.

Several people called out to Mick as he passed, but he didn't stop. He didn't feel like shooting the shit. Not tonight. As he moved down the hall toward the back door, an old high school girlfriend stopped him.

'Hey, Mick,' Pam Puckett said as she stepped out of the ladies' room.

He supposed pushing past her would have been rude. 'Hey, Pam.' He stopped and she took it as an invitation to wrap her arms around his neck and give him a friendly hug that lingered a few seconds beyond friendly.

'How're you doing?' she asked next to his ear.

'Good.' Since high school, Pam had been married and divorced three times. Mick could have predicted divorce in her future. He pulled back and looked into her face. 'How about yourself?'

'Not bad.' She dropped onto her heels, but kept one hand on his chest. 'I haven't seen you in here for a while.'

'I've been spending a lot of time at the other bar.' Pam was still attractive, and he knew that all he had to do was take her by the hand and he could take her home. He kept his palm on her waist, waiting to feel the first pull of interest behind his fly. 'Are you still working in the sheriff's office?'

'Yeah. Still dispatching calls. I threaten to quit every other day.' Her palm slid up and down his chest.

He had three hours before closing. It wasn't like he had to haul ass to Mort's. He'd been with Pam before and they both knew that it was just sex. Just two adults getting together and having a good time. 'You here by yourself?' he asked.

Her hand slid to his waist and she hooked a finger through his belt loop. He should have felt a spark of interest, but he didn't. 'With a few girlfriends.'

Tell me Mick, do all the women you sleep with know about each other? Sex was probably just what he needed to get Maddie out of his head. It had been a month since he'd gotten laid, and all he had to do was take Pam's hand and pull her behind him out the back door. 'You know I don't ever plan on getting married. Right?'

Her brows lowered. 'I think everyone knows that, Mick.'

'So I've never lied to you about that.'

'No.'

Once he got Pam naked, he'd let her take his mind off other things. Pam didn't like sex long and drawn out. She liked it quick and as many times as a man could get it up, and Mick was in the mood to accommodate her. He brushed his thumb up her ribs and felt a little spark of interest.

'I heard about that writer talking to everyone in town,' she said and snuffed out his spark.

He really wished she hadn't said that. 'See ya around.' He dropped his hand and took a step back toward the door.

'You're leaving?' What she meant was: *You're leaving without me?*

'Gotta work.'

It was still light out when he stepped from the bar and drove toward Mort's. He shoved his glasses on the bridge of his nose as a dull ache settled between his eyes. Maddie Dupree was messing with his past, talking to the town about his family, and affecting his sex life. With each passing moment, he felt the growing appeal of tying her up and stashing her someplace.

His stomach growled as he pulled his truck to a stop behind Mort's, and instead of walking into the back of his bar, he walked a few doors down to the Willow Creek Brewpub and Restaurant. It was a little after nine and he hadn't eaten since lunch. Small wonder that he had a headache.

The place was practically empty, and the

scent of pub wings made him even hungrier as he made his way from the back. He walked to the hostess stand and placed his order to go with a young waitress. The restaurant made the best pastrami on marbled rye and kettle chips in three states. If Mick'd had the time, he would have ordered a summer ale. The brewpub made a damn good summer ale.

The inside of the restaurant was decorated with beer posters from around the world, and sitting in a booth beneath a Thirsty Dog Wheat poster was the one woman he'd been fantasizing about tying up and tossing in a closet.

A big salad and an open folder sat on the table in front of Maddie Dupree. She'd pulled her hair back from her face and painted her lips a deep red. Her brown eyes looked up as he sat on the bench seat across from her. 'You've been busy,' he said.

'Hello, Mick.' She waved a fork toward him. 'Have a seat.'

Her orange sweater was left unbuttoned up the front and she wore it over a white T-shirt. A tight white T-shirt. 'I hear you've been talking to Bill Potter.'

'News travels fast.' She speared some lettuce and cheese and opened her mouth. Her red lips closed over the tines of the fork and she slowly pulled it back out of her mouth.

Mick pointed to the open folder. 'Is that my rap sheet?'

She watched him as she chewed. 'No,' she said after she swallowed. 'The sheriff mentioned that you were a pain in the ass, but he didn't mention a rap sheet.' She closed the folder and put it on the seat beside her. 'What did he arrest you for? Vandalism? Urinating in public? Window-peeking?'

Smart-ass. 'Fighting, mostly.'

'He mentioned a fire. You wouldn't know about that, would you?' She took a bite of her salad and washed it down with iced tea.

He smiled. 'I don't know anything about any fires.'

'Of course not.' She set her fork on her plate, then sat back and folded her arms beneath her large breasts. Her T-shirt was so thin he could clearly see the white outline of her bra.

'Did you have a nice chat with Harriet Landers?'

She bit the side of her lip to keep from laughing. 'It was interesting.'

Mick sank down on the seat and lowered his brows. The toe of his boot brushed her foot and she tilted her head to one side. Like smooth shiny silk, her hair fell across one shoulder as she looked at him. For several moments she stared into his eyes before she sat up straight and pulled her feet back.

'Harriet screwed my grandfather to death in the back of her car,' he said. 'That's hardly a crime.'

She pushed her plate aside and folded her arms on the table. 'That's true, but it's juicy stuff.'

'And you're going to write about it.'

'I hadn't thought to mention your grandfather's . . . ill-timed departure.' She turned her head a little to one side and looked at him out of the corners of her big brown eyes. 'But I do need to fill pages with family background.'

'Uh-huh.'

'Or I could fill pages with photos.'

He sat up, placed his elbows on the table, and leaned forward. 'You want me to give you photos? Nice happy family Polaroids? Maybe at Christmas or Thanksgiving or the summer we all went to Yellowstone?'

She took a drink of her tea, then set it back down. 'That would be great.'

'Forget it. I can't be blackmailed.'

'It's not blackmail. More like both of us getting what we want. And what I really want is to take pictures of the inside of Hennessy's.'

He leaned even farther across the table and

said, 'How does it feel to want?' A waitress set his plastic sack of food on the table and he said without removing his gaze from Maddie, 'Stay out of my bar.'

She leaned toward him until his face was just a few inches from hers. 'Or?'

She was gutsy as hell, and he almost liked that about her. Almost. He stood and reached into his back pocket for his wallet. He tossed a twenty on the table. 'I'll throw you out on your ass.'

9

'You're crazy.'

'It'll be fine.' Maddie looked over her shoulder at Adele and opened the door to Mort's.

'Didn't he say he was going to throw you out on your ass?'

'Technically, we were talking about Hennessy's.'

They stepped inside and the door closed behind them. Adele leaned close to Maddie and asked above the noise and the music pouring from the jukebox, 'Do you think he's going to care about technicalities?'

Maddie figured that was pretty much a rhetorical question and her gaze scanned the crowd inside the dimly lit bar, looking for the owner. It was eight-thirty on a Friday night and Mort's was once again packed. She'd had no intention of setting foot inside the cowboy bar again until Mick had told her not to. She had to let him know that he didn't intimidate her. He had to know she wasn't afraid of him. She wasn't afraid of anything.

She recognized Darla from the last time she'd been in Mort's and her neighbor Tanya from the Allegrezzas' party. She didn't see Mick and breathed a little easier. She wasn't afraid. She just wanted to get more than three feet inside the bar before he laid eyes on her.

Earlier, she'd curled her hair on big rollers that gave it lots of volume and loose curls. She wore more makeup than usual and a white cotton jersey halter dress and sandals with two-inch heels. If she was going to get escorted out, she wanted to look good on the way. She carried her red angora cardigan because she knew that as soon as the clock struck nine she would freeze without it.

The juke pumped out a song about redneck women as Adele and Maddie wove their way through the crowd toward an empty table in the corner. Adele, with her long curls, tight jeans, and SAVE A HORSE, RIDE A COWBOY shirt, drew her share of attention.

'Do you see him?' Adele asked as they slid into chairs facing the bar with their backs to the wall.

They'd gone over the plan. It was simple. Nothing risky: just walk into Mort's, have a few drinks, and walk out. Easy, cheesy, lemon squeezy, but now Adele was kind of acting spooked, casting her big-eyed gaze about as if she expected a SWAT team to swoop in, whip out their AK-47s, and force them spread-eagled on the floor.

'No. I don't see him yet.' Maddie placed her purse on the table by her elbow and looked out at the bar. Light from the jukebox and bar poured over the crowd but hardly penetrated the corner. It was the perfect spot to see without being seen.

Adele leaned her head close to Maddie and asked, 'What does he look like?'

She held up one hand and signaled the waitress. 'Tall. Dark hair and very blue eyes,' she answered. *Charming when he wants something, and one kiss could make a woman lose her mind.* Maddie thought about the day he'd brought her the Mouse Motel, about his kiss and his hands on her waist, and her stomach got a little tight. 'If the women in the bar start flipping their hair and reaching for a breath mint, you'll know he's here.'

A waitress with an atrocious perm, butt-tight Wranglers, and a Mort's T-shirt took their drink order.

'He's that prime?' Adele asked as the waitress walked away.

Maddie nodded. Prime was a fairly accurate description. He was certainly drool-worthy, and there had been a time or two when she'd been tempted to bite into him. Like when she'd looked up from her salad at the Willow Creek Brewpub and Restaurant and he'd been sitting across from her. One

164

moment she'd been minding her own business, reading her latest notes from Sheriff Potter, then, poof, there was Mick looking extremely hot and incredibly pissed off. Normally, she wouldn't consider an angry man in the least bit hot, but Mick wasn't a normal man. As he'd sat across from her, working himself up, warning her to stay out of his bar, his eyes had turned a deep, fascinating blue. And she'd found herself wondering what he'd do if she climbed across the table and planted her mouth on his. If she kissed his neck and bit him just below his ear.

'I talked to Clare today,' Adele said and pulled Maddie's attention away from the contemplation of Mick. The two friends talked about the upcoming wedding until the waitress returned with Adele's Bitch on Wheels and Maddie's extra-dry vodka martini. The waitress might have bad hair, but she was damn fine at her job.

'What is up with some of these women's hair?' Adele asked as the waitress walked away.

Maddie's gaze scanned the crowd and she figured the ratio of bad hair vs. good hair was about fifty-fifty. 'I've been trying to figure that out myself.' Maddie raised her glass to her lips. 'Half of them have good hair and the other half are an overprocessed mess.' Over the rim of her glass, she continued her surveillance. There was still no sign of Mick.

'Did I tell you about the guy I dated last weekend?' Adele asked.

'No.' Maddie put on her sweater and prepared for a dating disaster story.

'Well, he picked me up in a souped-up Pinto.'

'Pinto? Aren't those the cars from the seventies that explode?'

'Yeah. It was bright orange, like a moving target, and he drove like he thought he was Jeff Gordon.' Adele pushed several springy curls behind her ears. 'He even wore those fingerless racing gloves.'

'You have got to be shitting me. Where did you meet this guy?'

'At the raceway.'

Maddie didn't ask what Adele had been doing at the raceway. She didn't want to know. 'Tell me you didn't have sex with him.'

'No. I figure a guy who drove that fast had to do other things fast too.' Adele sighed. 'I think I've been cursed with bad dates.'

Maddie didn't believe in curses, but she couldn't disagree. Adele had the worst luck with men of any woman she'd ever known. And Maddie had had a lot of bad luck herself.

An hour and three more bad date stories

later, there was still no sign of Mick. Maddie and Adele ordered another drink and she began to wonder if he just might not show up at all.

'Hello, ladies.'

Maddie glanced up from her martini at the two guys standing in front of her. They were both tall and blond and very tan. The man who'd spoken had an Australian accent.

'Hello,' Adele said and took a sip of her Bitch on Wheels. Adele might have a lot of bad dates, but that was only because she attracted a lot of men. With her golden curls and big aquamarine eyes, Adele seemed to draw men in like bees to a barbeque. Obviously Adele's mojo worked on all nationalities. Behind her glass, Maddie glanced at Adele and laughed.

'Would you like to sit down?' Adele asked.

They didn't have to be asked twice and slid into the two empty chairs. 'M'name's Ryan,' the guy closest to Maddie introduced himself, flattening his vowels like he was Crocodile Dundee.

She set down her drink. 'Maddie.'

'That's Tom. He's m'mate.' He pointed to his friend. 'D'ya live in Truly?'

'Just moved here.' Good Lord, she half expected him to say 'G'day' and 'Crikey.' It was too dark to see the color of his eyes, but

167

he was cute. 'How about you?'

He scooted his chair closer so she could hear him better. 'We're just here for the summer fightin' fires.'

Foreign and cute. 'Are you a smoke jumper?'

He nodded and went on to explain that the fire season in Australia was the exact opposite of the season in the U.S. As a result, a lot of Australian smoke jumpers worked in the American West during the summer. The longer he talked, the more fascinated Maddie became, not only by what he said but by the sound of his voice as he said it. And the longer he talked, the more Maddie began to wonder if this wasn't the perfect man for her to fall off the wagon with. He would be in Truly for a short time and then he'd leave. He wasn't wearing a wedding ring, but she knew that didn't mean anything. She leaned in a little closer and asked, 'Are you married?' just to make sure. But before he could answer, two hands grasped the backs of her arms and lifted her to her feet. She was turned slowly around until her gaze landed on a broad chest in a black Mort's T-shirt. Through the dark surrounding them, she recognized the chest even before she raised her gaze up a thick neck, strong chin, and compressed lips. She didn't have to see his eyes clearly to know they burned an angry blue.

Mick leaned close and said next to her ear, 'What are you doing here?'

He smelled like soap and skin. 'Apparently I'm talking to you.'

One of his hands slid to hers and grasped her like a hot vise. 'Let's go.'

She grabbed her purse from the table and looked over her shoulder at Ryan then Adele. 'I'll be right back,' she hollered.

'You sound sure about that,' said the man hauling her through the crowd toward the back of Mort's. 'Excuse us,' she said as she bumped into Darla. He kept a tight grip on her hand as he just kind of moved through the crowd like a linebacker. She was forced to issue a 'Pardon me' and another 'Excuse us' over the music pouring from the juke. They walked past the end of the bar, down a short hall, and he pulled her behind him into a small room.

He closed the door and dropped her hand. 'I told you to stay out of my bar.'

In one quick glance, Maddie's gaze took in an oak desk, a coatrack, a big metal safe, and a leather sofa. 'You were talking about Hennessy's at the time.'

'No. I wasn't.' His gaze narrowed and she could practically feel anger rolling off him in waves. 'Because I'm a nice guy, I'm going to give you the option of grabbing your friend and walking out the front door.'

Once again, she didn't fear his anger. Instead, she kind of liked the way it turned his eyes a deeper blue, and she leaned back against the door. 'Or?'

'I'll toss you out on your ass.'

She tilted her head to the side. 'Then I should probably warn you that, if you touch me again, I have a Taser and I'll shoot fifty thousand volts in *your* ass.'

He blinked. 'You pack a Taser?'

'Among other things.'

Again he blinked, kind of slow, like he couldn't believe he'd heard her right. 'What things?'

'Pepper spray. Brass knuckles. A hundred-and-twenty-five-decibel screecher alarm. Handcuffs and a Kubaton.'

'Is it even legal to pack a Taser?'

'It's legal in forty-eight states. This is Idaho. What do you think?'

'You're crazy.'

She smiled. 'So I've been told.'

He stared at her for several moments before he asked, 'Do you make it a habit of running around pissing people off?'

She occasionally did make people mad, but she never made a habit of it. 'No.'

'Then it's just me.'

'I don't mean to make you mad, Mick.'

One dark brow rose up his tan forehead.

'Well, I didn't mean to make you mad before tonight. But I kind of have a little problem with being told what I can and can't do.'

'No shit.' He folded his arms across his wide chest. 'Why do you need all that stuff?'

'I interview people who aren't very nice.' She shrugged. 'They're usually in belly chains and leg irons and cuffed to a table when I talk to them, though. Or we talk through Plexiglas. Of course, prisons never let me take in my safety devices, but I always get them back when I leave. I feel safer when I'm packing.'

He took a step back and his gaze raked her up and down. 'You look normal. But you're not.'

Maddie didn't know whether to take that as a compliment or not. He probably didn't mean it as a compliment, though.

He rocked back on his heels and looked down at her. 'Were you planning on zapping the blond guy coming on to you in the corner?'

'Ryan? No, but if he plays his cards right, I might cuff him.'

'He's a tool.'

If she didn't know better, she'd think he was jealous. 'Do you know him?'

'I don't have to know him to know he's a tool.'

Which made no sense at all. 'How can you say someone's a tool if you don't know him?'

Instead of answering he said, 'You were practically tongue-kissing him.'

'That's ridiculous. I haven't made out with a stranger in a bar since college.'

'Maybe you're tired of being 'kind of celibate'.'

That was an understatement. She was really tired of it, but when she thought of having hot, down-and-dirty, animal sex, she thought of Mick. Ryan was cute, but ultimately he was a stranger in a bar, and she no longer made out or picked up strangers in bars. 'Don't worry about my celibacy.'

His gaze slid to her mouth and lower, down her chin and throat, and got hung up on her breasts. It was past nine, so of course she was cold. 'Honey, your body isn't made for celibacy.' Her hard nipples made two sharp points in the front of her dress. 'It's made for sex.' He raised his gaze to hers. 'Lots of rough, sweaty sex that lasts all night long and into the next morning.'

Normally she might have been tempted to Mace a guy for saying that, but when Mick said it, she felt hot little tugs in her stomach and her body urged her to raise her hand to volunteer for sweaty sex duty. 'Celibacy is a state of mind.'

'Which explains why you've gone insane.'

'Now who's the tool?' She adjusted her purse to keep it from falling off her shoulder, but her fingers barely touched the bag before Mick pinned her wrists to the door beside her head.

She looked up into his face an inch above hers. 'What are you doing?'

'I'm not going to just stand here and let you shoot my ass with fifty thousand volts.'

She tried not to smile and failed. 'I was adjusting my bag on my shoulder.'

'Call me paranoid, but I don't believe you.'

'You really thought I was going to zap you?' Zapping him had been the furthest thing from her mind.

'You weren't?'

She chuckled. 'No. You're too pretty to get shot with fifty thousand volts.'

'I'm not pretty.' He let out a breath and it touched the side of her face and neck. 'You smell like strawberries.'

'It's my lotion.'

'You smelled like strawberries that day in Handy Man Hardware.' He buried his nose in her hair and she was so shocked, she felt like *she'd* been zapped. 'You always smell so good. It's been driving me crazy.' He pressed the length of his body into hers. 'When I saw you across the bar, I wanted to do this.' He lowered his face to the side of her throat.

'I thought you wanted to toss me out on my ass.' How had it suddenly gotten so hot? A few minutes ago, she'd been cold. Now she felt hot little tingles rushing across her skin.

'I'll get to that. Later.' He let go of her hands, but his hips held hers against the door. He'd definitely dressed left. He was long and hard and a dull ache settled between her thighs. Harriet had been right. The Hennessy men were blessed. 'First I wanted to smell you right here.' He pushed her sweater away and kissed her bare shoulder. 'Where you're soft and taste good.'

'I like soft skin.' She took a shallow breath and closed her eyes. She wanted him to taste a little lower. 'I'm kind of a hedonist that way.'

'How can you be a hedonist and celibate?' he asked against her neck.

'It's not easy.' And becoming more difficult by the second. If she wasn't careful, her hedonist side would rule her celibate side, and she would go down in a blaze of orgasmic glory. Which didn't sound so horrible. Just not with him. She lifted her hand to the side of his face and brushed her thumb across the slight stubble of his cheek. 'Especially when you're around.'

He chuckled. A low masculine sound that came from the center of his chest. He raised his face and his gaze had gone all half-mast with lust and his lashes looked very long. Desire shone bright blue in his eyes and his hands moved to her waist.

'You're the last man on the planet I can have.' She raised her mouth to his and he lifted his weight. 'And the one I want most.'

'Ain't life a bitch,' he whispered against her lips.

She nodded and rose to the balls of her feet. Her hand slid to the back of his head and she pressed her mouth to his. His hands on her waist tightened, and for several agonizing heartbeats, he remained perfectly still. His warm palms glued to her waist, his mouth against hers. Then a deep groan sounded low in his throat, and he slid one hand to the small of her back and the other between her shoulders on the outside of her sweater. He brought her against his chest and he kissed her. Soft, sweet. His lips created a delicious suction and he drew her tongue into his mouth, his cheeks sucking lightly.

Maddie's purse fell to the floor and she moved her free hand up the hard muscles of his arm and shoulder. Heat radiated from him and warmed her breasts where she was pressed against his chest. Maddie had never been a passive lover, and while he sweetly made love to her mouth, her fingers combed through his hair and her free palm roamed the hard contours of his chest and back. If he wasn't Mick Hennessy, she would have pulled his shirt from his Levi's and felt his bare skin.

Mick slid his mouth to the side of her throat. 'You're the last woman I should want,' he said between short gasps. 'The only woman I can't stop thinking about.' His hands moved to cup her behind and her hips cradled his erection. 'What is it about you that drives me so crazy?' Pressed against her lower belly, he was enormous and so hard the pressure against her pelvis almost hurt.

Almost. She rocked against him as he pushed her sweater down her arms. He tossed the red angora somewhere behind him, but she didn't need it. She was too hot. Her fingers curled in the front of his shirt and her mouth moved to his neck. He tasted good beneath her tongue. Like warm flesh and aroused man, and she sucked his skin. She grasped handfuls of shirt and swayed against his stiff penis. It had been four years since she'd felt anything so delectable, and she'd missed it. She'd missed the touch of a man's hands, his hot mouth, and the sounds of arousal deep in his throat.

His fingers found the bow at the back of her neck and he tugged until her halter came untied in his hands. He pulled down the white straps as his lips once again sought hers. This time there was nothing soft or sweet in his kiss. It was all carnal and feeding, with hungry mouths and tongues, and she ate it up. She could have stopped him. She didn't want him to stop. Not yet. Not when she wanted more. The top of her dress slid to her waist and Mick's hands cupped her breast through the white strapless bustier. Under-wires and metal corseting kept her double-Ds front and center, and his thumbs brushed her nipples through the stiff cotton. She pressed her belly against him, touching the aching places, and he groaned into her mouth. She was so hot, dizzy. Her skin tingled, her breasts felt heavy and her nipples painfully tight. It had been so long since she'd felt such delicious pleasure, and she slid her hand down his chest, over the waistband of his jeans, and pressed her palm against his turgid erection.

'Touch me,' he groaned into her mouth. And she did. While his fingers brushed her nipples through her corset, she slid her hand up and down the length of him, from the bottom of his zipper up the long rock-hard length to the swollen tip. The man had heft, and the wet ache between her thighs urged her to take one of his hands and slide it between her legs to cup her crotch and touch her through her panties and . . . She dropped her hands. 'Stop!'

He raised his head. 'In a minute.'

In a minute she'd be in the throes of orgasm. 'No.' She took a step back and his hands fell to his sides. 'You know we can't do this. We can't ever have sex.' She kept her gaze on his as she tied her dress behind her neck. 'Not together.'

He shook his head and his eyes looked a little wild. 'I've been rethinking that.'

'There's nothing to rethink.' He was Mick Hennessy and she was Maddie Jones. 'Believe me, you're the last man on earth I can have sex with, and I'm the last woman you should have sex with.'

'Right now I can't remember why.'

She should tell him. All of it. Who she really was and who he was to her. 'Because . . .' She licked her lips and swallowed, her throat suddenly dry. Sexual tension pulled between them, an almost irresistible hot pulsing force. His neck was red from where she'd marked him, and he looked at her through blue eyes all shiny with lust. The last thing she wanted was to see all that fiery need replaced with disgust. Not now. Later. 'Because I'm writing a book about your parents and Alice Jones, and making love to you won't change that. It will only make it worse.'

He took a few steps back and sat on the edge of his desk. He took a deep breath and ran his fingers through the sides of his hair. 'I forgot about that.' His hands fell to his sides. 'For a few minutes, I forgot you're in town to dig up the past and make my life hell.'

Maddie bent down and picked up her purse. 'I'm sorry.' And she was, but being sorry didn't change anything. She almost wished it did.

'Not sorry enough to stop.'

'No,' she said and reached for the door handle behind her. 'Not that sorry.'

'How long, Maddie?'

'What do you mean?'

He took a deep breath and let it out. 'How long are you going to be in town messing with my life?'

Good question. 'I don't know. Next spring, maybe.'

He looked down at his feet. 'Shit.'

She slid her purse on her shoulder and looked across at him, sitting there with his dark hair sticking out from being finger-combed. She resisted the urge to smooth his hair.

He lifted his gaze. 'Obviously, we can't be within ten feet of each other without tearing at each other's clothes. And since telling you to stay out of my bars is like waving a red flag in the face of a bull, I'm going to ask you to stay the hell out of my bars.'

Her chest did some sort of constrict-and-expand thing, which was not only impossible, but alarming. 'You won't see me in here again,' she assured him and opened the door. She stepped out into the bar, with its loud country music and beer smells, and wove her way toward Adele. When she'd first entered Mort's she'd wondered if Mick would throw her out on her ass as he'd threatened.

Now she wondered if it wouldn't have been better if he had.

⋆　⋆　⋆

Mick shut the door to his office and leaned back against it. He closed his eyes and pressed a palm against his aching erection. If Maddie hadn't stopped him, he would have slid his hand up her thigh. He would have pulled off her panties and had sex with her right there, against the door. He would like to

180

think he'd have had the presence of mind to lock the door first, but he wouldn't bet on it.

He dropped his hand and circled his desk. Her red sweater was thrown on the floor and he picked it up before sitting in his chair to stare at the safe across the office from him. Earlier, looking across his bar and seeing Maddie sitting at a table, sipping a martini as if he hadn't told her to stay out of his bars, had shocked the hell right out of him. Shocked him like that Taser she carried in her purse. On the heels of all that shock came a big dose of anger and an urge to smell the side of her neck.

Seeing her chatting it up with the Aussie, he'd felt something else too. Something a little uncomfortable. Something that felt a bit like he wanted to rip the man's head off. Which was absolutely ridiculous. Mick didn't have anything against the Aussie, and he certainly didn't have any sort of relationship with Maddie Dupree. He didn't feel anything for her. Well, except anger. And raging lust. A burning desire to bury his nose in the side of her neck while he buried himself between her soft thighs. Again and again.

There was something about Maddie. Something other than her beautiful body and pretty face. Something beyond the scent of her skin and her smart mouth. Something that drew his gaze across a crowded bar to a table in a dark corner. Something that recognized her dark outline as if he knew her. Some indefinable thing that made him kiss her and touch her and hold her tight against his chest as if that's where she belonged, when in reality, she didn't belong anywhere near him. A fact he tended to forget when she *was* near him.

He brought the sweater to his face. It smelled like her. Sweet, like strawberries, and he tossed it onto his desk.

A few weeks ago, his life had been fairly good. He had a plan for the future that didn't include thinking about his past. A past that he'd done a pretty good job of forgetting.

Until now. Until Maddie had driven her black Mercedes into town and run his life off the road.

10

It took Maddie a little over a week to track down her mother's friend and neighbor from the Roundup Trailer Court. Shortly after her mother's death, Trina Olsen-Hays sold her trailer and moved to Ontario, Oregon. She'd married a fireman in the mid-'80s, had three grown children, and two grandchildren. Now, sitting across from her at a local café, Maddie had a slight recollection of the plump woman with red poufy hair, freckles, and painted-on eye-brows. She remembered staring at those brows and being somewhat frightened. Seeing Trina also brought back the fuzzy memory of a pink polka-dot quilt. She didn't know why or what it meant. Just that she'd felt warm and secure wrapped up in it.

'Alice was a real nice girl,' Trina said over coffee and pecan pie. 'Young.'

Maddie glanced at the tape recorder sitting on the table between them, then returned her gaze to Trina. 'She was twenty-four.'

'We used to share a bottle of wine and talk about the future. I wanted to see the world. Alice just wanted to get married.' Trina shook her head and took a bite of pie. 'Maybe because she had a little girl. I don't know, but she just wanted to find a man, get married, and have more kids.'

Maddie hadn't known that her mother thought about having other children, but she supposed it made sense. If her mother had lived, she'd no doubt have a brother or sister or both. Not for the first time, she was struck by how different her life would have been if not for Rose Hennessy. Maddie loved her life. She loved the woman she'd become. She wouldn't change it for anything, but sometimes she did wonder about how differently she might have turned out.

'Did you know either Loch or Rose Hennessy?' As she looked across the table at Trina, she wondered if her mother would have time-warp hair or if she would have kept up with changing styles.

'They were older than me, but I knew them both. Rose was ... unpredictable.' Trina took a drink of her coffee. 'And Loch was a natural-born charmer. It was really no wonder Alice fell in love with him. I mean, everyone did. Even though most of us knew better.'

'Do you know how Loch felt about Alice?'

'Only that she thought he was going to leave his wife and family for her.' Trina shrugged one shoulder. 'But every woman he ever got involved with thought that too. Only Loch never did. Sure, he had affairs, but he never left Rose.'

'Then what do you think made the affair between Loch and Alice different? What sent Rose over the edge and made her load a gun and drive to Hennessy's that night?'

Trina shook her head. 'I always figured she'd finally had enough.'

Maybe.

'Or it could have been that Alice was so much younger and prettier than the others. Who knows? What I remember most was how quickly Alice fell in love with Loch. You wouldn't believe how fast it was before she was madly in love.'

After reading her mother's diaries, Maddie actually could believe it.

Trina took another bite of pie and her gaze dropped to Maddie's mouth as she chewed. Her painted brows lowered and she looked up into Maddie's eyes. 'I recognize your mouth. You're Alice's little girl, aren't you?'

Maddie nodded. It was almost a relief to have it out.

Trina smiled. 'Well, how about that? I've always wondered what happened to you after your aunt took you away.'

'She was my great-aunt and I moved to Boise with her. She died last spring. That's when I came across my mother's diaries and your name.'

Trina reached across the table and patted Maddie's hand. The touch felt cool and a bit awkward. 'Alice would be very proud of you.'

Maddie liked to think so, but she would never know for sure.

'So, are you married? Have any kids?'

'No.'

Trina patted her hand one last time, then reached for her fork. 'You're still young. There's time.'

Maddie changed the subject. 'I have a faint memory of a polka-dot quilt. Do you recall anything about that?'

'Hmm.' She took a bite of pie and looked up at the ceiling in thought. 'Yes.' She returned her gaze to Maddie and smiled. 'Alice made it for you, and she used to roll you all up in it like — '

'A burrito,' Maddie finished as a recollection of her mother whispered across her memory. *You're my polka-dot burrito.* If Maddie were an emotional woman, the little pinch to her heart would have brought tears to her eyes. But Maddie had never been an emotional person, and she could count on one hand the number of times she'd cried as an adult. She didn't consider herself a cold person, but she'd learned early on that tears never changed a thing.

She interviewed Trina for another forty-five minutes before packing up her notes and tape recorder and heading for Boise. She had another bridesmaid dress fitting that afternoon, and she met her friends at Nan's Bridal before grabbing a late lunch with them and heading home to Truly.

She stopped at the Value Rite to pick up some toilet paper and a six-pack of Diet Coke. The drug-store had a display of wind chimes and hummingbird feeders and she chose a simple chime made of green tubes. She'd never had a humming-bird feeder, and she reached for one and read the instructions. It was silly, really. More than likely she wouldn't be living in Truly next summer. No use in making the house homey. She placed the feeder in the cart next to her Coke. She could always take it with her when she sold the place. She'd bought the house as an investment. She was one woman. One woman did not need two homes, but she supposed there was no hurry to sell.

Carleen Dawson stood in the dog food aisle shelving collars and leashes and talking to a woman with long black hair. Maddie smiled as she wheeled her cart past and Carleen stopped in midsentence.

'That's her,' she heard Carleen say. She

kept on walking until she felt a hand on her arm.

'Just one minute.'

She turned and looked into a pair of green eyes. The tiny hairs on the back of her neck tingled as if she should know her. The woman wore some kind of uniform as if she worked in a restaurant or diner. 'Yes?'

The woman dropped her hand. 'I'm Meg Hennessy and I hear you're writing about my parents.'

Meg. That's how she knew her. From photos of Rose. If Mick was the image of Loch, Meg looked a lot like her mother. The tingles on the back of her neck spread down her spine as if she were looking into the eyes of a killer. Her mother's killer, but of course Meg was as innocent as she was herself. 'That's right.'

'I've read your books before. You write about serial killers. The real sensational stuff. My mother wasn't a serial killer.'

Maddie didn't want to do this here. Not in the middle of a drugstore with Carleen looking on. 'Perhaps you'd like to talk about this somewhere else.'

Meg shook her head and her dark hair swung about her shoulders. 'My mother was a good person.'

That was open for debate, but not in the

middle of Value Rite. 'I'm writing a fair account of what happened.' And she was. She'd written some hard truths about her mother that she could have easily glossed over.

'I hope so. I know Mick doesn't want to talk to you about this. I understand how he feels, but you're obviously going to write this book with or without our input.' She dug around in her purse and pulled out a pen and a silver gum wrapper. 'I don't get why you think my parents' deaths are worthy of a novel, but you do,' she said as she wrote on the white side of the gum wrapper. 'But call me if you have questions.'

Maddie wasn't easily shocked, but when Meg handed her the wrapper, she was so stunned that she didn't know what to say. She glanced at the telephone number and folded the paper in half.

'You've probably talked to that waitress's relatives.' Meg shoved her pen back inside her purse and her black hair fell across her pale cheek. 'I'm sure they told you lies about my family.'

'Alice only has one living relative. Her daughter.'

Meg looked up and pushed her hair behind one ear. 'I don't know what she could tell you. Nobody around here even remembers her. She probably turned out just like her home-wrecking mother.'

Maddie's grasp tightened on the handle of her shopping cart, but she managed a pleasant smile. 'She's as much like her mother as I imagine you are like yours.'

'I'm nothing like my mother.' Meg stood up straighter and her voice got a bit more strident. 'My mother killed her cheating husband. I divorced mine.'

'Too bad your mother didn't consider divorce a better option.'

'Sometimes a person is pushed too far.'

Bullshit. Maddie had heard that excuse from every sociopath she'd ever interviewed. The old 'she pushed me too far so I stabbed her a hundred and fifty times' excuse. She slid the gum wrapper into her pants pocket and asked, 'What was it about your father's affair with Alice Jones that pushed your mother too far?'

Maddie expected the same response she'd gotten every time she asked that question. A shrug of the shoulders. Instead Meg got busy digging in her purse once more. She pulled out a set of keys and folded her arms across her chest.

'I don't know.' She shook her head.

She's lying. Maddie looked into Meg's green eyes and Meg turned her gaze to a bag of Purina ONE and Beggin' Strips. She knew something. Something she didn't want to talk about.

'Only three people know what really happened that night. My dad, my mom, and that waitress. They're all dead.' Meg stuck one finger through the ring and closed her fingers around the keys. 'But if you want to know the truth about my mom and dad's life, call me and I'll clear things up for you,' she said and turned to walk away.

'Thank you. I will,' Maddie answered even though she wasn't a bit fooled by Meg's eagerness to help, and she doubted that she'd get the entire truth about Rose and Loch's life. She'd get Meg's version, which Maddie was sure would be shaded and glossed over.

She pushed her cart to the checkout line and put her items on the counter. Mick had mentioned that his sister could be difficult. Did she suffer the same mental instability as Rose? Maddie had felt Meg's hostility and resentment toward Maddie's mother and even herself. Meg had refused to even say Alice's name, but she knew something about that night. Maddie was sure of it. Whatever it was, Maddie would find out. She'd extracted secrets from people a hell of a lot smarter and with more to lose than Meg Hennessy.

* * *

When Maddie walked into the house after being gone all day, the carcass of a dead mouse greeted her. Last week, Ernie's Pest Control had finally made it out and laid bait. As a result, Maddie kept finding dead mice all over the place. She set her Value Rite bags on the kitchen counter, then tore off some paper towels. She grabbed the mouse by its tail and carried it outside to the garbage cans.

'What're you doing?'

Maddie looked over her shoulder, into the deep shadows created by towering ponderosas, and her gaze landed on two boys dressed up like mini-commandos.

She held up the mouse. 'Throwing this in the trash.'

Travis Hennessy scratched his cheek with the barrel of a green Nerf gun. 'Did its head pop off?'

'Sorry. No.'

'Bummer.'

She dropped the carcass into the garbage.

'My mom and dad are going to Boise,' Pete informed her. ''Cause my aunt had her babies.'

Maddie turned and looked at Pete. 'Really? That's great news.'

'Yeah, and Pete is spending the night at my house.'

'My dad's taking us to Travis's in three

shakes. He says my uncle Nick needs a drink.'
Pete loaded his plastic camouflaged rifle with
an orange rubber dart. 'The babies' names
are Isabel and Lilly.'

'Do you know if — '

Louie called for the boys and interrupted
Maddie. 'See ya,' they said in unison, then
turned on the heels of their sneakers and took
off through the trees.

''Bye.' She replaced the garbage can lid
and walked back into the house. She washed
her hands and disinfected the floor where
she'd found the carcass. It was after seven
and she threw a chicken breast on her George
Foreman Grill. She made a salad and drank
two glasses of wine with her meal. She'd had
a long day, and after she ate and put the
dishes in the dishwasher, she changed out of
her clothes and into a pair of blue Victoria's
Secret lounging pants with the word PINK
printed across her butt. She zipped up a blue
hooded sweatshirt and pulled her hair back in
a ponytail.

A yellow legal pad sat on her desk, and she
grabbed it before turning on a few lamps and
relaxing on her sofa. As she reached for the
remote, she thought about Meg and their
conversation in the middle of Value Rite. If
Meg had lied about knowing what had set her
mother off, she'd lie about other things too.

Things that Maddie might not be able to prove or disprove.

Cold Case Files on A&E flashed on the television screen and Maddie tossed the remote on the sofa beside her. She put her feet up on the coffee table and jotted down her impressions of Meg. Then she wrote a list of questions she intended to ask and got as far as 'What do you recall about the night your parents died?' when the doorbell rang.

It was nine-thirty, and she looked through the peephole at the only man who'd ever been in her house or stood on her porch. It had been over a week since she'd kissed Mick inside his office at Mort's. Eight days since he'd untied her dress and made her ache for him. Tonight he wasn't wearing his happy face, but her body didn't seem to mind. A sharp tug pulled deep in the pit of her belly as she opened the door.

'I just talked to Meg,' he said as he stood there with his hands on his hips, all male belligerence and seething testosterone.

'Hello, Mick.'

'I thought I made it clear that you stay away from my sister.'

'And I thought I made it clear that I don't take orders from you.' Maddie folded her arms beneath her breasts and simply looked at him. The first pale shadows of night painted him in a faint gray light and made his eyes appear a startling blue. Too bad he was so bossy.

They stared at each other for several prolonged moments before he dropped his hands to his sides and said, 'Are we going to stand here all night staring at each other? Or are you going to invite me in?'

'Maybe.' She'd invite him in eventually, but she wasn't going to be all happiness and sunshine about it. 'Are you going to be rude?'

'I'm never rude.'

She lifted a brow.

'I'll try to be nice.'

Which was kind of half-assed, Maddie thought. 'Are you going to *try* and keep your tongue out of my mouth?'

'That depends. Are you going to keep your hands off my dick?'

'Jerk.' She turned and walked into the living room, leaving him to let himself in.

The yellow legal pad sat face up on the coffee table and she turned it over as he came into the room.

'I know Meg told you to call her.'

Maddie reached for the remote and turned off *Cold Case*. 'Yes, she did.'

'You can't.'

She straightened. It was so typical of him to think he could tell her what to do. He stood in her house, tall and imposing, as if he were king of *her* castle. 'I thought you might have learned by now that I don't follow your orders.'

'This isn't a game, Maddie.' He wore a black Mort's polo shirt tucked into a pair of Levi's resting low on his hips. 'You don't know Meg. You don't know how she gets.'

'Then why don't you tell me?'

'Right,' he scoffed. 'So you can write about her in your book?'

'I told you that I'm not writing about you or your sister.' She sat on the arm of the sofa and put one foot on the coffee table. 'Frankly, Mick, you're just not that interesting.' Lord, that was such a lie she was surprised her nose didn't grow.

He looked down at her. 'Uh-huh.'

She placed a hand on her chest. 'I stayed away from Meg just like you wanted me to, but she approached me. I didn't approach her.'

'I know that.'

'She's a grown woman. Older than you, and she can certainly decide whether or not to talk to me.'

He moved to the French doors and looked out at the deck and the lake beyond. Light from the lamp near the sofa touched his shoulder and the side of his face. 'She might be older, but she's not always predictable.' He was silent a few moments, then he turned his head and looked at her over his shoulder. His voice changed: gone was the demanding tone when he asked, 'How do you know my mother's footprints were all over the bar that night? Is it in a police report?'

Maddie slowly rose. 'Yes.'

She barely heard his next question. 'What else?'

'There are photographs of her footprints.'

'Jesus.' He shook his head. 'I meant, what else was in the report?'

'The usual. Everything from time of arrival to positions of the bodies.'

'How long did my father live?'

'About ten minutes.'

He rested his weight on one foot and folded his arms across his big chest. He was silent for several more seconds before he said, 'She could have called an ambulance and maybe saved his life.'

'She could have.'

Across the short distance, he looked at her. This time a wealth of emotion burned in his blue eyes. 'Ten minutes is a long time for a wife to watch her husband suffer and bleed to death.'

She took a few steps toward him. 'Yes.'

'Who called the police?'

'Your mother did. Right before she shot herself.'

'So she made sure my father and the waitress were dead before she called.'

Maddie stopped. 'The waitress had a name.'

'I know.' A sad smile curved one corner of his lips. 'Growing up, my grandmother always called her 'the waitress'. It's just a habit.'

'You didn't know any of this?'

He shook his head. 'My grandmother didn't talk about things that were unpleasant. Believe me, my mother murdering my father and Alice Jones were at the top of the list of things we didn't talk about.' He turned his gaze outside. 'And you have photographs.'

'Yes.'

'Here?'

She thought about her answer and decided to tell the truth. 'Yes.'

'What else?'

'Besides the police reports and crime scene photos, I have interviews, newspaper accounts, diagrams, and the coroner's report.'

Mick opened the French doors and stepped outside. Soaring ponderosa pines cast black shadows across the deck, chasing away the muted grays of dusk. A slight breeze scented the night with pine and lifted strands of Mick's hair where it touched his forehead. 'I went to the library when I was about ten, thinking I'd get a look at old newspaper reports, but the librarian was a friend of my grandmother's. So I left.'

'Have you seen any accounts of that night?'

'No.'

'Would you like to see them?'

He shook his head. 'No. I don't have a lot of memories of my parents, and reading about what happened that night would ruin those that I do have.'

She didn't have a lot of memories of her mother either. Recently, with the help of the diaries, a few had come back. 'Maybe not.'

He laughed without humor. 'Until you blew into town, I didn't know that my mother watched my father die. I didn't know she hated him that much.'

'She probably didn't hate him. Both love and hate are very powerful emotions. People kill the people they love all the time. I don't understand it, but I know that it happens.'

'That isn't love. It's something else.' He walked to the dark edge of the deck and his hands gripped the wood railing. Across the lake, the moon began to rise over the mountains and reflected a perfect mirror image into the smooth water. 'Until you came to town, everything was buried in the past where it belonged. Then you started digging and prying and it's all anybody around here can talk about now. Just like when I was growing up.'

She moved toward him and leaned her butt into the rail. She folded her arms beneath her breasts and looked up into the darkening outline of his face. She was so close, his hand rested next to her behind on the railing. 'Other than in your own house, I take it the subject of your mother and father used to come up a lot.'

'You could say that.'

'Is that why you fought all the time?'

He looked into her eyes and laughed without sound. 'Maybe I just liked fighting.'

'Or maybe you didn't like people saying unkind things about your family.'

'You think you know me. You think you have me all figured out.'

She shrugged one shoulder. Yeah, she knew him. In some regards, she imagined they'd lived mirror lives. 'I think it must have been hell to live in a town where everyone knows that your mother killed your father and his young lover. Children can be very cruel. That's not just a cliché, it's true. Believe me, I know. Kids are mean.'

The breeze blew a few long strands of hair across Maddie's cheek and Mick raised a hand and brushed them from her face. 'What did they do? Not pick you for kickball?'

'I didn't get picked for anything. I was a little pudgy.'

He pushed her hair behind her ear. 'A little?'

'A lot.'

'How much did you weigh?'

'I don't know, but in the sixth grade I got a really awesome pair of black boots. My calves were too big and I couldn't zip them up all the way. So I folded them down, deluding myself that everyone would think they were supposed to be worn that way. They weren't fooled and I never wore the boots again. That was the year they started calling me Cincinnati Maddie. At first I was just so happy they weren't calling me Fattie Maddie anymore. Then I found out why they called me that and I wasn't so happy.' Through the dusky space that separated them, he raised an inquiring dark brow and she explained, 'They said I was so fat because I ate Cincinnati.'

'The little bastards.' He dropped his hand. 'No wonder you're so ornery.'

Was she ornery? Maybe. 'What's your excuse?'

She felt his gaze touch her face for several moments before he answered, 'I'm not as ornery as you.'

'Right,' she scoffed.

'Well, I wasn't until you moved to town.'

'Long before I moved to town you were giving Sheriff Potter hell.'

'Growing up in this town was sometimes hell.'

'I can imagine.'

'No, you can't.' He took a deep breath and let it out. 'People have wondered my whole life if I was going to lose it like my mom and kill someone. Or if I'd grow up and be like my dad. That's a hard thing for a kid to live with.'

'Do you ever worry about that?'

He shook his head. 'No. I never do. My mother's problem, one of them, was that she never should have put up with a guy who repeatedly cheated on her. And my old man's problem was he never should have married at all.'

'So your solution is to avoid marriage?'

'That's right.' He sat beside her on the railing and took her hand into his. 'Kind of like you solved your fat problem by avoiding carbs.'

'It's different. I'm a hedonist and I have to avoid more than just carbs.' At the moment, her hedonist nature felt the warmth of his palm spread up her arm and across her chest.

'You're avoiding sex too.'

'Yes, and if I fall off either of those wagons, it could get ugly.'

'How ugly?'

He was suddenly too close and she stood. 'I'd binge.'

'On sex?'

She tried to pull her hand away, but he tightened his grasp. 'Or carbs.'

He grabbed the bottom of her sweatshirt with his free hand. 'On sex?'

'Yeah.'

Through the darkness that separated them, he flashed a white seductive smile. 'How ugly will you get?' Slowly, he drew her toward him until she stood between his thighs.

The warmth of his hand, the touch of his thighs, and his wicked smile conspired to pull her in, suck out her will to resist, and shove her headfirst off the wagon. Her breasts felt heavy, her skin tight, and the relentless ache that Mick had created the first time he had kissed her hit her now, sharp, painful, and overwhelming.

'You don't want to know.'

'Yeah,' he said. 'I think I do.'

11

'I thought you were going to keep your tongue out of my mouth.'

Mick glanced up into Maddie's face bathed in moonlight, and he reached for the zipper on the front of her sweatshirt. 'I guess I'll just have to put my tongue somewhere other than your mouth.' He pulled the zipper down, and the sweatshirt parted to give him a glimpse of her deep cleavage. She wasn't wearing anything beneath, and his testicles tightened as the pale swells of her naked breasts were revealed a few inches from his face.

'Someone will see us,' she said and grabbed his wrist.

'The Allegrezzas are in Boise.' He pulled until the zipper parted at her waist.

'What about the neighbors on the other side?' she asked, but she didn't stop him from pushing the edges of the sweatshirt aside. Her breasts were firm and pale white in the moonlight, her puckered nipples an erotic outline in the darkness.

'No one is out, but even if they were, it's too dark to see anything.' He slid his hands around her waist to the small of her back and brought her closer. 'No one can see me do this.' He bent forward to kiss her belly. 'Or this.' He kissed her cleavage.

'Mick.'

'Yeah?'

She combed her fingers through the sides of his hair; her nails scraping his scalp sent a tingling pleasure down his spine. She took short choppy breaths and said, 'We probably shouldn't do this.'

'Do you want me to stop?'

'No.'

'Good. I've found a place to put my tongue.' He opened his mouth and rolled her puckered nipple beneath his tongue. She smelled like sugar cookies tonight and she tasted a bit like sugar cookies too.

'Mmm,' she moaned and pulled him closer. 'That feels good, Mick. It's been so long.' She was a talker, but then, he could have guessed that about her. 'Don't stop.'

Mick had no intention of stopping, not when he was doing exactly what he'd wanted to do to her since the day he saw her at the hardware store. He slid one hand from around her back to cup her breast. 'You're a beautiful woman.' He pulled back far enough to look up into her face, at her parted lips and the desire shining in her dark eyes. 'I want to put my tongue all over you. Starting here.' He sucked her into his mouth and drew lightly. Her flesh puckered even more and he loved the feel and the taste of her. His palm cupping her breast moved down her smooth flat stomach and slid beneath her loose pants. Since that night he'd kissed her at Mort's, he'd had wild fantasies of what he'd do to her if he got her alone again. He slipped his hand between her thighs and cupped her through her thin panties. She was incredibly hot, and wet, and lust twisted and tightened painfully in his groin. He wanted her. He wanted her as he hadn't wanted a woman in a very long time. He'd tried to stay away from her, but at the first excuse to see her, here he was with his mouth on her breast and his hand in her pants, and he wasn't going anywhere this time until he satisfied the lust pounding through his body. She wanted him and he was beyond ready to give her what she wanted. He wasn't going anywhere until both of them were too exhausted to move.

'Yes, Mick,' she said just above a whisper, 'touch me there.' Her sweatshirt fell to her feet and he pulled back to look up past her breasts and into her face. He slid his fingers beneath her panties and stood.

'Right here?' He parted her slick flesh and touched her there. She was incredibly wet, and he wanted to put more than his fingers there.

'Yes.' Her breathing was rapid and her hands clung to his shoulders.

'I love knowing I get you this wet,' he said just above her mouth. 'I want to use my tongue on you.' He brushed his fingers across her small feminine bump. 'Here.' She nodded. 'You don't mind, do you?' She shook her head, then nodded, and then combined the two.

'Mick,' she whispered as her grasp on his shoulders tightened. 'If you don't stop . . . ' She sucked in a breath. 'Oh, my God, don't stop,' she moaned as a powerful orgasm buckled her knees. He wrapped an arm around her waist to keep her from falling as his fingers touched and stroked and felt her pleasure in his hand. He kissed the side of her throat and ached to be inside her, feeling her tight walls gripping him with each pulsation.

When it was through, she said, 'I didn't mean for that to happen.'

He pulled his hand from her pants and pressed his erection into her. 'Let's make it happen again. Only next time, I'm going to join you.' He brushed his wet fingers across the tip of her breast and lowered his mouth to her lips and fed her his need and greed and uncontrolled lust.

She pulled back from the kiss and gasped. 'You have condoms? Right?'

'Yes.'

Bare from the waist up, she took his hand and led him into the house. 'How many do you have on you?'

How many? How many? 'Two. How many do you have?'

'None. I've been celibate.' She closed the door behind them, then turned to face him. 'We're going to have to make those two condoms last all night.'

'What do you have planned?'

She pushed him against the closed door, pulled his shirt over his head, and tossed it aside. 'Something you should not have started.' She took control and her impatience got him so hard, he thought he might burst the buttons on his Levi's. 'But something you *are* going to finish.' Her breasts brushed his chest as she kissed his neck and her hands worked his fly. 'I'm going to use you for your body.' She sucked the side of his neck and shoved his pants and boxer briefs to his knees. 'You don't mind. Do you?'

'God, no.' His dick poked her belly and she took him into her warm hand. She cupped his balls and stroked him up and down, pressing her thumb into the corded vein of his shaft.

'You're a beautiful man, Mick Hennessy.'

She brushed her thumb over the head. 'Hard.'

No shit.

'Big.'

Mick sucked in a breath. 'You can handle it.'

'I know I can.' She bit the hollow of his throat, then slowly sank to her knees, kissing his belly and abdomen on the way down. 'Can you?'

Oh, God. She was going to use her gorgeous mouth on him. His 'Yes' came out on a rush of pent-up breath.

'You don't mind if I use my tongue on you?' She knelt before him and looked up, a little smirk on her red lips. 'Do you?'

'Christ, no.'

Her gaze locked with his as she ran her velvet tongue up his thick shaft, and he locked his knees to keep from falling on her. 'Do you like my tongue here?'

'Yes.' God, was she going to talk the whole time?

She licked the cleft in the head of his cock. 'Like it here?'

She was driving him insane, but he had a feeling she knew that. 'Yes.'

She smiled. 'Then you'll love this.' She parted her lips and she took him into her warm, wet mouth, drawing him to the back of her throat. 'Holy shit,' he whispered and placed his hands in her hair. Most women were hesitant to take a man into their mouths. Obviously she wasn't one of them. She sucked him into a sexual vortex that left him oblivious to anything but her. Anything but her warm hands, hot liquid mouth, and soft tongue giving him raw carnal pleasure. The glass door was cool against his back and his eyes slid shut. He expected her to stop at some point. Women always stopped, but she didn't. She stayed with him as he came, an intense, powerful climax that squeezed the breath from him and hit him like a freight train. She stayed with him until the last flush of orgasm stopped and he was able to breathe. Most women thought they knew how to pleasure a man with their mouths. Some were better than others, but he'd never experienced anything like the intense pleasure Maddie had just given him.

'Thank you,' he said, his voice rough and his breathing rapid.

'You're welcome.' She stood in front of him and touched a finger to the corner of her mouth. 'So, you liked that?'

He reached for her. 'You know I did.'

She wrapped her arms around his shoulders and her nipples brushed his chest. 'Now that we both got the first one out of the way,

I hope you weren't planning on going to work, because I have plans for you here.'

No, he didn't have to go to Mort's. The new manager he'd hired was doing a good job. He kissed the side of her throat and raised a hand to her breast. In the pit of his belly, the lust that had been thoroughly sucked out of him a moment ago caught fire once again.

He had plans of his own.

* * *

She should not have fallen off the wagon. Having sex with Mick was wrong of her on so many levels, but the time to stop things before they got out of control had passed an hour ago. She should have stopped him before he put his mouth on her breast and slid his hand into her pants. But of course she hadn't. Once she'd felt his moist mouth and skilled fingers, she'd become selfish and greedy. She'd wanted to feel his hands all over her body. To feel him touch her in places she hadn't been touched in a long time. To look into his eyes and see how much he wanted her.

Within the spill of lamplight pouring across the gold and red quilt, Mick kissed the small of Maddie's bare back and continued up her spine. 'You always smell so good.' His hands and knees were planted on her bed on both sides of her body and his erection brushed the inside of her bare thigh as he leaned down to kiss the back of her shoulder.

No, she should not have fallen off the wagon with Mick, but she wasn't sorry. Not yet. Not when he made her feel things. Wonderful things she hadn't even known she missed. Tomorrow she would be sorry when she thought about all the ways she'd just complicated her life and his, but tonight she was going to be completely selfish and enjoy the naked man in her bed.

Maddie turned onto her back and looked up into Mick's lusty blue eyes surrounded by thick black lashes. 'You feel good,' she said and ran her hands up his arms and across the hard muscles of his shoulders. 'You make me feel good too.'

He bent down, lightly bit the ball of her shoulder, and his penis touched her between her legs. 'Tell me all the ways you're going to use my body.'

She turned her head and said next to his ear, 'It's a surprise.'

'Should I be afraid?'

'Only if you can't get it up.'

He pressed his erection into her. 'That's not going to be a problem.' And it wasn't. He kissed and teased and tortured her with his hands and mouth, bringing her to the point of climax, then backing off. Just when she thought she might have to pin him to the bed and jump on him, he reached for the condom on the nightstand. Maddie took it from him and put it on while she kissed his belly. Then he pinned *her* to the bed and knelt between her thighs. He wrapped his hand around the thick shaft of his penis and brought the broad head to her slick opening. He pressed into her, hot and enormous, and she gasped from the sheer pleasure of his entry.

'Are you okay?'

'Yes. I love this part,' she said.

He pulled out and plunged a little deeper. 'This part?'

She licked her lips and nodded. She wrapped one leg around his waist and forced him even deeper. His nostrils flared slightly as he pulled out, then buried himself to the hilt, thrusting into her and shoving them up the bed.

She cried out, whether in pain or in intense pleasure, she wasn't quite sure. She only knew that she didn't want it to end.

'Sorry.' He spread kisses across her cheek. 'I thought you were ready.'

'I am,' she moaned. 'Do it again.' And he did. Again and again. Maddie hadn't had sex in a long time, but she didn't remember it feeling so good — if it had been this good, she was positive she would not have given it up for so long.

He groaned deep, deep within his chest and placed his hands on the sides of her face. 'You feel tight around me.' He kissed her lips and said just above her mouth, 'And so good.'

Heat flushed her skin, radiating outward from where they were joined, and she slid her fingers up his warm shoulders and into his hair. 'Faster, Mick,' she whispered. She loved the feeling of him touching her deep inside, the plump head of his penis rubbing her G-spot, then pushing into her cervix. She loved the press of his moist skin against her and the intensity of his blue eyes. Without missing a beat of his pumping hips, he ran a hand down her side and bottom to the back of her thigh.

'Put this leg around my back,' he said just above a whisper. He pressed his forehead into hers and his breathing rasped against her temple. He plunged faster. Harder.

'Mick,' she cried out as he thrust in and out, pushing her closer and closer toward climax. 'Please don't stop.'

'Not a chance.'

Like a flash fire, heat spread from the apex of her thighs, across her body, and she was completely mindless of anything but Mick and the pleasure of his body. She called his name once, twice, maybe three times. She tried to tell him how good it felt, how much she loved and missed sex, but her words came out short and abbreviated as he relentlessly thrust his erection into her, and slammed her into a pleasure so intense she opened her mouth to scream. The sound died in her throat as wave after luscious wave rolled through, and her vaginal muscles pulsed and contracted, gripping him hard. On and on it went as he plunged into her, his labored breath hot against her cheek until finally he shoved into her one last time and a long tortured groan died in his throat.

'Oh . . . my . . . God,' she said when she could catch her breath.

'Yeah.' He raised up onto his elbows and looked into her face.

'I don't remember sex being that good.'

'It usually isn't.' He pushed a few strands of her hair off her forehead. 'In fact, I don't think it's ever been that good.'

'You're welcome.'

He laughed, and his two dimples dented his cheeks. 'Thank you.' When she didn't reciprocate, he lifted one brow up his forehead.

She smiled and unwrapped her legs from

around his waist. 'Thank you.'

He pulled out of her and moved off the bed. 'You're welcome,' he said over his shoulder as he walked into the bathroom.

Maddie rolled on her side and closed her eyes. She sighed and settled within a nice comfy bubble of afterglow. She didn't have a tense muscle in her body and couldn't recall ever being so relaxed. She heard the toilet flush, and she wrapped her arms around the pillow under her head. She should probably have sex more often, as a sort of stress reducer.

'Who's Carlos?'

Maddie opened her eyes and her afterglow bubble popped. 'What?'

Mick sat on the bed and looked at her over his shoulder. 'You called me Carlos.'

She didn't remember that. 'When?'

'When you were coming.'

'What did I say?'

A little scowl turned down the corners of his mouth. ' "Yes. Yes. Carlos." '

Heat rose up her neck to her cheeks. 'I did?'

'Yeah. I've never been called another man's name.' He thought a moment, then added, 'I don't think I like it.'

She sat up. 'Sorry.'

'Who's Carlos?'

He obviously wasn't going to let it drop and she was forced to confess, 'Carlos isn't a man.'

He blinked and stared at her for several moments. 'Carlos is a woman?'

She laughed and pointed to the bedside dresser. 'Open that top drawer.'

He leaned forward and pulled the drawer open. His brows lowered, then slowly rose up his forehead. 'Is that a . . . ?'

'Yes, that's Carlos.'

He looked at her. 'You named it?'

Maddie sat up. 'I thought since we're intimately acquainted he should have a name.'

'It's purple.'

'And glows in the dark.'

He chuckled and shut the drawer. 'It's big.'

'Not as big as you.'

'Yeah, but I can't . . . ' He scratched his cheek. 'What does it do?'

'It can pulse, vibrate, throb, and get hot.'

'All that and glows in the dark too?' He dropped his hand to the bed.

'You're better than Carlos.' She moved to kneel behind him and slid her hands down his chest. 'I'd much rather spend time with you.'

He looked up into her face. 'I don't glow in the dark.'

'No, but your eyes get all sexy, and I love the way you kiss and touch my body.' She pressed her breasts into his warm back. 'You make me vibrate and you make me hot.'

He turned and pushed her down on the bed. 'You make me feel like the last time I was in this room. Like I can't get enough. Like I'm fifteen and can go at it all night.'

A lock of dark hair fell over his forehead and she reached up and smoothed it back. 'Is this room a lot different from the last time you were here with . . . what was her name?'

'Brandy Green.' He glanced about the bedroom. At the mahogany dressers and bedside tables and lamps. 'To tell you the truth, I don't remember what it looked like.'

'Too long ago?'

He returned his gaze to her. 'Too busy to notice.' Laugh lines creased the corners of his eyes. 'Brandy was a senior and I was a sophomore and I was just trying to impress the hell out of her.'

'Did you?'

'Impress her?' He thought a moment, then shook his head. 'I don't know.'

'Well, you've impressed me.'

'I know.' He moved over the top of her onto his back, then pulled her across his chest.

'How do you know?'

'You're a moaner.'

She pushed her hair over her shoulder. 'I am?'

'Yeah. I like it.' He brushed his hand up and down her arm. 'It lets me know you're into what I'm doing to you.'

She shrugged. 'I like sex. I've liked sex since my first time when I was a sophomore at UCLA and lost my virginity to my first boyfriend, Frankie Peterson.'

His hand stilled. 'You waited until you were, what . . . twenty?'

'Well, I was Cincinnati Maddie, remember? But once I moved out of my aunt's house and went away to college, I dropped sixty pounds by virtue of being so poor I didn't have money to spend on food. In those days, I used to work out a lot too. So much so that I burned myself out, and now I refuse to work up a sweat on anything that is painful and boring.' She ran her fingers up the thin line of hair on his belly.

'You don't need to work out.' He slid his hand down her back to her behind. 'You're perfect.'

'I'm too soft.'

'You're a woman. You're supposed to be soft.'

'But I'm — '

He rolled her onto her back and looked down at her. 'I look at you and there isn't anything I can tell myself that makes me not want to be with you.' His gaze moved over her face. 'I've tried to stay away. Tried to keep my hands off you. I can't.' He looked into her eyes. 'Maybe after tonight I can.'

Maddie's breath got caught in her chest. She didn't want one night. She wanted several nights, but he was Mick Hennessy and she was Maddie Jones. She would have to tell him. Soon.

'We better make it good, then.' She slid her hand to the back of his head and ran her fingers through his short hair. 'And tomorrow you can go back to being mad at me, and I'll go back to being celibate. Everything will go back the way it was before tonight.'

One corner of his mouth lifted. 'You think?'

She nodded. 'Neither of us is looking for love, nor even a commitment beyond this room. We both want the same thing, Mick.' She brought his mouth down to hers and whispered against his lips, 'No strings. Just a one-night stand.' Since it was the last time she figured she'd have sex before she jumped back on the wagon, she made sure it was memorable.

She left him long enough to turn on the jetted tub and pour mango-scented bubble bath into the water. Then she took him by the hand and led him into the bathroom. They played within the foamy bubbles, and when it was time, she rode him like a seahorse. This time when she hit her peak, she made sure she called out his name.

Once it was over and Mick flushed the last condom, she fell asleep with her back pressed against his chest and his hand on her breast. He'd been talking to her about something, and she'd nestled her bottom against his groin and passed right out. She'd meant to put on a robe and walk him to the door, but it had been a long time since she'd let herself feel safe and secure and protected. It was an illusion, of course. It had always been an illusion. No one except Maddie could keep her safe and secure and protected, but it had felt so good.

When she woke in the morning, she was alone. Just as she wanted. No strings. No commitment. No demands. He hadn't even said good-bye.

She rolled onto her side and looked at the morning shadows playing across her wall. She placed her hand in the indent on the pillow next to hers and curled her fingers into a fist. It was better this way.

Even if she never told him who she was, if she just left town and never set eyes on him again, he'd find out eventually. He'd find out when the book hit the stores.

Yes, it was better that he'd left without a goodbye. One night was bad enough; anything more would be impossible.

12

The voice of Trina Olsen-Hays filled Maddie's office as she scribbled notes on index cards in an attempt to try and make some sort of order out of the taped conversation. Once she finished transcribing the pertinent information, she would shuffle and mix them with other cards she'd made in order to make a timeline she would then pin across her office wall. She'd learned after her first book that it was easier to move things around if they were written on cards as opposed to a straight line.

After an hour of writing notes, she turned off the tape and leaned back in her chair. She yawned and knitted her fingers together on the top of her head. It was Sunday and she figured the citizens of Truly were just getting out of church. Maddie hadn't been raised in any one religion. As with most everything else while she was growing up, when Maddie had attended church, it had been totally arbitrary and dependent on her aunt's fickle whims or one of her 'programs'. If Great-Aunt Martha saw a *60 Minutes* episode about religion, it reminded her that she might be falling down on the job in the God department, and she'd drop Maddie off at a random church and reassure herself on the way home that she was being a good guardian. After a few Sundays, Martha would forget about church and God and move on to something else.

If Maddie had to choose a religion, she'd probably choose Catholicism. For no other reason than the stained glass, rosary beads and Vatican City. Maddie had visited Vatican City several years ago, and it was definitely awe-inspiring. Even to a heathen like herself. But if she was Catholic, she'd have to go to church and confess the many sins she'd committed upon the body of Mick Hennessy. If she understood confession, she should feel repentant, but she didn't. She might get away with lying to a priest, but God would not be fooled.

Maddie stood and moved into the living room. She'd had a great time with Mick last night. They'd had sex. Good sex, and now it was over. She knew she should feel bad that she hadn't told him her mother was Alice Jones, but she didn't. Okay, maybe a little, but probably not as bad as she should feel. She might feel worse if she had any sort of relationship with Mick, but she didn't. Not even a friendship, and if she felt bad about anything it was that she and Mick could never be friends. She would have liked that. Not just for the sex, but because she liked him.

She moved to the French doors and looked out at the lake. She thought of Mick and his sister and his insistence that she not speak with Meg. Why? Meg was a grown woman. A single mother who supported herself and her son. What was Mick afraid would happen?

'Meow.'

Maddie looked down at her feet. On the other side of the glass door sat a small kitten. It was pure white and had one blue eye and one green. Its head looked almost too big for its body, like maybe it was inbred or something. Maddie pointed at it and said, 'Go home.'

'Meow.'

'I hate cats.' Cats were nasty creatures. They shed all over your clothes, shredded the furniture with their claws, and slept all day.

'Meow.'

'Forget it.' She turned and walked through the house and into her bedroom. Her sheets, pillow-cases, and duvet cover lay in a heap on the floor and she carried them to the laundry room off the kitchen. She needed to get all reminders of Mick out of her house. No indents in her pillows. No empty condom wrappers on the nightstand. Mick was like cheese-cake, and she just couldn't have anything around to remind her how much she liked and missed cheese-cake. Especially when it was so good she'd just gorged herself into a coma the night before.

She stuffed her sheets and pillowcases into the washing machine, loaded it up with soap, and turned it on. As she shut the lid, the doorbell rang, and her stomach kind of got light and heavy at the same time. There had only ever been one person who rang her doorbell. She tried to ignore the feeling in her stomach and the sudden spike in her heartbeat as she moved toward the front of the house. She looked down at her green Nike T-shirt and black shorts. They were old and comfy and not the sort of clothes to inspire lust, but neither had the sweatshirt and pants she'd had on last night, and Mick hadn't seemed to mind.

She looked through the peephole, but it wasn't Mick. Meg stood on her porch wearing dark sun-glasses, and Maddie wondered how Meg knew where she lived. Maybe from Travis. She also wondered what Meg could possibly want on a Sunday afternoon. The obvious answer was she wanted to talk to Maddie about the book. But Meg looked so much like her mother that another answer came to mind; she'd come over for some kind of confrontation. Maddie wondered if she should break out her Taser, but she'd hate to shoot Meg with fifty thousand volts if she'd just come over to talk about what had happened twenty-nine years ago. That wouldn't be very nice, and would be counterproductive, since she wanted to hear what Meg had to say. She opened the door.

'Hi, Madeline. I hope I'm not disturbing you,' Meg began. 'I just dropped Pete off next door, and I was wondering if I could talk to you a moment or two.'

'The Allegrezzas are back so soon?'

'Yes. They came home this morning.'

A slight breeze played with the ends of Meg's dark hair, but she didn't appear agitated or crazy, and Maddie stepped back. 'Come in.'

'Thank you.' Meg pushed her sunglasses to the top of her head and stepped inside. She wore a khaki skirt and a black short-sleeved blouse. She looked so much like her mother it was spooky, but Maddie supposed it was no more fair to judge her by her mother's behavior than it was for people to judge Maddie by hers.

'How can I help you?' Maddie asked as the two moved into the living room.

'Was my brother here last night?'

Maddie's footsteps faltered a fraction before she continued across the living room.

While she'd been wondering what brought Meg to her porch, it hadn't occurred to her that Meg was here to talk about last night's debauchery. Perhaps she'd need the Taser after all. 'Yes.'

Meg sighed. 'I told him not to come here. I'm an adult and I can take care of myself. He's worried that if I talk to you about Mom and Dad, I'll get upset.'

Maddie smiled with relief. 'Please sit,' she said and indicated the couch. 'Would you like something to drink? I'm afraid I only have Diet Coke or water.'

'No, thank you.' Meg sat and Maddie took the chair. 'I'm sorry that Mick felt he needed to come to your house and order you not to talk with me.'

He'd done more than that. 'Like you, I'm an adult, and I don't take orders from your brother.' Except for when they'd been in the spa tub, and he'd looked at her through those gorgeous eyes of his and said, 'Come over here and sit on my lap.'

Meg set her purse on the coffee table. 'Mick isn't a bad person. He's just protective. Growing up, he had it rough and doesn't like talking about our parents. If you'd met him under different circumstances, I'm sure you'd like him.'

She liked him more than was wise under

the current circumstances. She didn't even want to think about how much she might like sitting in his lap if he wasn't a Hennessy. 'I'm sure that's true.'

A frown wrinkled Meg's brow. 'There's a rumor going around town that a movie is going to be made out of your book.'

'Really?'

'Yeah. Carleen came into my work yesterday and told me that Angelina Jolie is going to play my mother, and Colin Farrell my dad.'

Colin Farrell made a little sense because he was Irish. But Angelina Jolie? 'I haven't been offered a movie deal.' Hell, she hadn't even told her agent about the book. 'So you can tell everyone that there isn't going to be a film crew arriving anytime soon.'

'That's a relief,' Meg said, then turned her attention toward the French doors. 'Your cat wants in.'

'It's not mine. I think it might be a stray.' Maddie shook her head and leaned back into her chair. 'Do you want a kitten?'

'No. I'm not really a pet person. I've promised my son a dog if he behaves for a month.' She chuckled. 'I don't think I'll have to make good on that promise anytime soon.'

When Meg laughed, she looked a bit like Mick. 'I'm not really a pet person either,'

Maddie confessed and wondered if Meg had come over for a chat about pets or to talk about her parents. 'They're a lot of bother.'

'Oh, I wouldn't mind that. I'm not a pet person because they die.'

As far as Maddie was concerned, that was the only good thing about cats.

'Growing up, we had a poodle named Princess. She was mostly Mick's dog.'

Mick had a poodle? Not only could she not see Mick owning a poodle, she couldn't imagine him naming it Princess. 'Did he name her?'

'Yes, and she died when he was about thirteen. The only time I've seen Mick cry was when he had to bury that dog. Even at our parents' funeral, he was a stoic little man.' Meg shook her head. 'I've had too many people die in my life. I don't want to get attached to a pet and have it die on me. Most people don't understand that, but it's how I feel.'

'I understand.' And she did. More than Meg would ever know. Or at least know for now.

'You're probably wondering why I stopped by instead of waiting for you to contact me.'

'I assume you are anxious to talk about your mother and father and what happened on that night in August.'

Meg nodded and pushed her hair behind

her ears. 'I don't know why you want to write about what happened, but you do. So I think you should hear it from my family's side. And Mick's not going to talk to you. That leaves me.'

'Do you mind if I tape-record the conversation?'

Meg took such a long time to answer, Maddie thought she might refuse. 'I guess that would be okay. As long as I get to stop if I feel uncomfortable.'

'That's perfectly fine.' Maddie rose from the chair and walked to her desk. She popped a new cassette into the tiny recorder, grabbed a folder and pen, then returned to the living room. 'You don't have to say anything you don't feel like saying,' she said, although it was her job to get Meg to spill it all. Maddie held the recorder in front of her mouth, gave Meg's name and the date, then set it on the edge of the coffee table.

Meg looked at the tape recorder and asked, 'Where do I begin?'

'If you feel comfortable, why don't you talk about what you recall of your parents?' Maddie sat back in her chair and rested her hands lightly on her lap. Patient and nonthreatening. 'You know, the good times.' And after Meg talked about those, they would get to the bad.

'I'm sure you heard that my parents fought.'

'Yes.'

'They didn't fight all the time, it was just that when they did . . . ' She paused and looked down at her skirt. 'My grandmother used to say that they were passionate. That they fought and loved with more passion than other people.'

'Do you believe that?'

A wrinkle furrowed her brow and she clasped her hands in her lap. 'I just know that my dad was . . . bigger than life. He was always happy. Always singing little songs. Everyone loved him because he just had a way about him.' She looked up and her green eyes met Maddie's. 'My mother stayed at home with Mick and me.'

'Was your mother happy?'

'She . . . she was sad sometimes, but that doesn't mean she was a bad mother,' Meg said and proceeded to talk about wonderful picnics and birthday parties. Big family gatherings and Rose reading bedtime stories that made the family sound like one big Hallmark card of happiness.

Bullshit. After about thirty minutes of listening to Meg cherry-pick her stories, Maddie asked, 'What happened when your mother was sad?'

Meg sat back and folded her arms across her chest. 'Well, it's no secret that things got broken. I'm sure Sheriff Potter told you about the time my mother set my father's clothes on fire.'

Actually, the sheriff hadn't mentioned it. 'Mmm.'

'She had the fire under control. There was no need for the neighbors to call the fire department.'

'Perhaps they were concerned because this area is a forest and it doesn't take much to start it on fire.'

Meg shrugged. 'It was May. So it wasn't likely. The fire season isn't until later.'

Which didn't mean the fire wouldn't have caused serious damage, but Maddie figured it was pointless and counterproductive to argue, and time to move things along. 'What do you recall of the night your parents died?'

Meg looked across the room at the empty television screen. 'I remember that it had been hot that day and Mom took Mick and me to the public beach to swim. My dad usually went with us, but he didn't that day.'

'Do you know why?'

'No. I suspect he was with the waitress.'

Maddie didn't bother reminding her that the waitress had a name. 'After you went to the public beach what happened?'

'We went home and had dinner. Dad wasn't home, but that wasn't unusual. I'm sure he was at work. I remember we had 'whatever night', meaning we could have whatever we wanted for dinner. Mick had hot dogs and I had pizza. Later we ate ice cream and watched *Donny & Marie*. I remember what we watched because Mick was really mad that he had to watch Donny and Marie Osmond. But later he got to watch *The Incredible Hulk*, so he cheered up. My mom put us to bed, but sometime around midnight, I woke up because I heard her crying. I got out of bed and went into her room, and she was sitting on the side of her bed and she had all her clothes on.'

'Why was she crying?' Maddie leaned forward.

Meg turned to Maddie and said, 'Because my father was having another affair.'

'Did she tell you that?'

'Of course not, but I was ten years old. I knew about the affairs.' Meg's gaze narrowed. 'Daddy wouldn't have left us for her. I know he wouldn't have really done that.'

'Alice thought he was going to.'

'They all thought that.' Meg laughed without humor. 'Ask them. Ask Anna Van Damme, Joan Campbell, Katherine Howard, and Jewel Finley. They all thought he was going to leave my mother for them, but he never did. He never left her and he wouldn't have left her for the waitress either.'

'Alice Jones.' Maddie had almost felt sorry for Meg, rattling off the names of her father's lovers.

'Yes.'

'Jewel Finley? Wasn't she friends with your mother?'

'Yeah,' Meg scoffed. 'Some friend.'

'Did something happen that day out of the ordinary?'

'I don't think so.'

Maddie put her forearms on her knees, leaned forward, and looked into Meg's eyes. 'Usually when you see an otherwise sane woman kill her husband and then herself, there is something that has added stress to the relationship. Usually it's the belief that the person feeling the most stress feels powerless, like she's losing everything and therefore she has nothing else to lose. If it wasn't your father's infidelity, then it had to be something else.'

'Maybe she just planned to frighten them with the gun. Maybe she wanted to scare them and things got carried away.'

That was usually the excuse, but rarely the case. 'Is that what you believe?'

'Yes. Maybe she found them naked together.'

'They were both clothed. Alice was behind the bar and your father was in front of it. They were at least ten feet apart.'

'Oh.' She bit her thumbnail. 'I still think she went there to scare Dad and things got out of control.'

'You *think* that, but you don't know.'

Meg dropped her hand and stood. 'My mother loved my father. I just don't think she went there with the intention of killing anyone.' She put her purse over her shoulder. 'I've got to get home.'

Maddie stood. 'Well, thanks for your help,' she said and walked Meg to the door. 'I appreciate it.'

'If I can clear anything up, give me a call.'

'I will.' After Meg left, Maddie moved into the living room and turned off the tape. She felt sorry for Meg. She truly did. Meg was a victim of the past just like she was, but Meg was older than both Mick and Maddie and recalled more of that horrible night. Meg also recalled more than she was willing to talk about too. More than she wanted Maddie to know, but that was okay — for now. Maddie had written the first chapter of the book but had stopped to work on the timeline. When she got the sequence of —

'Meow.'

Maddie leaned her head back. 'For the love

of God.' She moved to the door and looked down at the kitten on the other side. 'Go away.'

'Meow.'

She pulled the cord to her vertical blinds and turned them so that she could no longer see the annoying cat. She moved into the kitchen and made a low-carb dinner. She ate in front of the television with the sound turned way up. After dinner, she took a leisurely bath and scrubbed her skin with a vanilla body scrub. A white jar of Marshmallow Fluff body butter sat on the counter next to a towel. She'd received it in the mail at her house in Boise yesterday and had tossed it into her purse.

Lord, had it only been yesterday that she'd met with Trina, had a bridesmaid fitting, and had sex with Mick? She unplugged the bathtub drain and stood. She'd been a busy girl.

Maddie dried herself, then rubbed the creamy lotion into her skin. She pulled on her striped pajamas pants and PINK T-shirt then moved to the living room and picked up the tape recorder from the coffee table where it still sat. A cell phone commercial blared from the television and she hit the off button on the remote control. She wanted to replay Meg's recollections of the evening her mother had killed two people and then herself.

'Meow.'

'Damn it!' She pulled the cord to the blinds and there, sitting like a white snowball in the darkening shadows of evening, sat her tormentor. She put her hands on her hips and glared at the kitten through the glass. 'You have gotten on my last nerve.'

'Meow.'

How such a racket could come from such a tiny mouth was beyond Maddie. 'Go away!' As if it understood, the kitten stood, walked around in a circle, then sat in the same exact spot.

'Meow.'

'I've had it.' Maddie went to the laundry room, shoved her arms into a jean jacket, then stomped across the floor to the French doors. She threw them open and scooped up the kitten. The kitten was so small its entire torso fit in one hand. 'You probably have fleas or ringworm,' she said.

'Meow.'

She held the kitten out at arm's length. 'The last thing I need is a big-headed *inbred* cat.'

'Meow.'

'Shh. I'm going to find you a good home.' The dang kitten started to purr like they were going to be friends or something. As quietly as possible, she moved down the steps and tiptoed across the cold grass to the Allegrezzas' yard. A light in the kitchen burned and through the sliding glass door, she watched Louie make a sandwich. 'You're going to love these people,' she whispered.

'Meow.'

'Really. They have a kid, and kids love kittens. Act cute and you're in.' She set it on the deck, then ran like hell back to her house. As if she were escaping a demon, she closed the door, locked it, and shut the blinds. She sat on the couch and leaned her head back. Quiet. Thank God. She closed her eyes and told herself she'd just performed a very good deed. She could have chased it off by throwing something at it. Little Pete Allegrezza was a nice kid. He probably wanted a cat and would give it a good home. It obviously hadn't eaten in a while and Louie would no doubt hear it and feed it a hunk of lunch meat. Maddie was practically a friggin' saint.

'Meow.'

'Are you shitting me?' She sat up and opened her eyes.

'Meow.'

'Fine. I tried to be nice.' She stormed into her bedroom and shoved her feet into a pair of black flip-flops. 'Stupid cat.' She returned to the living room, threw open the back door, and scooped up the kitten. She held it up in front of her face and glared into its spooky eyes. 'You're too stupid to know I found you a good home.'

'Meow.'

This was karma. Bad karma. Definitely a pay-back for something she'd done. She grabbed her purse with her free hand and flipped on the outside lights by the laundry room door. Once she was outside, the transponder in her purse unlocked the car's door. 'Don't you even think about scratching this leather,' she said as she set the cat on the passenger seat. It was Sunday night and the animal shelter was closed. So dropping off the cat was not an option. If she drove to the other side of the lake and dumped it on a doorstep over there, the damn thing would not be able to find its way back.

She hit the start button on the gearshift. She wasn't totally heartless. She wouldn't dump it somewhere with a big pit bull chained in the yard. She didn't want that kind of karma.

She put the car into reverse and glanced over at the kitten sitting on her expensive leather seat and staring straight ahead. '*Hasta la vista*, baby.'

'Meow.'

★ ★ ★

Mick drove his Dodge into the parking lot of the D-Lite Grocery Store and parked in a slot a few rows from the front doors. Pulling in, he'd seen the black Mercedes parked beneath one of the lot's bright lights. Although he'd never personally seen the car, everyone in town knew Madeline Dupree drove a black Mercedes like Batman. Within the slightly tinted windows, Mick could just see the outline of her head and face. He walked to the car and knocked on the driver's-side window. Without a sound, the glass lowered inch by inch. The parking lot light shone into the window and suddenly he was staring into the dark brown eyes of the woman who'd wrung him out the night before.

'Nice car,' he said.

'Thanks.'

'Meow.'

He looked down past her face to a white ball of fur in her lap. 'Why, Maddie, you have a pussycat on your — '

'Don't say it.'

He laughed. 'When did you get a cat?'

'It's not mine. I hate cats.'

'Then why's it on your . . . lap?'

'It wouldn't go away.' She turned and looked ahead; her hands gripped the steering wheel. 'I tried to find it a home across the lake. I even had a house all picked out. A nice one with yellow shutters.'

'What happened?'

She shook her head. 'I don't know. I was sneaking up to the porch, ready to toss the cat up there and run, but the damn thing purred and rubbed its head on my chin.' She looked up at him as a frown settled between her brows. 'And here I am, thinking about all the cat food commercials on TV and wondering if I should buy Whiskas or Fancy Feast.'

He chuckled. 'What's its name?'

She closed her eyes and whispered, 'Snowball.'

His chuckle turned to laughter, and she opened her eyes and glared at him. 'What?'

'Snowball?'

'It's white.'

'Meow.'

'It's so girly.'

'This from a guy who named his poodle Princess.'

His laughter died. 'How do you know about Princess?'

Maddie opened her car door and he stepped back. 'Your sister told me.' She rolled up the window, grabbed the kitten with her free hand, and got out of the car. 'And before you get all bossy, your sister showed up on my porch this afternoon and wanted to talk to me about your parents.'

'What did she say?'

'A lot.' She locked the door and shut it. 'Mostly, though, I think she wanted *me* to think that growing up you were all happy as clams until Alice Jones moved to town.'

'Do you believe her?'

'Of course not.' She shoved the kitten inside her jean jacket and hung a big purse over one shoulder. The same big purse that carried her Taser. 'Especially when she let it slip that your mother set a pile of your father's clothes on fire.'

'Yeah. I remember that.' It was certainly no secret. 'I remember the grass in the front yard didn't grow back for a long time.' He'd probably been five at the time. A year before his mother had completely lost it.

'And in case you've heard the rumor, no, there is not going to be a movie starring Colin Farrell and Angelina Jolie.'

He'd heard the rumor and was relieved to hear it wasn't true. 'Are you wearing your pajamas?'

The kitten poked its head out of her jacket as Maddie looked down. 'I don't think anyone will notice.'

'I noticed.'

'Yeah, but I was wearing pajama pants like this last night.' She looked up and a sexy little smile teased the corners of her lips. 'For a little while anyway.'

And she didn't think they were going to have sex again. Right. 'Is that you?' he asked.

'Is what me?'

'I smell Rice Krispies treats.' He took a step toward her and dipped his head. 'Of course it's you.'

'That's my Marshmallow Fluff body butter.'

'Body butter?' Oh, God. Did she really think they wouldn't end up in bed together again? 'I've thought about you all day.' He put his hand on the side of her throat and pressed his forehead to hers. 'Come home with me.' Beneath his thumb, her pulse pounded through her veins almost as hard as his beat through his body.

'I'm back on the wagon.'

'You're back to being sort of, kind of, celibate?'

'Yes.'

'I can change your mind.' He was trying to convince a woman to go home with him, something he didn't normally do. Either they wanted to or they didn't.

'Not this time,' she said, although she didn't sound particularly convinced.

But when it came to Maddie, nothing was normal. 'You love the way I kiss and touch your body. Remember?'

'I, ahh . . . ' she stammered.

Normally he didn't think and obsess about a woman all day. He didn't wonder what she was doing. If she was working or finding dead mice or how he was going to get her naked again. 'You're already dressed for bed.' He brushed his mouth across hers and her lips parted on a little gasp. Normally he didn't waste his time because there were others he didn't have to try and convince. 'You know you want to.'

'Meow.'

She took a step back and his hand dropped to his side. 'I have to buy cat food.'

Mick lowered his gaze to the white furry head poking out of Maddie's jean jacket. That cat was pure evil.

'Good girl, Snowball,' she said and patted her kitten's head. She looked up at him, then turned toward the front of the store. 'Watch out for him. He's a very bad man.'

13

The little collar had pink sparkles and a tiny pink bell and when Maddie had walked to the road to check her mail at around three, she'd found it in her mailbox. No note. No card. Just the collar.

Mick was the only other person who knew about Snowball. She hadn't told any of her friends for fear they'd all die of shock. Maddie Jones — cat owner? Impossible. She'd spent most of her life hating cats, but here she stood, pink collar in hand and staring down at a white ball of fur curled up in her office chair.

She scooped the kitten up in both hands and brought it face level. 'This is my chair,' she said. 'I made you a bed.' She carried the kitten to the laundry room and set her on a folded towel inside an Amazon box. 'Rule number one: I'm the boss. Number two: you can't get on my furniture and get it all hairy.' She knelt down and placed the collar around Snowball's neck.

'Meow.'

Maddie scowled.

'Meow.'

'Fine. You look cute.' She stood and pointed a finger in the kitten's direction. 'Rule number three: I let you in and gave you some food. That's where it ends. I don't like cats.' She turned on her heel and walked out of the laundry room. The tinkling of a bell followed her into the kitchen and she looked down at her feet. She sighed and pulled a local telephone book out of a drawer. She turned to the yellow pages, reached for her cell phone, and punched in the seven numbers.

'Mort's,' a man answered, but it wasn't Mick.

'Is Mick available?'

'He usually doesn't show up until eight.'

'Could you give him a message for me?'

'Let me grab a pen.' There was a pause and then, 'Okay.'

'Mick, thanks for the pink collar. Snowball.'

'Did you say 'Snowball'?'

'Yeah. Sign it 'Snowball'.'

'Got it.'

'Thanks.' Maddie disconnected and closed the phone book. At ten minutes after eight while Maddie glanced through a crime magazine, her phone rang.

'Hello.'

'Your cat called me.'

Just the sound of Mick's voice made her smile, which was a very bad sign. 'What did she want?'

'To thank me for her collar.'

Maddie glanced at Snowball lying in the red chair, licking her leg and in flagrant disregard of rule number two. 'She has good manners.'

'What are you doing tonight?'

'Teaching Snowball which fork to use.'

He chuckled. 'When is she going to bed?'

She flipped a page in the magazine and her gaze scanned an article about a man who'd killed three of his trophy wives. 'Why?'

'I want to see you.'

She wanted to see him too. Bad. And that was the problem. She didn't *want* to feel all happy inside just at the sound of his voice on her telephone. She didn't *want* to see him in a parking lot and remember the touch of his hands and mouth. The more she saw him, thought about him, wanted him, the more their lives became entangled. 'You know I can't,' she said and flipped a few more pages.

'Meet me at Hennessy's and bring your camera.'

Her hand stilled. 'Are you offering to let me take photos inside your bar?'

'Yes.'

She didn't usually take the photos for her

books, but there wouldn't be a problem if she did.

'I want to see you.'

'Are you bribing me?'

There was a pause on the line and then he asked, 'Is that a problem?'

Was it? 'Only if you think I'll have sex with you for a few photos.'

'Honey,' he said through what sounded like a sigh of exasperation, 'I wish getting you naked was that easy, but no.'

Just because she went to Hennessy's and took some photographs didn't mean anyone was going to end up naked. She'd lived without sex for four years. Clearly she did have some self-control.

'Why don't you come here around midnight? The place will be cleared out and you can take as many pictures as you want.'

If she went, she'd be using the undeniable attraction between them to get what she wanted. Just as he was using her desire to photograph the inside of the bar to get what he wanted. She wondered if her conscience should rise up and decline the tempting offer, but as had happened from time to time in her life when it came to her work and her scruples, her conscience was silent.

'I'll be there.' After she hung up the phone, she took a deep breath and held it in.

Entering that bar would not be the same as every other crime scene she'd walked and explored and stood within. This was personal.

She let out her pent-up breath. She'd viewed the crime scene photos and read the reports. Twenty-nine years after the fact would not be a problem. She'd sat across a mesh barrier from killers who told her exactly what they'd do to her body if they ever got the chance. Compared to that nightmare, walking into Hennessy's was going to be a piece of cake. No sweat.

★　★　★

Hennessy's was painted a nondescript gray and was bigger than it looked from the outside. Inside it had two pool tables and a dance floor on either side of the long bar. In the middle, three steps led down to the sunken floor surrounded by a white railing and fitted with ten round tables. Hennessy's had never had the unruly-girls-gone-bad reputation of Mort's. It was more laid-back and was known for good drinks and music. And for a time, murder. Hennessy's had finally lived down the latter — until a certain true crime writer had blown into town.

Mick stood behind the bar and poured South Gin into a cocktail shaker. He glanced up at Maddie, at the light shining in her hair, picking out reddish gold strands in her ponytail. He returned his gaze to the tall clear bottle in his hand. 'My great-grandfather built this bar in 1925.'

Maddie set her camera on the bar and glanced about her. 'During Prohibition?'

'Yeah.' He pointed to the sunken middle. 'That part was a restaurant dining room,' he said. 'He made and sold grain alcohol out of the back.'

Maddie looked at him through those big brown eyes that turned all warm and sexy when he kissed her neck. At the moment her eyes were a little wide, like she was seeing ghosts. 'Was he ever caught?' she asked but looked about once again, her mind clearly not on his masterful attempt at conversation. When he'd opened the back door and seen her standing there, she'd looked so tense, he'd had to check his first impulse to push her against the wall and kiss the breath out of her.

'Nah.' Mick shook his head. They both knew she was there to take photographs, and Mick was surprised at how uptight she was about being inside the bar. He thought she'd be happy. He was giving her what she wanted, but she didn't look happy. She looked ready to break. 'The town was too small and unimportant in those days, and Great-Grandfather was too well liked by everyone. When Prohibition ended, he gutted most of the place and turned it into a bar. Except for maintenance and a few necessary renovations, it's been like this since.' He added a splash of vermouth, then put the lid on the cocktail shaker. 'My grandfather turned the area over there into a dance floor and my father brought in the pool tables.' He shook the premium gin and vermouth with one hand and reached below the bar with the other. 'I've decided to leave it as is.' He set first one and then another frosted martini glass on the bar. He added a few olives on toothpicks, and as he poured, his gaze lowered from the firm set of her jaw down her throat to her white blouse and the top button that looked perilously close to popping open and giving him a great view of her cleavage. 'I've put my money and energy into Mort's. Next week my buddy Steve and I have a meeting with a couple of investors to talk about starting a business giving helicopter tours in the area. Who knows if it will pan out? Owning bars is what I know, but I really want to branch out and have other interests. That way I don't feel as if I'm standing still.' He pushed the martini glass toward her and wondered if she was even listening to him.

Her fingers touched the stem. 'Why do you feel as if you're standing still?'

He guessed she had been listening. 'I don't know. Maybe because as a kid I couldn't wait to get the hell out of here.' He reached for the toothpick in his martini and bit an olive off the end. 'But here I am.'

'Your family is here. I don't have family — well, except for a few cousins I've met briefly. If I had a brother or sister, I'd want to live by them. At least I hope I would.'

He recalled that her mother had died when she'd been young. 'Where's your father?'

'I don't know. I never met him.' She stirred her martini with the olives. 'How do you know what I drink?'

He wondered if she'd purposely changed the subject. 'I know all your secrets.' She looked a bit alarmed and he laughed. 'I remember what you were drinking the first night I saw you.' He walked around the end of the bar and sat next to her. She turned to face him and he planted one of his feet between hers on the rungs of her stool. She wore a black skirt and his knee forced the material up her smooth thighs.

'Really?' She picked up the drink and gazed at him over the top of the glass. She drained half of her drink. Sucking down his best gin as if it were water, and if she wasn't careful, he'd have to drive her home. Which wasn't a bad idea. 'I'm surprised you remember anything beyond Darla's tempting offer to show you her bare bottom,' she said and licked her bottom lip.

'I remember you were being a smart-ass that night too.' He took her hand and brushed his thumb across the backs of her knuckles. 'I wondered what it would be like to kiss your smart mouth.'

'Now you know.'

'Yes.' He moved his gaze across her face, her cheeks, and jaw and wet lips. He looked back up into her eyes. 'Now that I know, I think about all the places I didn't get to kiss you the other night.'

She set her glass on the bar. 'Lord, you're good.'

'I'm good at a lot of things.'

'Especially at saying just the right thing to make a woman feel like you really mean it.'

He dropped her hand. 'You don't think I mean it?'

She grabbed her camera and spun around on her stool. Mick moved his foot and she stood. 'I'm sure you do mean it.' She turned her back on him and raised her camera. 'Every time you say it and to every woman you say it to.'

Mick picked up his glass and also stood.

'You think I've said that to other women?'

She adjusted the focus and snapped a picture of the empty tables. The strobe flashed and she said, 'Of course.'

That stung, especially since it wasn't true. 'Well, honey, you don't give yourself enough credit.'

'I give myself a lot of credit.' Another click and flash, then she said, 'But I know how things are.'

He took a drink and the cool gin warmed a path down his throat and settled next to a spot of irritation. 'Tell me what you think you know.'

'I know I'm not the only woman you spend time with.' She lowered her camera and moved to one end of the bar.

'You're the only woman I'm seeing right now.'

'Right now. You'll move on. I'm sure we're all interchangeable.'

Mick walked away as the strobe flashed. 'I didn't think you had a problem with that.' He moved into the dark shadows and leaned a hip into the jukebox.

'I don't. I'm just saying that I'm sure we're all the same in the dark.'

She was really starting to piss him off, but he had a feeling that was her point. He wondered why the hell he'd wanted to see her so damn bad. She believed the gossip about him, and he wondered why he cared. She didn't mind if he saw other women, and he wondered why that bothered him. Maybe he should. Maybe he should kick her ass out and call someone else. The problem was he didn't want to call someone else, and that ticked him off almost as much as her attitude.

She took several photos of the floor in front of the bar from different angles, then he said, 'You're wrong about that. Not all pussy is the same in the dark.'

She glanced over at him. He'd meant to offend her, but typical of Maddie, she didn't act like other women. Instead, she took a deep breath and let it out slowly. 'Are you trying to make me mad?'

'It seems fair. You're trying to make me mad.'

She thought a moment and then confessed, 'You're right.'

'Why?'

'Maybe because I don't want to think about what I'm doing.' She moved to the end of the bar and looked at the no-skid mats on the floor. She snapped a few photos, then lowered her camera. Just above a whisper, barely loud enough for him to hear, she said, 'This is harder than I thought it would be.'

He straightened.

'It's the same bar and mirrors and lighting and old cash register.' She set the camera down and grasped the end of the bar. 'The only things that are different are the blood and the bodies.'

Mick walked toward her and set his glass on the railing as he passed it.

There was a catch in her voice when she said, 'She died here. How can you stand it?'

He placed his hands on her shoulders. 'I don't think about it anymore.'

She turned and looked up at him, her eyes wide and stricken. 'How is that possible? Your mother killed your father right at the top of the stairs.'

'It's just a place. Four walls and roof.' He slid his hands down her arms and back up again. 'It happened a long time ago. Like I said, I don't think about it.'

'I do.' She bit her lip and turned her head away to wipe at her eyes.

Mick had never met a writer before Maddie, but it did seem to him as if she were awfully emotional for a woman writing a book about people she didn't even know.

'This has just been so much harder than I thought it was going to be. I don't take my own photos for the books, and I thought I could do this.'

Maybe she had to immerse herself in the

details and feel them in order to write about them. Hell, what did he know? He didn't even read books that often.

She looked up at him. 'I have to go.' She grabbed her camera off the bar and walked around him. On her way out, she picked up her jacket and purse off one of the stools where she'd set them earlier.

This evening had turned to shit and he did not know why. He didn't know what he'd done or hadn't done. He'd thought she'd take a few photos. They'd have a drink, talk, and, yeah, hopefully get naked. He followed Maddie through the back and out into the alley.

'Are you going to be okay to drive?' he asked as he stepped from the back door.

She stood just inside the pool of light and fumbled to shove her arms into the sleeves of her jacket. She nodded, and her purse dropped to the ground by her foot. Instead of picking it up, she covered her face with her hands.

'Why don't I take you home?' He moved toward her, then bent down and picked up her purse. He'd been raised by females, but he did not understand Maddie Dupree. 'You're too upset to drive.'

She looked up at him through liquid eyes as a tear spilled over her bottom lashes.

'Mick, I have to tell you something about me. Something I should have told you weeks ago.'

He didn't like the sound of that. 'You're married.' He put her bag on the hood of her car and waited.

She shook her head. 'I . . . I'm . . . ' She let out a breath and brushed the tears from her cheeks. 'I'm not . . . I'm afraid . . . I can't . . . ' She wrapped her arms around his neck and glued her body to his. 'I can't get the crime scene photos out of my head.'

That was it? That's why she was so upset? He didn't know what to say. What to do. He felt helpless and he slid his hands around her sides and held her. The skin across his abdomen got tight, and he knew what he'd like to do. He figured it was a good thing she couldn't read his mind, but it was her fault, really. She shouldn't have pressed into him and clung to his neck.

'Mick?'

'Hmm?' Tonight she smelled like vanilla again and he ran his hands up and down her back. Holding her was almost as good as sex.

'How many condoms do you have on you?'

His hand stilled. He'd bought a box of Trojans yesterday. 'I have twelve in the truck.'

'That ought to be enough.'

He pulled back to look into her face, her profile lit by the light at the back of

Hennessy's. 'I don't understand you, Maddie Dupree.'

'Lately, I don't understand myself.' She ran her fingers through his hair and brought his mouth down to hers. 'And where you're concerned, I just can't seem to do the right thing.'

★   ★   ★

Late the next morning, Maddie stood in her kitchen and raised a steaming cup of coffee to her lips. She wore her white bathrobe and her wet hair was slicked back from her shower. Last night she'd almost told Mick that Alice Jones was her mother. She should have told him, but each time she opened her mouth, she couldn't say the words. She hadn't been afraid to tell him. She wasn't afraid of anything, but for some reason, she just couldn't tell him. Maybe the timing was off. Another time would be better.

More than anything, she'd needed him to help clear her head of the horrible images. She'd been to her mother's grave and she hadn't fallen apart. But standing in the exact spot where her mother had died, she'd felt like someone had reached inside her chest and ripped out her heart. Perhaps if she hadn't seen the photos of her mother's blood and her blond hair stained a dark brown. Perhaps her world wouldn't have flipped upside down and she wouldn't have gotten so emotional.

She hated getting emotional, especially in front of other people. Most specifically in front of Mick, but he'd been there and seen it and she'd needed someone to hold on to and focus on when everything seemed so unbalanced.

He'd followed her home and she'd taken his hand and led him into the bedroom. He'd kissed her in all those places he'd said he'd been thinking about. He set every nerve ending in her body on fire, and she knew she should feel bad about being with him again. It was wrong of her, but being with him felt too good to feel really bad.

'Meow.'

Snowball wove a figure eight between her feet and she looked down at her cat. How had her life come to this? She had a cat in her house and a Hennessy in her bed.

She set her cup on the counter and moved to the pantry to grab a bag of kitten food. A dead mouse lay on the floor and Snowball sniffed its tail. 'Don't eat that or you'll get sick.' She grabbed Snowball and carried her into the laundry room. Snowball purred and butted her head against Maddie's chin. 'And

I know for a fact you did not sleep in your bed. I found white fur on my office chair.' She set the kitten in her Amazon box and poured food onto a little dish. 'I do not want to walk around with white fur on my butt.' Snowball jumped out of her box and attacked her food as if she hadn't eaten in a week. Last night as Mick had walked from the bathroom, a smug, satisfied smile tilting one corner of his lips, the kitten had stalked him across the carpet and attacked his leg.

'What the hell?' he'd yelped and danced around as Snowball had dashed back under the bed. 'I can't believe I wasted money buying that damn thing a collar.'

Maddie had laughed and patted the bed next to her. 'Come here so I can make you feel better after the big bad cat attack.'

He'd moved to the bed and pulled her up so she knelt before him. 'I'm going to make you pay for laughing at me.' And he had. All night long, and when she'd woke this morning, she was alone. Again. She would have liked to have woken and seen his face, his blue eyes looking at her, all sleepy and sated, but it was better this way. Better to keep a distance even though they'd shared a night as physically close as two people could possibly get.

While Snowball chowed, Maddie picked up

the mouse with a paper towel and carried it to the garbage outside. She called a local veterinarian and made Snowball an appointment for the first week in August. Her low-carb granola bars had teeth marks on the outside of the box, but the bars looked okay. As she took a bite, her doorbell rang.

Through the peephole she gazed at Mick, standing on her porch, looking showered and shaved and relaxed in a pair of Levi's and an untucked striped shirt over a wife beater. She ignored the little tumble in her stomach and opened the door.

'How'd you sleep?' he asked as a knowing little smile brought out his dimples.

She opened the door wide and he stepped inside. 'I think it was around three when I finally passed out.'

'It was three-thirty.' He walked past her and she shut the door behind him. 'Where's your cat?' he asked as they moved into the living room.

'Eating breakfast. Are you scared of a little kitty?'

'Of that Tasmanian furball?' He made a rude scoffing sound and pulled a little stuffed mouse from the front pocket of his jeans. 'I got her some catnip to mellow her out.' He tossed it on the coffee table. 'What are your plans?'

She planned to work. 'Why?'

'I thought we could drive to Redfish Lake and get a bite to eat.'

'Like in a date?'

'Sure.' He reached for the terrycloth belt and pulled her toward him. 'Why not?'

Because they weren't dating. They shouldn't even be having sex. Dating couldn't happen no matter how her stomach tumbled or her skin tingled.

'I'm hungry and I thought you might be hungry too.' He dipped his head and kissed the side of her neck.

She moved her head to one side. She did have to eat, though. 'Why Redfish Lake?'

'Because they have a good restaurant in the lodge there, and I want to spend the whole day with you.' He kissed the side of her throat. 'Say yes.'

'I'll need to get dressed.' She pulled her belt from his grasp and turned away. As she entered her bedroom she called out, 'How far is Redfish Lake?'

'About an hour and a half,' he answered from the doorway.

She hadn't expected him to follow her and she looked over at him as she grabbed a pair of underwear from a drawer. He leaned against the doorframe, and his eyes watched her, moving with her hands as she pulled up a pair of pink silky panties. His gaze felt very intimate. More intimate than when he kissed the insides of her thighs and his eyes turned that certain sexy blue. Intimate like they were a couple and it was normal for him to watch her dress. Like this relationship was more than it really was and more than he was ever going to be. As if there were a chance at tomorrows and the day afters. She raised her brows up her forehead. 'Do you mind?'

'You're not going to get all modest, are you? Not after last night.' She continued to stare at him until he sighed and pushed away from the doorframe. 'All right. I'll go get your cat stoned.'

She watched him leave and tried not to think about tomorrow or the days after and things that could never be. She dressed quickly in a pink cotton sundress. She pulled her hair back in a claw and gazed in the mirror as she put on a little mascara and lip gloss.

In the harsh light of day, with her sexual desire sated and her emotions tightly under control, she knew she had to tell him she was Madeline Jones. He deserved to know.

The thought of telling him cramped her stomach and she wondered if he really had to be told at all. Last night she might not have been real tactful when she'd brought up other women. She'd obviously made him mad, but the fact was, Mick Hennessy was no more a one-woman man than his father had been. Or his grandfather. Even if he wasn't seeing anyone else right now, he would get tired of Maddie. He'd move on sooner or later, so why tell him today?

If anything, she should clear up her mortifying outburst last night. She wasn't a woman who got all weepy and cried on a man's neck. Perhaps she hadn't broken down like some women were apt to do, but for her, it was a loss of control that embarrassed her. Even twelve hours later.

A half hour into their drive to Redfish, she decided to clear it up. 'Sorry about last night,' she said above the country music filling the cab of Mick's truck.

'You don't have anything to be sorry about. You got a little loud, but I like that about you.' He grinned and glanced at her through the lenses of his blue mirrored sunglasses before returning his gaze to the road. 'Sometimes I don't always understand everything you say, but you sound real sexy while you're saying it.'

Somehow she suspected they weren't talking about the same thing. 'I was talking about getting all emotional at Hennessy's.'

'Oh.' His thumb tapped against the

steering wheel, keeping time to a song about a woman liking chrome. 'Don't worry about it.'

She wished she could take his advice, but it wasn't that easy for her. 'There are just certain girls I've never wanted to be. One of them is the emotional girl who cries all the time.'

'I don't think you're an emotional girl.' Air from the vents touched the dark hair about his forehead. 'What are the other girls?'

'What?'

'You said there are girls you never wanted to be.' Without taking his eyes from the road, he turned off the CD player and spoke into the suddenly silent cab. 'One is the emotional girl. What are the others?'

'Oh.' She counted them off on her fingers. 'I don't ever want to be the stupid girl. Nor the get-drunk-and-slutty girl. The stalker girl or the butt girl.'

His looked over at her. 'The butt girl?'

'Don't make me explain it to you.'

He returned his gaze to the road and smiled. 'Then you're not talking about a girl with a big butt.'

'No.'

'Oh, so I guess I don't ever . . . '

'Forget it.'

He laughed. 'Some women say they like it.'

'Uh-huh. Some women say they like to be paddled, but I'll never know the pleasure of either.'

Mick reached across the center console and took her hand. 'What about being tied to a bed?'

She shrugged. 'I kind of like that.'

He brought her hand to his mouth and smiled against her skin. 'I guess I know what we're doing after I get off work.'

Maddie laughed and turned her attention to the scenery. To the pines and thick brush and the South Fork of the Payette River. Idaho might grow famous potatoes, but it also had spectacular wilderness areas.

At the lodge, they sat at a table that looked out at the blue-green water of Redfish Lake and at the snow-covered peaks of the Sawtooth Mountains. They ate lunch and talked about the people in Truly. She told him about her friends, and about Lucy's wedding last year and Clare's impending nuptials. They talked about everything from the weather to world events, sports to the latest West Nile virus outbreaks.

They talked about almost everything but the reason she moved to Truly. By tacit agreement they avoided talking about the book she was writing and about the night his mother had killed two people and then herself.

The day was relaxing and fun and during those rare moments when Maddie looked into his blue eyes and her conscience reminded her that he would not be with her if he knew who she really was, she shoved it down and ignored it. She turned a deaf ear, and by the ride home, she'd buried her conscience so deep, it was just a faint whisper that was easily ignored.

14

After he got off work that night, Mick showed up on Maddie's doorstep with silk neckties in one hand and another catnip mouse in the other. While he tied Maddie's wrists, Snowball batted the mouse around, then once again flagrantly disregarded the rules and passed out in Maddie's office chair. Disregarding the rules was becoming a bad habit for Snowball. Just as Mick Hennessy was becoming a habit for Maddie. A habit she was eventually going to have to break, but there was a problem. Maddie liked spending time with him. In and out of bed, and that created another problem. She wasn't getting a lot of work done. She hadn't finished her notes or completed the timeline, and she really needed to do that before she sat down to write Chapter Two. She needed to remember why she was in Truly and get to work. No more dropping everything to have a good time with Mick, but when he called the next night and asked her to meet him at Mort's after he closed for the night, she didn't think twice. At twelve-thirty, she knocked on the back door wearing a red trench coat, four-inch pumps, and one of Mick's blue neckties nestled between her bare breasts.

'Like the tie,' Mick said as he opened her coat.

'I thought I'd return it.'

He put his hands on her bare waist and brought her against his chest. 'There's something about you, Maddie,' he said as he looked into her eyes. 'Something more than the way you make love. Something that makes me think about you when I'm pouring drinks or watching Travis strike out in T-ball.'

She put her arms around his neck and her nipples brushed the front of his polo shirt. Against her pelvis, he was enormous and ready. This was the part where she should tell him that she thought about him too, but she couldn't. Not because it wasn't true. It was true, but it was best to keep things platonic until he moved on.

Instead of talking, she brought his mouth down to hers and her hand slid to the front of his pants. What had started as a one-night stand had turned into more nights. He wanted to see more of her. She wanted to see more of him, but it wasn't love. She did not love Mick, but she liked him a whole lot. Especially when he laid her on his bar and, between the bottles of alcohol, she caught glimpses in the mirror of his long hard body moving, driving, pushing her toward a release that curled her toes inside her pumps.

It was sex. Just sex. Ironically, the kind of relationship she'd waited four years to find. Nothing more, and if she were to ever forget that fact, she had only to remind herself that while she knew his body intimately, she didn't even know his home phone number or where he lived. Mick might say that there was something about her, but whatever that something was, it wasn't enough to want her in his life.

★   ★   ★

The morning of Snowball's vet appointment, Maddie packed up her kitten and drove into town. August was the hottest month of summer, and the weatherman predicted that the valley would heat up to a scorching ninety-three degrees.

Maddie sat in an examination room and watched as veterinarian John Tannasee checked out her kitten. John was a tall man with hard muscles beneath his lab coat and a Tom Selleck moustache. His voice was so deep it sounded as if it came from his feet. He gently looked in Snowball's ears and then checked her bottom, determining that Snowball was indeed a girl.

He took her temperature and gave her a clean bill of health.

'Her heterochromia doesn't appear to affect her vision.' He scratched her between the ears and pointed out her other genetic defect. 'And her malocclusion isn't so bad that it will affect her eating.'

Maddie understood what he'd meant by heterochromia, but, 'Malocclusion?'

'Your cat has an overbite.'

Maddie had never heard of such a thing in a cat and didn't quite believe it until he tipped the kitten's head back and showed her Snowball's upper jaw was a bit longer than the bottom. For some strange reason, the kitten's oral affliction made Maddie kind of like Snowball.

'She's bucktoothed,' Maddie said in astonishment. 'She's a hillbilly.' She made a follow-up appointment to get Snowball spayed so that she couldn't produce any more big-headed hillbilly cats, then she and Snowball drove to the grocery store.

'Behave,' she warned her kitten as she pulling into the D-Lite Grocery Store's parking lot.

'Meow.'

'Behave and maybe I'll get some Whisker Lickin's.' She groaned as she got out of the car and locked the door. Had she just said

Whisker Lickin's? She was embarrassed for herself. As she moved across the parking lot, she wondered if she was destined to become one of those women who doted on their cats and told boring cat stories to people who didn't give a flying crap.

Once inside the grocery store, she loaded up on chicken breasts, salad, and Diet Coke. She couldn't find Whisker Lickin's, so she tossed in Pounce Caribbean Catch. She wheeled her cart to the front of the store and register five. A clerk by the name of Francine scanned the Pounce while Maddie dug around in her purse.

'How old's your cat?'

Maddie looked up and into Francine's long face surrounded by eighties *Flashdance* hair.

'I'm not sure. She just showed up on my deck and wouldn't go away. I think she's inbred.'

'Yep. That happens around here a lot.'

Francine's eyes were slightly googly and Maddie wondered if she was talking about the cat or herself.

'I heard there's a second suspect in your book,' Francine said as she scanned the chicken breasts.

'Pardon?'

'I heard you found a second suspect. That maybe Rose didn't shoot Loch and the waitress and then herself. That maybe someone else came in and killed all three of them.'

'I don't know where you heard that, but let me assure you it isn't true. There is no other suspect. Rose shot Loch and Alice Jones, then turned the gun on herself.'

'Oh.' Francine looked a bit disappointed, but that could have been her uneven eyes. 'Then I guess the sheriff isn't going to reopen the investigation and call that *Cold Case* show.'

'No. There isn't a second suspect. No *Cold Case* show, no movie deal, and Colin Farrell isn't coming to town.'

'I heard it was Brad Pitt.' She scanned the last item and hit total.

'Good Lord.' Maddie handed over the exact cash and grabbed her groceries. 'Brad Pitt,' she scoffed as she put the bags in the backseat.

When she got home, she fed Snowball brightly colored shaped fish and cooked herself lunch. She worked on the timeline for the book, writing down events as they unfolded minute by minute, moving them around, and tacking them to the wall behind her computer screen.

At ten that evening, Mick called and asked her to meet him at Mort's. Her first instinct was to say she would. It was Friday night and she wouldn't mind getting out, but something held her back. And that something had everything to do with the way her stomach got light at the sound of his voice.

'I'm not feeling well,' she lied. She needed to put some time and distance between them. A little breathing room. A break from what she feared was becoming more than casual sex. At least for her.

In the background she could hear the muffled sound of the jukebox competing with several dozen raised voices. 'Are you going to be okay?'

'Yeah, I'm just going to bed.'

'I could come by later and check up on you. We don't have to do anything. I could just bring you soup or some aspirin.'

She'd like that. 'No, but thank you.'

'I'll call you around noon tomorrow to check up on you,' he said, but he didn't. Instead he showed up at her boat dock, wearing a white Cerveza Pacifico T-shirt, a pair of navy blue swim trunks that hung low on his hips, and driving a twenty-one-foot Regal.

'How're you feeling?' he asked as he stepped into her house through the French doors.

He removed his sunglasses and she gazed

up into his handsome face. 'About what?'

'You were sick last night.'

'Oh.' She'd forgotten. 'It was nothing. I'm over it now.'

'Good.' He gathered her up against his chest and kissed her hairline. 'Change into your swimsuit and come with me.'

She didn't ask where they were going or how long she'd be gone. As long as she was with Mick, she didn't care. She pulled on her one-piece swimsuit and tied a blue wrap with red sea horses around her hips.

'Aren't you getting tired of me yet?' she asked him as they walked toward his yellow and white boat.

His brows lowered and he looked at her as if the thought hadn't entered his head. 'No. Not yet.'

Mick gave her a tour of the lake and some of the truly spectacular cabins that could not be seen from the road. He handed Maddie a Diet Coke from the cooler and pulled out a bottle of water for himself.

Set in the cloudless August sky, the relentless sun warmed Maddie's skin. At first it felt nice, but after an hour, trickles of sweat slid between her breasts and down the back of her neck. Maddie hated to sweat. It was one of the reasons she didn't exercise. That and she didn't believe in 'no pain, no gain'.

She was a believer in 'no pain is a good thing'.

Mick dropped anchor in Angel Cove and shucked his white T-shirt. 'Before the Allegrezza boys developed this area, we used to come here to swim every summer. My mom would bring us here and later Meg or I would drive.' He stood in the middle of the boat and looked out at the sandy shoreline, now dotted with big homes and docks filled with boats and Jet Skis. 'I remember lots of bikinis and baby oil. Sand in my shorts and my nose peeling like crazy.' He kicked off his flip-flops and moved to the back. 'Those were some good times.'

Maddie dropped the wrap from her hips and followed him. They stood side by side on the swimming platform. 'Sand in your shorts doesn't sound like a good time.'

He laughed. 'No, but Vicky Baley used to come up out of the water in a string bikini that kind of slid around, and she had this amazing rack that — '

Maddie shoved him and as he teetered, he grabbed her wrist and they both went into the lake. He surfaced with a loud, 'Whaaaa, that's cold,' while Maddie surfaced, trying to catch her breath. The icy water stole the air from her lungs and Maddie grabbed on to the ladder at the back of the boat.

Mick's quiet laugher skimmed along the

rippled surface as he swam toward her.

She pushed her wet hair from her eyes. 'What's so funny?'

'You, getting all jealous over Vicky Baley.'

'I'm not jealous.'

'Uh-huh.' He grabbed the edge of the swimming platform and said, 'Her rack isn't as good as yours.'

'Gee, thanks.'

Droplets of water fell from a strand of hair touching his forehead and ran down his cheek. 'You have no reason to be jealous of anyone. Your body is beautiful.'

'You don't have to say that. My breasts aren't — '

He placed a finger on her lips. 'Don't do that. Don't dismiss what I feel as if I'm just saying something to get into your pants. I'm not. I've already been in your pants and you're amazing.' He placed his free hand behind her head and gave her a kiss that was all hot mouths and cool lips, drips of water and smooth gliding tongues.

When he kissed her like that, she felt amazing.

'I missed you last night,' he said as he pulled back. 'I wish I didn't have to work late tonight, but I do.'

She licked the taste of him from her lips and swallowed. 'I understand.'

'I know you do. I think that's why I like you so much.' He smiled at her. A simple little curve of his mouth that felt anything but simple. It pinched her chest and stole her breath and she knew she was in trouble. Big bad trouble, with a way of saying things that made her feel like she was drowning in his beautiful blue eyes. She dunked herself under and came up with her head tilted back and her hair out of her face. 'We both work inconvenient hours,' she said and climbed up the ladder. She stood on the back of the boat and squeezed water from her hair. 'But it works for us because we're nocturnal and can sleep late.'

'And because you want me.' He climbed out of the water.

She looked at him out of the corners of her eyes. At his hard chest muscles and the line of wet, dark hair trailing down his abdomen and belly and disappearing beneath the waistband of his swimming trunks. 'True.'

'And Lord knows I want you too.' He pulled up the anchor and put it in a side compartment. Then he moved to the captain's chair and looked over at her while she tied her sarong around her hips.

'What?'

He shook his head and started the motor, a deep throaty churning of the prop. The boat rocked from side to side and Maddie took the companion seat. For several more seconds, Mick gazed at her before he finally looked away and pushed the throttle forward.

Maddie held her hair with one hand as they shot across the lake. Conversation was impossible, but she wouldn't have known what to say. Mick's behavior was a little odd. She'd thought she knew how to read most of his expressions. She knew how he looked when he was angry, when he was teasing and charming, and she certainly knew how he looked when he wanted sex. He was oddly quiet, as if he were thinking about something, and didn't say much until they stood on her deck twenty minutes later.

'If I didn't have to go to work tonight, I'd stay here and play with you,' he said.

'You can come back later.'

He sat in an Adirondack chair facing her and pulled the sarong from her hips. It fluttered to her feet. 'Or you could come over tonight when I get off work.' He placed his hands on the backs of her thighs and brought her between his knees.

'To Mort's?'

He shook his head and nibbled the side of her leg. 'Throw some stuff in a bag and come over to my house. I know you like to fall asleep and have me gone in the morning, but

I think we've moved beyond pretending this is nothing more than sex. Don't you?'

Did she? It couldn't be more. It could never be more. She closed her eyes and ran her fingers through his hair. 'Yes.'

He softly bit the outside of her thigh. 'I should probably pick you up so you don't have to drive at night.'

This was bad. Wrong, but it felt so good. So right. 'I can drive.'

'I know you can, but I'll pick you up.'

From somewhere behind Maddie, a little voice asked, 'What are you doing?'

Mick lifted his head and froze. 'Travis.' He dropped his hands and stood. 'Hey, buddy. What's up?'

'Nothin'. What were you doing?'

Maddie turned to see Mick's nephew standing on the top stair of the deck.

'I was just helping Maddie with her swimming suit.'

'With your mouth?'

Maddie laughed behind her hand.

'Well, ah . . . ' Mick paused and looked at Maddie. It was the first time she'd ever seen him flustered. 'Maddie had a thread,' he continued and pointed vaguely at her thigh, 'and I had to bite it off for her.'

'Oh.'

'What are you doing here?' Mick asked.

'Mom dropped me off to play with Pete.'

Mick looked toward the neighbors' deck. 'Is your mother still at the Allegrezzas'?'

Trevor shook his head. 'She left.' He looked from his uncle to Maddie. 'You got more dead mice?'

'Not today. But I did get a cat and she'll be old enough in a few months to kill them for me.'

'You have a cat?'

'Yeah. Her name is Snowball. She has different colored eyes and an overbite.'

Mick looked at her. 'Seriously.'

'I'll show you two boys.'

'What's an overbite?' Travis asked as the three of them moved into the house.

★　★　★

Mick was home half an hour before his sister knocked on the door. She didn't wait for him to answer.

'Travis told me he saw you kissing Maddie Dupree's butt,' she said as she walked into the kitchen, where she found Mick fixing a sandwich before work.

He looked up. 'Hello, Meg.'

'Is it true?'

'I wasn't kissing her butt.' He'd been biting her thigh.

'Why were you there? Travis saw your boat at her dock. What is going on between the two of you?'

'I like her.' He sliced the ham sandwich and put it on a paper plate. 'It's not a big deal.'

'She's writing a book about Mom and Dad.' She grabbed his wrist to get his attention. 'She's going to make us all look bad.'

'She says she's not interested in making anyone look bad.'

'Bull. She's digging up dirt to make money off our pain and suffering.'

He looked into his sister's deep green eyes. 'Unlike you, Meg, I don't dwell on the past.'

'No.' She let go of his wrist. 'You just choose to not think about it as if it didn't happen.'

He picked up half the sandwich and took a bite. 'I know what happened, but I don't live it every day like you do.'

'I don't live it every day.'

He swallowed and took a drink from a bottle of Sam Adams. 'Maybe not every day, but every time I think you've finally moved on, something happens and it's like you're ten again.' He took another bite. 'I'm going to live my life in the present, Meg.'

'You don't think I want you to live your

life? I do. I want you to find someone, you know I do, but not her.'

'You talked to her.' He was getting bored with the conversation. He liked Maddie. He liked everything about her, and he was going to keep seeing her.

'Only because I wanted her to hear that our mother wasn't a crazy woman.'

He took another drink and set the bottle on the counter. 'Mom was crazy.'

'No.' She shook her head and grabbed his shoulder to turn him toward her. 'Don't say that.'

'Why else would she kill two people and then herself? Why else would she leave her two children orphaned?'

'She didn't mean to.'

'You say that, but if she'd just wanted to scare them, why did she load the .38?'

Meg dropped her hand. 'I don't know.'

He set his sandwich back on the plate and crossed his arms over his chest. 'Do you ever wonder if she gave us a thought?'

'She did.'

'Then why, Meg? Why was killing Dad and then herself more important than her children?'

Meg looked away. 'She loved us, Mick. You don't remember the good things. Just the bad. She loved us and she loved Dad too.'

He wasn't the one with the faulty memory.

He remembered the good and the bad. 'I never said she didn't. Just not enough, I guess. You can stick up for her for another twenty-nine years, but I'll never understand why she felt her only option was to kill Dad and then herself.'

She glanced at her feet and said just above a whisper, 'I never wanted you to know, but . . . ' She returned her gaze to his. 'Dad was leaving us.'

'What?'

'Dad was leaving us for that waitress.' She swallowed hard, as if the word were stuck in her throat. 'I heard Mom talking about it on the telephone to one of her friends.' She laughed bitterly. 'Presumably one of her friends who hadn't slept with Dad.'

His father had planned to leave his mother. He knew he should feel something, anger and outrage, maybe, but he didn't.

'She'd put up with so much from him,' Meg continued. 'The humiliation of the whole town knowing about all the sordid affairs. Year after year.' Meg shook her head. 'He was leaving her for a twenty-four-year-old cocktail waitress and she couldn't take it. She couldn't let him do that to her.'

He looked at his sister, with her pretty eyes and black hair. The same sister who'd protected him as he'd protected her. Or as much as they'd been able. 'And you've known about this for all these years and you didn't tell me?'

'You wouldn't have understood.'

'What's not to understand? I understand that she killed him rather than let him divorce her. I understand that she was sick.'

'She wasn't sick! She was pushed too far. She loved him.'

'That isn't love, Meg.' He grabbed his plate and beer and walked out of the kitchen.

'Like you would know.'

That stopped him, and he turned back and looked at her from the small dining room.

'Have you ever been in love, Mick? Have you ever loved someone so much that the thought of losing her ties your stomach up in knots?'

He thought of Maddie. Of her smile and her dry humor and the bucktoothed kitten that she'd taken into her house even though she professed to hate cats. 'I'm not sure, but I am sure of one thing. If I ever did love a woman like that, I wouldn't hurt her, and I sure as hell wouldn't hurt any children I had with her. I might not know a lot about love, but I do know that.'

'Mick.' Meg moved toward him with her hands palms up. 'I'm sorry. I shouldn't have said that.'

He set his plate on the table. 'Just forget it.'

'I want the best for you. I want you to get married and have a family because I know you'd be a good husband and father. I know you would because I know how much you love me and Travis.' She wrapped her arms around his waist and rested her cheek on his shoulder. 'But even if you don't ever find someone, you'll always have me.'

Mick drew breath into his lungs even as he felt as if he were suffocating.

15

Maddie sat on her sofa, Snowball curled up in her lap, and stared into the blank screen of her television. Her stomach ached and her chest was so tight it hurt to breathe. She was going to be sick. She thought about calling her friends and getting their advice, but she couldn't. She was the strong, fearless one of the group, but at the moment she didn't feel so strong or fearless. Far from it.

For the first time in a very long time, Maddie Jones was afraid. There was no denying it. She couldn't call it apprehension and move on. It was too real. Too deep, and too terrifying. Worse than sitting across from a serial killer.

She'd always assumed that falling in love would be like getting slammed into a brick wall. That you'd just be going along as usual and you'd get knocked on your ass and think, *Gee, I guess I'm in love*. But it hadn't happened that way. It had just kind of snuck up on her before she'd realized it. It had happened one smile and one touch at a time. One look. One kiss. One pink cat collar. One pinch to the heart and one breathless anticipation after another until she was in so deep there was no denying it. No turning back before it was too late. No more lying about what she felt.

Maddie slid her hand down Snowball's small back and didn't care that the cat's fur clung to her black shirt and the lap of her skirt. She'd always thought that she couldn't lie to herself about anything. Apparently she'd gotten better at it.

She'd fallen in love with Mick Hennessy and the minute he found out who she really was, she would lose him. And she didn't have a clue what she was going to do about it.

Her doorbell rang and she looked at the clock sitting on a shelf above the television. It was eight-thirty. Mick was at work and she didn't expect to see him until sometime around one.

She set Snowball on the floor and moved to the door. The kitten chased after her and she scooped her up rather than step on her. She looked through the peephole and got that little heated flush she now recognized. Evidently Mick had skipped work. He stood on her porch wearing jeans and his Mort's polo. She opened the door and stared at him standing there with the first shadows of night bathing him in a light gray and making his eyes a vibrant blue. As he stared at her across the short distance, elation and despair collided in her heart and twisted her stomach.

'I needed to see you,' he said and stepped across the threshold. He wrapped one arm around Maddie's waist and placed his free hand on the back of her head. His mouth swooped down and he kissed her. A long drugging kiss that made her want to attach herself to him and never let go.

He pulled back and looked into her face. 'I was at work pulling beer and listening to the same old stories, and all I could think about was you and the night we had sex on the bar. I can't get you out of my head. Put your cat down, Maddie.'

She bent down to set Snowball on the floor and he shut the door behind him. 'I didn't want to be there. I wanted to be here.'

She straightened and looked into his face. She'd never felt love like this in her life. Not really, not the stomach-lifting and skin-tingling kind of love. Not the kind that made her want to hold his hand forever. To leach herself into his body so she didn't know where he stopped and she began. 'I'm glad you came back.' But she had to tell him she was Maddie Jones. Now.

He pushed her hair behind her ear. 'I can breathe here with you.'

At least one of them could. She rubbed her

cheek into his hand, and before she told him who she was, before she lost him forever, she wrapped her arms around his neck and kissed him one last time. She poured her heart and soul into it, her ache and joy, showing him without words what she felt inside. She kissed his mouth and jaw and the side of his throat. She ran her hands over him, touching and memorizing the feel of him beneath her hands.

Mick slid his warm palms to her behind and then the backs of her thighs. He lifted until she wrapped her legs around his waist. A deep groan vibrated through his chest as he returned her hungry kisses, and he carried her into the bedroom.

She would tell him. She would. In a minute. Her legs slid from his waist and he pulled her shirt over her head. She just wanted a few more minutes, but the more she poured her heart into each kiss, the more he wanted from her. The more he sucked the breath from her lungs and made her light-headed. He slid his hands all over her, her shoulders and arms, her back and behind, until she was left wearing nothing but her bra, unhooked and open in the back.

Mick took a step back from the kiss and gasped. He looked at her through eyes so far gone, there was no thought to stopping him when he slowly pulled her bra straps and the blue satin cups slid down the slopes of her breasts, shimmered across her nipples, then fell down her arms to the floor.

'We've only known each other for a short time.' He lightly brushed the tips of his fingers across the tips of her breasts and her breathing became shallow. 'Why does it feel longer?' He moved behind her and Maddie looked down at his big hands on her breasts, touching her, squeezing her puckered nipples. Her back arched and she raised her arms. Her hands cupped the sides of his face as she brought his mouth down to hers. She gave him a hot, greedy kiss as she tilted her hips and pressed her naked behind into his erection. He groaned deep within his chest as he played with her breasts. He still wore his jeans and his shirt, and the feeling of worn denim and soft cotton against her skin was erotic as hell. His mouth left hers and trailed hot little kisses down the side of her throat, and he slid one hand down her stomach. He placed one of his feet between hers, then he slipped his hand between her parted thighs, and he touched her. Her insides melted, pooling deep and low in her pelvis, and she let her herself savor the touch of the only man she'd ever loved. She'd always wondered if there was a difference between sex and making love. And now she knew. Sex started with physical desire. Making love started in a person's heart.

She didn't know what would happen after this, after she told him who she was, but perhaps it wouldn't matter. She turned and looked up at him as her hands drifted down his stomach to the end of his polo shirt. She pulled the stretchy cotton from the waistband of his pants and Mick raised his arms. She yanked it over his head and tossed it aside. Maddie lowered her gaze from his passion-filled eyes to his strong chest. The tips of her breasts touched him a few inches below his flat brown nipples. A trail of fine hair ran down his chest, between her cleavage, to his waistband.

His voice was husky with lust when he said, 'Why did I ever think I would get enough of you?'

Maddie pulled at his button fly and slipped her hands inside his jeans and cupped him through his boxer briefs. 'I'll never get enough of you, Mick. Whatever happens, I'll always want you.' She closed her eyes and kissed the side of his throat. 'Always,' she whispered.

His breath whooshed from his lungs as she slipped her hand inside his underwear and wrapped her palm around his hot shaft. He grabbed his wallet out of his pants and tossed it on the bed.

'I'll never get enough of the way you feel in my hand,' she whispered. 'Hard and smooth at the same time. I will never forget what it feels like to touch you like this.'

'Who says you have to forget?' He walked her to the side of the bed and pushed her shoulders until she sat.

Who? He would. She laid down and watched him quickly undress until he stood completely naked in front of her, a tall, beautiful man who made her heart and soul ache. She raised a hand to him and pulled him on top of her. The voluptuous head of his hot penis touched between her legs. 'I've loved being together,' she whispered as she sucked his earlobe and rubbed against his warm body. She delivered little nibbling bites to his neck and shoulder.

Mick pushed her onto her back. 'We have a lot more time to be together.' He kissed her chin and throat. 'A lot more.' He sucked her nipple into his warm mouth while his other hand slid down her stomach to touch her with his fingers. As she watched him kiss her breast, raw emotion pumped through her veins. This was Mick, the man who could make her feel beautiful and desired. The man she loved and would probably lose.

Mick raised his head and the cool night air brushed across her breasts where his mouth had left her wet and shining. He reached into his wallet and pulled out a condom, but Maddie took it from his hands and stretched the thin latex down the length of him. She could feel his pulse in her hand, strong and steady. She pushed him onto his back and straddled his hips. His lids lowered over his blue eyes and the breath left his body as he watched her lower herself and take him inside her.

'You look good up there,' he said, his voice low, rough. His hands grasped her waist. 'Feel good too.' He slid his hands up her sides to her breasts.

Maddie rocked her pelvis as she raised a little and slid back down. The head of his penis stroked her inside and she moaned deep in her throat. Up and down she moved, tilting her hips as she rode him. Tingling heat flowed outward from where his body touched hers. 'Mick. Oh, God.' He moved with her, matching her with powerful thrusts, until the sensations swamped her completely and her head fell back as a hot liquid orgasm washed through her, starting at her pelvis and spreading to her fingers and toes. 'Mick. I love you,' she said as new emotions wrapped around her pounding heart, squeezing her chest in its fiery grasp.

Just as the climax ended, Mick wrapped an arm around her back and bottom, and turned with her so that she lay on the bed looking up at him. He was still buried deep inside her and she automatically wrapped her legs around his waist as she knew he liked. She brought his mouth down to her and gave him wet wild kisses as he withdrew and thrust deep inside her again. She clung to him as he drove into her over and over. His chest heaved and he placed his hands on the bed beside her face. With each stroke, he pushed her toward a second climax, and she cried out as her body milked him hard for a second time.

Mick's eyes drifted shut, and his breath hissed between his teeth. 'Holy shit,' he swore, then groaned his satisfaction. He drove into her one last time, then collapsed on top of her.

His weight pushed down on her, heavy and welcome. His face rested on the pillow next to hers and he kissed her shoulder.

'Maddie?' he asked, breathless.

'Yeah?' She slid her hands across his back.

He raised onto his elbows and looked into her face, his breathing still heavy. 'I don't know what was different this time, but that was the hottest sex I've ever had.'

She knew what was different. She loved him. Her face got hot and she shoved at his shoulders. She loved him and she'd told him so too.

He rolled off her and lay on his back.

'I need some water,' she said as she crawled off the bed and stood. Her ears were ringing from embarrassment and she moved to her closet and grabbed her robe.

'Where's your cat?' he asked.

'Probably on my office chair.' She looked down at her shaking hands as she tied the terrycloth around her waist.

'If she attacks me, I'm getting her some GHB.'

Maddie had no idea what he was talking about. 'Okay,' she called from the closet.

'I have more condoms in my pants pocket,' he said, all chipper as he walked to the bathroom. 'But you're going to have to give me some time to get up to speed again.'

While Mick used the bathroom, Maddie walked to the kitchen. She opened the refrigerator and pulled out a bottle of Diet Coke. She placed it against her burning cheeks and closed her eyes. Maybe he hadn't heard her. He'd told her on the way to Redfish that sometimes he didn't understand everything she said during sex. Perhaps she hadn't spoken as clearly as she'd thought.

She unscrewed the cap and took a long drink. She hoped like hell it had been one of those times, which only took care of one problem. The bigger problem loomed ahead, black and devastating and unavoidable.

Mick walked from the bedroom and made his way into the kitchen. He wore his Levi's low on his hips and his hair was tousled from her fingers. 'Are you embarrassed about something?' he asked as he moved behind Maddie and wrapped his arms around her.

'Why?'

He took the bottle from her hands and raised it to his lips. 'You practically ran out of the bedroom and your cheeks are red.' He took a long drink, then handed it back to her.

She looked down at her feet. 'Why would I be embarrassed?'

'Because you shouted, 'I love you,' in the throes of passion.'

'Oh, God.' She covered the side of her face with her free hand.

He turned her and placed his fingers beneath her chin and brought her gaze to his. 'It's okay, Maddie.'

'No, it's not. I didn't mean to fall in love with you.' She shook her head and insisted, 'I don't *want* to be in love with you.' Her chest felt raw and tears stung the backs of her eyes, and she didn't think it was possible to be in any worse pain. 'My life sucks.'

'Why?' He softly kissed her lips and said, 'I'm in love with you too. I didn't think I would ever feel for a woman what I feel for you. These past few days, I've been wondering how you felt.'

She took a few steps back and his hands fell to his sides. This should be the best, most euphoric time of her life. This wasn't fair, but as she'd discovered as a five-year-old child, life was not fair. She opened her mouth and forced the truth past the horrible clog in her throat. 'Madeline Dupree is my pen name.'

His brows rose up his forehead. 'Madeline is not your real name?'

She nodded. 'Madeline is my name. Dupree is not.'

He tilted his head to one side. 'What is your name?'

'Maddie Jones.'

He looked at her, his eyes clear. He shrugged one bare shoulder and said, 'Okay.'

She didn't for one second believe he meant 'okay' like he was okay with who she was. He wasn't connecting the dots. She licked her dry lips. 'My mother was Alice Jones.'

A slight frown creased his brow and then he jerked back like someone had shot him. His gaze moved across her face as if trying to see something he'd never noticed before. 'Tell me you're making a joke, Maddie.'

She shook her head. 'It's true. Alice Jones isn't some face in a newspaper article that caught my attention. She was my mother.' She reached a hand toward him, but he took a step back and her hand fell to her side. She hadn't thought she could be in more pain; she'd been wrong.

His eyes stared into hers. Gone was the man who'd just told her that he loved her. She'd seen Mick angry, but she'd never seen him so coldly furious. 'Let me see if I'm getting this right. My father fucked your mother and I've been fucking you? Is that what you're telling me?'

'I don't see it that way.'

'There's no other way to see it.' He turned on his heels and moved from the kitchen.

Maddie followed him through the living room and into her bedroom. 'Mick — '

'Have you gotten some sort of sick pleasure out of all this?' he interrupted her as he picked up his shirt and shoved his arms through the sleeves. 'When you came to town, was it your intention from the beginning to totally screw with my head? Is this some sort of twisted revenge for what my mother did to yours?'

She shook her head and refused to give in to the tears that threatened to fill her eyes.

She would not cry in front of Mick. 'I didn't want to get involved with you. Ever. But you kept pushing. I wanted to tell you.'

'Bullshit.' He pulled the shirt over his head and down his chest. 'If you'd wanted to tell me, you'd have found a way. You had no problem sharing every other detail of your life. I know you grew up fat and lost your virginity at twenty. I know you wear different scented lotion every day, and that you keep a vibrator named Carlos next to your bed.' He bent forward and picked up his socks and shoes. 'For Christ's sake, I even know you're not a butt girl.' He pointed one of his shoes at her and continued, 'And I'm supposed to believe that you couldn't work the truth into any conversation at some point before tonight!'

'I know that it's no consolation, but I never wanted to hurt you.'

'I'm not hurt.' He sat on the edge of the bed and shoved his feet into a pair of white socks. 'I'm disgusted.'

She felt her anger rise up and she was amazed she could feel anything beyond the deep mortal pain in her chest. She reminded herself that he had a right to be furious. He had a right to know early on whom he was getting involved with instead of after the fact. 'That's harsh.'

'Baby, you don't know harsh.' He glanced up at her, then looked down as he put on his black boots and tied the laces. 'I spent an hour tonight trying to defend you to my sister. She tried to tell me not to get involved with you, but I was thinking with my cock.' He paused to let his gaze rake her up and down. 'And now I have to go tell her about you. I have to tell her you're the daughter of the waitress who ruined her life and watch her come apart.'

He might have more right to be angry than she did, but hearing him call her mother 'the waitress' and worrying more about his sister than her scraped her raw emotions and pushed her over the top. 'You. You. You. I am so sick of hearing about you and your sister. What about me?' She pointed to herself. 'Your mother killed my mother. At the age of five, I moved in with a great-aunt who never wanted children. Who showed more love and affection for her cats than she ever did for me. Your mother did that to me. I've never been given so much as a second thought by you or your family. So I don't want to hear about you and your poor sister.'

'If your mother hadn't been sleeping around — '

'If your father hadn't been sleeping around with about every woman in town and your

303

mother hadn't been a vindictive bitch with a healthy dose of psychosis, then we'd all be happy as clams, wouldn't we? But your father was sleeping with my mother and your mother loaded a pistol and killed them both. That's our reality. When I moved to Truly, I expected to hate you and your sister for what your family has done to me. You look so much like your father that I expected to loathe you on sight, but I didn't. And as I got to know you, I realized that you are nothing like Loch.'

'I used to believe that until tonight. If you are anything in the sack like your mother, then I get why my dad was ready to walk out the door and leave us for her. You Jones women drop your clothes and the Hennessy men get stupid.'

'Wait!' Maddie interrupted him and held up one hand. 'Your dad was going to leave? For my mother?' Her mother had been right about Loch.

'Yeah. I just found out. Guess you have something to put in your book.' He smiled, but it wasn't pleasant. 'I'm just like my dad, and you're just like your mother.'

'I am nothing like my mother, and you are nothing like your father. When I look at you, I just see you. That's how I fell in love with you.'

'It doesn't matter what you see, because when I look at you, I don't know who you are.' He stood. 'You aren't the woman I thought you were. When I look at you, I feel sick that I fucked the waitress's daughter.'

Maddie's hands clenched into fists. 'Her name was Alice and she was my mother.'

'I don't really give a shit.'

'I know you don't.' She stormed out of the room and into her office, only to return a few moments later with a file and photograph. 'This was her.' She held up the old framed picture. 'Look at her. She was twenty-four and beautiful and had her whole life ahead of her. She was flighty and immature and made horrible choices in her young life. Especially when it came to men.' She pulled the crime scene photo from the files. 'But she didn't deserve this.'

'Jesus.' Mick turned his head away.

Maddie dropped everything onto the dresser. 'Your family did this to her and to me. The least you could do is say her goddamn name when you talk about her!'

Mick looked at her, his brows lowered over his beautiful eyes. 'I've spent most of my life not talking or thinking about her. I'm going to spend the rest of it not thinking about you.' He reached for his wallet on her bed, then walked out of the room.

Above the sound of her beating heart, Maddie heard the front door slam and she flinched. That had gone worse than she'd imagined. She'd thought he'd be angry, but disgusted? That had hit like a punch to the stomach.

She walked to the front door and, through the peephole, watched his truck pull out of her driveway. She locked the deadbolt and leaned her back against the solid door. The tears she'd refused to shed filled her eyes. A sound she almost didn't recognize as coming from her broke past the emotion in her chest. Like a puppet whose strings had been cut, she slid down until her butt hit the floor.

'Meow.'

Snowball climbed into her lap and scaled the front of her robe. Her tiny pink tongue licked the tears from Maddie's numb cheek.

How was it possible to hurt so much but feel absolutely hollow inside?

16

Meg raised her fingers to her temples and pushed, like she had as a kid. 'She shouldn't be allowed to get away with this.' The ends of her pink robe flapped about her ankles as she paced her small kitchen. It was nine A.M. and luckily her day off work. Travis had spent the night with Pete and was blissfully unaware of the turmoil brewing within his home.

'She shouldn't be allowed to live here,' Meg ranted. 'Our lives were fine until she showed up. She's just like her mother. Moving to town and messing up our lives.'

After Mick had left Maddie's house, he'd gone back to work and tried to ignore the anger and chaos in his soul. After the bar closed, he stayed and worked on business. He'd looked over his bank records and wrote out payroll checks. He checked inventory and made notes on what he needed to order, and after the clock struck eight, he drove to his sister's.

'Someone should do something.'

Mick set his coffee on the old oak table where he'd eaten dinner as a kid and sat in a chair. 'Tell me you're not going to do anything.'

She stopped and looked over at him. 'Like what? What can I do?'

'Promise you won't go anywhere near her.'

'What is it you think I'm going to do?'

He simply looked at her, and she seemed to deflate before his eyes.

'I'm not like Mom. I'm not going to hurt anyone.'

No, just herself. 'Promise,' he insisted.

'Fine. If it will make you feel better. I promise that I'm not going to burn her house down.' She laughed quietly and sat in the chair next to him.

'That's not funny, Meg.'

'Maybe not, but no one got hurt that night, Mick.'

Only because he'd shown up in time to pull her out of their farmhouse the night she'd torched it. She'd always insisted that she hadn't meant to kill herself. To this day, he wasn't sure he believed her.

'I'm not crazy, you know.'

'I know,' he said automatically.

She shook her head. 'No, you don't. Sometimes you look at me and I think you see Mom.'

That was so close to the truth that he didn't even bother denying it. 'I just think that sometimes your emotions are over the top.'

'To you they are, but there is a big difference between being an emotional person who rants and raves as opposed to a person who takes a gun and kills herself or anyone else.'

He thought calling her outbursts 'being an emotional person' an understatement, but he didn't want to argue. He stood and walked to the sink. 'I'm tired and going home,' he said and poured his coffee down the drain.

'Get some sleep,' his sister ordered.

He grabbed his keys off the kitchen table and Meg rose to hug him good-bye.

'Thanks for coming by and telling me everything.'

He hadn't told Meg everything. He hadn't mentioned that he'd had sex with Maddie, nor that he'd fallen for her. 'Tell Travis I'll come by tomorrow morning and take him fishing.'

'He'll like that.' She rose and walked him to the door. 'You've been so busy with work lately that you boys haven't had much time together.'

He'd been busy, but mostly busy chasing after Maddie Dupree. No. Maddie Jones.

'Take a shower,' she called after him as he made his way to his truck. 'You look like crap.'

Which he figured was perfect, since he felt

like crap. He jumped in his truck and ten minutes later he stood in his bedroom, wondering how his life had gone to complete hell.

He pulled his shirt over his head and caught a scent of Maddie. Last night she'd smelled like coconut and lime and this morning was the first time since he'd met her that he didn't want to bury his face in her neck. No, he wanted to wring her neck.

He tossed the shirt in the laundry basket in his closet and knelt to take off his shoes. Standing in her kitchen last night, realizing who she was, had hit him like a blow to the side of the head. If that hadn't been good enough for her, she'd held up the bloody photo of her mother, which finished him off with a roundhouse kick to the gut. She'd beat the hell out of him and he'd gone down for the count.

He took off his shoes and undressed. He was a fool. For the first time in his life, he'd truly fallen hard for a woman. So hard it ate at his chest like acid. Only she wasn't who she'd led him to believe she was. She was Maddie Jones. Daughter of his father's last girlfriend. It didn't matter that she didn't see Loch when she looked at him or that she looked nothing like her mother. It really didn't matter that she'd lied to him, or at least not as much as *knowing* who she really was mattered. He'd spent most of his life fighting to free himself from the past, only to fall for a woman deeply tangled up in it.

Mick walked into the bathroom and turned on the shower. Evidently he was more like Loch than he'd ever thought, and that just pissed him off. From almost the beginning, he'd known there was something about Maddie. Something that drew him in. He hadn't known what it was and couldn't have even guessed. Now he understood, and it sat in his gut like hot lead. He understood that it was the same singleminded attraction his father must have felt for her mother. The same fascination that made him want to see her smile, watch her laugh, and listen to her whisper his name as he gave her pleasure. The same sort of calm his father must have felt when he was near her mother. As if everything else dropped away and his vision cleared, and he saw what he wanted even before he knew he'd wanted anything.

He stepped into the shower and let the warm water run over his head. For his father to have been planning to leave his mother for Alice Jones, Loch must have been in love with her. Mick understood that too. He was in love with Maddie Jones. He hated to admit it now. He was ashamed and embarrassed, but when she'd opened her door last night and he'd seen her standing there holding her cat, his heart had felt like the sun was warming him up from the inside. And he'd known. Known what it felt like for a man to love a woman. Known it in every cell in his body. Every beat of his heart. Then he'd carried her to her bed, and he'd known what it felt like to make love to a woman, and he'd been amazed.

Then she'd ripped his heart from his chest.

Mick tipped his head back and closed his eyes. He'd seen and done things in his life that he regretted. Experienced heart-wrenching pain at the deaths of fellow soldiers. But the things he'd done and experienced were not as bad as the regret and pain he felt over loving Maddie.

There was only one thing to do. He'd told her that he hadn't thought about her mother and that he wasn't going to think about her, and that was exactly what he planned to do. He was going to forget about Maddie Jones.

★　★　★

Meg opened her front door and looked into Steve Castle's calm blue eyes. She'd taken a shower and he'd arrived just as she'd finished drying her hair. 'I didn't know who else to call.'

'I'm glad you called me.'

He stepped inside and followed her into the kitchen. He wore a pair of jeans and a T-shirt with a cornucopia and the words EVERYBODY HATES VEGETARIANS across his chest. Over a fresh pot of coffee, she told him what she'd learned from Mick.

'The whole town is going to find out, and I don't know what to do.'

Steve wrapped his big hand around the mug and raised it to his mouth. 'Doesn't sound like there is anything you can do except hold your head up,' he said, then took a drink.

'How can I?' The last time she'd talked with Steve about Maddie Dupree Jones, he'd given good advice and made her feel better. 'This is just going to keep everyone talking about what my mother did and all my father's affairs.'

'Probably, but that isn't your fault.'

She stood and moved to the coffeepot. 'I know, but that won't keep people from talking about me.' She reached for the coffee then refilled Steve's mug and hers.

'No. It won't, but while they're talking, you just keep telling yourself that you didn't do anything wrong.'

She returned the coffeepot and leaned a hip against the counter. 'I can tell myself that, but it won't make me feel better.'

Steve placed a hand on the kitchen table and stood. 'It will if you believe it.'

'You don't understand. It's so humiliating.'

'Oh, I understand about humiliation. When I returned from Iraq, my wife was pregnant and everyone knew the baby wasn't mine.' He moved toward her, his limp barely noticeable. 'Not only did I have to deal with the loss of my leg and my wife, but I had to deal with her being unfaithful with an army buddy.'

'Oh, my God, I'm sorry, Steve.'

'Don't be. My life was hell for a while, but it's good now. Sometimes you have to go taste the shit to appreciate the sugar.'

Meg wondered if that was some sort of army saying.

He reached for her hand. 'But you can't appreciate the sugar until you let go of all the bad shit.' He brushed his thumb across the inside of her wrist and the hair on her arms tingled. 'What your parents did, didn't have anything to do with you. You were a kid. Just like my wife screwing my buddy didn't have anything to do with me. Not really. If she was unhappy because I was gone, there were other, more honorable ways to handle it. If your mama had been unhappy because your daddy was having affairs, there were other ways to handle that too. What my wife did wasn't my fault. Just like what your mama did wasn't your fault. I don't know about you, Meg, but I don't plan on paying the rest of my life for other people's dumb-ass mistakes.'

'I don't want to.'

He squeezed her hand and somehow she felt it in her heart. 'Then don't.' He pulled her toward him and placed his free hand on the side of her neck. 'One thing I know for sure is that you can't control what other people say and do.'

'You sound like Mick. He thinks I can't get over the past because I dwell on it.' She turned her face into his palm.

'Maybe you need something in your life to take your mind off the past.'

When she'd been married to Travis's daddy, she hadn't let it bother her as much as it did these days.

'Maybe you need someone.'

'I have Travis.'

'Besides your son.' He lowered his face and spoke against her lips. 'You're a beautiful woman, Meg. You should have a man in your life.'

She opened her mouth to speak, but she couldn't remember what to say. It had been a very long time since a man had told her she was beautiful. A long time since she'd kissed anyone but her son. She pressed her mouth against Steve's and he kissed her. A warm gentle kiss that seemed to go on forever within the sunlight spilling into the kitchen. And when it was over, he cupped her face in his rough hands and said, 'I've wanted to do that for a long time.'

Meg licked her bottom lip and smiled. He made her feel beautiful and wanted. Like more than just a waitress, a mom, and a woman who'd just hit forty. 'How old are you, Steve?'

'Thirty-four.'

'I'm six years older than you.'

'Is that a problem?'

She shook her head. 'No, but it might be a problem for you.'

'Age is not a problem.' He slid his hands to her back and pulled her against his chest. 'I just have to figure out a way to tell Mick that I want his sister.'

Meg smiled and wrapped her arms around his neck. She knew there were a lot of things Mick kept to himself. Most recently his relationship with Maddie Jones. 'Let him figure it out on his own.'

17

Maddie lay curled up on her in bed. She didn't have the energy to get up. She was drained and empty except for the ball of regret sitting in her stomach. She regretted not telling Mick sooner. If she'd told him who she really was the first night she'd walked into Hennessy's, he never would have shown up at her door with mousetraps and catnip. He never would have touched her and kissed her, and she never would have fallen in love with him.

Snowball climbed onto the bed and picked her way across the quilt toward Maddie's face.

'What are you doing?' she asked her kitten, her voice raw from the emotion she'd expended all night. 'You know I don't like cat hair. This is completely against the rules.'

Snowball crawled beneath the covers, then stuck her head back out just beneath Maddie's chin. Her soft fur tickled Maddie's throat. 'Meow.'

'You're right. Who gives a shit about the rules?' She stroked the cat's fur as her eyes filled with tears. She'd cried so much the night before, she was surprised she had any water left in her body, that she wasn't all dehydrated and wrinkled like a raisin.

Maddie rolled to her back and looked up at the shadows spread across her ceiling. She could have lived her entire life quite happy if she'd never fallen in love. She'd be happy to never know the high dopamine rush or the heart-wrenching anguish and despair of having loved and lost. Lord Tennyson was wrong. It was not better to have loved and lost than to have never loved at all. Maddie would have much preferred to have never loved at all than to love Mick only to have lost him.

I'm not hurt, he'd said. *I'm disgusted*. She could take his anger and even the hate she'd seen in his eyes. But disgust? That hurt to the core. The man she loved, the man who'd not only touched her heart but her body, was disgusted by her. Knowing how he felt made her want to curl up in a ball and cover her head until it didn't hurt anymore.

Around noon her back began to ache, so she grabbed her kitten and a quilt off her bed. She and Snowball lay on the couch and watched mindless television all day and into the evening. She even watched *Kate & Leopold*, a movie she'd always hated because she'd never understood why any sane woman would jump off a bridge for a man.

However, this time her dislike of the movie didn't keep her from crying into a Kleenex. After *Kate & Leopold*, she watched *Meerkat Manor* and *Project Runway* reruns. When she wasn't crying over Leopold, the poor Meerkats, or the abomination of Jeffrey's rocker pants, she was thinking about Mick. What he'd said, his face when he'd said it, and what he'd told her about his father leaving his mother for Alice. Alice had been right about Loch's feelings. Who would have thought it? Not Maddie, or rather she had *thought* of it, but given Alice's history with men, especially married men, and Loch's history with women, Maddie had dismissed the possibility.

Rose's reasoning for what she'd done was a classic case of loss of control and the feeling of loss of self. The typical 'if I can't have you, no one can' that had been analyzed and studied and found throughout history.

It had been so simple, and right in front of her the whole time. Knowing the truth made writing the book easier, but on a personal level, it really didn't change anything. Her mother had still made a bad choice that ended in her death. Three people died and three children were left devastated. Motive didn't really matter a whole lot.

At around midnight she fell asleep and

woke the next morning feeling as bad as ever. Maddie had never been a whiner or a crier. Most likely because she'd learned at an early age that whining and crying and feeling sorry for yourself didn't get you anywhere. Even though she still felt like emotional road-kill, she took a shower and moved into her office. Lying around and feeling bad wasn't going to get her work done. That was the thing about writing her books, she was the only one who could do it.

Her timeline was pinned to the wall and everything was ready. She sat down and began to write:

At three p.m. on July ninth, Alice Jones put on her white blouse and black skirt and sprayed Charlie on her wrists. It was the first day of her new job at Hennessy's, and she wanted to make a good impression. Hennessy's had been built in 1925 during Prohibition and the family had prospered by selling grain alcohol out of the back . . .

At around noon, Maddie got up to fix lunch, feed Snowball, and grab a Diet Coke. She wrote until midnight, when she fell into bed, and woke the next morning with Snowball under the covers and curled beneath her chin.

'This is a bad habit,' she told her cat. Snowball purred, a steady rattling of love, and Maddie couldn't quite bring herself to kick the kitten out of bed.

During the next several weeks, Snowball developed other bad habits as well. She insisted on lying in Maddie's lap while she wrote or the kitten walked on the desk and batted off paper clips, pens, and blocks of sticky notes.

Maddie kept herself busy, writing ten hours a day, taking occasional breaks out on her back deck to feel the sun on her face, before getting back to work until she fell into bed exhausted. During those moments when she wasn't thinking about work, her mind always turned to Mick. She wondered what he was doing and who he was seeing. He'd said that he wasn't going to think about her, and she believed him. If not thinking about the past was easy for him, not thinking about her would be even easier.

On those occasions when her mind wasn't filled with work, she recalled their conversations, their lunch at Redfish, and the nights he'd spent in her bed.

She wished she could hate Mick. Or even dislike him. It would be so much easier if she could. She'd tried to recall all the mean and nasty things he'd said the night she'd told him who she was, but she couldn't hate Mick. She loved him and was fairly sure she'd love him forever.

On the anniversary of her mother's death, she wondered if Mick was alone, remembering that night that had changed their lives. If he felt as alone and sad as she did. As the clock struck a minute after midnight, her heart sank as she realized she'd been holding on to a tiny shred of hope that he might show up on her porch. He didn't, and she was forced to accept all over again that the man she loved didn't love her.

The last day of August, she dressed in a pair of khaki shorts and a black cotton tank and took Snowball for her vet appointment. Leaving her kitten in the big hands of Dr Tannasee was more traumatic than Maddie was willing to admit. She ignored the little burst of panic as she walked out of the examining room without the crazy-eyed, bucktoothed, rule-breaking ball of white fur, and she was forced to face an inconceivable fact. Somehow, Maddie had become a cat person.

When she returned home, the house seemed intolerably still and empty, and she forced herself to work for a few hours before moving out onto the deck to take a break in the fresh air and sunshine. She sat in an

Adirondack chair and tilted her face to the sun. Next door, the Allegrezzas stood on their deck, laughing and talking and barbequing something.

'Maddie, come over and see the twins,' Lisa called out to her. She stood and took a quick inventory, but she didn't spot a Hennessy. Her black flip-flops slapped the bottoms of her feet as she walked the short distance to the neighbors'.

Wrapped like burritos and lying in the same baby carriage shaded by a big ponderosa, Isabel and Lilly Allegrezza slept, oblivious to the fuss around them. The girls had dark glossy hair like their father and the most delicate faces Maddie had ever seen.

'Don't they look like little porcelain dolls?' Lisa asked.

Maddie nodded. 'They're so tiny.'

'They both weigh a little more than five pounds now,' Delaney said. 'They were early, but they're perfectly healthy. If there was the slightest concern, Nick would have them at home in a germ-free bubble.' She looked over at her husband manning the grill with Louie. She lowered her voice and added, 'He's bought every gadget imaginable. The baby book calls that nesting.'

Lisa laughed. 'Who would have thought he'd be a nester?'

'Are you talking about me?' Nick asked his wife.

Delaney looked over at the grill and smiled. 'Just saying how much I love you.'

'Uh-huh.'

'When are you going back to work?' Lisa asked her sister-in-law.

'I'll open the salon again next month.'

Maddie looked at Delaney and her smooth blond hair, cut straight across at her shoulders. 'A hair salon?'

'Yeah. I own the salon on Main.' Delaney looked at Maddie's hair and added, 'If you need a trim before next month, let me know and I'll bring over my shears. Whatever you do, don't go to Helen's Hair Hut. She'll fry your hair and make you look like a bad eighties rock video. If you want your hair done right, come to me.'

Which explained why half the town had badly fried hair.

The back door opened and Pete and Travis walked out, each with a hot dog bun in his hand. They waited patiently as Louie slid a hot dog in each bun and Nick provided a stream of ketchup. Seeing Travis reminded Maddie of his uncle. She wondered where Mick was, and if he was likely to show up. If he did, would he be alone or have some slut on his arm who expected more from Mick than he would give? He'd said he loved her, but she didn't believe him. As she'd learned all too painfully, love didn't go away just because you didn't want to think about it.

'Hey, Travis, how are you?' she asked as he moved toward her.

'Good. How's your cat?'

'She's at the vet's today, so it's fairly quiet around my house.'

'Oh.' He looked up at her and squinted against the glare of the sun. 'I'm going to get a dog.'

'Oh.' She remembered what Meg had said about getting Travis a pet. 'When?'

'Someday.' He took a bite of his hot dog and said, 'I went fishing with my uncle Mick on his boat. We got skunked.' He swallowed, then added, 'We drove by on the water and saw you. We didn't wave, though.'

Of course not. She said her good-byes and went home. The house was still much too quiet, and she drove to Value Rite Drug to do a little nesting of her own. It was time Snowball got a proper pet carrier, and she planned to look for a better bed for the kitten. Obviously the Amazon box wasn't a hit.

What Maddie hadn't planned was to run smack-dab into the middle of the Founders Day celebration. She vaguely recalled seeing something about it somewhere, but she'd forgotten all about it. The trip to Value Rite Drug, which normally took about ten minutes, took half an hour. The parking lot was packed with cars from the Founders Day Arts and Crafts Fair held in the park across the street.

Maddie had to circle the parking lot like a vulture until she finally found a slot. Normally she wouldn't have bothered, but she figured it would probably take her another half hour to get home anyway.

Once inside the store, she found a little cat bed but no carrier. She tossed it into her cart along with a catnip toy, and a cat DVD filled with footage of birds, fish, and mice. She was a bit embarrassed to find herself buying a DVD for a cat, but she figured Snowball might stay off the furniture if she was mesmerized by watching fish.

While at the store, she stocked up on toilet paper, laundry soap, and her most secret indulgence, the *Weekly News of the Universe*. She loved the stories of fifty-pound grasshoppers and about women who were having Big Foot's baby, but her favorites were always the Elvis sightings. She dropped the black-and-white magazine into her cart and headed for the checkout lanes.

Carleen Dawson was working register five

when Maddie set her items on the counter.

'I heard you're Alice's daughter. Or is that just a rumor like Brad Pitt comin' to town?'

'No, that's true. Alice Jones was my mother.' Maddie dug around in her purse and pulled out her wallet.

'I worked with Alice at Hennessy's.'

'Yes, I know,' she said and braced herself for what Carleen might say next.

'She was a nice girl. I liked her.'

Surprise curved Maddie's lips into a smile. 'Thank you.'

Carleen rung up everything and put it all, except the bed, into a bag. 'She shouldn't have been fooling around with a married man, but she didn't deserve what Rose did to her.'

Maddie swiped her card and entered her PIN number. 'I obviously agree.' She paid for her items and walked out of Value Rite feeling a lot better than when she'd walked in. She put everything in the trunk of her car and decided that since she was there, she'd check out the arts and crafts fair. She put her big black sunglasses on the bridge of her nose as she crossed the street and entered the park. She'd never been into arts and crafts, mostly because she didn't really decorate.

At the Pronto Pup stand, she splurged on a corn dog with extra mustard. She saw Meg and Travis with a tall bald man wearing a SPARROW IS MY CO-PIRATE T-shirt. She noticed right away that Mick wasn't with them, and she waited for them to pass before she moved to the PAWS booth and looked at pet collars, pet clothes, and feeders. The pink princess cat ottoman was over the top, but she did find a carrier in the shape of a bowling bag. It was red with black mesh hearts and lined in black fur. It also came with a matching wristlet for pet treats. She ordered Snowball a three-story kitty condo and an electronic litter box, to be delivered the following week. The carrier she took with her so that she could bring Snowball home in it the next day.

She hung the carrier on her shoulder and threw her corn dog stick away as she left the booth. As she hooked a right by the Mr Pottery stand, she practically ran headfirst into Mick Hennessy's chest. She looked up past the blue T-shirt covering his wide chest, past the throat she'd kissed so often and the stubborn set of his chin and angry press of his mouth, and up into his eyes covered by sunglasses. Her heart pounded and pinched, and heat flushed her body. Her first instinct was to run away from the anger rolling off him in waves. Instead she managed a very pleasant, 'Hello, Mick.'

He frowned. 'Maddie.'

Her gaze skimmed across his face, feeding images of him to the lonely places inside her, images of his black hair touching his brow and of the bruise on his cheek.

'What happened to your face?'

He shook his head. 'Doesn't matter.'

Panty-tossing Darla stood beside him and asked, 'Are you going to introduce me to your friend?'

Until that moment, Maddie had not realized they were together. Darla's big hair was as fried as ever, and she wore one of her sparkly tank tops and painfully tight jeans.

'Darla, this is Madeline Dupree, but her real name is Maddie Jones.'

'The writer?'

'Yes.' Maddie adjusted the cat carrier on her shoulder. What was Mick doing with Darla? Surely he could do better.

'J.W. told me that he heard you were trying to get the Hennessys and your mother exhumed.'

'Christ,' Mick swore.

Maddie glanced at Mick, then returned her gaze to Darla. 'That's not true. I would never do something like that.'

Mick pulled a wad of cash out of his front pocket and handed it to the other woman. 'Why don't you head over to the beer garden and I'll meet you there in a minute?'

Darla took the money and asked, 'Is Budweiser all right?'

'Fine.'

As soon as Darla walked away, Mick said, 'How much longer are you going to be in town?'

Maddie shrugged and watched Darla's big behind disappear into the crowd. 'Can't really say.' She looked back up into the face of the man who made her broken heart pound in her throat. 'Please tell me you aren't dating Darla.'

'Jealous?'

No, she was angry. Angry that he didn't love her. Angry that she would always love him. Angry that a part of her wanted to throw herself on his chest like some desperate high school girl and beg him to love her. 'Are you shitting me? Jealous of a low-exception dumb-ass? If you want to make me jealous, start dating someone with half a brain and a modicum of class.'

His gaze narrowed. 'At least she isn't running around pretending to be someone she's not.'

Yes, she was. She was running around pretending she was a size ten, but Maddie chose not to point that out in a crowded park because she *did* have a modicum of class.

Just above the noise surrounding them he said, 'Not everything that comes out of her mouth is a lie.'

'How would you know? You don't ever stick around long enough to get to know anyone.'

'You think you know me so well.'

'I do know you. Probably better than any other woman, and I'd be willing to bet that I'm the only woman you've ever really known.'

Slowly he shook his head. 'I don't know you.'

She looked into his mirrored sunglasses and said, 'Yes, you do, Mick.'

'Knowing your favorite sexual position is not what I call knowing you.'

He wanted to reduce what had been between them to just sex. It might have started out that way, but it had become so much more. At least to her. She took a step forward and raised onto the balls of her feet. He was so close she could feel the heat of his skin through his shirt and hers. So close she was sure he could feel her pounding heart as she said next to his ear, 'You know more than whether I like it on top or bottom. You know more than the smell of my skin or the taste of me in your mouth.' She closed her eyes and added, 'You know me. You just can't handle who I am.' Without another word she turned on her heels and left him standing there. She couldn't say that her first encounter with him had gone well, but at least he was going to be thinking about her after she was gone.

Instead of getting the hell out of the park and getting home to avoid seeing Mick again, she forced herself to take her time. She'd been down for a few weeks, but she was better now, stronger than her broken heart. She paused at the Mad Hatter stand and stopped at the Spoon Man booth. Mr Spoon Man had made everything from jewelry to clocks out of spoons, and Maddie bought a chime she thought would sound nice on the back deck.

She put the chime in the cat carrier and made her way out of the park. But like the pull of a magnet on a paper clip, her gaze was drawn to the beer garden and the man who stood at the entrance. Only this time Mick wasn't with Darla. Tanya King, with her little body and little clothes, stood in front of him, and his head was bent forward slightly as he listened to her every word. Her hand rested on his chest, and the corners of his mouth turned up as he smiled at something she said.

He didn't appear to be thinking about Maddie at all, and suddenly she didn't feel stronger than her broken heart.

* ★ *

Through the lenses of his sunglasses, Mick watched Maddie as she crossed the street and left the park. His gaze slid down her back to her butt. The memory of her legs around his waist and his hands on her behind flashed across his brain whether he wanted to remember or not. And he didn't. Hardly a day passed without something reminding him of Maddie. His truck. His boat. His bar. He couldn't walk into Mort's without remembering the night she'd arrived at his back door wearing a trench coat and one of his ties between her beautiful bare breasts. He'd like to believe that it had just been about sex with her, but she'd been right about that. It had been more than the smell of her skin and the taste of her in his mouth. At odd random moments he'd wonder where she was and if she'd gone to Boise for her friend's wedding. Or he'd remember her laugh, the sound of her voice and her smart mouth.

Are you shitting me? Jealous of a low-exception dumb-ass? If you want to make me jealous, start dating someone with half a brain and a modicum of class, she'd said, as if there were a chance in hell he'd ever date Darla. He hadn't had sex since that last night with Maddie, but he wasn't hard up. He'd never been that hard up.

You know more than whether I like it on top or bottom. You know more than the smell of my skin or the taste of me in your mouth. Seeing her and smelling the scent of her skin, the urge to feel her against his chest once again had been overwhelming, and for a fraction of one unguarded second, he'd actually raised his hands to pull her closer. Thank God he had stopped himself before he'd touched her.

You just can't handle who I am. She was right about that. She was a liar who'd used her body to get him to talk about the past, and he'd fallen for it.

Darla wasn't the only dumb-ass.

Maddie disappeared across the street and his gaze returned to Tanya. She was talking about . . . something.

'My new trainer is brutal, but he gets results.'

Oh, yeah. Tanya's exercise. No doubt about it, Tanya had a good body. Too bad her hand on his chest wasn't doing much for *his* body. He needed a distraction. His efforts to forget about Maddie, to put her out of his head and not think about her, were clearly not working.

Maybe, if he put his mind to it, sex with Tanya was exactly what he needed.

18

The night before Clare's wedding, the four friends got together at Maddie's house in Boise. They sat in Maddie's living room in front of a big fireplace made of river rock. The house in Boise was furnished in brown and beige tones, and moments earlier Maddie had cracked open a bottle of Moët. The four women raised their champagne glasses and toasted Clare's future happiness with her fiancé Sebastian Vaughan.

A little over a year ago, all four women had been single. Now Lucy was married and Clare was about to get married. Adele continued to believe she was cursed with bad dates, and Maddie had fallen in love and gotten her heart broken. Adele was the only one out of the four whose life hadn't drastically changed. Although Maddie had yet to confide to her friends about her feelings for Mick. This was Clare's night. Not a pity party for Maddie. It had been a week since she'd seen Mick in the park with Tanya, and the image still made her sick.

'My mother has invited half of Boise to the wedding. She has been in her . . . ' Clare paused and leaned to the left to look behind Maddie's chair. 'There's a cat in your house.'

Maddie turned around and looked at Snowball, flagrantly disregarding the rules as she climbed up the satin drapes. Maddie clapped her hands and stood. 'Snowball.' The cat looked over at Maddie and dropped to the floor.

'Do you know that cat?' Adele asked.

'I kind of adopted it.'

'Kind of?'

Lucy leaned forward. 'You hate cats.'

'I know.'

Clare covered her lips with two fingers. 'You named your cat Snowball. That's so cute.'

'So unlike you,' Lucy added.

Adele tilted her head to one side and looked concerned. 'Are you all right? You go away for a few months and come back with a cat. What else have you been doing up there in Truly that we don't know about?'

Maddie lifted her glass and finished off the champagne. 'Nothing.'

Lucy raised a suspicious brow. 'How's the book?'

'Actually, it's going fairly well,' she answered truthfully. 'I'm a little over halfway finished.' The next half was going to be the rough part. The part where she would have to write about the night her mother died.

'How's Mick Hennessy?' Adele asked.

Maddie rose and moved to the coffee table. 'I don't know.' She poured herself more champagne. 'He won't talk to me.'

'Did you finally tell him who you really are?'

Maddie nodded and refilled her friends' glasses. 'Yes, I told him, and he didn't take it very well.'

'At least you didn't sleep with him.'

Maddie looked away and took a drink from her glass.

'Oh, my God!' Clare gasped. 'You fell off the wagon with Mick Hennessy?'

Maddie shrugged and took her seat. 'I couldn't help myself.'

Adele nodded. 'He's hot.'

'A lot of men are hot.' Lucy took a sip as she studied Maddie. Her brows shot up her forehead. 'You're in love with him.'

'It doesn't matter. He hates me.'

Clare, the most kindhearted of the four, said, 'I'm sure that's not true. No one can hate you.'

That was so blatantly untrue, Maddie couldn't help a smile, while Lucy coughed on her champagne.

Adele sat back and laughed. 'Maddie Jones got a cat and fell in love. Hell has officially frozen over.'

* ★ *

The day after Clare's wedding, Maddie packed up her cat and headed to Truly. The wedding had been beautiful, of course. And at the reception, Maddie had partied and danced the night away. Several of the men she'd danced with had been good-looking and single, and she wondered if she'd ever get to a point in her life when she would not compare every man she met to Mick Hennessy.

She spent the rest of September writing and reliving the days before her mother's death. She inserted parts of interviews and diary entries, including the very last:

My baby will turn six next year and will go to first grade. I can't believe how big she is. I wish I could give her more. Maybe I can. Loch said that he loves me. I've heard that before. He says he's going to leave his wife and be with me. He says he doesn't love Rose, and he's going to tell her that he doesn't want to live with her anymore. I've heard that before too. I want to believe him. No, I do believe him!! I just hope he isn't lying. I know he loves his children. He talks about them a lot. He worries that when he tells his wife he wants a divorce his kids will have to witness a big scene. He's afraid she'll throw things or do something really crazy like start his car on fire. I worry that she will hurt Loch and I told him so. He just laughed and said Rose would never hurt anyone.

The hardest part of the book hadn't been reliving the death of her mother moment by moment, as she'd always thought. That had been hard, to be sure, but the most difficult part had been writing the end and saying good-bye. In writing the book, she realized that she'd never said good-bye to her mother. Never had any sort of closure. Now she did, and it felt as if one part of her life had ended.

When she was through with the book, it was mid-October and she was physically and emotionally drained. She fell into bed and slept for almost twenty hours. When she woke, she felt as if a thorn had been taken from her chest. A thorn that she'd never even known was embedded there. She was free from the past and she hadn't even known she'd needed freeing.

Maddie fed Snowball, then jumped in the shower. Her cat had yet to sleep in the bed Maddie had bought for her. She liked the video, and the carrier not at all. Maddie had given up on any sort of rules. Snowball liked to spend most of her time lying on the windowsill or in Maddie's lap.

Maddie washed her hair and scrubbed her body with watermelon-scented sugar scrub and wondered what she was going to do with her life. Which was such an odd question, really, when she thought about it. Until she'd finished the book, she hadn't realized how much of her life had been wrapped up in the past. It had dictated her future without her even knowing it.

Maybe she'd take a vacation. Someplace warm. Just pack a swimsuit and a pair of flip-flops and hit a nice beach. Maybe Adele needed a break from her cycle of cursed dating.

As Maddie toweled herself dry, she thought of Mick. She was thirty-four, and he was her first real love. She would always love him even though he could never love her back. But perhaps there was something she could do for him. She could give him the same gift that she'd given herself.

★　★　★

Mick's gaze rose from the bottle in his hand to the woman walking in the front door. He set the Corona on the bar and watched her as she moved between the tables. Mort's was slow, even for a Monday night, and he'd been about to leave and have the bartender close.

Her hair curled about her shoulders like the first time he'd seen her, and she wore a black bulky sweater that hid the wonders of her body. He hadn't seen her since Founders Day when she'd told him that he couldn't handle the truth about her. She'd been right. He couldn't, but that didn't mean he hadn't missed her every damn day. Didn't mean that his gaze didn't drink up everything about her. Trying to forget about her hadn't worked. Nothing had worked.

Above Trace Adkins on the jukebox, she said, 'Hello, Mick.' Her voice poured through him like warmed brandy.

'Maddie.'

'May I talk to you somewhere private?'

He wondered if she'd come to tell him good-bye and how he'd feel about that. He nodded and the two of them moved to his office. Her shoulder touched his, adding need to the warm mix spreading across his flesh. He wanted Maddie Jones. Wanted her like he was starving, wanted to jump on her and eat her up. She shut the door, and the urge got stronger. He moved behind his desk, as far away from her as possible. 'Maybe you should leave the — '

'Please let me talk,' she interrupted and

held up a hand. 'I have something to say and then I'll leave.' She swallowed hard and stared directly into his eyes. 'The first time I recall being afraid, I was five. I'm not talking about Halloween and boogeyman afraid. I am talking sick-to-my-stomach afraid.

'A sheriff's deputy woke me up to tell me my great-aunt was coming to get me and that my mother was dead. I didn't understand what had happened. I didn't understand why my mother had gone away, but I knew she was never coming back. I cried so hard I threw up all over the back-seat of my great-aunt Martha's Cadillac.'

He remembered that night too. Remembered the backseat of the cop car and Meg sobbing beside him. What was the point of remembering?

'When I met you,' she continued, 'I didn't expect to like you, but I did. I certainly didn't expect to like you so much that I ended up in bed with you, but I did. I didn't expect to fall in love with you, but I did that too. From the beginning, I knew I should have told you who I was. I knew I should have told you a hundred different times. I knew it was the right thing to do, but I also knew that I'd lose you if I did. I knew when I told you, you'd leave and never come back. And that's what happened.'

She set a Xerox copier-paper box on his desk. 'I want you to have this. It's the book I moved here to write, and I want you to read it. Please.' She looked down at the box. 'The disk is with it, and I've deleted it from my computer. This is the only copy. Do what you want with both. Throw them away, run over them with your truck, or have a bonfire. It's up to you.'

She looked back at him. Her brown eyes steady, calm. 'I hope that someday you can forgive me. Not because I personally need your forgiveness. I don't. But I've learned something in the past few months, and that is just because you refuse to acknowledge something, refuse to look at it or think about it, doesn't mean it's not there, that it doesn't affect you and the choices you make in your life.'

She licked her lips. 'I forgive your mother. Not because the Bible tells me I should forgive. I guess I'm not that good a Christian, because I'm just not that magnanimous. I forgive her because, in forgiving her, I am free of all the anger and bitterness of the past, and that is what I want for you too.

'I've thought about what I've done since I moved to Truly, and I'm sorry that I hurt you, Mick. But I'm not sorry that I met you and fell in love with you. Loving you has broken my heart and caused me pain, but it made me a better person. I love you, Mick, and I hope that someday you find someone you can love. You deserve more in life than a string of women you don't really care about and who don't care all that much for you. Loving you taught me that. It taught me how it feels to love a man, and I hope that someday I can find someone who will love me the way that you can't. Because I deserve more than a string of men who don't really care about me.' Her gaze moved over his face, then returned to his eyes. 'I came here tonight to give you the book and because I wanted to say good-bye.'

'You're leaving?' He didn't have to wonder how he'd feel about her good-bye. Now he knew.

'Yes. I have to.'

Her leaving was best, no matter that it felt like she was reaching into his chest and ripping out his heart all over again. 'When?'

She shrugged and walked to the door. 'I don't know. Soon.' She looked over her shoulder one last time and said, 'Good-bye, Mick. Have a good life.' Then she was gone and he was left with the scent of her skin in the air and a big emptiness in his chest. The red sweater she'd worn the night she'd come into his office wearing a white halter dress still hung on a hook behind the door. He knew that it still smelled like strawberries.

He sat in his chair and leaned his head back. He thought of old drunk Reuben Sawyer spending three decades sitting on a barstool, sad and pathetic and unable to move beyond the pain of losing his wife. Mick wasn't that pathetic, but he understood old Reuben in a way that he never had before he'd loved Maddie Jones. He hadn't picked up the bottle. He owned two bars and knew where that path led, but he had gotten into a fight or two. A few days before he'd seen Maddie in the park, he'd kicked the Finley boys out of Mort's. Usually he called the cops to deal with assorted assholes and numb nuts, but that night he'd taken on both Scoot and Wes. No one had ever accused the Finley boys of being smart, but they were fighters, and it had taken both Mick and his bartender to shoved them out into the alley, where a knock-down free-for-all had ensued. The kind Mick hadn't enjoyed since high school.

Mick raked his fingers through the sides of his hair and sat forward. Since the night he'd found out who Maddie really was, he'd been in hell and he didn't know how to get out. His life seemed to be one miserable day after another. He thought things would get better, but his life wasn't heading in the direction of better, and he didn't know what to do about it. Maddie was who she was, and he was Mick Hennessy, and no matter how much he loved her, real life wasn't a made-for-TV movie on that women's channel Meg liked to watch.

He leaned forward and pulled the Xerox box toward him. He took off the top and looked inside at the orange disk and a stack of paper. In big type across the first page was written: *Till Death Us Do Part*.

Maddie said this was the only copy. Why would she give it to him? Why go to so much trouble and spend so much time doing something, only to give it to him when she was through?

He didn't want to read it. He didn't want to get sucked back in time. He didn't want to read about his unfaithful father and his sick mother and the night she'd gone over the edge. He didn't want to see the photographs or read the police reports. He'd lived through it once and didn't feel like revisiting the past, but as he picked up the lid to replace it on the box, the first sentence caught his eye.

'I promise it's going to be different this time, baby.' Alice Jones glanced at her young daughter, then returned her gaze to the road. 'You're going to like Truly. It's a little like heaven, and it's about damn time Jesus dropkicked us into a better life.'

Baby didn't say anything. She'd heard it before . . .

Maddie plugged Snowball's DVD into the player and sat her on the cat bed in front of the television. It wasn't even ten A.M., and she'd had enough of Snowball. 'If you don't behave, I'm going to throw you in your carrier and toss you into the trunk of my car.'

'Meow.'

'I mean it.' Snowball was going through some sort of passive-aggressive phase. She meowed to go out. Meowed to come in, but when Maddie opened the door, she'd run the opposite way. You'd think the cat would be more grateful.

She pointed at her kitten's nose. 'I'm warning you. You've just gotten on my last nerve.' She rose and tiptoed away. Snowball didn't follow, for the moment transfixed by the parakeets chirping on the screen.

The doorbell rang and Maddie moved to the front of the house and looked through the peep-hole. Last night when she'd said good-bye to Mick, she hadn't expected to see him again. Now here he was, looking a bit rough. The lower half of his face was covered in stubble like all the times they'd stayed up late making love. She opened the door and saw the Xerox box in his hand. Her heart dropped. All that work and he hadn't read it.

'Are you going to invite me in?'

She opened the door wider and shut it behind him. He wore a black North Face fleece jacket and, beneath the black stubble, his cheeks were pink from the cold morning chill. He followed her into the living room, bringing the scent of October air and of him into her house. She loved the way he smelled and had missed it.

'Is your cat watching television?' His voice was kind of rough too.

'For the moment.'

He set the box on her coffee table. 'I read your book.'

She glanced at the clock above the television just to make sure of the time. She'd given it to him to read and destroy because she loved him, and he'd probably skimmed it. 'That was fast.'

'I'm sorry.'

'Don't be sorry. Some people are just fast readers.'

He smiled, but it didn't reach his blue eyes or bring out his dimples. 'No. I'm sorry for what my mother did to yours. I don't believe anyone in my family has ever apologized to you. We were all too wrapped up in what it did to us to even stop and think about what it did to you.'

She blinked and managed a stunned, 'Oh. You don't have to apologize. You didn't do anything wrong.'

He laughed without humor. 'Don't let me off the hook, Maddie. I've done a lot of things wrong.' He unzipped his jacket, and he wore the same Mort's polo shirt he'd had on the night before. The man must have dozens of them. 'Believing that just because I don't think about what had happened in the past meant it doesn't bother or affect me was not only wrong, it was stupid. If I'd truly gotten over it, who you are wouldn't have mattered to me. It would have surprised me, maybe even shocked the shit out of me, but it wouldn't matter.'

But it had mattered to him. So much so that he'd cut her out of his life.

'I've been up all night reading your book. At first I didn't want to read it because I thought it would be a long laundry list of the things my parents had done, complete with grisly photos. But it wasn't.'

She wanted to reach out and touch him. To run her hands up his chest and bury her face in his neck. 'I tried to be fair.'

'You were surprisingly fair. If your mother had shot mine, I don't know if I would have been as fair. I felt a kind of weird connection to my parents. To my life as a kid, and I understand how everything went so wrong. And I understand that you don't always get a second chance to do it right.'

She wanted him to reach out and touch her. To put his hands on the sides of her face and lower his mouth to hers. Instead he stuck his fingers in the front pocket of his Levi's.

'When I saw you in the park, I said I didn't know you, but that was a lie. I know you. I know that you're funny and smart and that you're freezing when it's seventy degrees outside. I know that you crave cheesecake but settle for cake-scented lotion instead. I know you have a problem with people telling you what to do. And I know that you want everyone to think you're a hard-ass, but that you take in a bucktoothed cat and give her a home. Everything I know about you makes me want to know more.'

Her chest got that familiar ache, and she looked down at her feet, not trusting the emotion expanding in her chest.

'Since I moved back to Truly,' he said, 'I've felt as if I were standing in one place, unable to move. But I wasn't standing still. I was waiting. I think I was waiting for you.'

The backs of her eyes stung and she bit her bottom lip.

'When I'm with you, I feel a kind of calm I've never felt in my life. I'm tangled up in you and you're tangled up in me and it feels right. Like it was meant to be. I love you, Maddie, and I'm sorry it's taken me so long to say it to you again.'

She looked up at him and smiled. 'I've missed you.'

He laughed, and his dimples finally dented his cheeks. 'You haven't missed me any more than I've missed you. I've been one miserable shithead.' He bent his knees and wrapped his arms around her behind. He rose and lifted her off the ground. 'I've never believed that death happens for a reason,' he said as he looked up into her face. 'But if our lives had been different, I wouldn't have fallen in love with you.' Slowly she slid down his body until her pelvis fit his. He was ready for love, and his hands slipped beneath her shirt and caressed her bare back.

'Who's to say? If your mother hadn't killed your father or my mother, we might be brother and sister.'

His hands stilled. 'Stepbrother and -sister. If you were my stepsister, I wouldn't do this.' He lowered his head and kissed her. His mouth was warm and wet and so welcome. Later she would take his hand and take him to her room. For now, she just wanted to feel his kiss again, and it was like walking into the sun after a long cold winter. An *ahh* that felt good clear to the marrow of her bones.

He pulled back and pressed his forehead to hers. 'Ever since that first night you came into Mort's, my eyes have been on you,' he said. 'You were the only thing I could see, even when I tried like hell to look someplace else.'

'Hmm. Look or touch? I saw you talking to Tanya in the park.'

'Just look. I don't want anyone else.'

She put her arms around his back and locked her hands together. 'What about Meg?'

He raised his head. 'What about my sister?'

'What are you going to tell her? She hates me.'

'Actually, she's been too busy with my friend Steve to think much about you.' He thought a moment, then said, 'I don't think she really hates you. She blames your mother for everything that happened, but she doesn't know you.'

Maddie laughed. 'Getting to know me isn't a guarantee that she'll like me.'

He shrugged. 'I think she'll get over it, because ultimately she does want me to be happy. She wants me to marry someone I love. To have a wife and a family. I never thought I wanted kids, but after I've seen the way you've raised your cat . . . ' He paused to look over at Snowball, who was mesmerized by goldfish. 'You're a natural.' He looked back at her and smiled. 'Let me know if any or all parts of that plan appeal to you. If not, we'll make adjustments.'

'This sounds a lot like a white wedding, picket fence, baby maker plan.'

He chuckled. 'Who would have thought?'

Certainly not her. She'd never thought she'd be some man's wife or that she'd be thinking about having a family. Of course, she never thought she'd fall in love or be a cat owner either. Her life had drastically changed since she'd moved to Truly. She'd changed.

She took Mick's hand and led him from the room. Maybe he was right. Maybe their lives had always been entwined and they were meant to be together. If that was the case, she'd happily spend the rest of her life tangled up in Mick Hennessy.

We do hope that you have enjoyed reading this large print book.

Did you know that all of our titles are available for purchase?

We publish a wide range of high quality large print books including:
Romances, Mysteries, Classics
General Fiction
Non Fiction and Westerns

Special interest titles available in large print are:
The Little Oxford Dictionary
Music Book
Song Book
Hymn Book
Service Book

Also available from us courtesy of Oxford University Press:
Young Readers' Dictionary
(large print edition)
Young Readers' Thesaurus
(large print edition)

For further information or a free brochure, please contact us at:
Ulverscroft Large Print Books Ltd.,
The Green, Bradgate Road, Anstey,
Leicester, LE7 7FU, England.
Tel: (00 44) 0116 236 4325
Fax: (00 44) 0116 234 0205